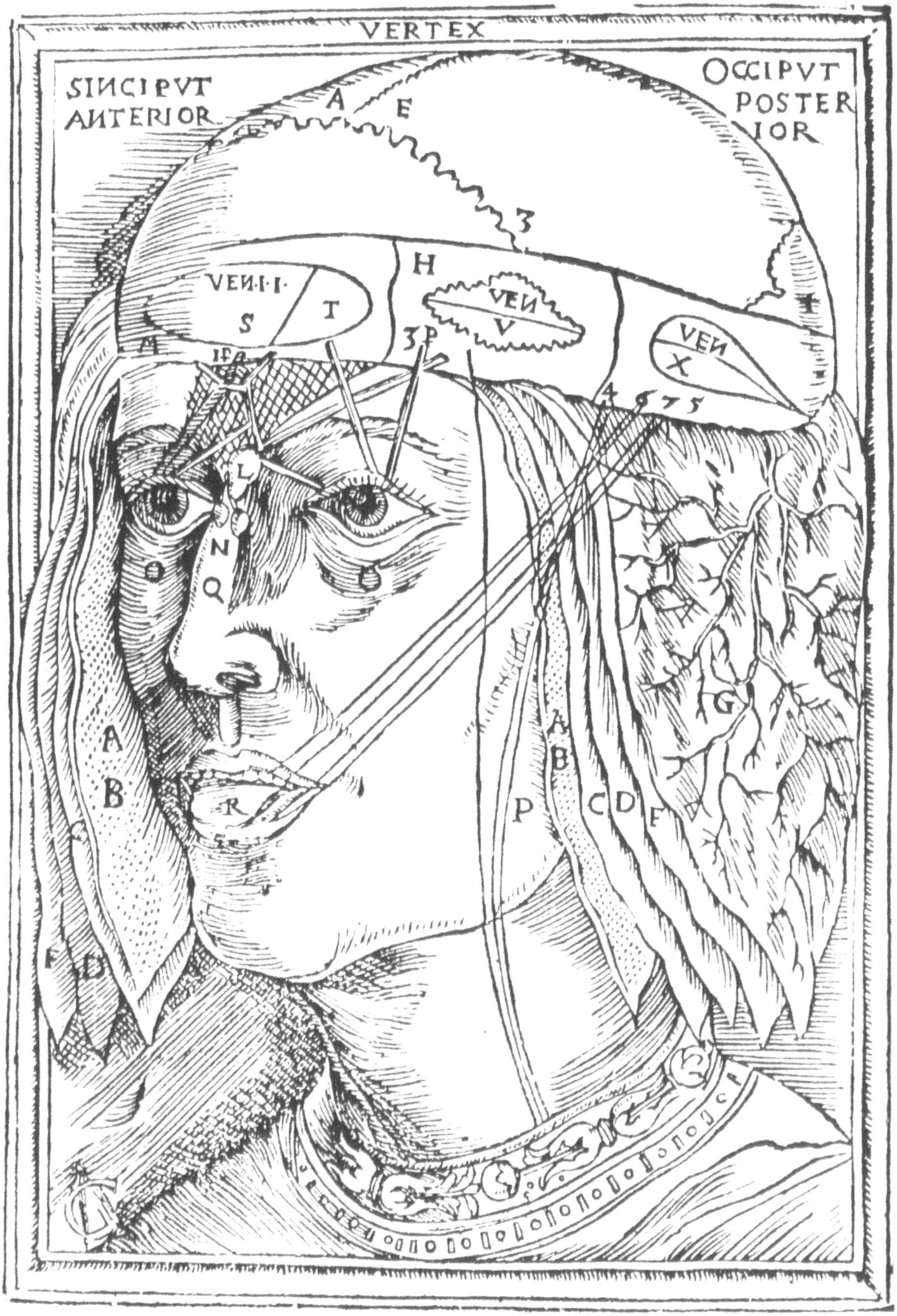

VERTEX
SINCIPVT ANTERIOR
OCCIPVT POSTERIOR
VEN.I.I.
VEN V
VEN X

G. Salamon   Y. P. Huang

Radiologic Anatomy of the Brain

In Cooperation with

P. Michotey, N. Moscow, Ch. Raybaud, Ph. Farnarier, G. Scialfa, W. O. Bank, and K. Hall

Department of Radiology
Hospital de la Timone
Marseille

B. S. Wolf, T. Okudera, K. Oana, S. Panichavatena, J. Ito, R. Kawai, S. Antin, J. Pinner, and N. Christoff

Department of Radiology
Mount Sinai Hospital and School of Medicine
of the City University of New York
New York

With 282 Figures in 463 Separate Illustrations

Springer-Verlag Berlin Heidelberg GmbH 1976

Prof. Georges Salamon
Neuroradiologie-Radiologie Vasculaire C.H.U. de la Timone, F-13 Marseille, France

Prof. Yun Peng Huang
Dept. of Radiology (Neuroradiology Section), Mount Sinai Hospital and School of Medicine of the City University of New York, New York, NY 10029/USA

ISBN 978-3-642-66275-1 ISBN 978-3-642-66273-7 (eBook)
DOI 10.1007/978-3-642-66273-7

Library of Congress Cataloging in Publication Data. Salamon, Georges, 1931–. Radiologic anatomy of the brain. Bibliography: p. Includes index. 1. Brain – Radiography. 2. Brain – Anatomy. I. Huang, Yun P., 1926–, joint author. II. Title. RC386.6.R3S24 616.8′04′752 75-45294.

Softcover reprint of the hardcover 1st edition 1976

Typeface: Monophoto Times 11/12. Paper: Phönix Imperial, Papierfabrik Scheufelen, Oberlenningen. Reproduction of the figures: Gustav Dreher, Württembergische Graphische Kunstanstalt GmbH, Stuttgart. Layout of the cover: W. Eisenschink, Heidelberg. Production managing: I. Oppelt, Heidelberg
Typesetting: Universitätsdruckerei H. Stürtz AG, Würzburg

Preface

Despite all recent advances, the most important progress in neuroradiology has been in our knowledge of the anatomy of the nervous system. DANDY's injection of ventricles and cisterns with air, SICARD's studies of the epidural and subarachoid space with lipiodol, MONIZ's work on cerebral arteries and veins, and, more recently, DJINDJIAN's and DI CHIRO's investigations of spinal arteries, have modified, refined and expanded current knowledge of anatomy of the central nervous system.

As described by LINDGREN, "the neuroradiologist dissects the region of interest with x-rays like a surgeon with a scalpel". In fact, neuroradiologic examination is nothing less than an anatomic survey *in vivo*, using multiple orthogonal projections.

The authors of this book are convinced that frequent reference to normal anatomy is currently the most useful and rewarding means of understanding neuroradiologic problems. Arteries and veins of the brain may be considered in terms of the sulci, gyri, cisterns, ventricles, basal nuclei, and cortical centers. In this book, efforts have been made to match anatomic elements of the ventricles, cisterns, and vessels to the region being studied. The foundation of this book lies in the detailed anatomico-radiologic correlations, demonstrated by numerous photographs of dissected specimens, radiographs of injected specimens, anatomic drawings, diagrams, and normal cerebral angiograms and encephalograms. Indeed, there is no region in the central nervous system which cannot be delineated by its relationships with arteries, veins, cisterns, and ventricles. Recent developments in computerized transaxial tomography have given us another means of investigating the anatomy of the central nervous system—this time in the horizontal plane.

Whenever a patient with neurologic disorders is investigated, the region of interest must first be localized by clinical history and examination. This is followed by properly selected neuroradiologic procedures to best demonstrate the anatomy of the suspected region or regions. For this reason, neuroradiology is one of the richest subdivisions of the neurologic and radiologic sciences.

This book was prepared with technical contribution of Mr. M. CAREN, Mr. J.M. CORBAZ, Mr. F. FINIDORI, Mr. J.F. LANDOU, Mrs. M. MAUREL, Miss J. PELOUX, Miss V. REDON, Mrs. F. RODRIGUEZ, Miss C. RUSSO, Mrs. A. YVANT, and Mrs. CL. VIDAL-NAQUET.

We wish to acknowledge Mrs. J. VIGNAUD and Dr. G. GIUDICELLI who kindly provided radiological documents.

We would like to express our sincere gratitude to Dr. P. ANDERSON for his assistance and encouragement in preparation of specimens for this study.

We wish to thank the National Institute of Health, US Public Health Service (5 Ro I HE09913–10), INSERM (National Institute for Health and Medical Research), Siemens Corporation, Compagnie Générale de Radiologie, and Kodak Eastman Co. for their generous support.

March 1976

G.S.
Y.P.H.

Contents

PART 1

CEREBRAL HEMISPHERE

Chapter 1

Fissures and Sulci

The terms fissure and sulcus as they are classically defined are: a fissure separates one lobe from another, while a sulcus is within a lobe and delimits gyri.
The fissures and sulci of the cerebral hemispheres can be arranged into three groups according to their location. They are divided into those found on the external, the internal and the inferior surfaces of the hemispheres.
The study of these structures has been the subject of anatomical works by ROLANDO, BROCA (1898), GRATIOLET (1839) and DEJERINE (1895). Other studies have been done in order to relate the principal fissures and sulci to the landmarks on the skull [LUCAS-CHAMPIONNIERE (1948), DOYEN (1951), HARTMANN (1956), POIRIER *et al.* (1921), MARIE, FOIX and BERTRAND (1915)]. The most accurate approach to the visualization and identification of the cerebral sulci in the patient is by means of pneumoencephalography or indirectly by the study of the relationships between vascular structures and the sulci.

I. Anatomic Study of the Fissures and Sulci of the External Surface of the Cerebral Hemisphere

1. Principal or Interlobar Fissures

Sylvian fissure (Figs. 2, 3, 4)
Central fissure (Figs. 2, 1)
Parieto-occipital fissure, external segment (Fig. 2)

The Sylvian fissure is directed from inferiorly to superiorly and anteriorly to posteriorly. It has considerable depth and separates the frontal and parietal lobes above from the temporal lobe below. The Sylvian fissure arises in the region of the anterior perforated substance and is related to the lesser wing of the sphenoid. It is transversely orientated and convex anteriorly.
At the level of the insula, the Sylvian fissure divides into two limbs. The principal limb is directed posteriorly and extends to the midportion of the parietal lobe, where it forms the anterior boundary of the supramarginal gyrus. The anterior limb is short and divides into two branches, the anterior horizontal and ascending limbs. The anterior horizontal limb represents the boundary between the external surface of the inferior frontal gyrus and its orbital portion, and is separated from the ascending limb by the pars triangularis. At the posterior extremity of the Sylvian fissure the supramarginal gyrus unites the parietal and temporal lobes.

The central fissure is directed obliquely, inferiorly and anteriorly. It arises along the interhemispheric fissure and terminates just above the Sylvian fissure from which it is separated by the thickness of the frontoparietal operculum. The degree of obliquity of the central fissure relative to the Sylvian fissure is variable. It presents two constant curves, both of which are convex anteriorly forming the superior and inferior "knees" described by BROCA. The central fissure separates the precentral gyrus from the postcentral gyrus. Superiorly it terminates on the medial surface of the brain, slightly posterior to the midfrontal plane, in the paracentral lobule.

The parieto-occipital fissure is found on both the internal and external surfaces of the hemisphere. Its external portion has also been called the external perpendicular fissure by GRATIOLET (1839). It is, however, rather short on this surface of the brain where it is represented only by a notch.

2. Sulci of the External Surface

a) Sulci of the Frontal Lobe

Superior frontal sulcus (Figs. 2, 1, 4)
Inferior frontal sulcus (Figs. 2, 1)
Precentral sulcus (Figs. 2, 1)

These three sulci divide the external surface of the frontal lobe into four gyri: the superior, middle and inferior frontal gyri, and the precentral gyrus.

b) Sulci of the Parietal Lobe

Postcentral sulcus (Fig. 2)
Intraparietal sulcus (Figs. 2, 1)
Sulcus of Jensen (Fig. 2)

The parietal lobe is divided into the postcentral gyrus and the superior and inferior parietal lobules by the postcentral and intraparietal sulci, respectively. The intraparietal sulcus begins posteriorly to the postcentral gyrus and has a vertical course passing along the posterior edge of this gyrus. It then describes a wide curve, concave inferiorly and becomes horizontal, where it continues into the occipital lobe as the intra-occipital sulcus.
At the site where intraparietal sulcus changes direction, a vertical sulcus, the postcentral sulcus continues its original course posteriorly to the postcentral gyrus. In the region of the inferior parietal gyrus, a descending sulcus, the sulcus of Jensen, separates the supramarginal gyrus anteriorly from the angular gyrus posteriorly.

c) Sulci of the Occipital Lobe

Anterior occipital sulcus (Fig. 2)
Superior, middle and inferior occipital sulci (Fig. 2)

The occipital lobe is separated from the parietal and temporal lobes by the parieto-occipital fissure and the occipital notch. An anterior occipital sulcus is sometimes present limiting the occipital lobe anteriorly. This sulcus is quite variable and has its inferior extent posterior to the occipital notch and its superior limit inferior to the intraparietal sulcus.
Three secondary sulci further subdivide the occipital lobe. These are the superior occipital sulcus or intra-occipital sulcus (which continues the course of the intraparietal sulcus), and the middle and inferior occipital sulci.

d) Sulci of the Temporal Lobe

Superior temporal sulcus (Figs. 2, 4)
Inferior temporal sulcus (Fig. 2)
Occipitotemporal sulcus (Fig. 3)

On the external surface of the brain, the temporal lobe is limited superiorly by the Sylvian fissure and is subdivided by the superior and inferior temporal sulci and the occipitotemporal sulcus. The superior temporal sulcus begins at the anterior aspect of the temporal lobe and follows a course parallel to the Sylvian fissure. It continues posteriorly around the Sylvian fissure to show the axis of the angular gyrus.
The two other temporal sulci, with the superior temporal sulcus, separate the superior, middle and inferior temporal gyri, and the fusiform gyrus.

II. Anatomic Study of the Fissures and Sulci of the Internal Surface of the Cerebral Hemisphere

1. Fissures of the Internal Surface

Callosomarginal fissure (cingulate sulcus) and its extensions (Figs. 5, 4)
Parieto-occipital fissure (Fig. 5)
Calcarine fissure (Figs. 5, 3)

The callosomarginal fissure or cingulate sulcus runs parallel to the corpus callosum and marks the superior limit of the cingulate gyrus. It begins beneath the rostrum of the corpus callosum and courses around the genu to follow the body of the corpus callosum. Posteriorly, it changes course to become vertical and forms the posterior limit of the paracentral lobule. Anteriorly, it serves as the boundary between the cingulate gyrus and the superior frontal gyrus. An anterior extension of the callosomarginal fissure, the subfrontal sulcus, separates the orbital surface (the gyrus rectus) from the remainder of the superior frontal gyrus. Another extension, the paracentral sulcus, is vertically orientated and forms the anterior border of the paracentral lobule. Lastly, the callosomarginal fissure may present a posterior extension, the subparietal fissure, which lies inferiorly to the parietal lobe and separates the precuneus from the cingulate gyrus.

The parieto-occipital fissure is represented on the internal surface of the brain as a perpendicular fissure which separates the precuneus from the cuneus. It is very deep and is directed obliquely, inferiorly and anteriorly.

The calcarine fissure separates the cuneus from the lingual gyrus. It is horizontally orientated and extends anteriorly to meet the parieto-occipital fissure. The calcarine fissure produces an impression on the medial wall of the occipital horn, the calcar avis.

2. Sulci of the Internal Surface

Transverse parietal sulcus (Fig. 5)
Lingual sulcus (Fig. 5)

The transverse parietal sulcus divides the precuneus into superior and inferior gyri. The inferior boundary of the precuneus is formed by the subparietal sulcus, which is generally considered a fissure.

The lingual sulcus partially subdivides the lingual gyrus posteriorly. This gyrus is separated superiorly from the cuneus by the calcarine fissure, and inferiorly from the fusiform gyrus by the collateral sulcus.

III. Anatomic Study of the Fissures and Sulci of the Inferior Surface of the Cerebral Hemisphere

1. Fissure of the Inferior Surface—Sylvian Fissure (Fig. 3)

The only fissure identifiable on the inferior surface of the cerebral hemisphere is the initial portion of the Sylvian fissure. It arises in the region of the anterior perforated substance and follows the lesser wing of the sphenoid describing a course convex anteriorly.

2. Sulci of the Inferior Surface

a) Sulci of the Orbital Surface of the Frontal Lobe

Medial orbital sulcus or olfactory sulcus (Fig. 3)
Orbital sulci or H-shaped sulcus (Fig. 3)
External orbital sulcus (Fig. 3)

Medially, the olfactory bulb is directly applied to the medial orbital sulcus or olfactory sulcus. The olfactory sulcus divides longitudinally the orbital portion of the superior frontal gyrus. The orbital sulci, or H-shaped sulcus, form the boundaries of the orbital surface of the middle frontal gyrus. The orbital portion of the inferior frontal gyrus is divided longitudinally by the external orbital sulcus.

b) Sulci of the Inferior Surface of the Temporal and Occipital Lobes

Collateral sulcus (Fig. 3)
Hippocampal sulcus
Inferior temporal sulcus (equally well included with sulci of external surface of temporal lobe) (Fig. 2)

The ***collateral sulcus*** begins in the occipital lobe and is directed towards the anterior extremity of the temporal lobe. It is constant, prominent, and may join the inferior temporal sulcus in the anterior part of the temporal lobe. In the occipital lobe the collateral sulcus separates the lingual gyrus from the fusiform gyrus, while in the temporal lobe it separates the fusiform gyrus from the hippocampal gyrus. The collateral sulcus produces an impression on the temporal horn of the lateral ventricle, the collateral eminence.
The ***hippocampal sulcus*** extends from the region of the splenium of the corpus callosum to the uncus of the hippocampus. Deep anteriorly, this sulcus is crossed by secondary sulci. These hippocampal digitations produce the rather characteristic appearance of the impression of Ammon's horn. Ammon's horn indents the medial aspect of the temporal horn of the lateral ventricle anteriorly. More posteriorly, the hippocampal sulcus follows an ascending course and limits the deep surface of the subcallosal gyrus. In the region of the splenium of the corpus callosum, the hippocampal sulcus is continuous with the pericallosal cistern.
The collateral sulcus and callosomarginal fissure laterally, and the pericallosal cistern and hippocampal sulcus medially, form the boundaries of the limbic lobe.

IV. Radiologic Study of the Fissures and Sulci

Many anatomists have studied the topographic relationships between the bony landmarks of the cranial vault and the superficial fissures and sulci of the brain. Several of their anatomic observations maintain their validity for radiologic purposes. Included among these are the works of Poirier *et al.* (1921), Lucas-Championniere (1948), Kronlein (1964), and Doyen (1951) (Fig. 9).
During World War I the radiologic examination of patients with cranial injuries inspired Marie, Foix and Bertrand (1915) to investigate further the relationships between convolutions and the cranial vault (Fig. 10). An analogous study was performed by Taylor and Haughton (1900).
The simplest of these relationships are the following:
For Poirier *et al.* (1921) (Fig. 9A) the central fissure (of Rolando) is located by constructing a perpendicular to the zygomatic arch anteriorly to the tragus. The inferior end of the central fissure, or inferior Rolandic point, is situated 7 cm above the tragus on this line. The superior end of this fissure, or superior Rolandic point, is located 2 cm posteriorly to the circumferential midpoint of a line from the nasofrontal suture to the external occipital protuberance.
Using the method of Lucas-Championniere (1948) (Fig. 9B), the superior Rolandic point is found by measuring 5 cm posteriorly to the coronal suture—or more precisely, 5 cm posteriorly to that point on the inner table crossed by a true coronal plane through the anterior margin of the external auditory canal.
Ruggiero (1961) (Fig. 9C) suggests that the superior Rolandic point can be localized, without measurement, by constructing a perpendicular to the clivus which passes through the external occipital protuberance. A second line, perpendicular to the first and originating at the external occipital protuberance, defines the superior Rolandic point where it crosses the inner table.
Lucas-Championniere (1948) localized the Sylvian fissure (Fig. 9D) with a line 5 cm above and parallel to the zygomatic arch. The anterior end of the fissure is

situated 3 cm behind the posterior aspect of the frontal process of the zygoma.

Pneumoencephalographic studies of the cerebral sulci have been performed by many authors [ROBERTSON (1957), RUGGIERO (1956, 1966), DI CHIRO (1961)]. The most precise localization of the sulci, in relationship to the bicommissural base line, however, has been developed by neurosurgeons [TALAIRACH (1967), BAUCAUD *et al.* (1973), SZIKLA *et al.* (1976)] interested in the stereotactic approach to the telencephalon.

The Sylvian fissure, callosomarginal fissure, and pericallosal cistern are usually visualized during pneumoencephalography (Figs. 6, 7, 8). On the other hand, the central, calcarine and parieto-occipital fissures are difficult, if not impossible, to demonstrate in this manner.

The superimposition of the internal and external fissures of both hemispheres on a lateral radiograph, and the obliquity of the sulci, make pneumoencephalography suboptimal for topographic study of most cerebral convolutions, with the exception of those such as the insula and cingulate gyrus.

The interpretation of radiographs is always impaired by the superimposition of the sulci of the two surfaces of both hemispheres. For this reason the lateral projection provides more information regarding the location of the fissures and sulci of the medial surface of the brain than it does for those on the convexities.

Angiographic study of the cerebral arteries and veins reveals many characteristic relationships between vessels, fissures, and sulci. The earliest works in this regard were those concerning the insula [SCHLESINGER (1939), VLAHOVITCH (1965, 1966), TAVERAS and WOOD (1964)].

On the lateral surface of the brain, angiography readily reveals the location of the Sylvian and central fissures, and the precentral, inferior frontal, intraparietal, superior temporal and inferior temporal sulci. Vascular relationships on the medial surface of the hemispheres define the pericallosal cistern, the callosomarginal and calcarine fissures, the collateral sulcus and the margins of the paracentral lobule. It is probable that angiotomography will permit evaluation of the depth and direction of the sulci.

Currently, evaluation of the cerebral vasculature provides the most reliable method for studying gyral topography *in vivo*.

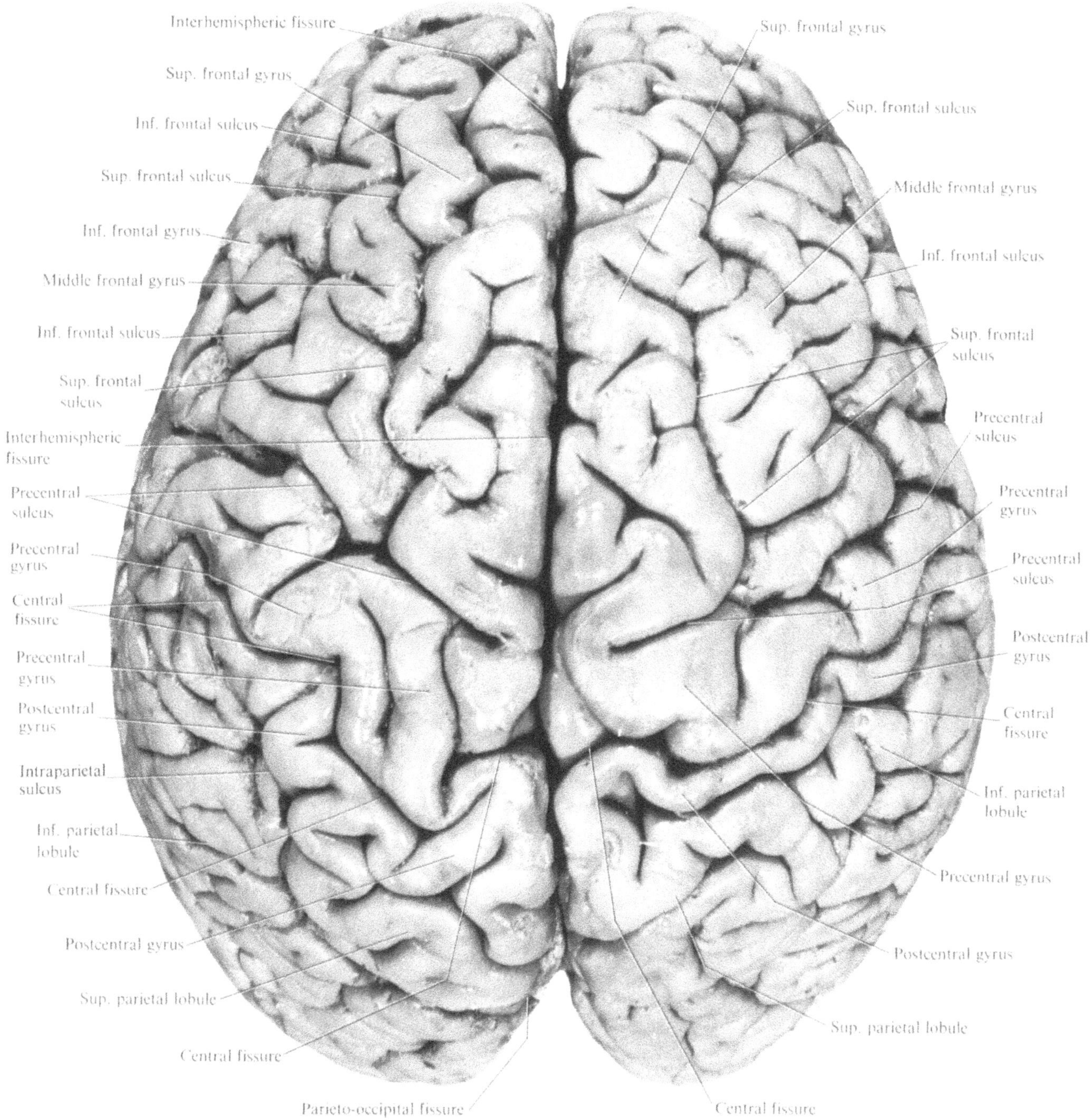

Fig. 1. Fissures and sulci of the superior surface of the cerebral hemisphere

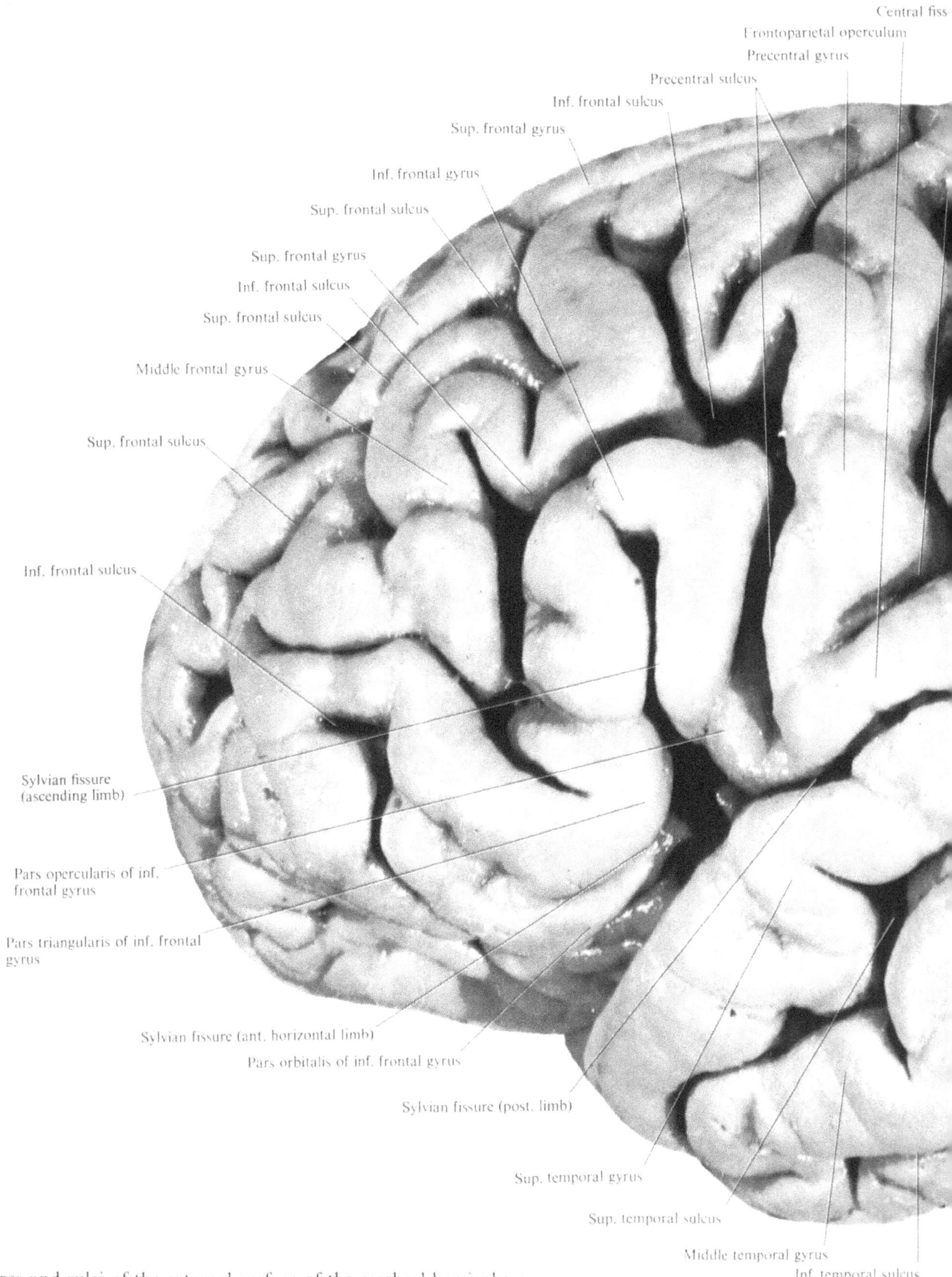

Fig. 2. Fissures and sulci of the external surface of the cerebral hemisphere

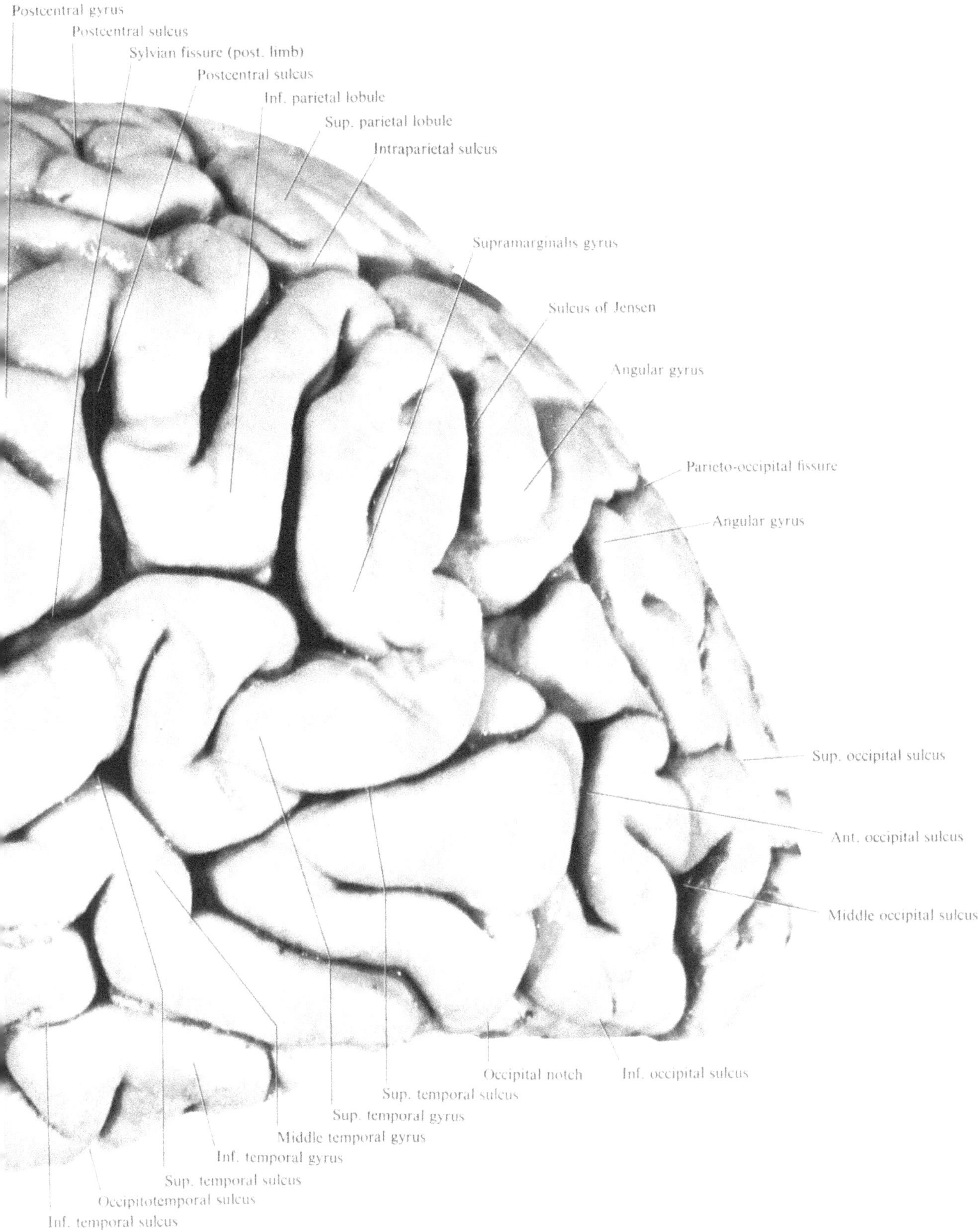

Postcentral gyrus
Postcentral sulcus
Sylvian fissure (post. limb)
Postcentral sulcus
Inf. parietal lobule
Sup. parietal lobule
Intraparietal sulcus
Supramarginalis gyrus
Sulcus of Jensen
Angular gyrus
Parieto-occipital fissure
Angular gyrus
Sup. occipital sulcus
Ant. occipital sulcus
Middle occipital sulcus
Occipital notch
Inf. occipital sulcus
Sup. temporal sulcus
Sup. temporal gyrus
Middle temporal gyrus
Inf. temporal gyrus
Sup. temporal sulcus
Occipitotemporal sulcus
Inf. temporal sulcus

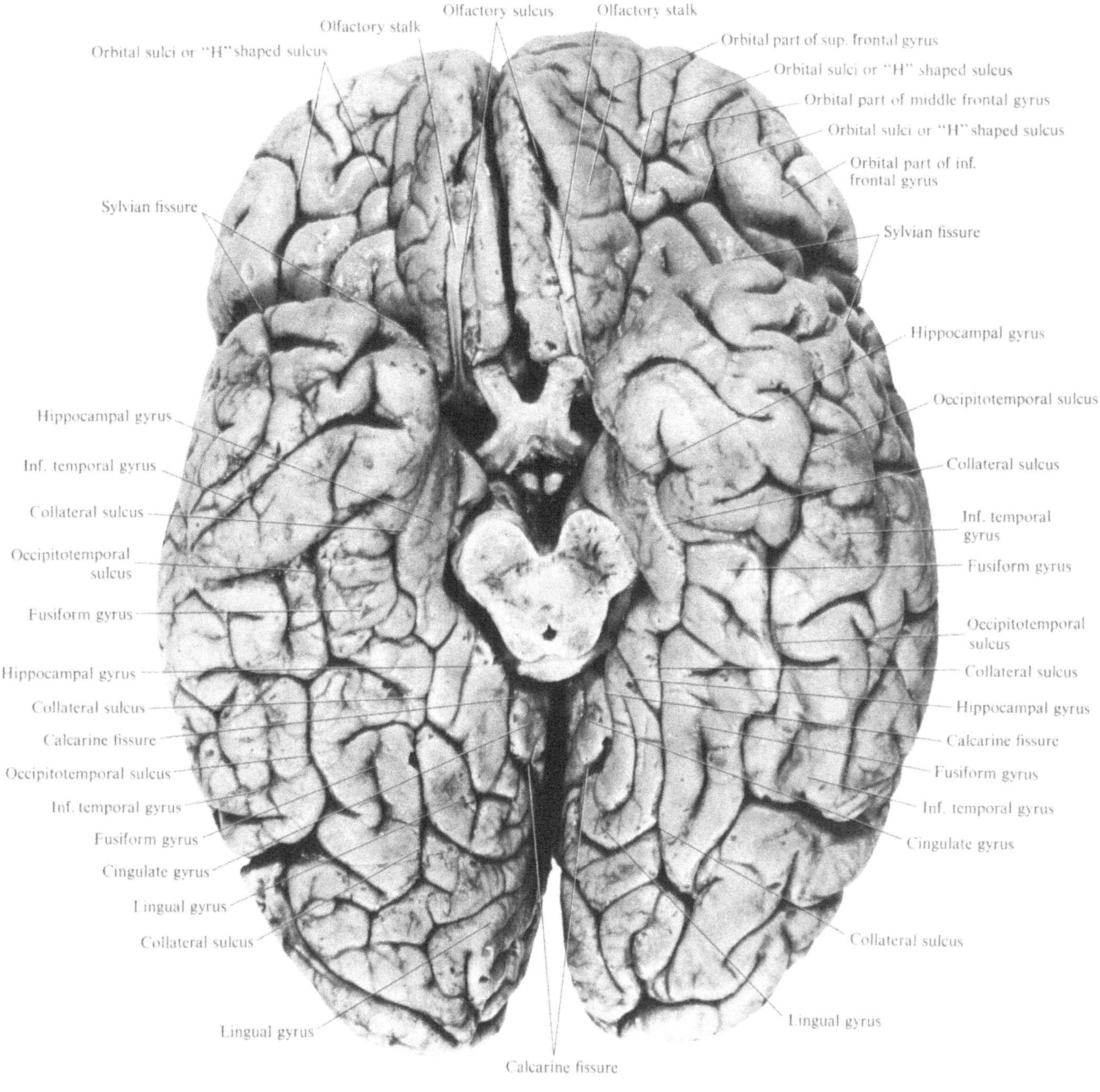

Fig. 3. Fissures and sulci of the inferior surface of the cerebral hemisphere

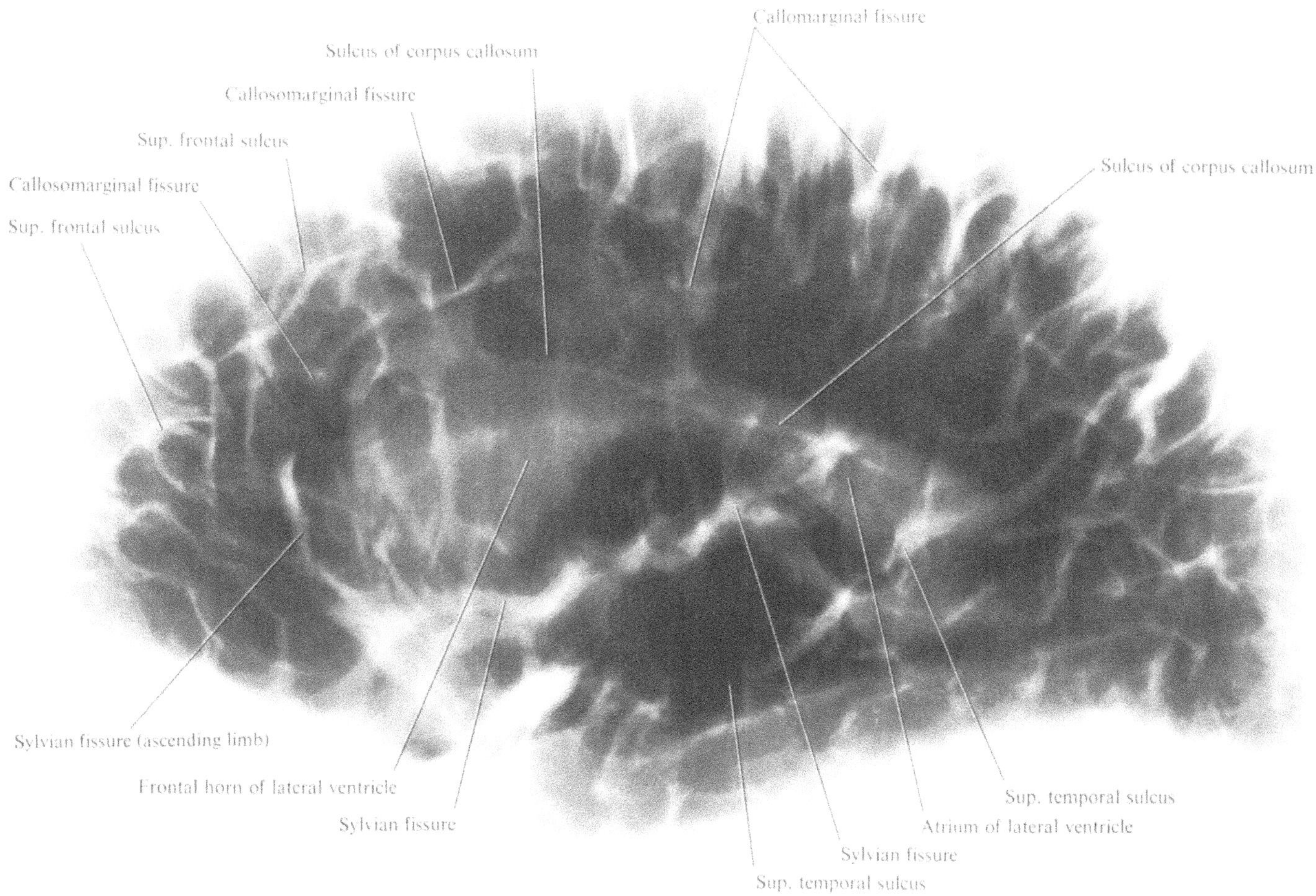

Fig. 4. Lateral radiograph of an uninjected cadaver brain with air outlining the fissures and sulci of the internal and external surfaces of the hemispheres

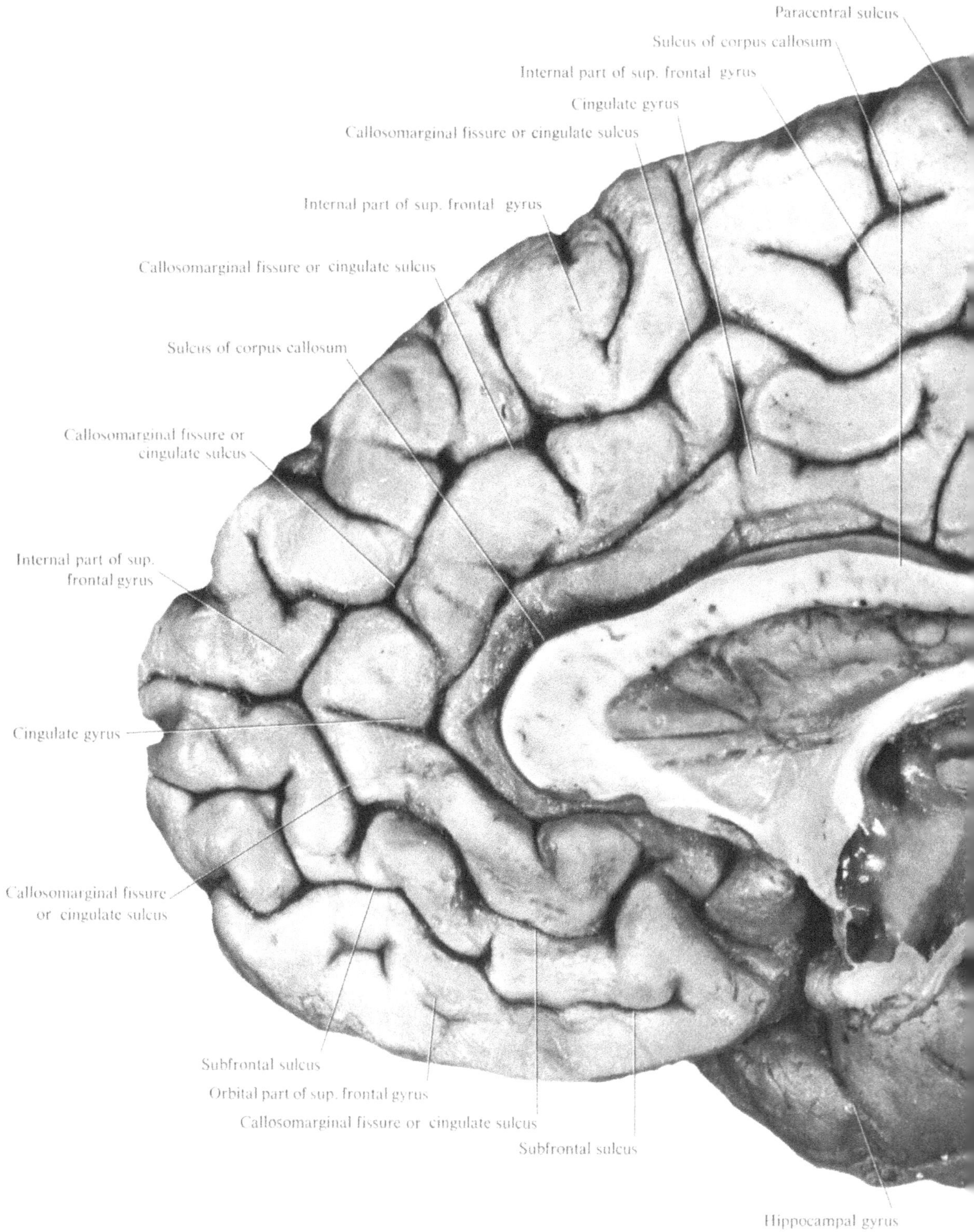

Fig. 5. Fissures and sulci of the internal surface of the cerebral hemisphere

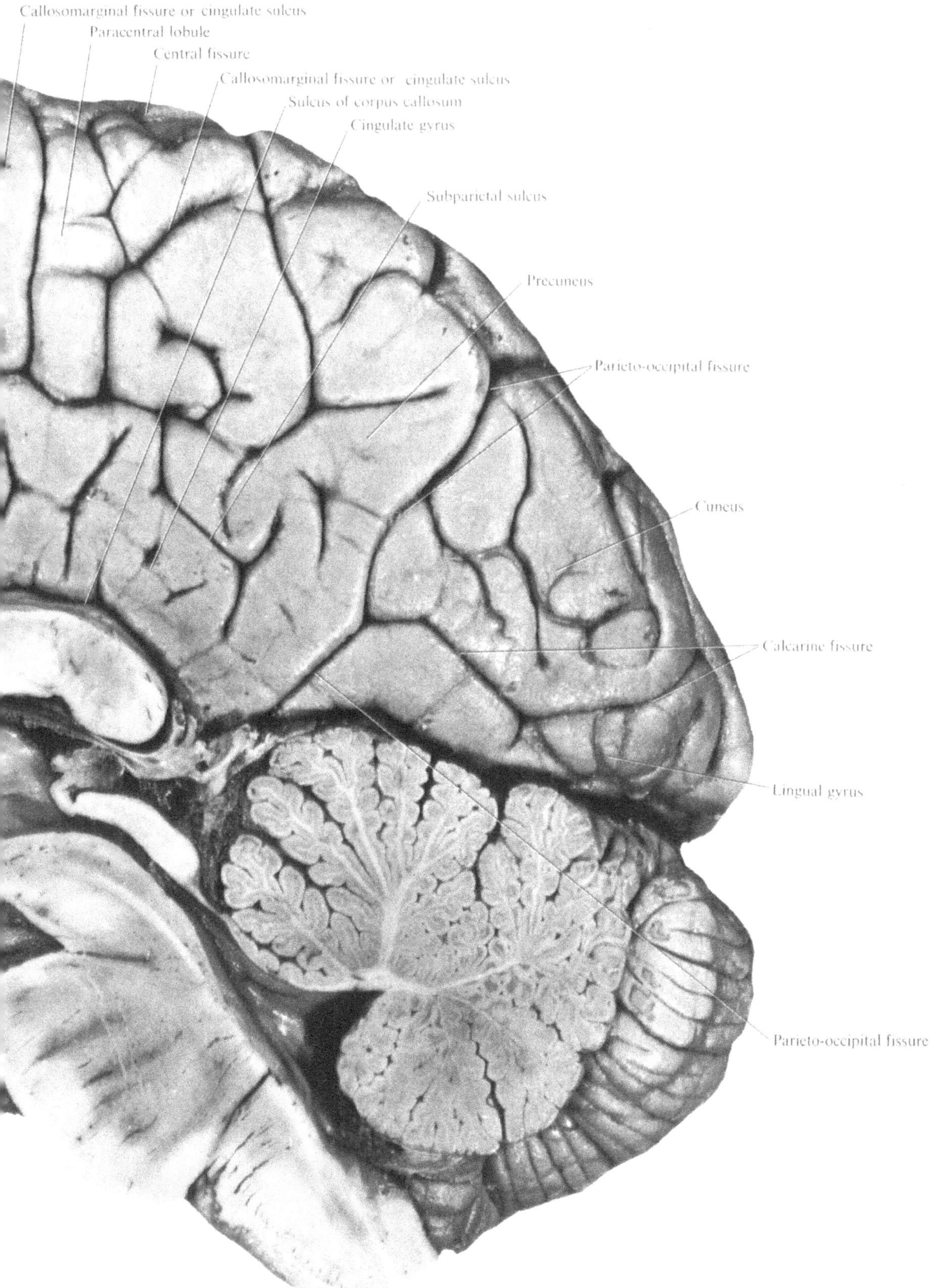

Callosomarginal fissure or cingulate sulcus
Paracentral lobule
Central fissure
Callosomarginal fissure or cingulate sulcus
Sulcus of corpus callosum
Cingulate gyrus
Subparietal sulcus
Precuneus
Parieto-occipital fissure
Cuneus
Calcarine fissure
Lingual gyrus
Parieto-occipital fissure

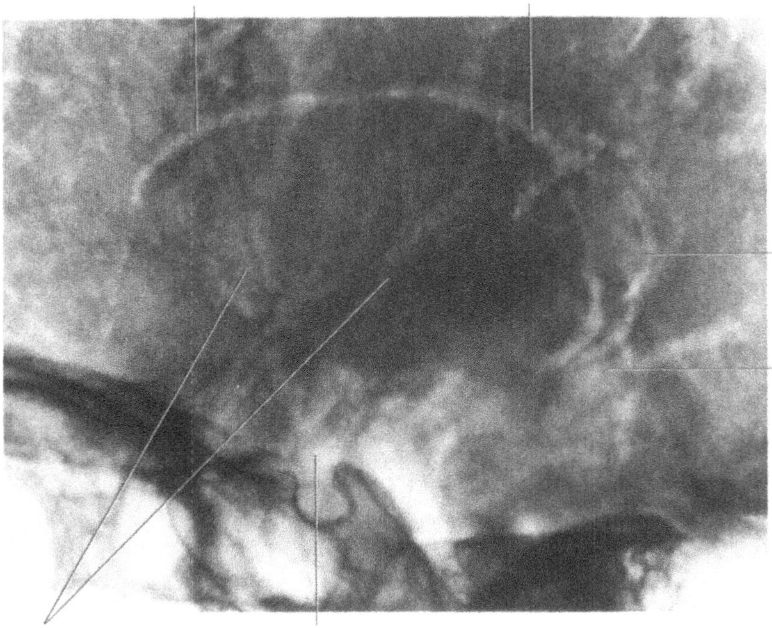

◁ Fig. 6. Pneumoencephalogram, lateral projection

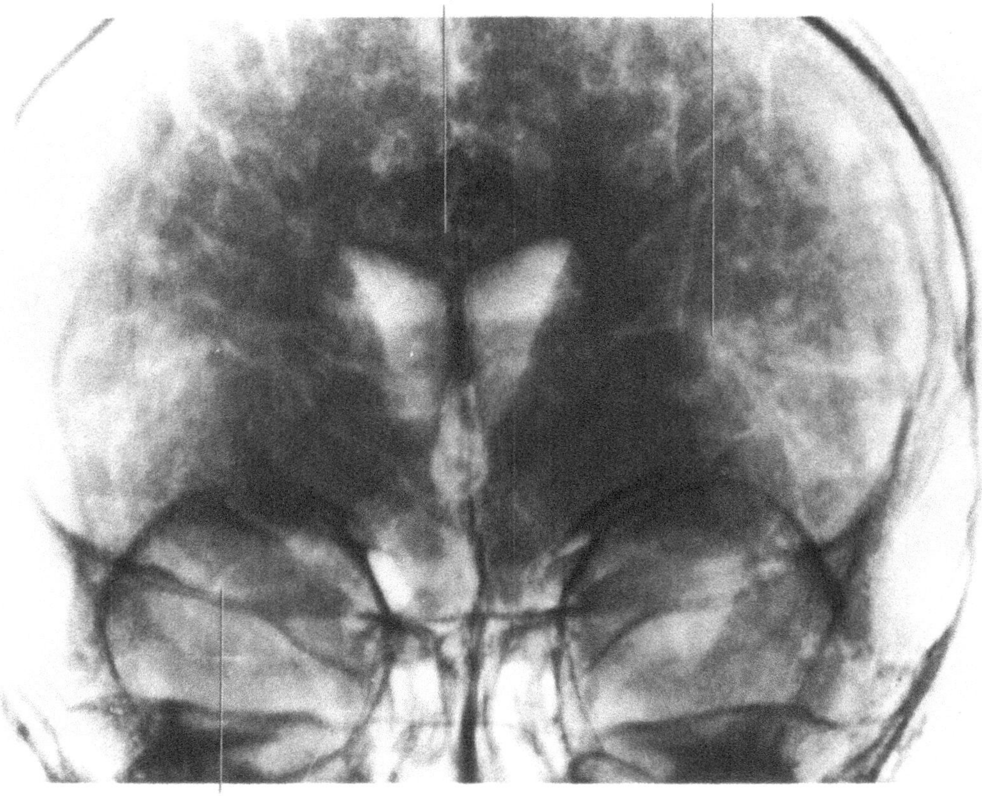

Fig. 7. Pneumoencephalogram, frontal projection

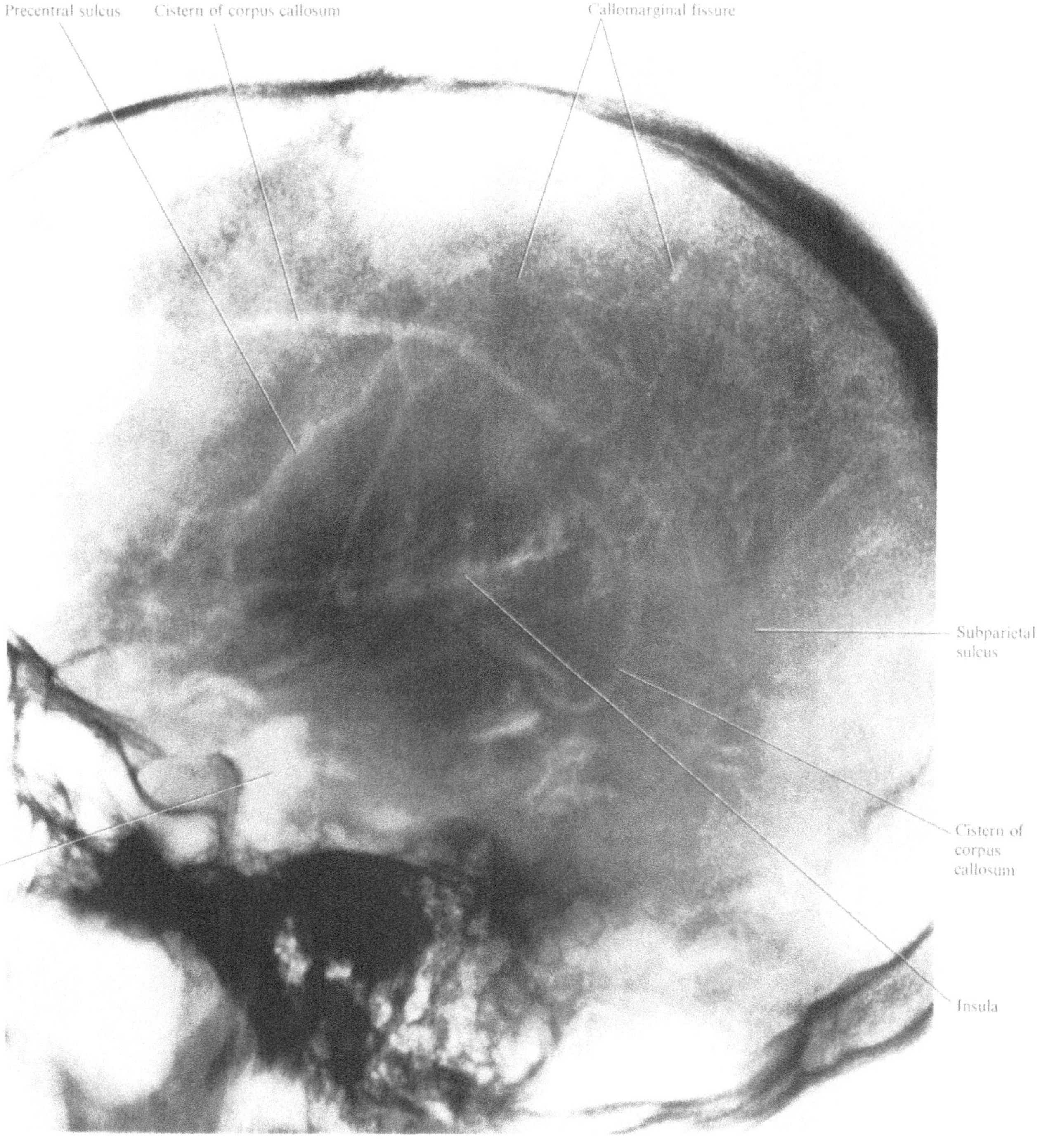

Fig. 8. Pneumoencephalogram, lateral projection

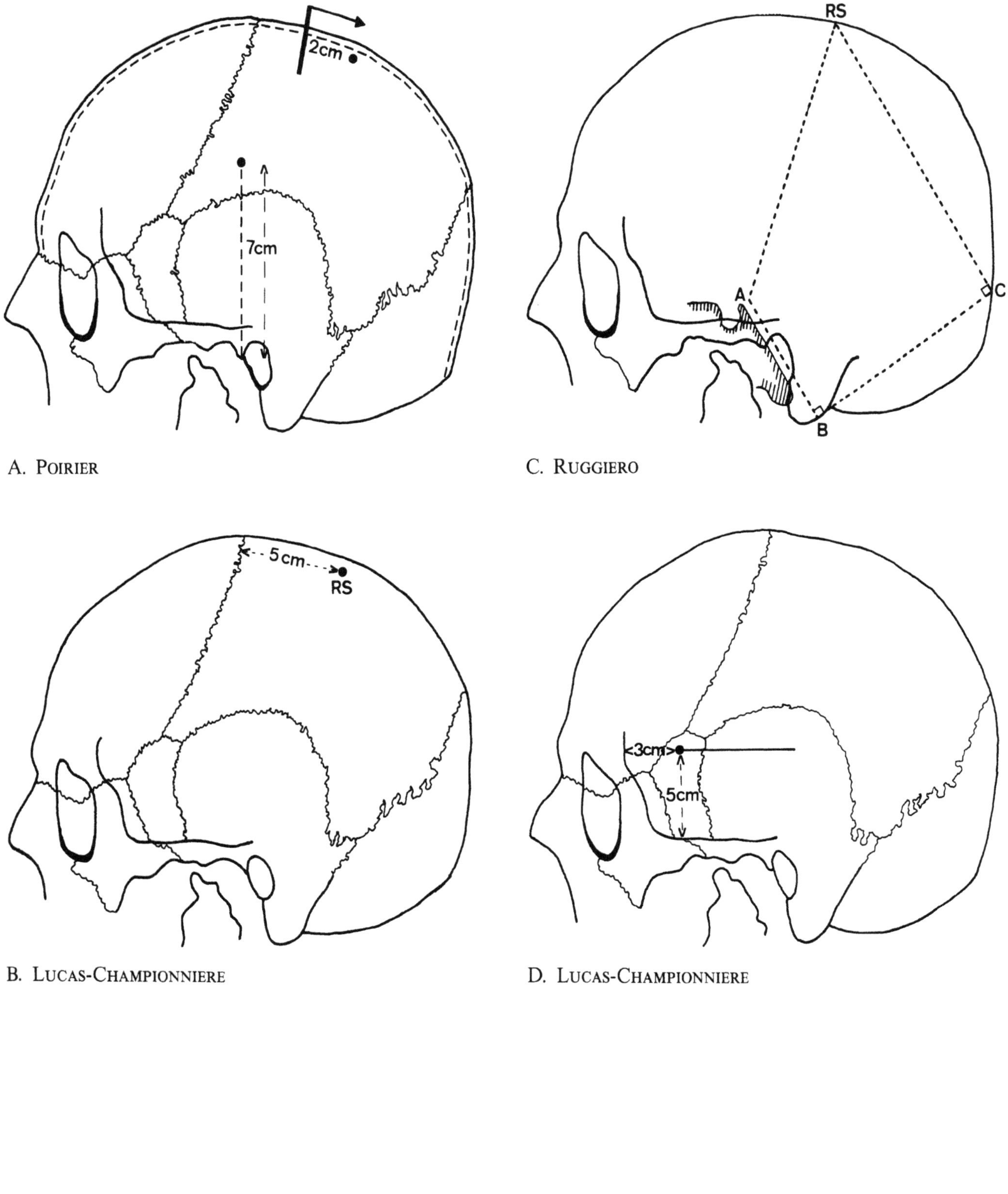

Fig. 9. Schematic representation of the methods of Poirier *et al.* (1921) (A), Lucas-Championniere (1948) (B) and Ruggiero (1958, 1966) (C) for localization of the central fissure (superior and inferior Rolandic points) and the method of Lucas-Championniere (D) for defining the Sylvian fissure

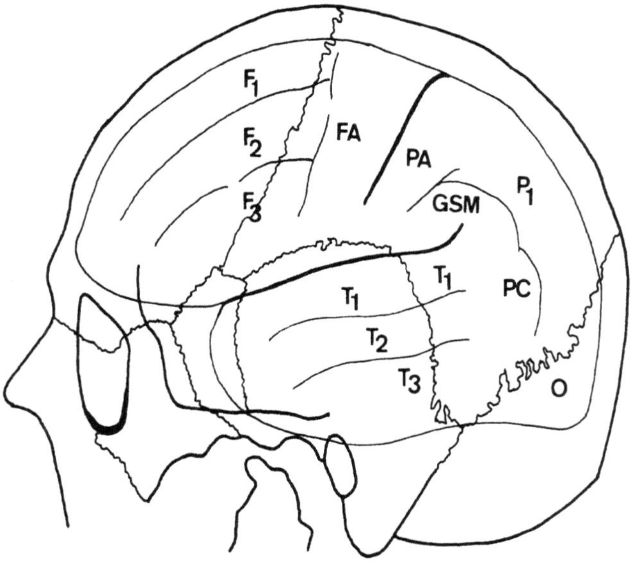

Fig. 10. Schematic representation of the relationships observed by MARIE, FOIX and BERTRAND (1915) between the gyri and the bony landmarks of the cranial vault (F_1, F_2 and F_3 superior, middle and inferior frontal gyri, *FA* precentral gyrus, *GSM* supramarginal gyrus, *O* occipital lobe, P_1 superior parietal lobule, *PA* postcentral gyrus, *PC* angular gyrus, T_1, T_2 and T_3 superior, middle and inferior temporal gyri)

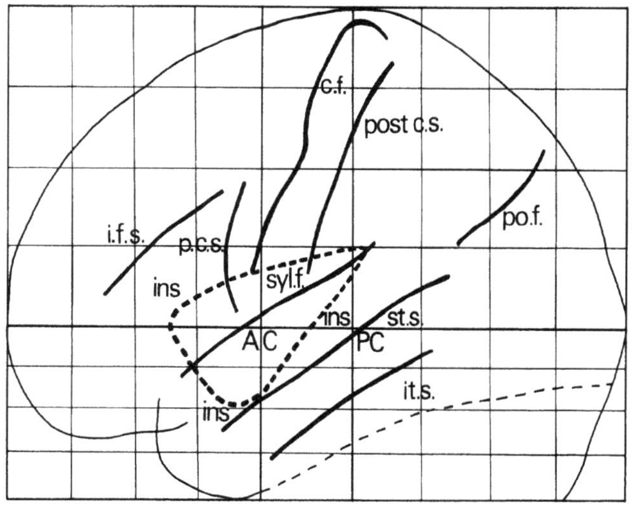

Fig. 12. Illustration of the fissures and sulci of the external surface of the hemisphere as related to the bicommissural line by TALAIRACH and SZIKLA (1967) (*AC* anterior commissure, *c.f.* central fissure, *ins* insula, *i.f.s.* inferior frontal sulcus, *it.s.* inferior temporal sulcus, *PC* posterior commissure, *p.c.s.* precentral sulcus, *post. c.s.* postcentral sulcus, *po.f.* parieto-occipital fissure, *st.s.* superior temporal sulcus, *syl.f.* Sylvian fissure)

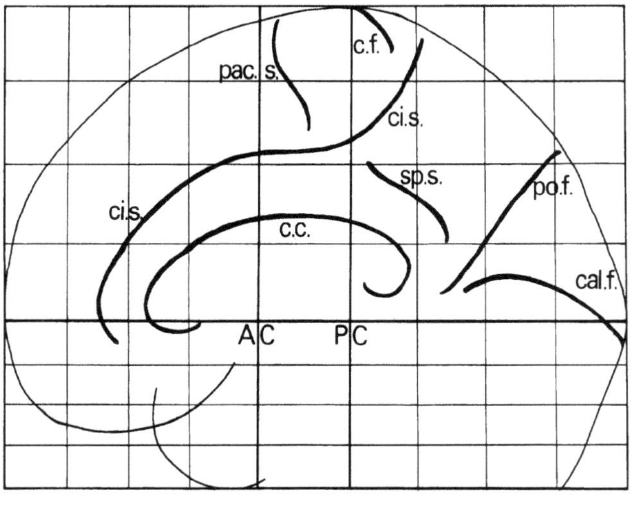

Fig. 11. Illustration of the fissures and sulci of the internal surface of the hemisphere as related to the bicommissural line by TALAIRACH and SZIKLA (1967) (*AC* anterior commissure, *cal.f.* calcarine fissure, *c.c.* corpus callosum, *c.f.* central fissure, *ci.s.* cingulate or callosomarginal sulcus, *pac.s.* paracentral sulcus, *PC* posterior commissure, *po.f.* parieto-occipital fissure, *sp.s.* subparietal sulcus)

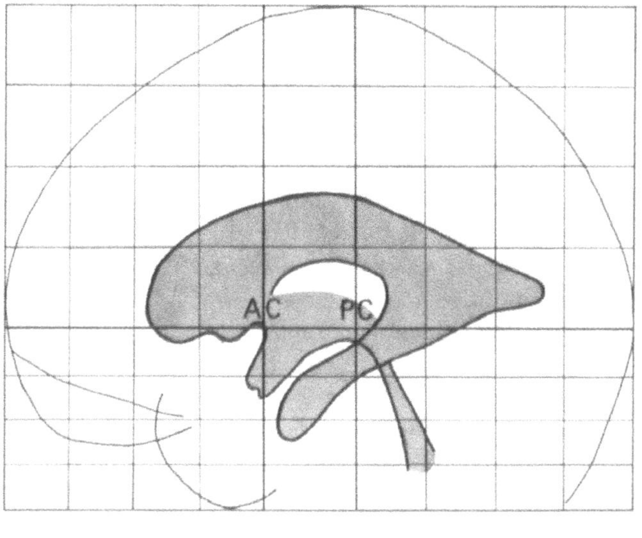

Fig. 13. Illustration of the cerebral ventricles as related to the bicommissural line by TALAIRACH and SZIKLA (1967) (*AC* anterior commissure, *PC* posterior commissure)

Chapter 2
Lateral Ventricles

Historically, the ventricles were considered a clinically insignificant part of cerebral anatomy. With the advent of pneumoencephalography and ventriculography, their central location and their relative ease of visualization, has made their study a most important part of the evaluation of lesions in the cerebral hemispheres and basal ganglia.

The discovery, by HOUNSFIELD (1973), of computerized axial tomography, gives to the lateral ventricles, so easily seen in this examination, an important role.

I. Anatomic Study of the Lateral Ventricles

The two lateral ventricles lie on either side of the midline, separated by the septum pellucidum and they communicate with the third ventricle through the foramina of Monro (the interventricular foramina). The lateral ventricles approach each other anteriorly, then deviate posteriorly around the thalamus and the cerebral peduncles, describing an open curve directed inferiorly and anteriorly. The anterior parts of the frontal horns are located anterior to the genu of the corpus callosum. The frontal horns, which are concave laterally, continue medially and superiorly to become the bodies of the lateral ventricles.

The ventricular cavities arch around the thalamus to extend into the temporal lobes. The temporal horns are directed from superiorly to inferiorly and posteriorly to anteriorly. Anteriorly they reach a position approximately 2 cm from the temporal poles. The lateral ventricles also extend posteriorly and horizontally to form the occipital horns. The junctions between the bodies of the lateral ventricles and their temporal and occipital horns form the atria of the lateral ventricles.

1. Frontal Horn of the Lateral Ventricle
(Figs. 14, 15, 16, 17, 18, 19)

The largest components of the ventricular system are the two frontal horns which are situated in the concavity of the genu of the corpus callosum. Viewed from above the frontal horns deviate from the midline in their anterior portions, while more posteriorly they are separated only by the septum pellucidum. Anteriorly to the septum pellucidum the frontal horns are shaped like vertical clefts with their superior, medial and inferior limits established by the corpus callosum. At this level the head of the caudate nucleus forms the lateral boundary. At the level of the septum pellucidum the frontal horns have a triangular configuration with superior, medial, and lateral surfaces. The superior surface is bounded by the corpus callosum, while the medial surface is formed by the septum pellucidum and the anterior columns of the fornix. The lateral surface corresponds to the head and body of the caudate nucleus.

2. Body of the Lateral Ventricle
(Figs. 14, 15, 16, 19, 20)

The shape of the body of the lateral ventricle is quite different from that of the frontal horn. It has a quadrangular configuration, flattened in such a way that superior and inferior surfaces and medial and lateral walls can be identified.

The superior surface of the body of the lateral ventricle is formed by the corpus callosum. Its inferior surface is more complex, comprising the body and tail of the caudate nucleus, the ventricular surface of the thalamus, the superior aspect of the fornix and the choroid plexus of the lateral ventricle.

At the junction between the caudate nucleus and the thalamus, the thalamostriate sulcus is seen on the inferior surface. From superficial to deep at this level, one can identify the lamina affixa, a thickening of the ventricular ependyma, the thalamostriate vein which flows into the internal cerebral vein and the stria terminalis.

The medial wall of the body of the lateral ventricle corresponds to an angle formed between the fornix and the corpus callosum. The lateral wall is formed by the angle between the corpus callosum and the caudate nucleus.

3. Atrium of the Lateral Ventricle
(Figs. 14, 15, 16, 21)

The atrium of the lateral ventricle is formed by the junction of the body, the temporal horn and the occipital horn. It is located behind the pulvinar and represents a region shared by the most anterior part of the occipital horn and the most posterior part of the temporal horn.

4. Occipital Horn of the Lateral Ventricle
(Figs. 15, 16, 22)

The occipital horn extends posteriorly from the atrium, invaginates the occipital lobe and terminates approximately 3 cm from the occipital pole. Its size, and particularly its diameter, present numerous variations. Generally the left occipital horn has a characteristic shape, orientated obliquely from superiorly to inferiorly and medially to laterally.

Two surfaces of the occipital horn can be described: the superolateral and inferomedial. The superolateral surface is convex laterally and corresponds with the medial part or forceps major of the corpus callosum. More laterally, it is related to the fibers of the tapetum, the optic radiations and the inferior longitudinal fasciculus. The inferomedial aspect has two sulci and three impressions of variable size. The forceps of the corpus callosum forms a fold, the bulb of the occipital horn, which produces the superior impression. The middle impression, or calcar avis, is the largest and corresponds with the invagination of the calcarine fissure. The inferior impression into the occipital horn is the collateral eminence, which is produced by the collateral fissure, located between the lingular and fusiform gyri. The two sulci which form the borders of these impressions are the lingual diverticulum and the diverticulum of the cuneus.

5. Temporal Horn of the Lateral Ventricle
(Figs. 14, 15, 23, 24, 25, 26, 27)

The temporal horn is that portion of the ventricular system which extends into the temporal lobe. Its direction is from superiorly to inferiorly, posteriorly to anteriorly, and medially to laterally. It arches around the cerebral peduncles and the thalamus, extending from the atrium of the lateral ventricle to approximately 2 cm posterior to the tip of the temporal pole.

As with the occipital horns, two surfaces can be described; a superolateral and an inferomedial. The former is flat or slightly convex laterally, while the latter is clearly concave along its medial aspect. The superolateral wall of the temporal horn is continuous with the superolateral wall of the occipital horn. It is related laterally to the tapetum. More medially the borders of the superolateral wall are formed by the optic radiation and the tail of the caudate nucleus. The inferomedial wall is modified by two impressions. The medial one is produced by Ammon's horn, an invagination of the hippocampal sulcus. The lateral one, the collateral eminence, represents the invagination of the collateral sulcus.

Ammon's horn forms a large impression in the temporal horn which is smooth posteriorly but undulates anteriorly. It is covered by white matter, the alveus, and is related to the concavity of the hippocampus, the subiculum. Ammon's horn is joined posteriorly by the fimbria or posterior columns of the fornix. The dentate gyrus is medial to Ammon's horn.

The lateral impression is produced by the invagination of the collateral sulcus into the temporal horn. This sulcus separates the lingual and fusiform gyri. A sulcus, the diverticulum of the subiculum, is located between Ammon's horn and the collateral eminence.

Childe and Penfield (1944) and later Lindgren (1948) divide this portion of the temporal horn into two parts. The medial one which corresponds to Ammon's horn is referred to as the supracornual portion or supracornual cleft. The lateral one, which relates to the collateral eminence, is termed the lateral portion or lateral cleft.

II. Radiologic Study of the Lateral Ventricles

All works dedicated to pneumoencephalography and ventriculography contain abundant illustrations of the morphology and variations of the various portions of the ventricular complex [Lysholm (1935), Robertson (1957), Lindgren (1948, 1954, 1957), Ruggiero (1957, 1966), Taveras and Wood (1964), di Chiro (1961), Fischgold (1972)].

Bull (1961) measured the volume of the lateral ventricles using Tomsett (1956) casts. The average volume of the two lateral ventricles is approximately 8 to 12 cc.

Radiologic nomenclature attempts to identify the same divisions of the lateral ventricles identified by anatomists; that is to say, one differentiates between the frontal horn, the body (sometimes subdivided into anterior and posterior parts), the atrium, and the occipital and temporal horns of the lateral ventricle.

The technical aspects of pneumoencephalography, which provide diagnostic information about the part of the ventricular system in question, have been simplified by the frequent use of apparatus derived from the principle of Pott's isocentric chair. Circulatory motion of the diagnostic arm, frequently motorized, readily permits frontal, lateral, and oblique radiography with the patient in the upright, brow-up and brow-down positions. The temporal horns are visualized after rotating 270°.

Simplification of the technique of pneumoencephalography has increased the time available for study of the images obtained and the categorization of normal and pathologic appearances.

Tomography, especially in the hypocycloidal mode, adds a method for enhancing the data obtained during conventional pneumoencephalography. The development of safe water-soluble media for contrast ventriculography provides another means for precisely outlining part, or all, of the ventricular system.

In the realm of pneumoencephalography, the morphology itself plays a more important diagnostic role than any of the diverse measurements proposed for evaluation of the ventricular system. However, neither method excludes the other, and it is interesting to note the different average diameters obtained for the various parts of the lateral ventricles.

1. Frontal Horn of the Lateral Ventricle

(Figs. 28, 29, 30, 31)

The frontal horn is readily demonstrated pneumoencephalographically by the air which collects in front of the foramen of Monro, in the brow-up position. In the lateral projection the roof of the frontal horn exhibits a convex superior curve which conforms to the radiations of the corpus callosum. A variation in the tonality of the image anterior to the foramen of Monro corresponds to the imprint of the head of the caudate nucleus.

Two distinct zones contribute to the composite image seen in the frontal projection; the area in front of the head of the caudate nucleus has an oval or quadrangular configuration; at the level of the nucleus the shape is triangular, limited by the head of the caudate nucleus laterally, the corpus callosum above, and the septum pellucidum in the midline. It is important to distinguish the two constituents of the image of the frontal horn in this projection from the quadrangular image of the anterior part of the body of the lateral ventricle, which may also be filled.

Slight asymmetry may be present in the transverse diameters of the lateral ventricles. For Davidoff and Dyke (1951), the total transverse diameter of the two frontal horns averages 40 mm. The anteroposterior length of the frontal horn averaged 25 mm for Orley (1949) and 35 mm for Taveras and Wood (1964) (Fig. 29A).

The angle formed by the roofs of the two frontal horns is about 130° [Le May and New (1970)] (Fig. 29B). The relationship between the transverse diameter of the two frontal horns and the transverse diameter of the cranial vault varies between 0.16 and 0.31 as measured by Evans (1942) (Fig. 29C).

In a series of 100 normal pneumoencephalograms, Ruggiero (1966) found the transverse diameter of the right frontal horn to be 15 to 32 mm and the left to be 17 to 33 mm.

It must always be remembered that the size of the ventricles, as measured immediately after insufflation, can vary during the subsequent hours, first increasing and later decreasing.

2. Body of the Lateral Ventricle

(Figs. 31, 32, 33, 34)

The body of the lateral ventricle is visualized with the patient in the upright position. In the lateral projection its roof corresponds to the convex superior curve of the corpus callosum. The latter can cause a corrugated appearance of the superior surface, especially in the anterior portion of the body of the lateral ventricle (Lindgren, 1957).

In the frontal projection the image of the body must be distinguished from that of the frontal horn or the atrium, depending upon the position of the patient and the degree of filling of the ventricle. The quadrangular bodies of the two lateral ventricles diverge progressively from anteriorly to posteriorly. If the relationships of the superior margins (corresponding to the corpus callosum) are simple, the inferior relationships are complex, being made up of the thalamus, the caudate nucleus (laterally) and the fornix (medially).

The anteroposterior length of the body of the ventricle is 45 mm according to Taveras and Wood (1964) and 50 mm according to Orley (1949). Slight asymmetry between the two sides may be tolerated.

3. Atrium of the Lateral Ventricle

(Figs. 32, 33, 34)

The atrium of the lateral ventricle is situated at the junction of the body with the occipital and temporal horns. In the lateral projection the choroid plexus of the lateral ventricle frequently protrudes into the anterior part of the atrium. In the frontal projection the image of the atrium is characteristic, corresponding to the bulge of the posterior pole of the thalamus which it envelopes. Taveras and Wood (1964) give 23 mm as the anteroposterior length of the atrium.

4. Occipital Horn of the Lateral Ventricle
(Figs. 33, 34, 35)

The occipital horn is the most variable portion of the ventricular system, not only from patient to patient, but also from one side to the other in the same patient. LAZORTHES and POULHES (1948) studied the form and degree of development of the occipital horns in great detail. When well-developed, the occipital horn terminates about 30 mm anterior to the inner table.

In the frontal projection there are three characteristic impressions on the inferomedial surface of the occipital horn. The most superior of these is the fold of the forceps major of the corpus callosum. The middle impression or calcar avis is largest and corresponds to the invagination of the calcarine fissure. The third and most inferior impression is the collateral eminence, produced by the collateral fissure.

5. Temporal Horn of the Lateral Ventricle
(Figs. 36, 37, 38, 39)

The temporal horn, comprehensively studied by LINDGREN (1948), is radiologically examined with frontal, lateral and semi-axial projections. Of the diverse maneuvers suggested for filling the temporal horn (LINDGREN, 1948; ROBERTSON, 1957), the easiest is the forward somersault.

In the lateral projection the temporal horn extends anteriorly from the atrium to the region of the dorsum sellae. Here, the temporal horn is adjacent to the amygdaloid body and exhibits an increase in its previously slight downward angulation. This results in a curve which is concave posteriorly and inferiorly.

In the frontal projection, the roof of the temporal horn is convex superolaterally. The inferomedial concavity of the floor is caused by two impressions. The medial and best-defined impression corresponds to Ammon's horn [the supracornual cleft of LINDGREN (1948), or CHILDE and PENFIELD (1944)]. The collateral sulcus produces the lateral impression (lateral cleft) which is more variable radiologically.

The semi-axial projection demonstrates the general direction of the temporal horn from posteriorly to anteriorly, superiorly to inferiorly, and medially to laterally.

The anteroposterior length of the temporal horn averages 50 mm for DAVIDOFF and DYKE (1951), and ORLEY (1949). The former authors state that the temporal horns are separated by 90 mm in the frontal projection. RUGGIERO (1966), SALAMON *et al.* (1963) and LE MAY and NEW (1970) have studied the variations in temporal horn dimensions during the time following injection of air.

The most complete study of the temporal horn is the work of TALAIRACH, DAVID and TOUNOUX (1958), performed to facilitate their exploration, by stereotactic surgery, of the temporal lobe in patients with temporal lobe epilepsy. In their study, TALAIRACH *et al.* (1958) used oily opaque contrast media to outline the temporal horn (Fig. 39). A base line LT is then constructed on the lateral radiograph from the most anterior point (A) of the temporal horn, tangentially to the floor of the posterior portion of the temporal horn. A posterior point (P) is located 40 mm behind (A), on LT. Anterior and posterior vertical lines (VA and VP, respectively) are then constructed perpendicular to LT at these points. In the frontal projection the most lateral aspect of the temporal horn gives information about the depth of different structures.

Using the previously described reference lines, TALAIRACH *et al.* (1958) have localized the hippocampal gyrus, the uncus, Ammon's horn, the amygdaloid body and the outer surface of the temporal lobe (T1, T2, T3).

TALAIRACH and SZIKLA (1967) have also proposed a system of coordinates derived from the bicommissural line for the stereotactic approach to the telencephalon. This method of quadrangulation provides an unique method for standardizing the image of the human ventricular system.

In yet another dimension, computerized axial tomography, even if it is not so precise, still provides information about the ventricular system as it is observed in the horizontal plane.

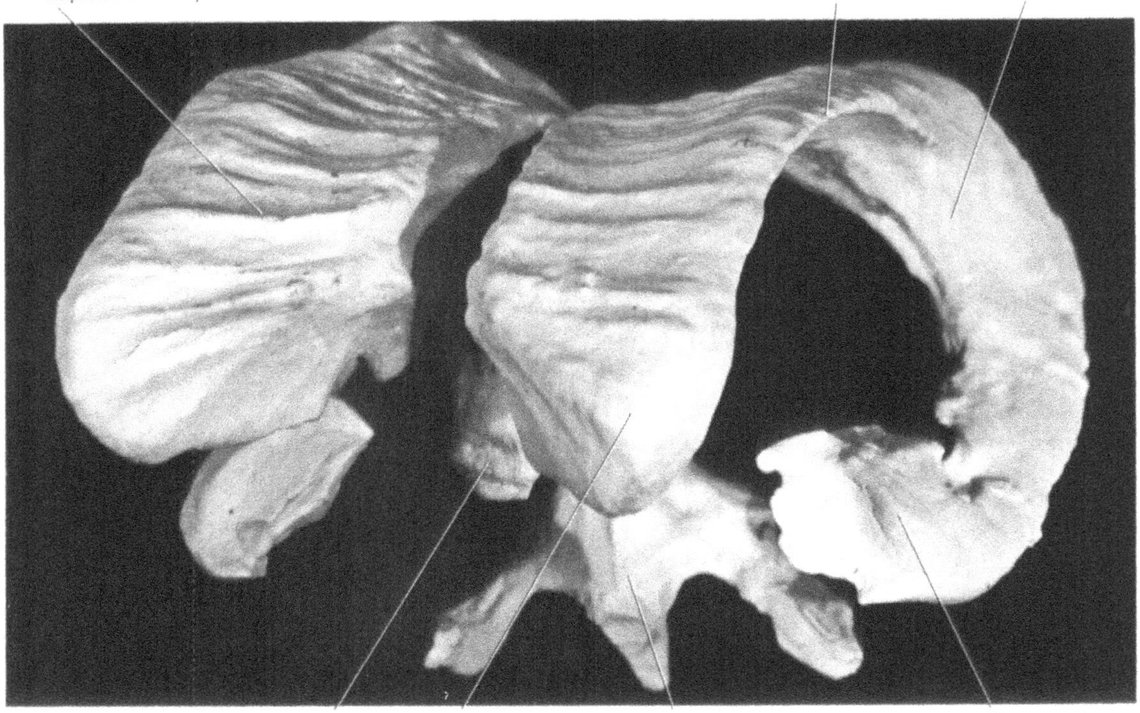
Impression of corpus callosum
Body of lateral ventricle
Atrium of lateral ventricle
Third ventricle
Frontal horn
Fourth ventricle
Temporal horn

Fig. 14

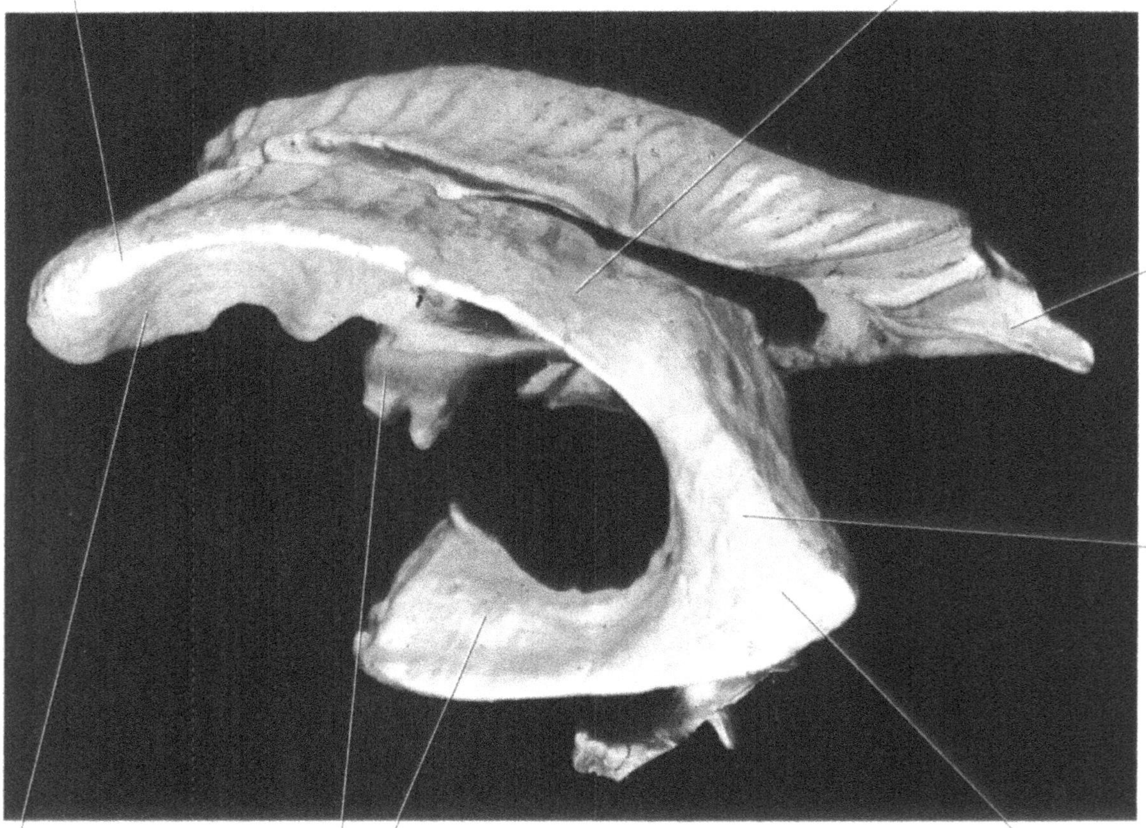
Frontal horn
Body of lateral ventricle
Occipital horn
Atrium of lateral ventricle
Impression of caudate nucleus
Third ventricle
Temporal horn
Occipital horn

Fig. 15

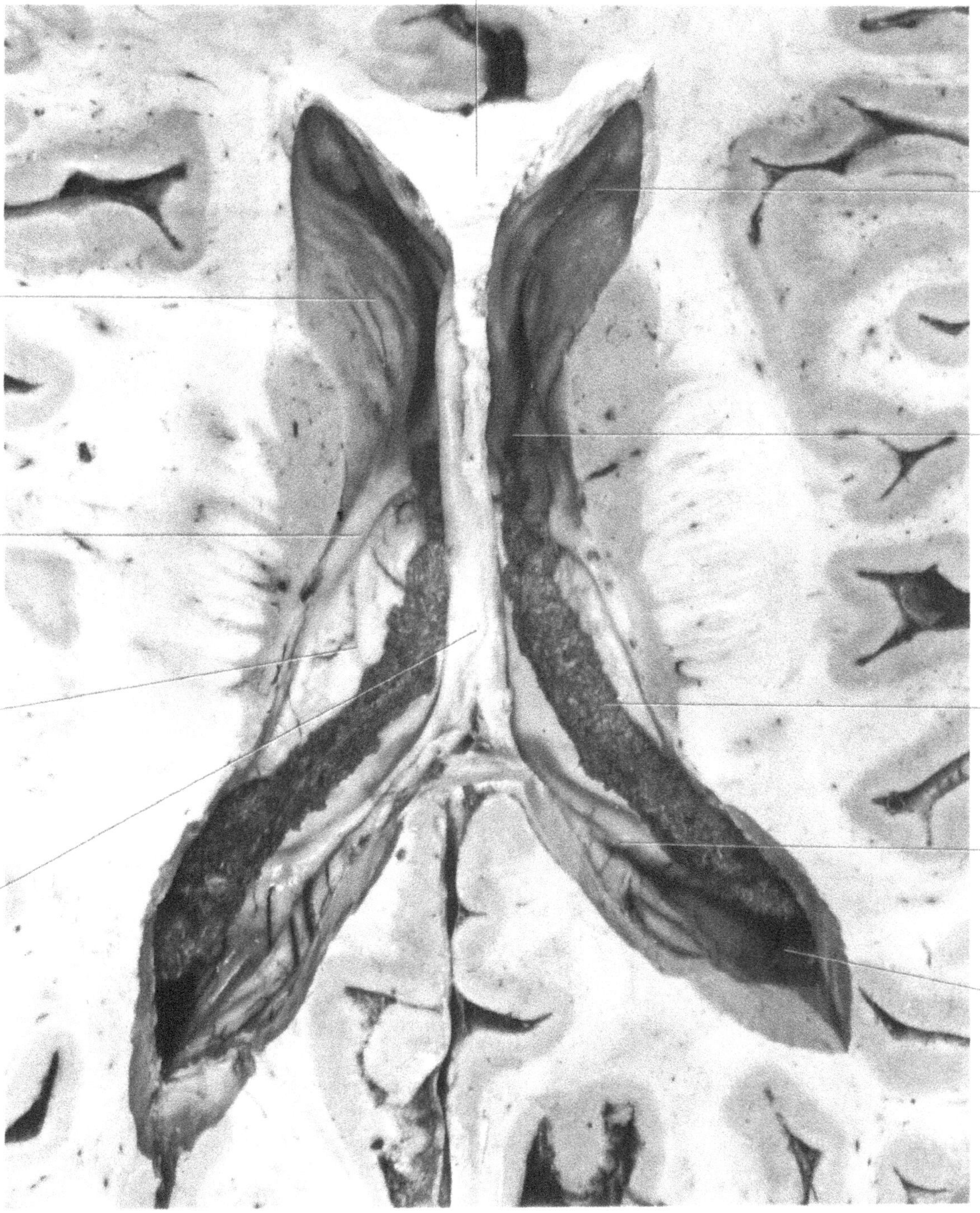

Fig. 16. Superior view of the floor of the lateral ventricles

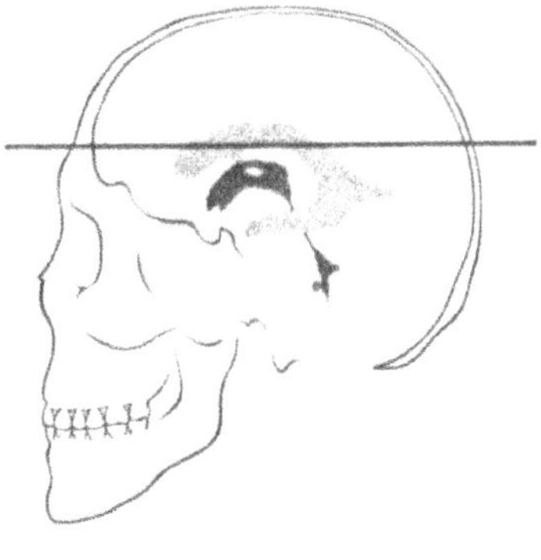

◁
Fig. 14. Cast of the ventricular system, anterolateral view

Fig. 15. Cast of the ventricular system, posterolateral view

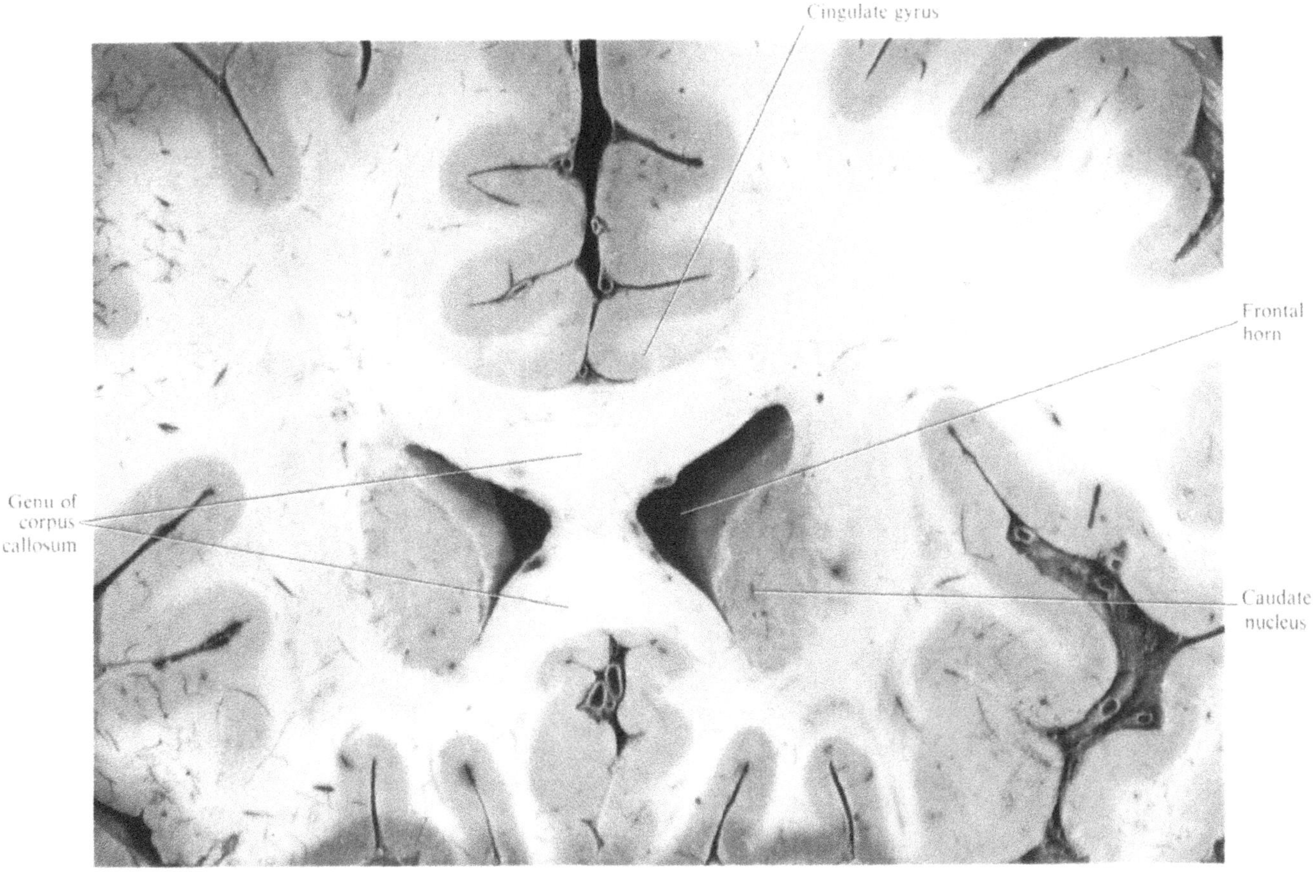

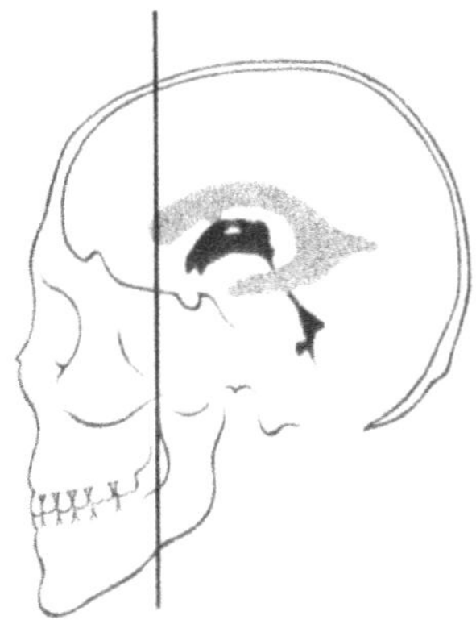

Fig. 17. Frontal section through the anterior part of the frontal horns

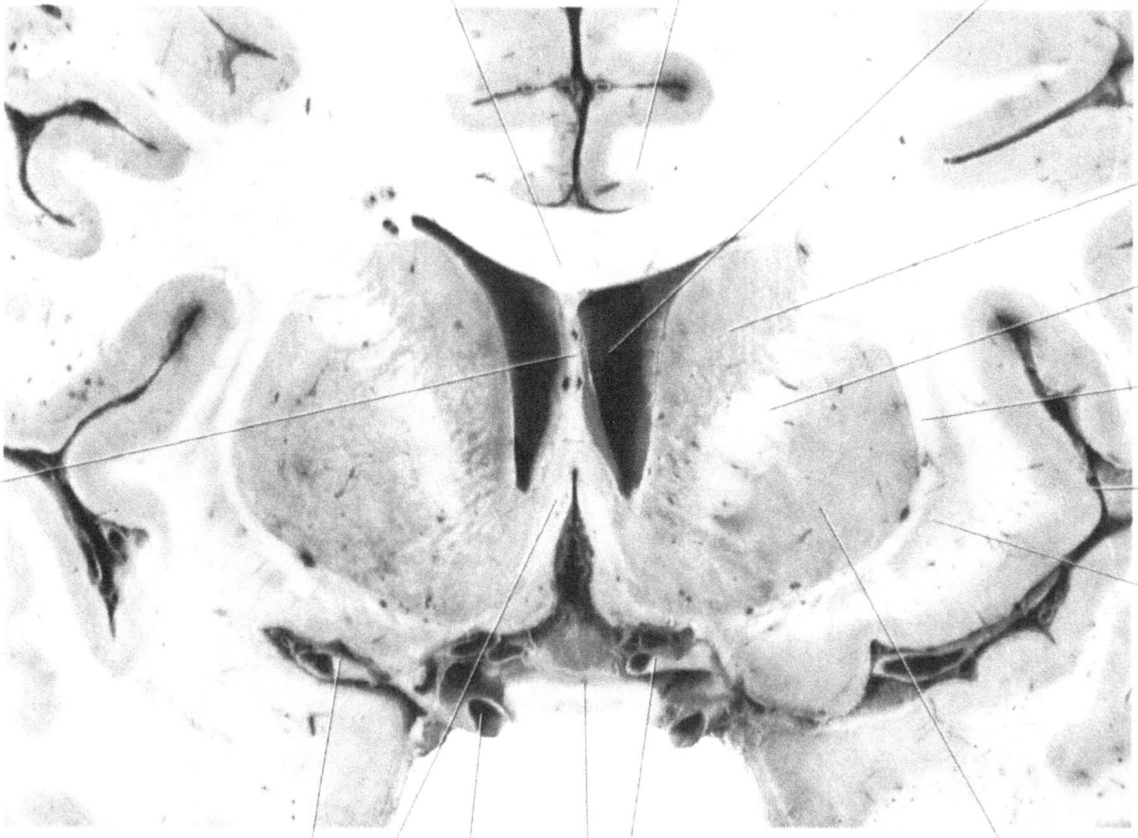

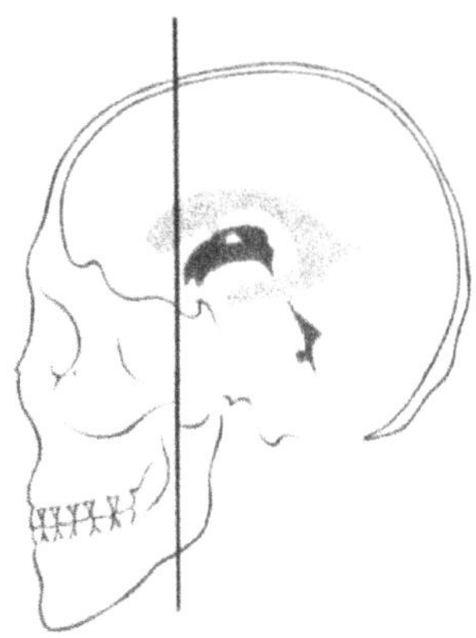

Fig. 18. Frontal section through the mid portion of the frontal horns

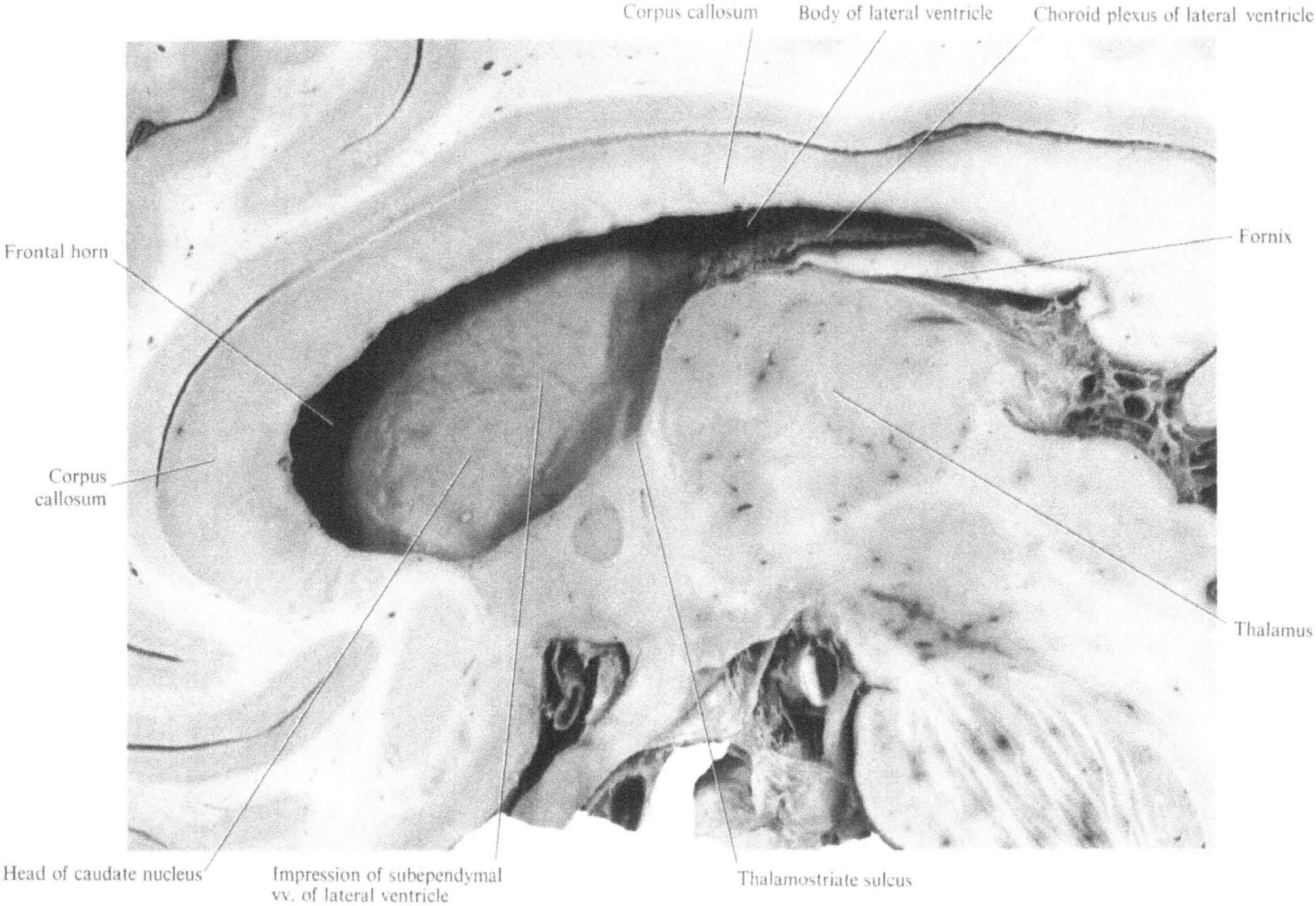

Fig. 19. Internal view of the frontal horn and anterior part of the body of the lateral ventricle

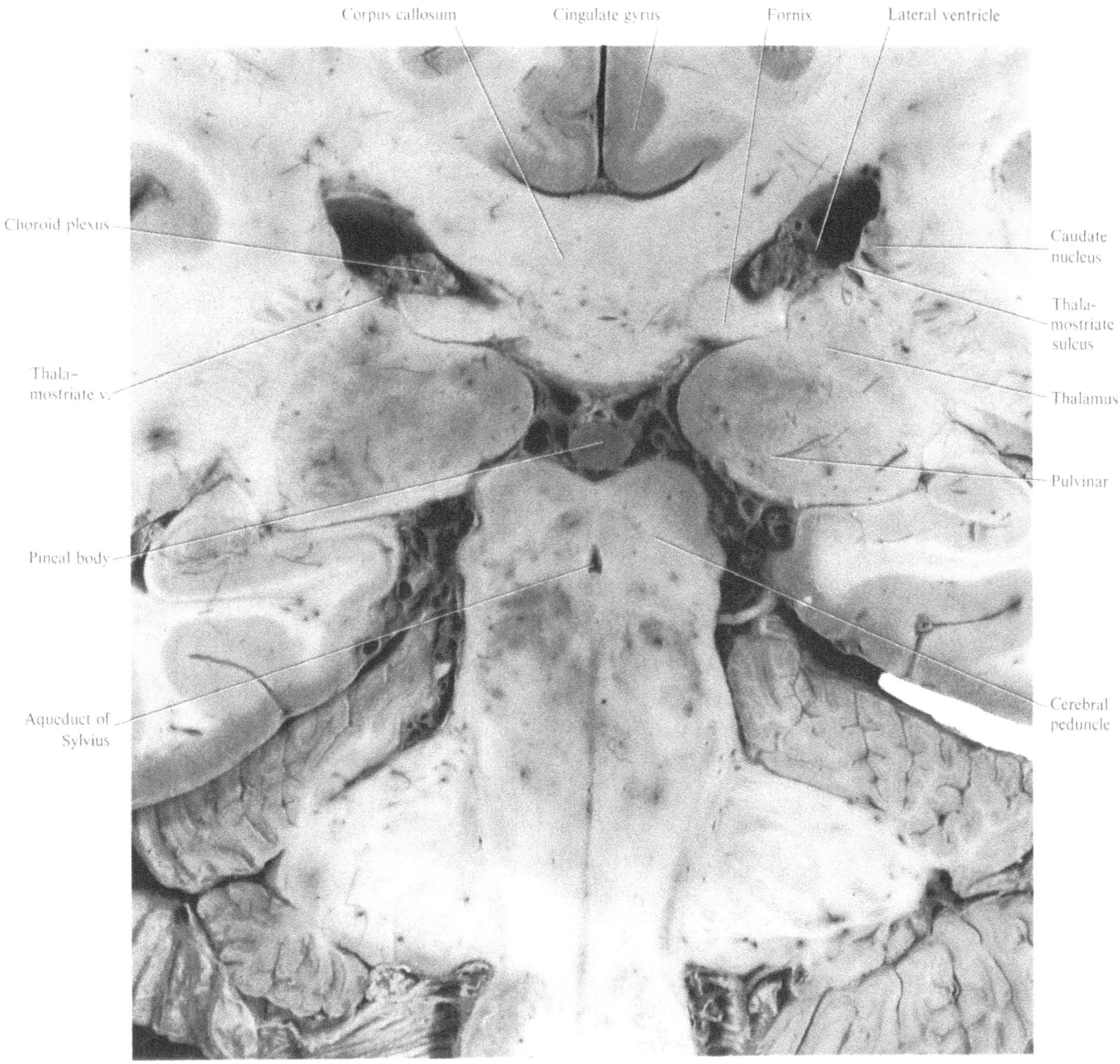

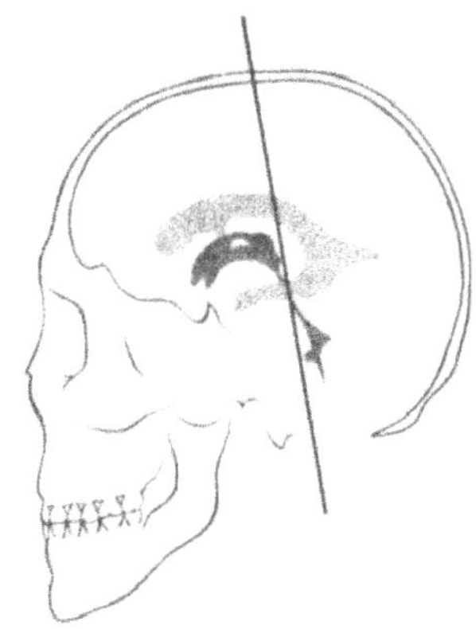

Fig. 20. Frontal section through the midportion of the bodies of the lateral ventricles

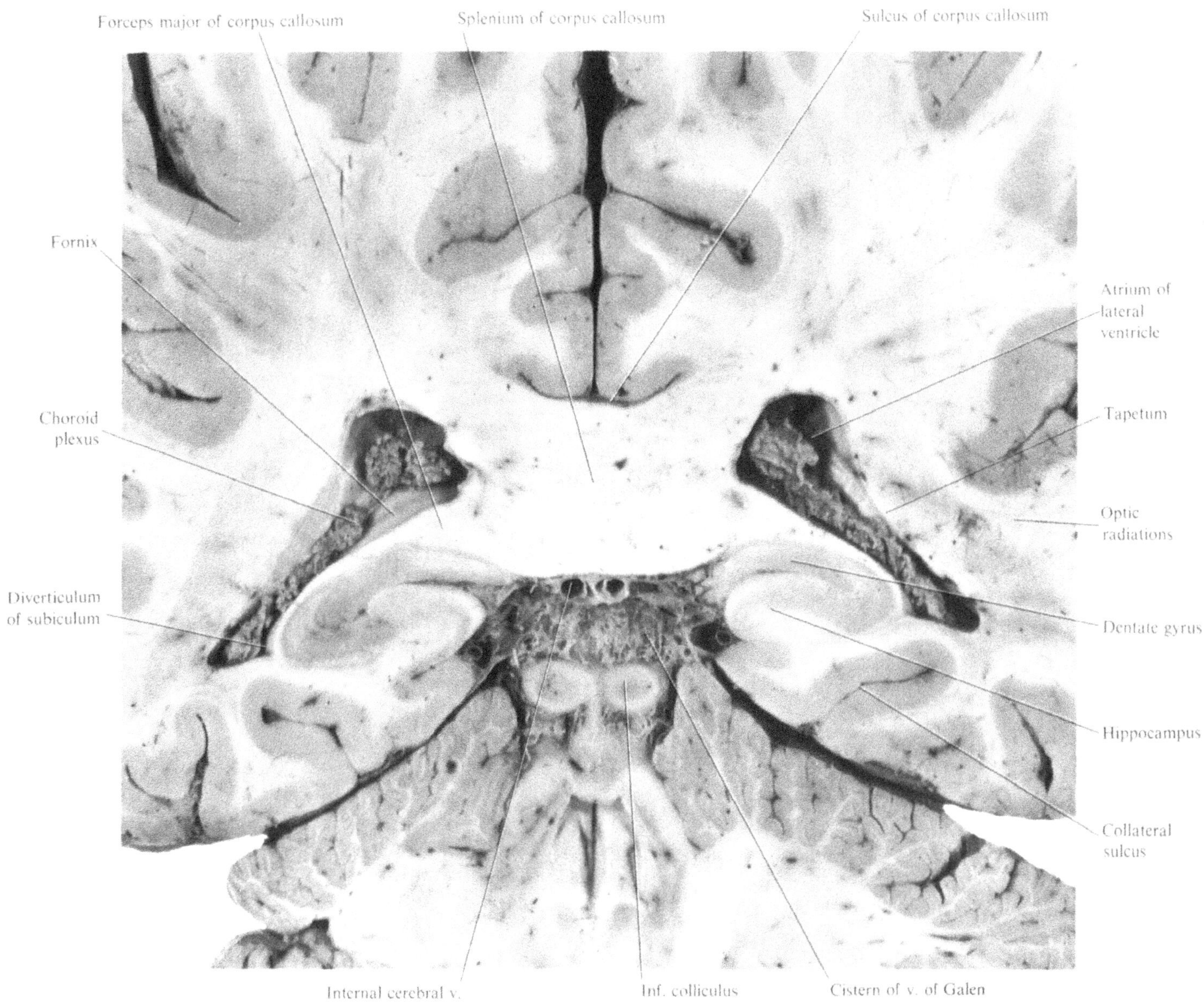

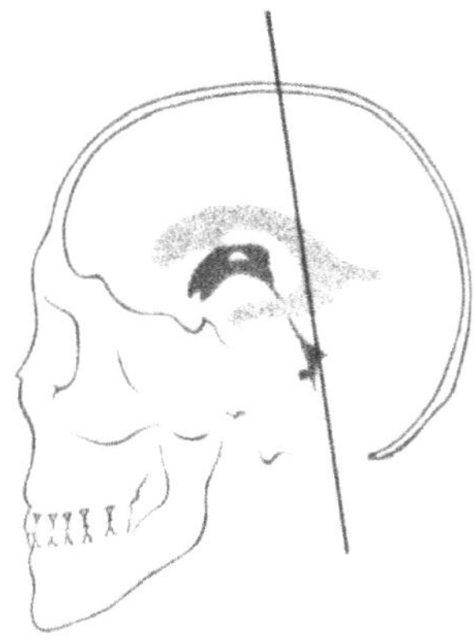

Fig. 21. Frontal section through the atria of the lateral ventricles

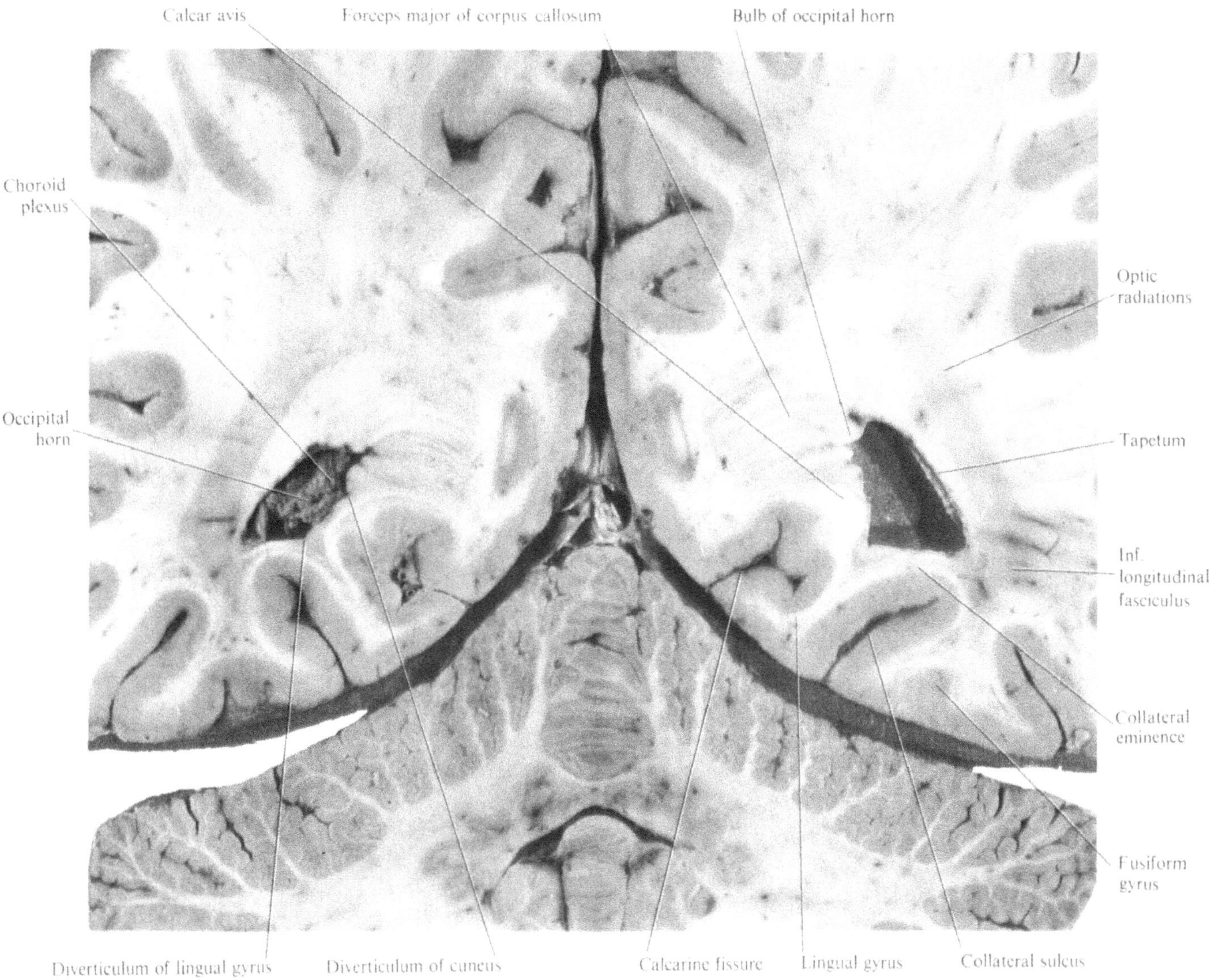

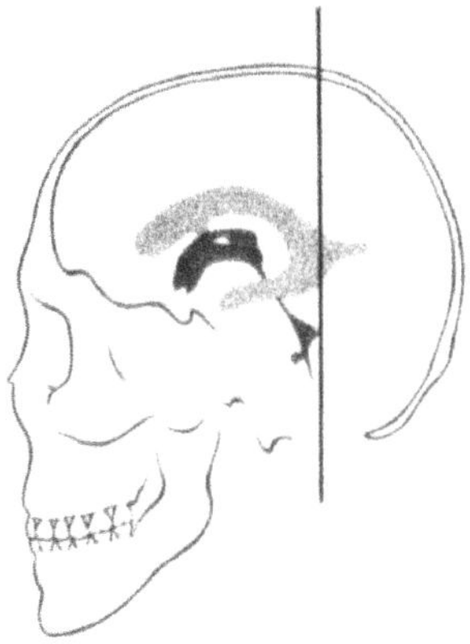

Fig. 22. Frontal section through the occipital horns

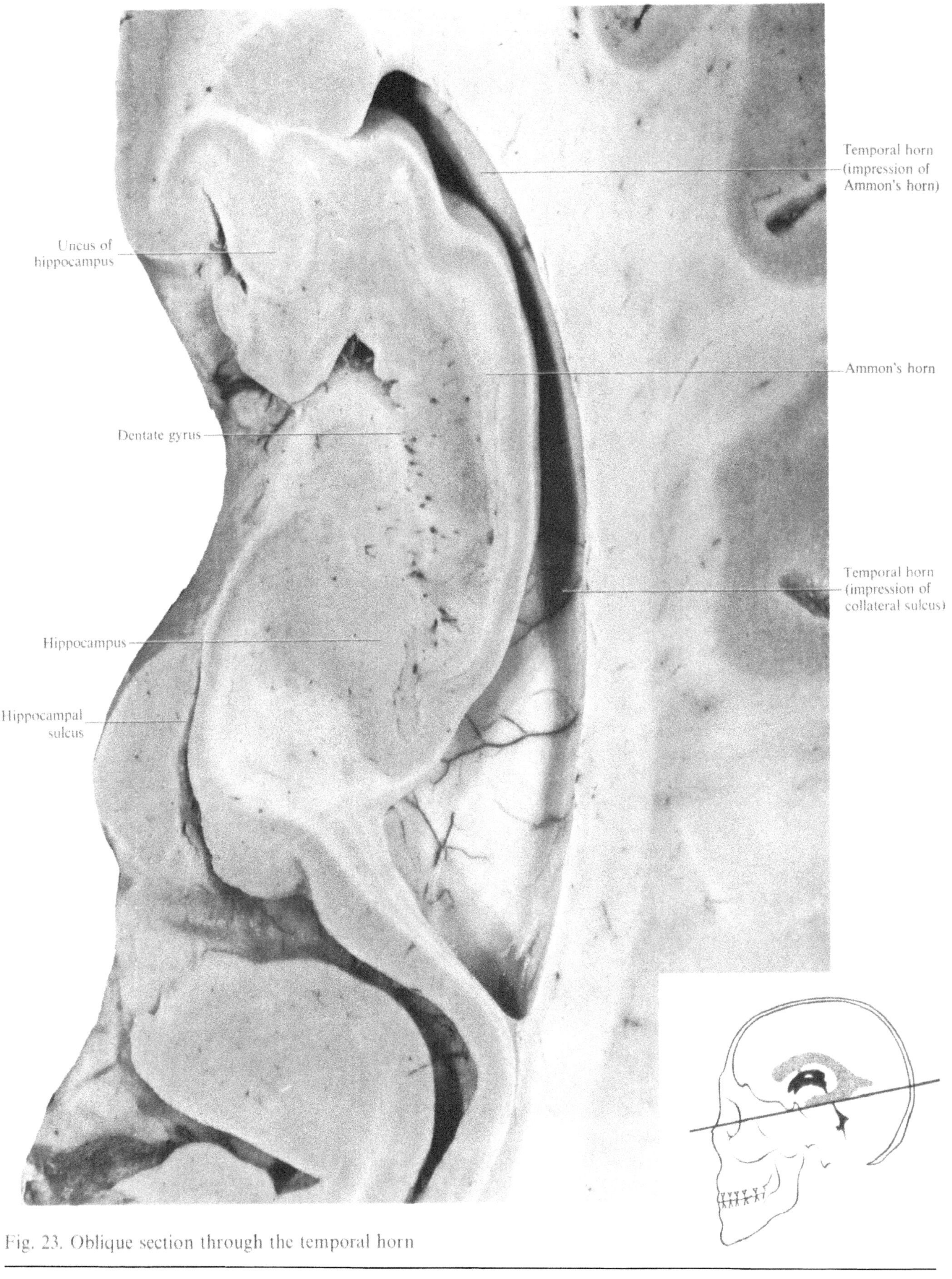

Fig. 23. Oblique section through the temporal horn

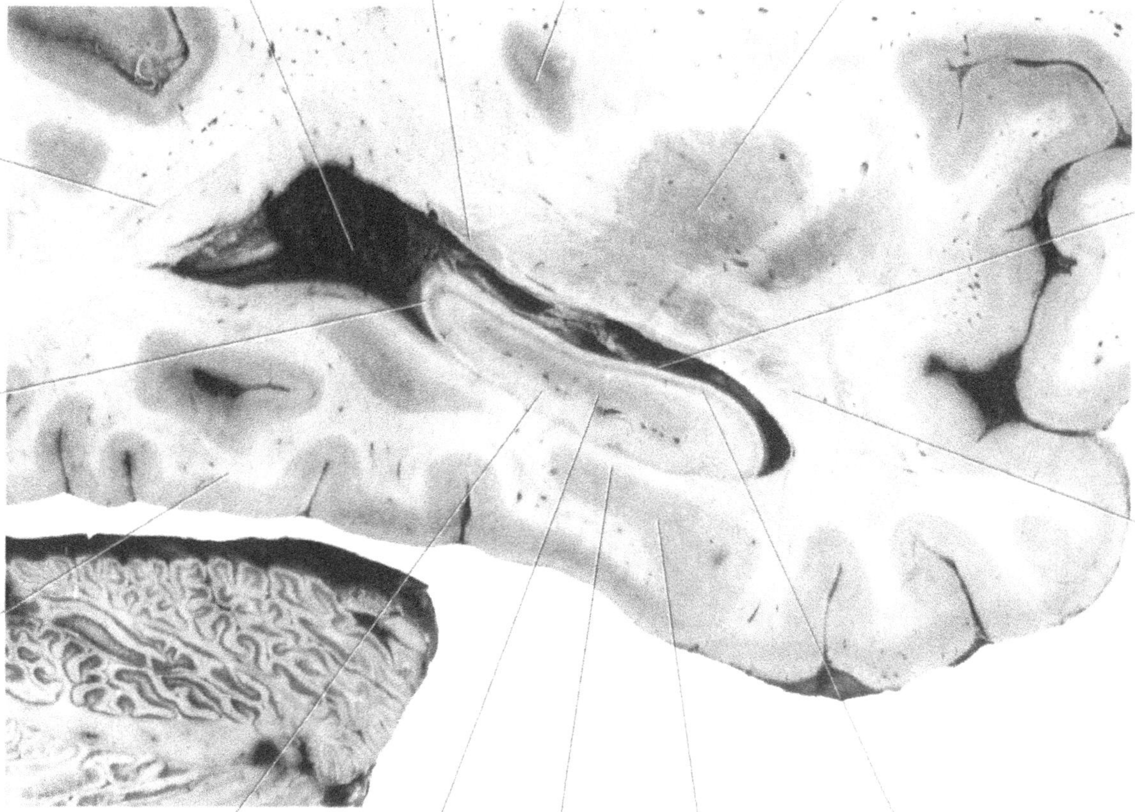

Fig. 24. Parasagittal section through the midportion of the temporal horn

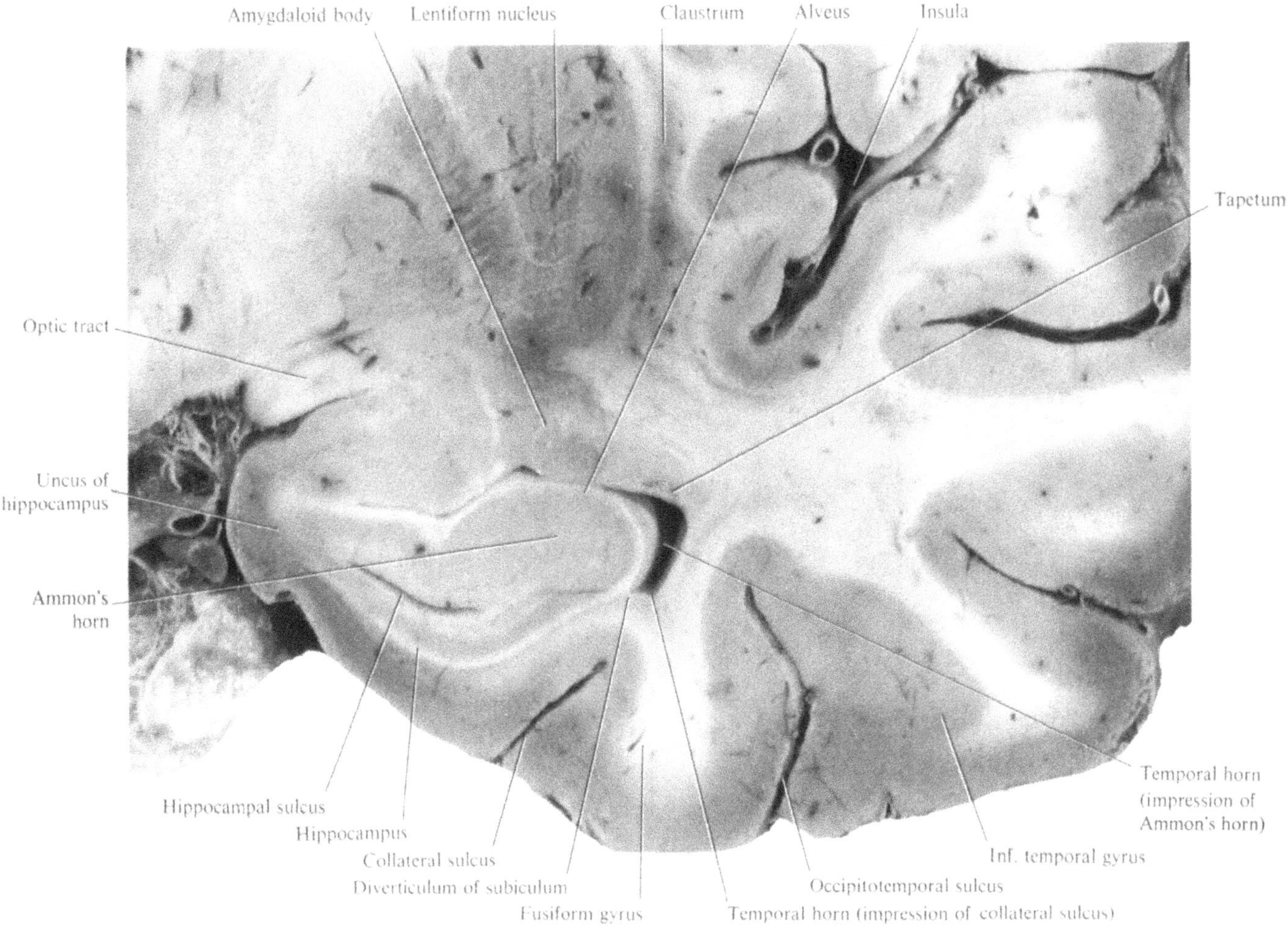

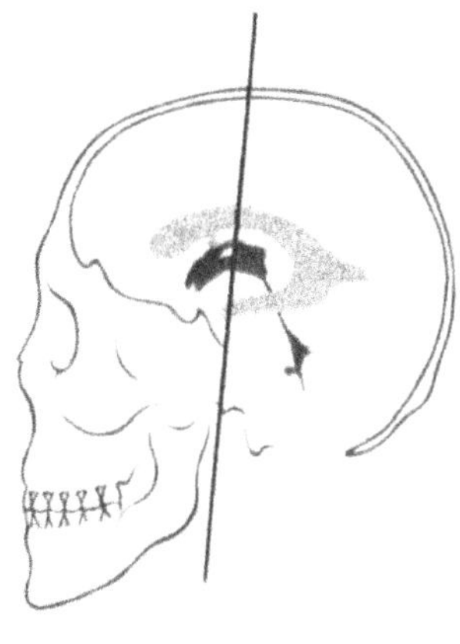

Fig. 25. Frontal section through the anterior part of the temporal horn

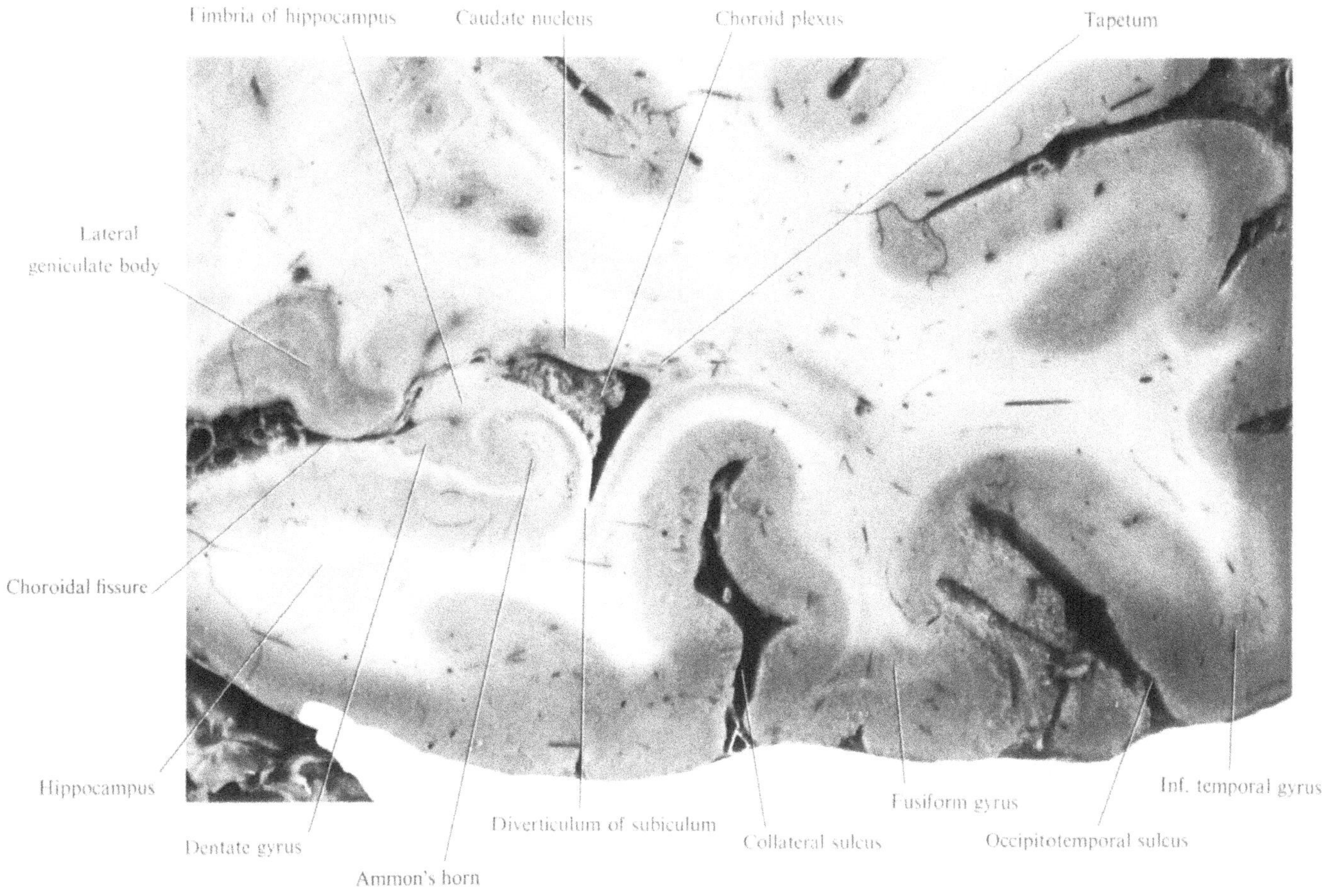

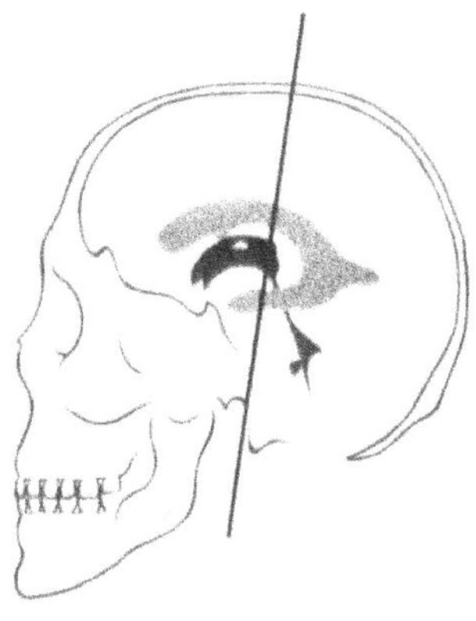

Fig. 26. Frontal section through the midportion of the temporal horn

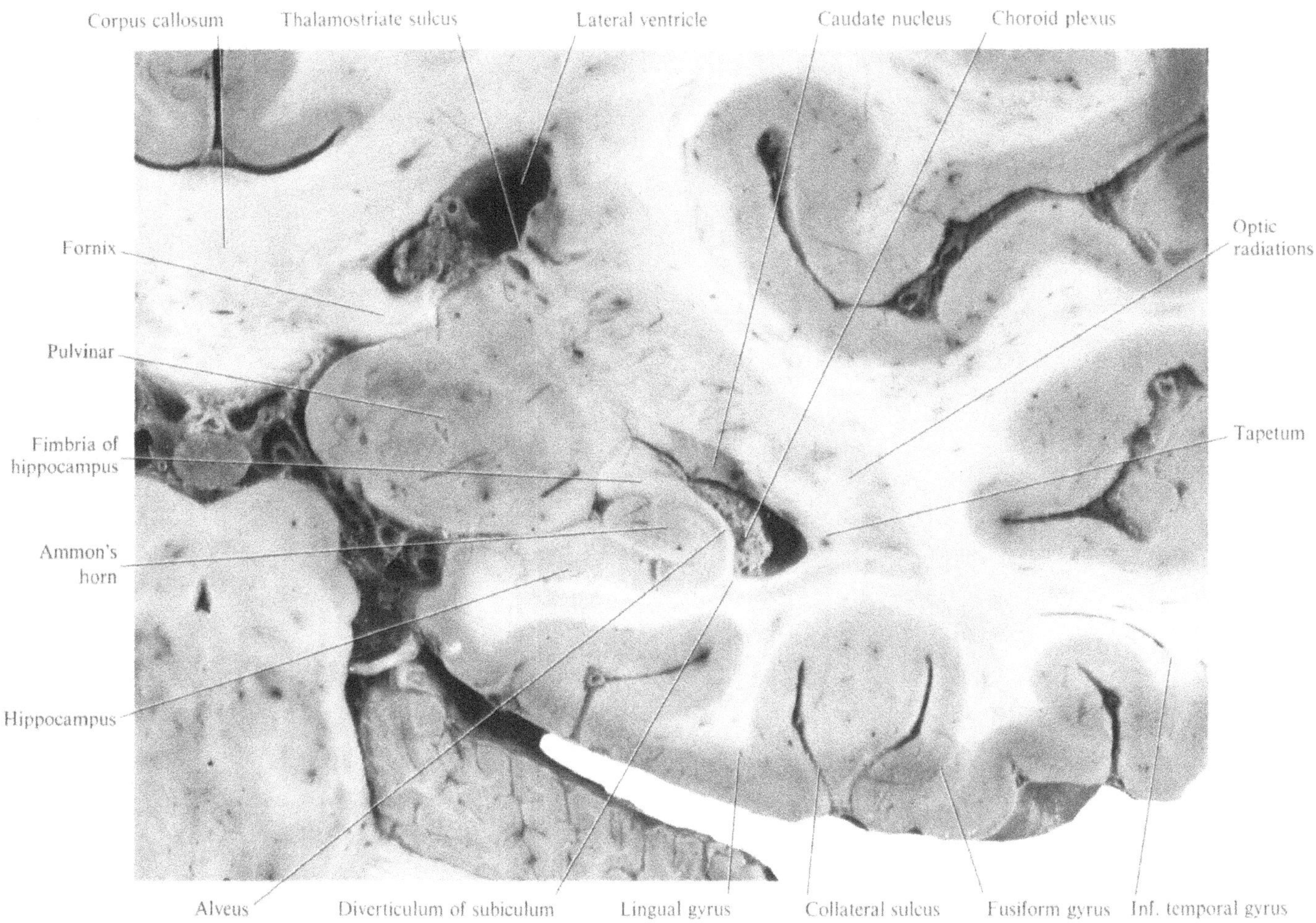

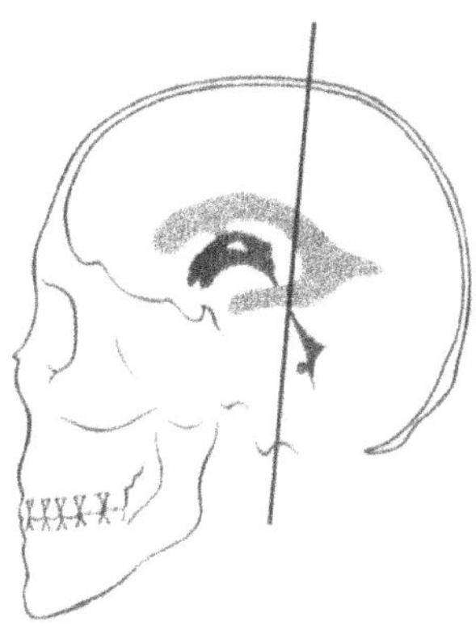

Fig. 27. Frontal section through the posterior part of the temporal horn

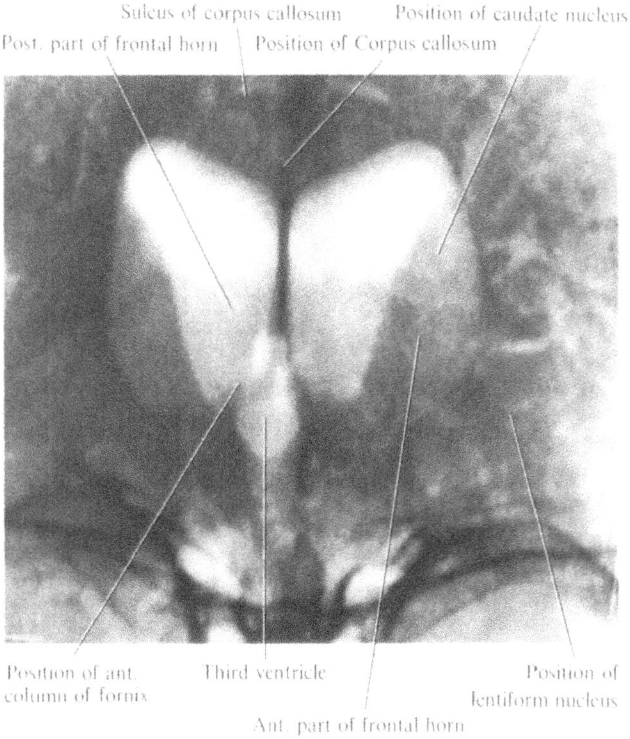

Fig. 28A

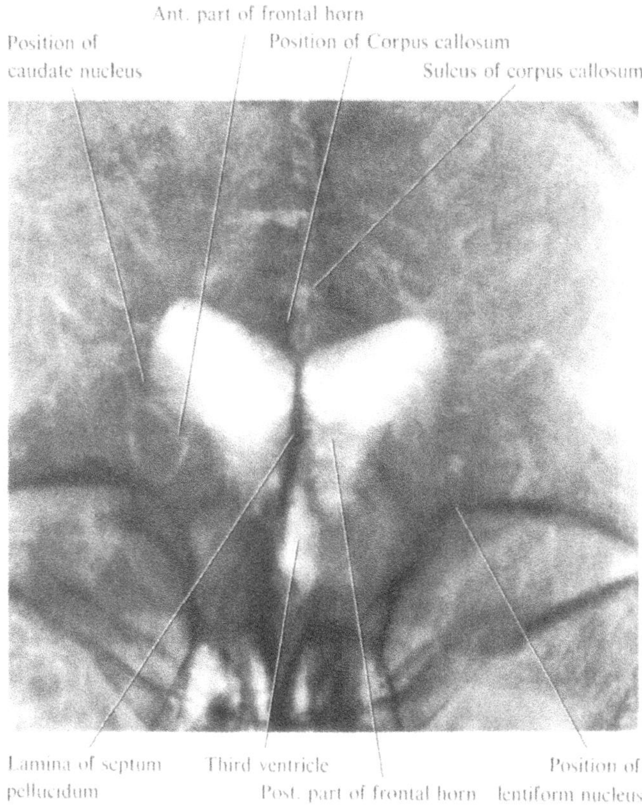

Fig. 28B

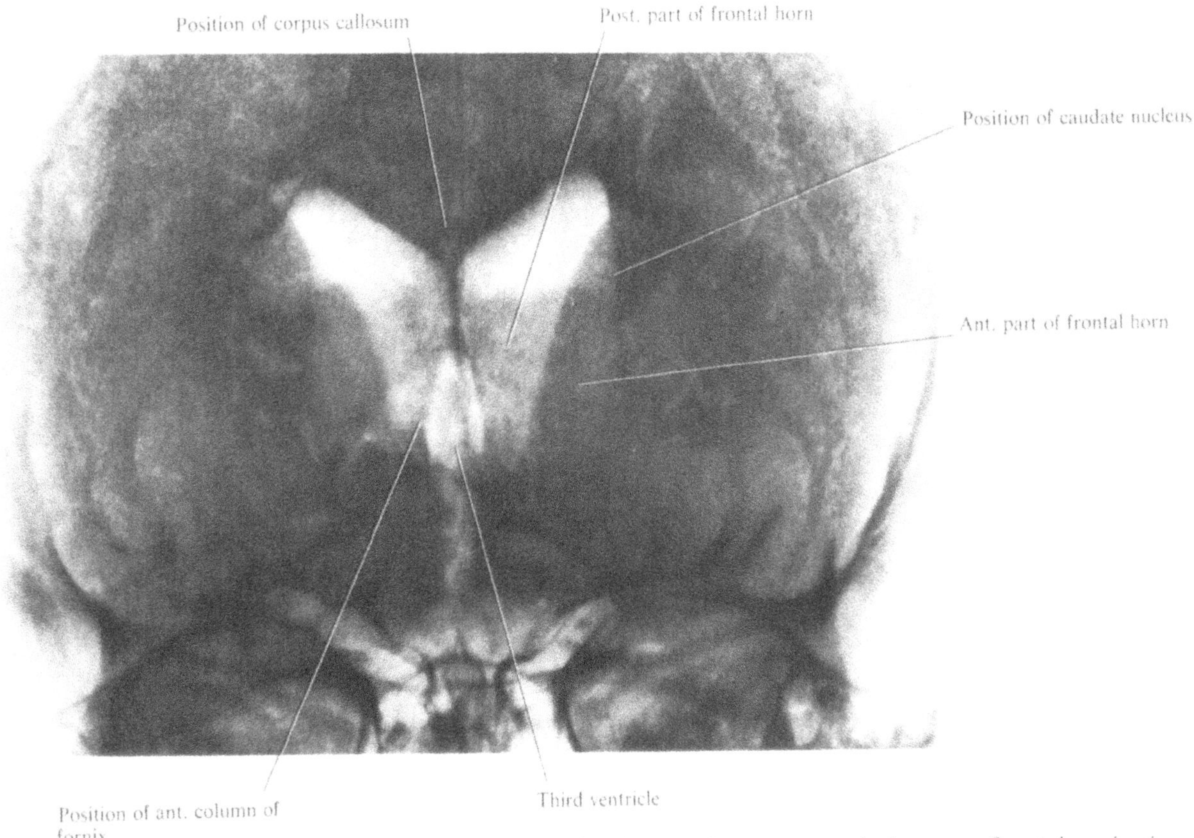

Fig. 28C

Fig. 28A–C. Pneumoencephalograms, frontal projections

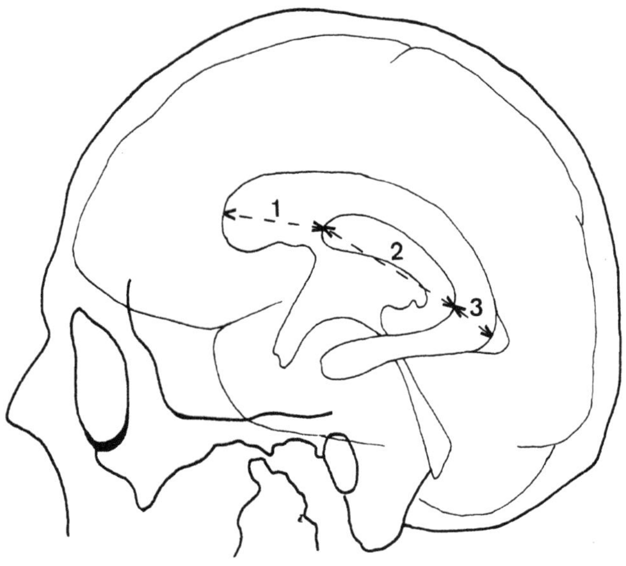

A. TAVERAS. 1=35 mm, 2=45 mm, 3=23 mm

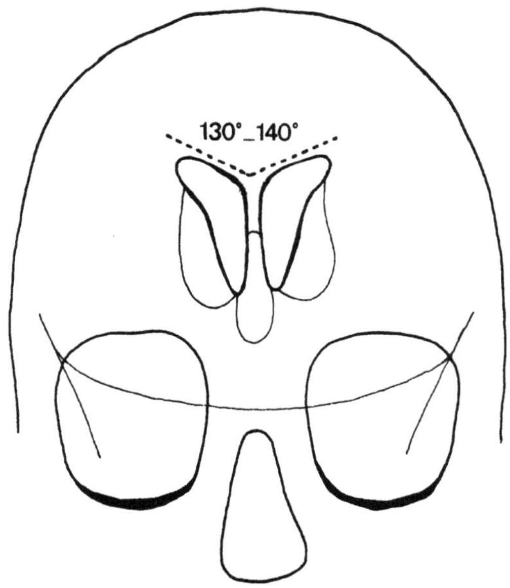

B. LE MAY and NEW

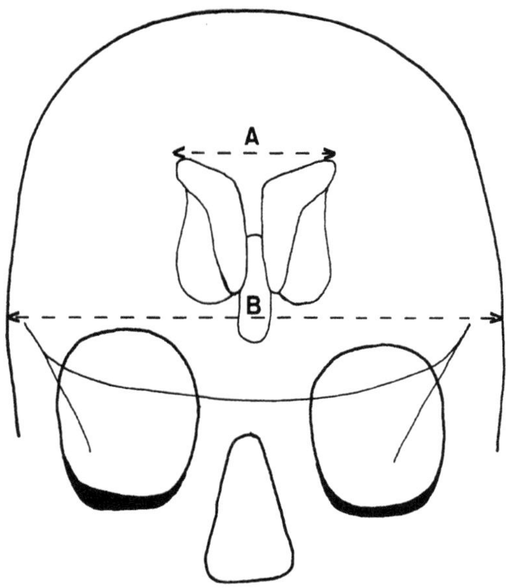

C. EVANS. A/B=0.16–0.31 mm

Fig. 29. Schematic representations of the various measurements of the ventricular system proposed by TAVERAS and WOOD (1964) (A), LE MAY and NEW (1970) (B) and EVANS (1942) (C)

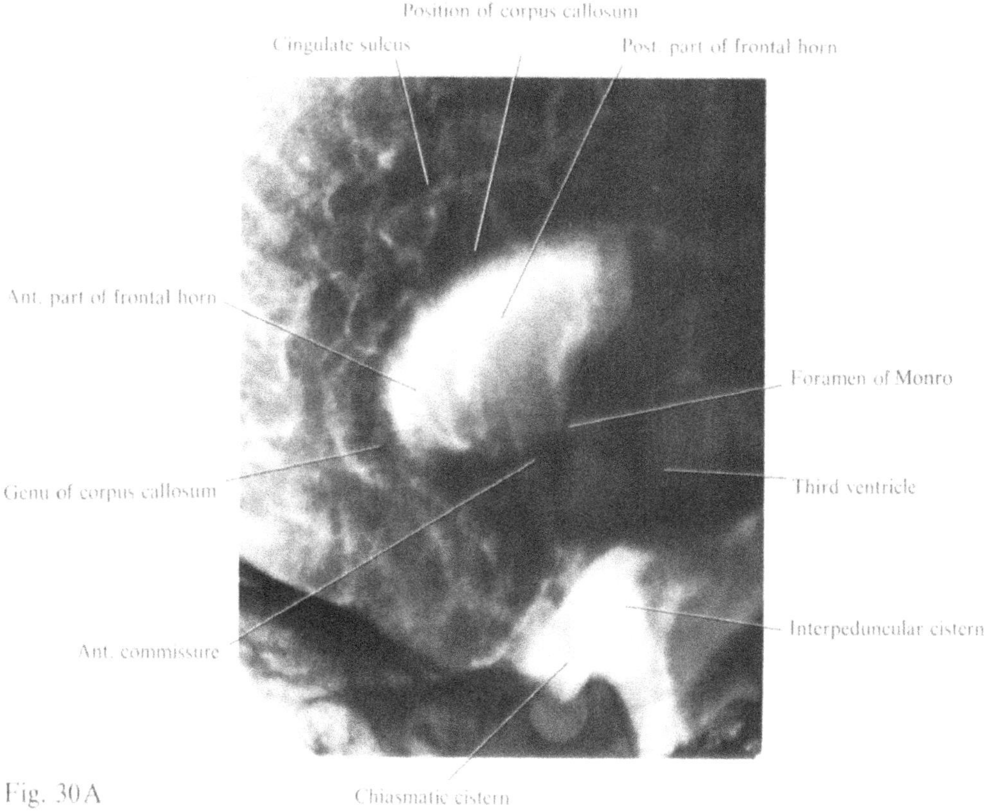

Fig. 30A

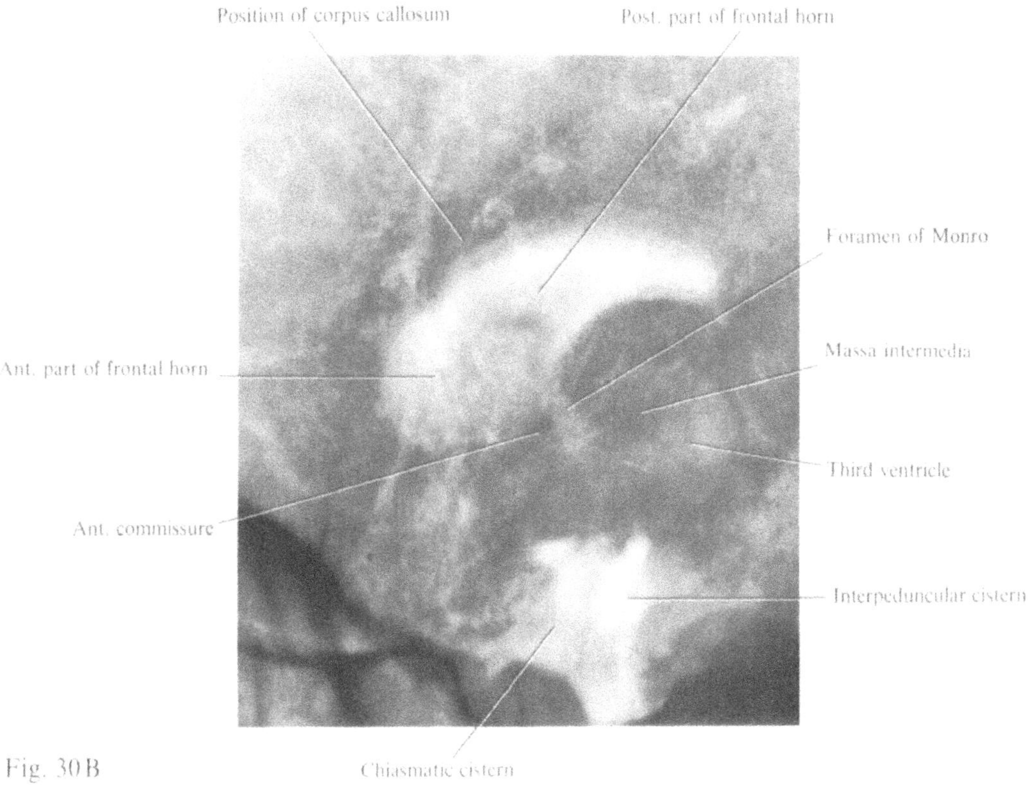

Fig. 30B

Fig. 30 A–B. Pneumoencephalograms, lateral projections

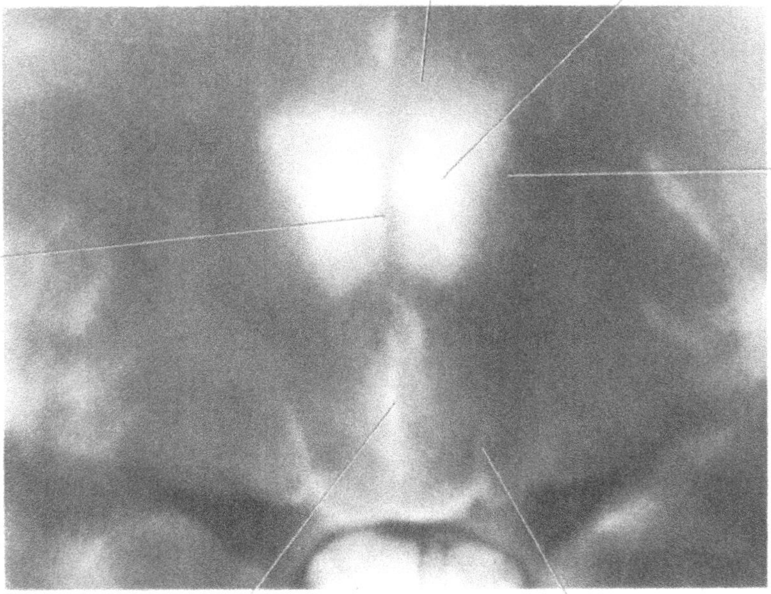

Fig. 31 A

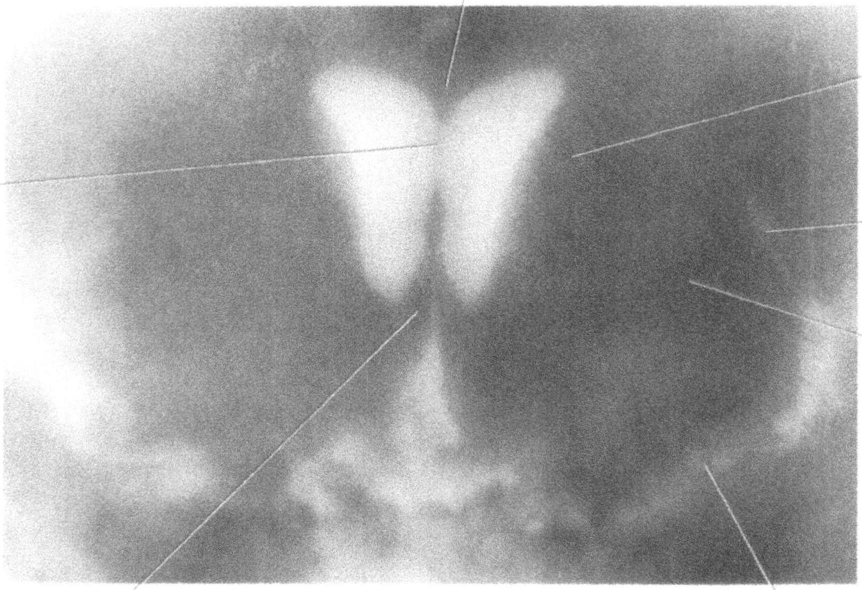

Fig. 31 B

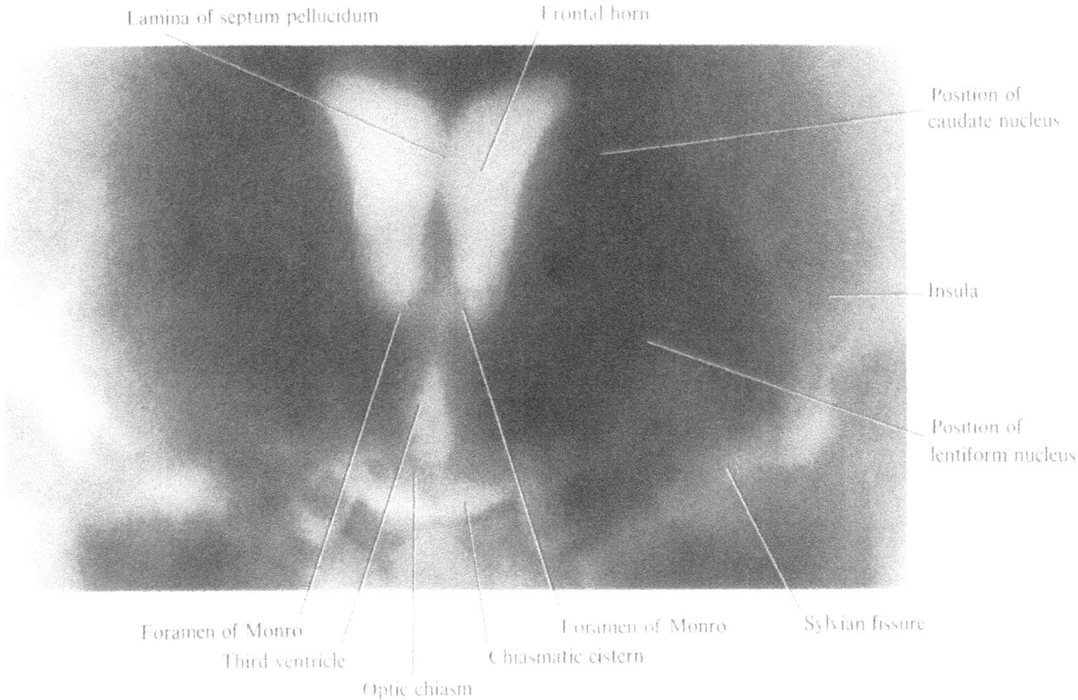

Fig. 31 C

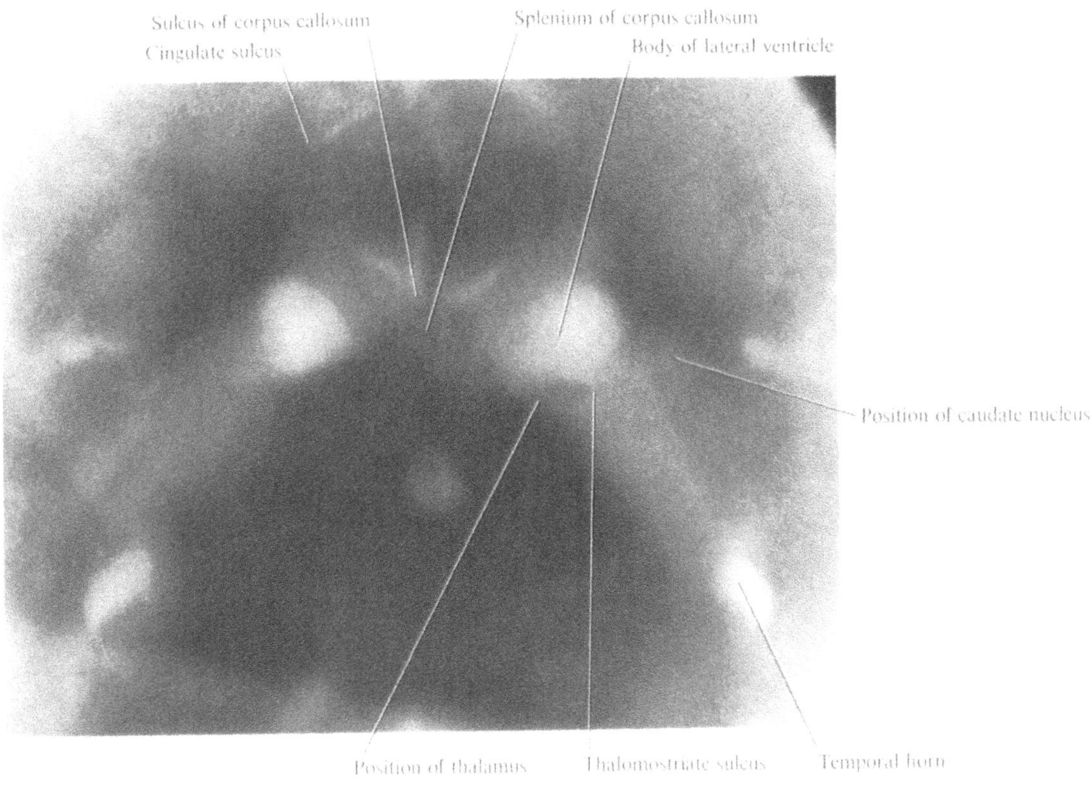

Fig. 31 D

Fig. 31 A–D. Pneumoencephalograms, frontal tomograms through the frontal horn and the body of the lateral ventricle

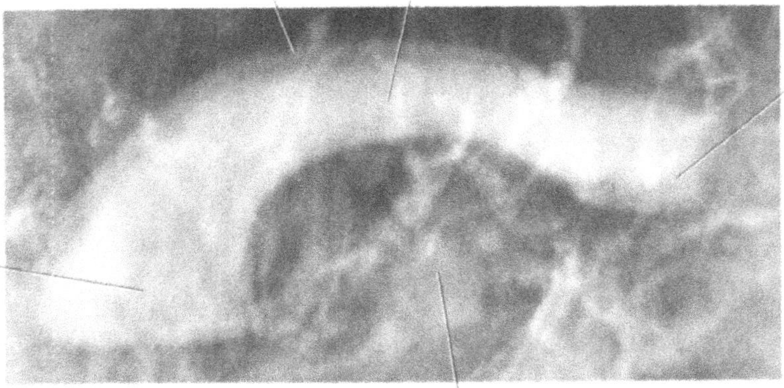

Fig. 32A

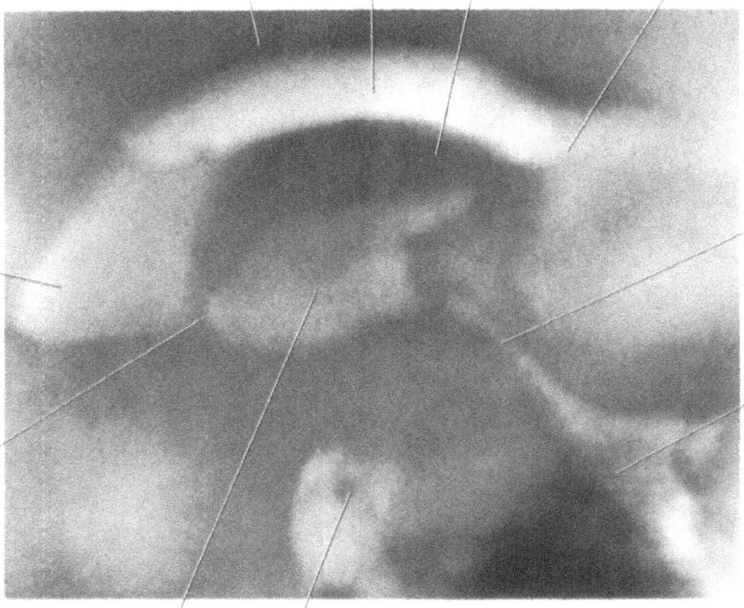

Fig. 32B

Fig. 32A–B. Pneumoencephalograms, lateral projection and sagittal tomogram through the body of the lateral ventricle

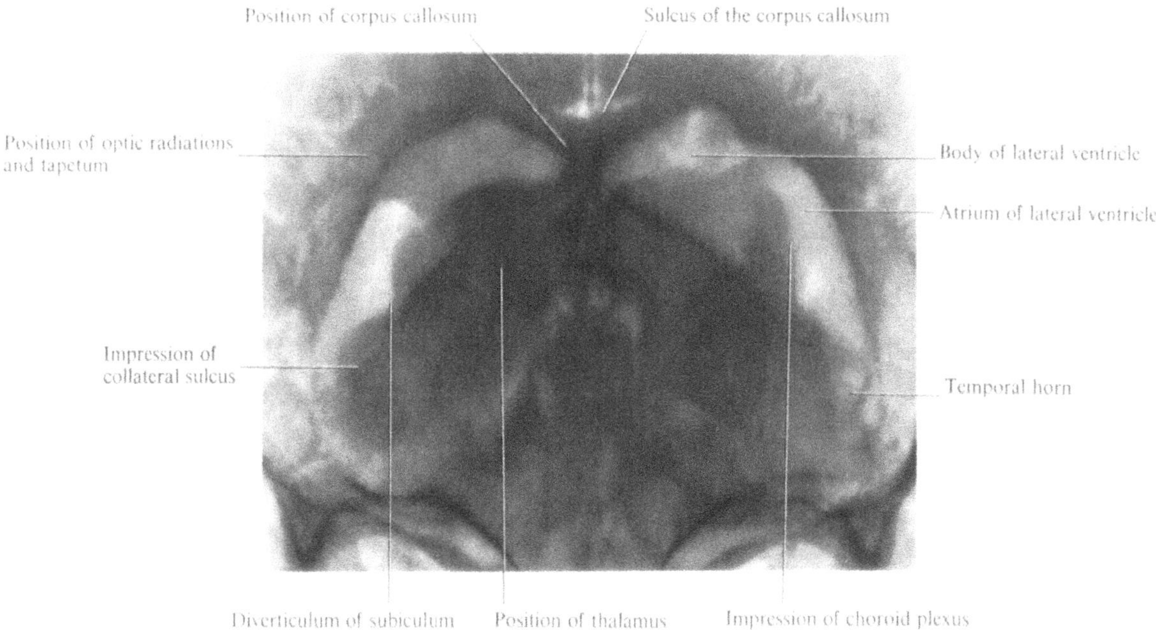

Fig. 33A

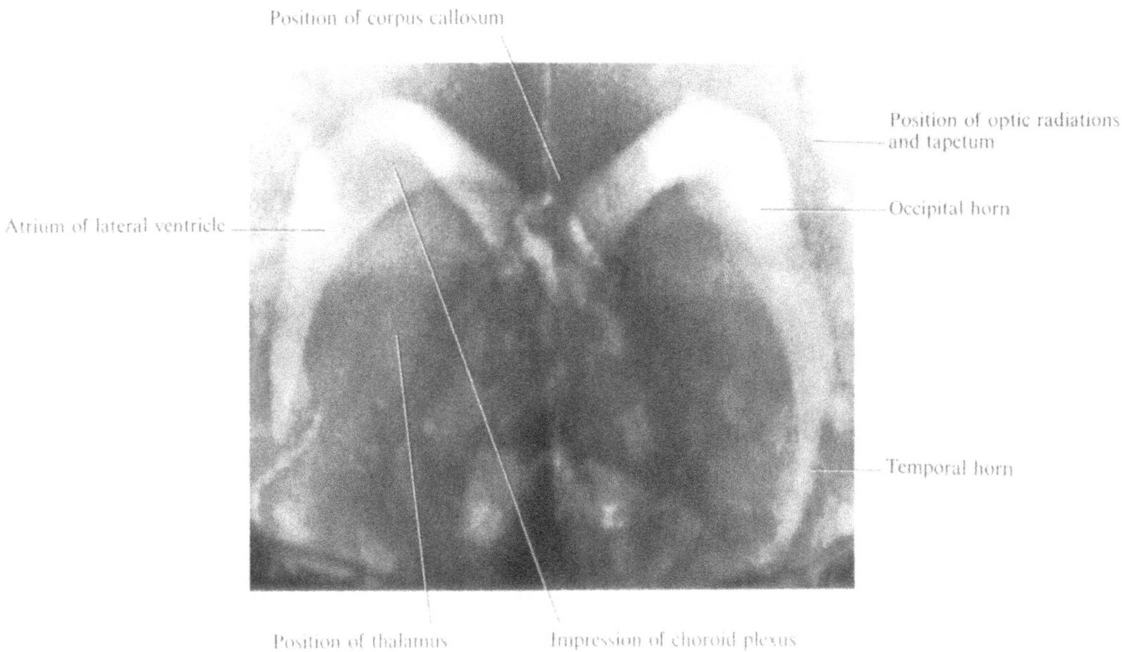

Fig. 33B

Fig. 33A–B. Pneumoencephalograms, frontal projections

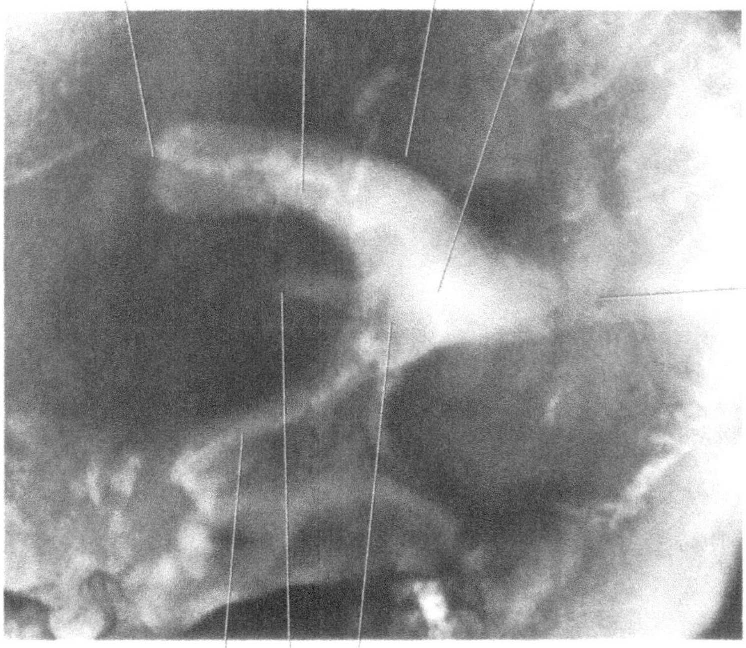

Fig. 34A

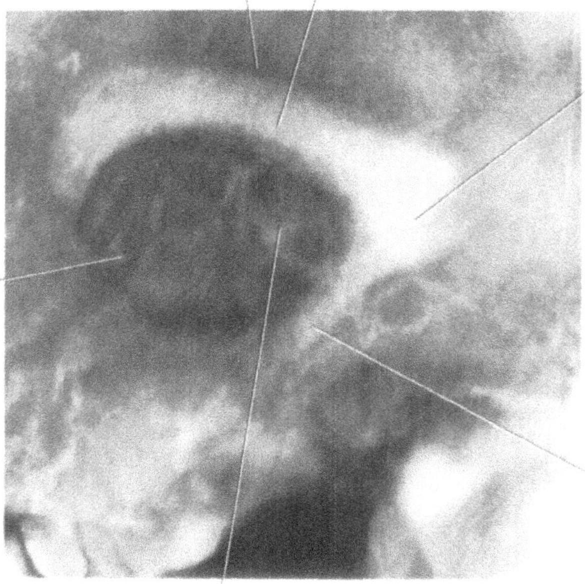

Fig. 34B

Fig. 34A–B. Pneumoencephalograms, lateral projections

Fig. 35. Schematic representation of the different types of occipital horns observed by LAZORTHES and POULHES (1948) ▷

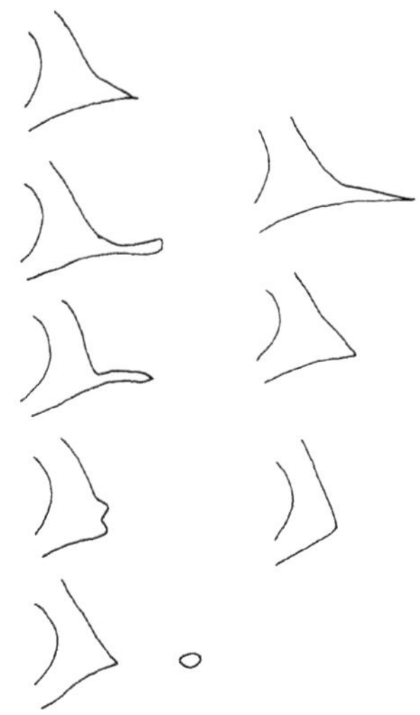

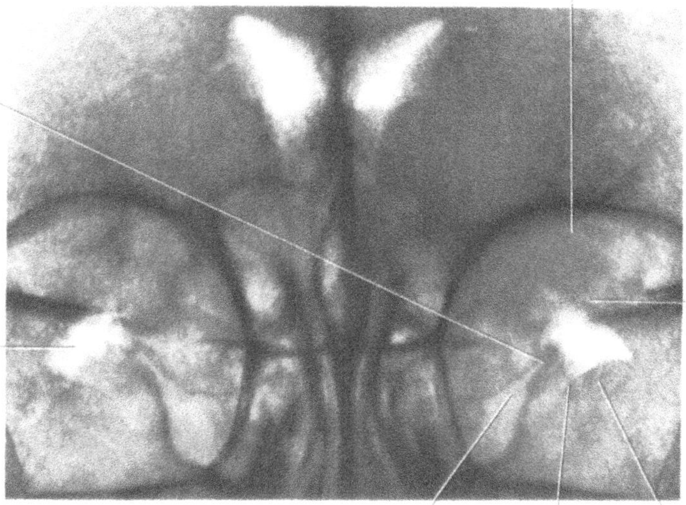

Fig. 36 A

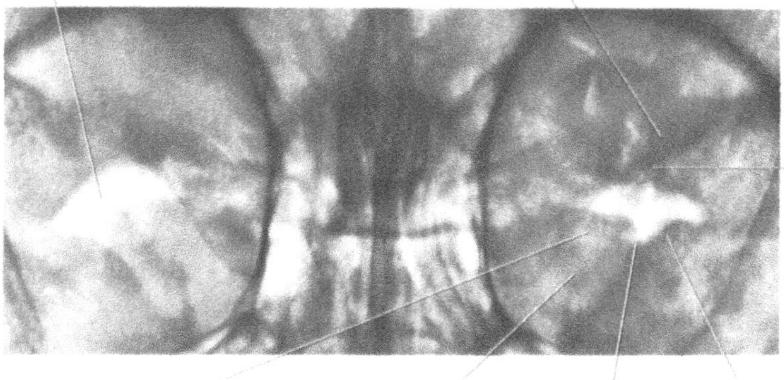

Fig. 36 B

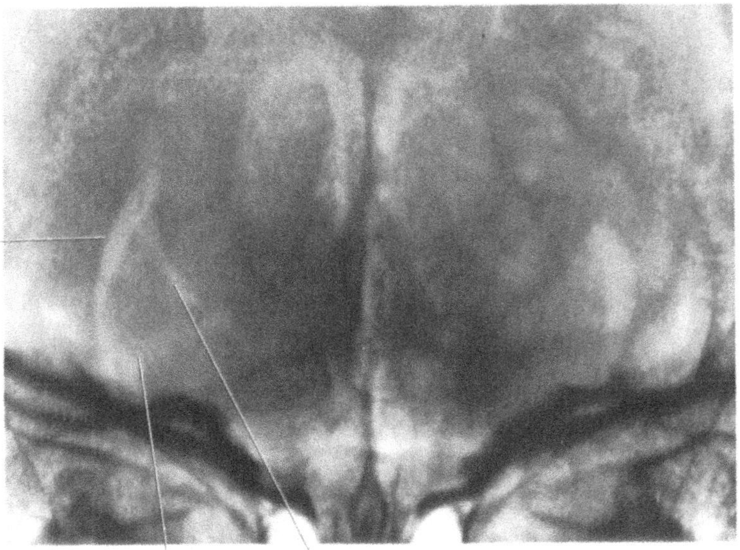

Fig. 36C

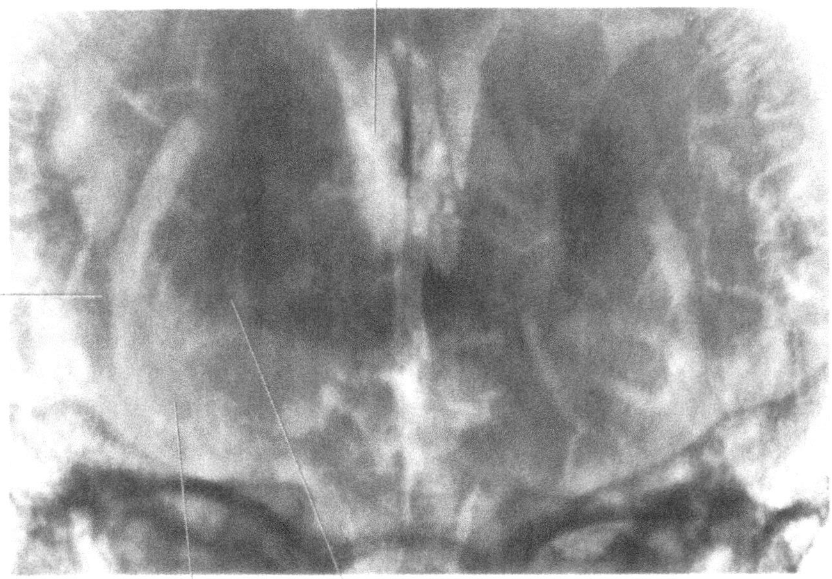

Fig. 36D

Fig. 36A–D. Pneumoencephalograms, frontal projections through the temporal horns

Fig. 37A–C. Pneumoencephalograms, frontal tomograms through the temporal horns ▷

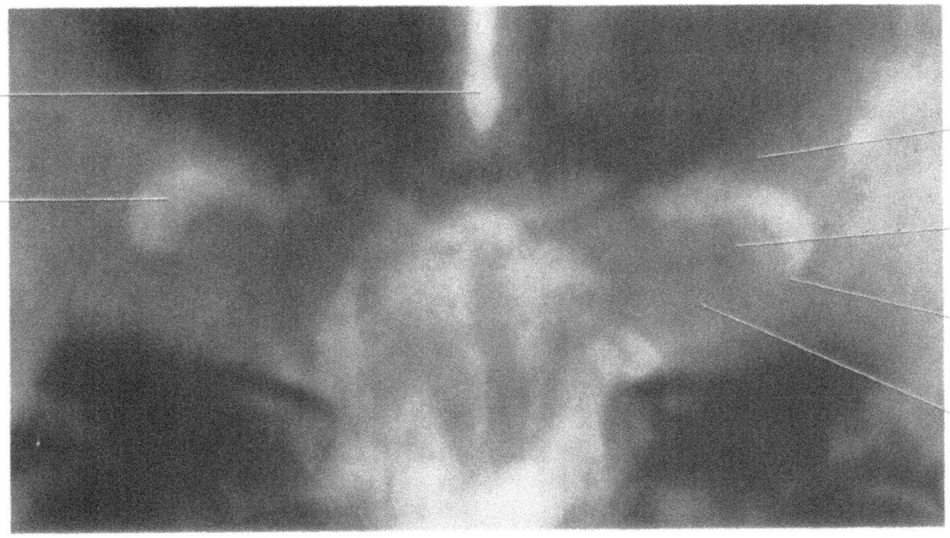

Fig. 37A

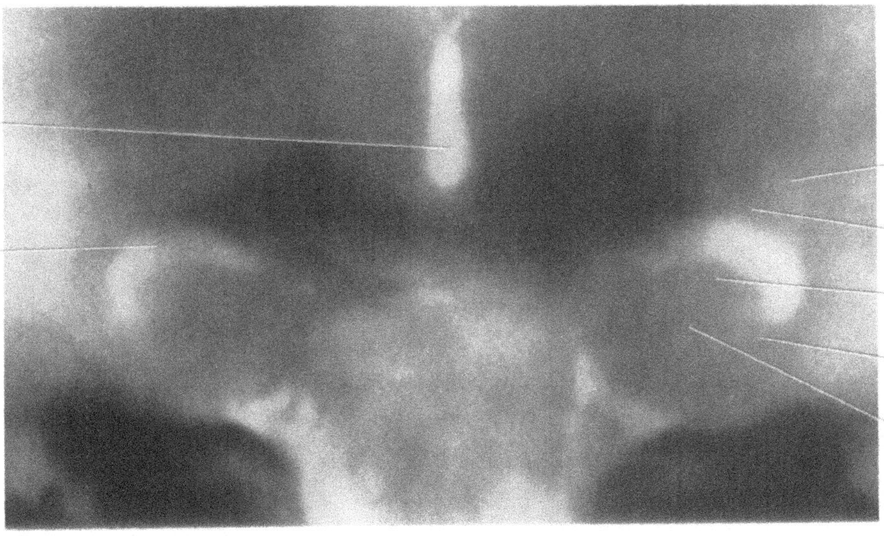

Fig. 37B

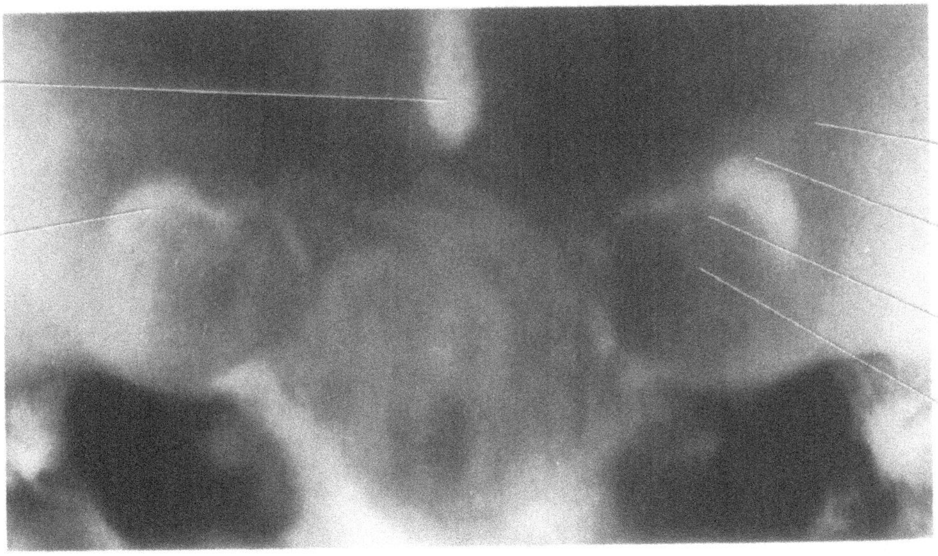

Fig. 37C

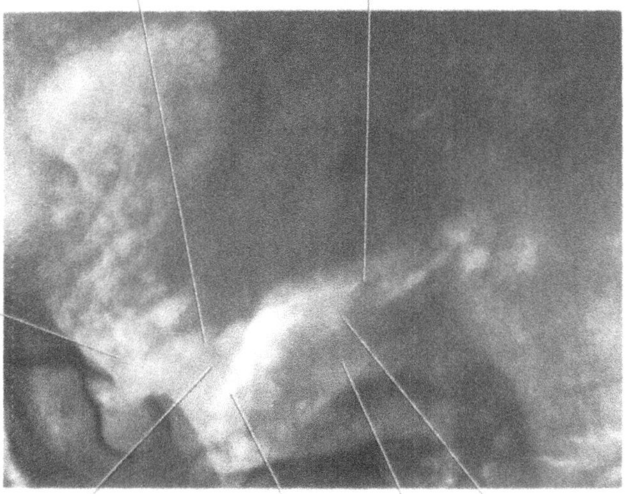

Fig. 38A

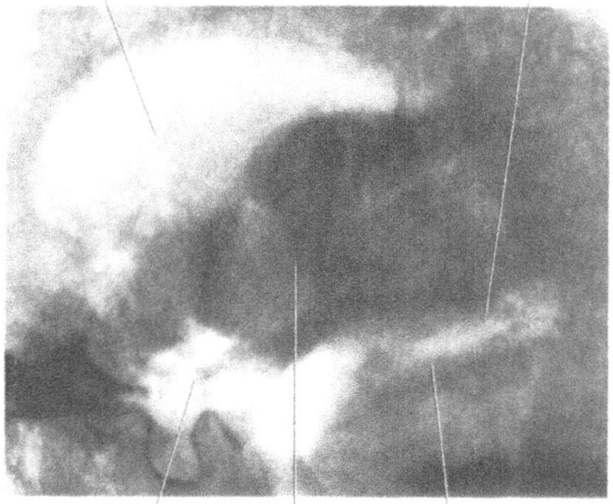

Fig. 38B

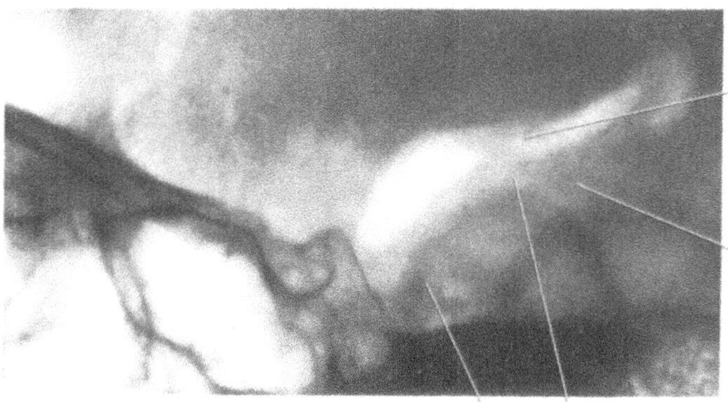

Fig. 38C

Fig. 38A–C. Pneumoencephalograms, lateral projections through the temporal horns

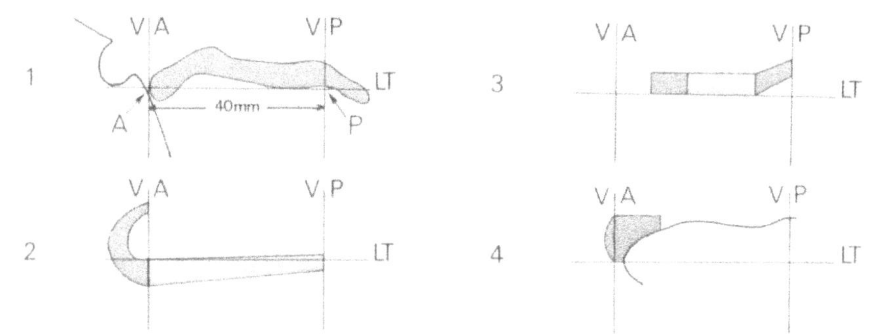

Fig. 39. Schematic drawings from the work of TALAIRACH *et al.* (1958)

1. Construction of line LT. Point (A) is at the most anterior end of the temporal horn, and LT is tangential to the posterior end of this horn. Point (P) is 40 mm behind (A) on LT. Lines VA and VP are perpendiculars to LT at (A) and (P)
2. Localization of the uncal gyrus (shaded area anterior to VA) and hippocampal gyrus (posterior to VA); these areas are 20–30 mm from the midsagittal plane
3. Localization of Ammon's horn (three shaded areas – anterior, middle and posterior); these areas are 22–34 mm from the midsagittal plane
4. Localization of the amygdaloid nucleus; this area is 20–30 mm from the midsagittal plane

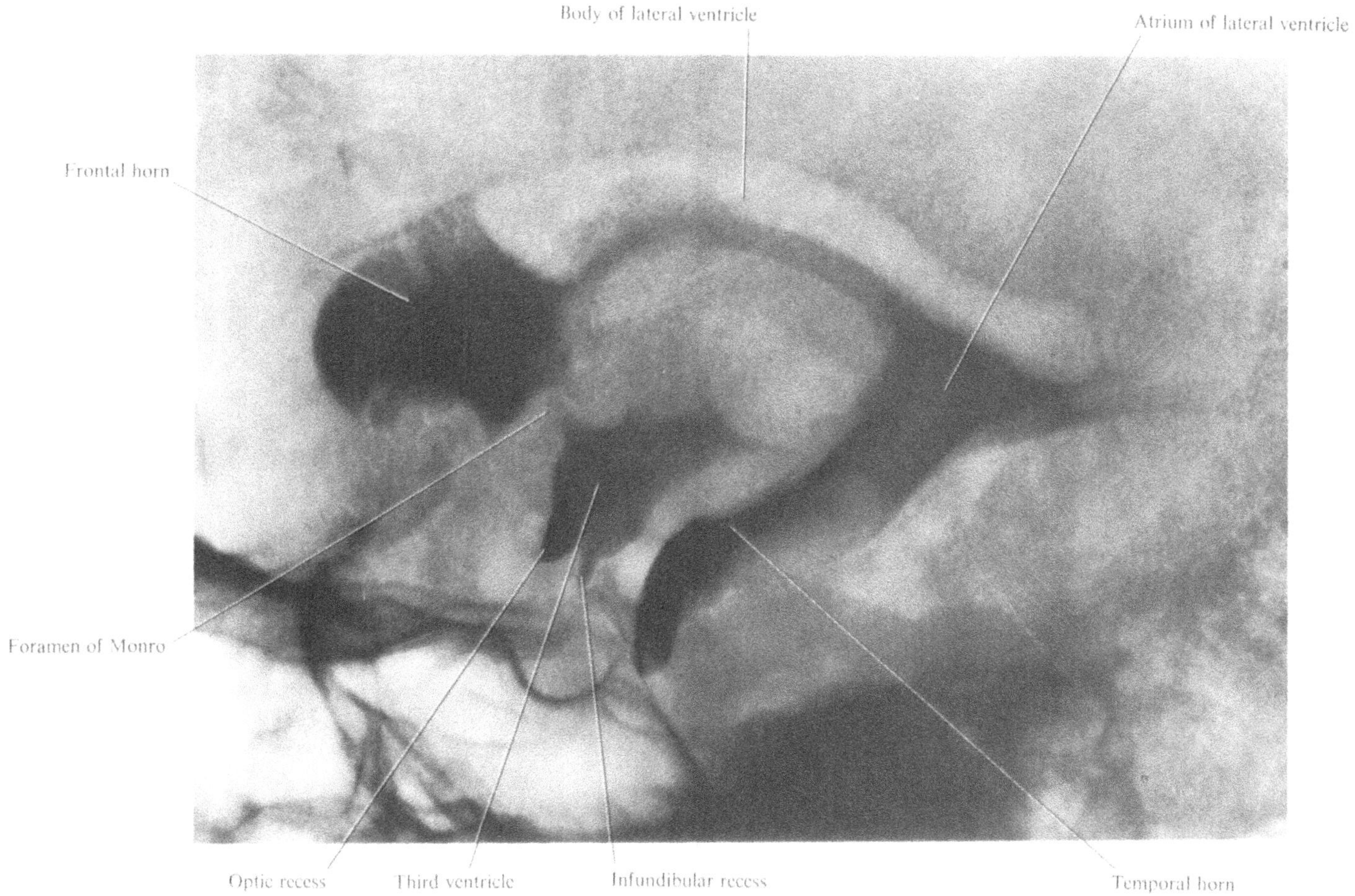

Fig. 40. Ventriculography with water-soluble contrast medium, lateral projection

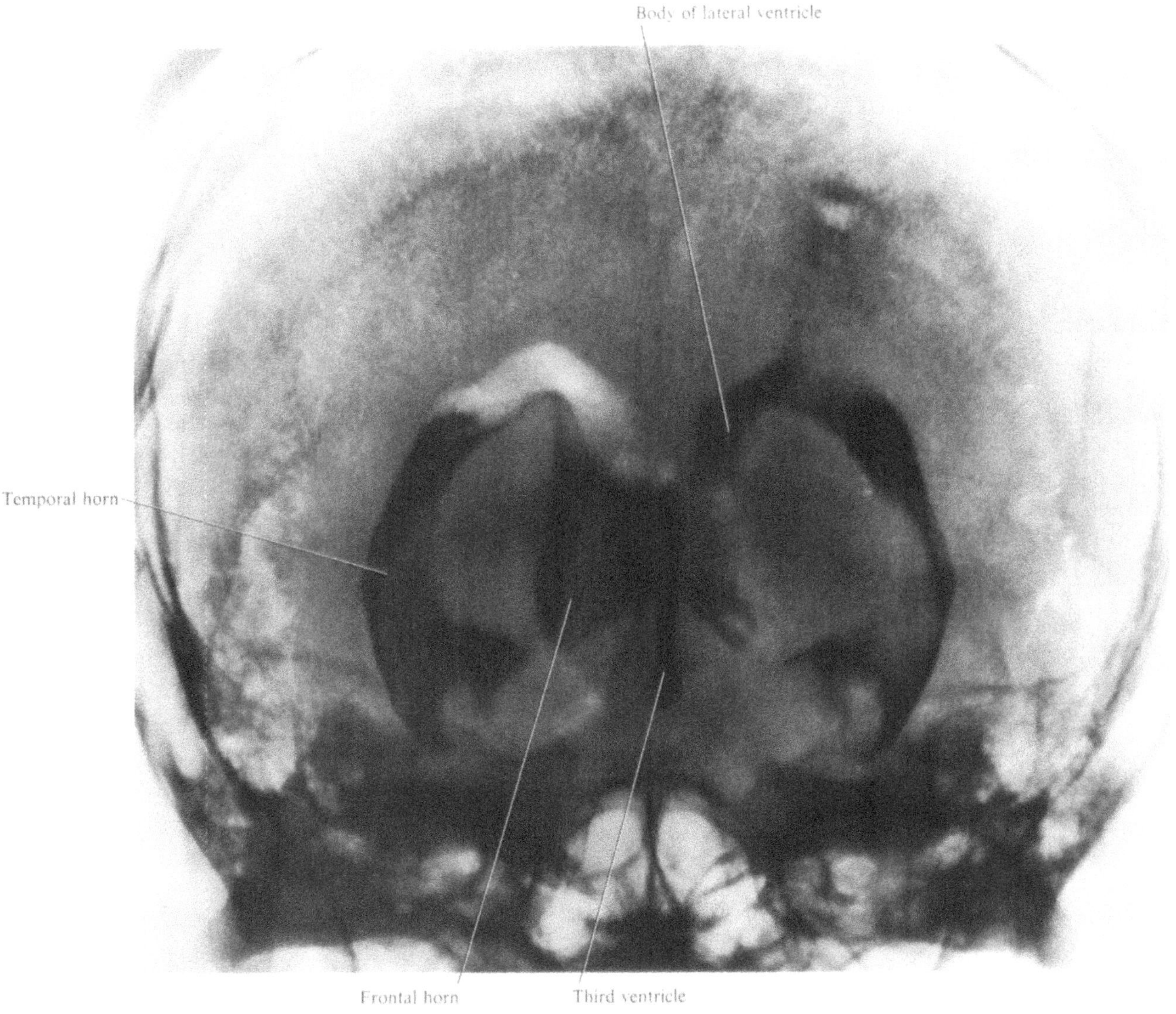

Fig. 41. Ventriculography with water-soluble contrast medium, frontal projection

Chapter 3
Cortical Arteries

Blood reaches the cerebral hemispheres via branches of the internal carotid arteries (the anterior and middle cerebral arteries, and the anterior choroidal arteries), and the terminal branches of the vertebrobasilar system (the posterior cerebral arteries).
The internal carotid and vertebrobasilar systems anastomose at the base of the brain via the circle of Willis. The anterior cerebral arteries are united by the anterior communicating artery, and the two internal carotid arteries are joined, via the posterior communicating arteries, with the proximal parts of the posterior cerebral arteries.
Large zones of anastomoses also exist in the terminal distribution of the various systems [van der Ecken (1953, 1959), Gouaze (1967)]. These anastomoses unite the finest ramifications of the anterior and middle cerebral arteries and also the terminal ramifications of the middle and posterior cerebral arteries. Branches of the anterior and posterior cerebral arteries anastomose around the splenium of the corpus callosum or on the internal surface of the parietal lobe. The anterior choroidal arteries communicate with the posteromedial and posterolateral choroidal arteries via the choroid plexuses.
The posterior cerebral arteries and the branches of the internal carotid arteries exhibit a mode of division illustrated by Foix and Hillemand (1925). Each major division provides a series of perforating branches destined for the basal ganglia:

- the recurrent artery of Heubner (1872) from the anterior cerebral artery;
- the lenticulostriate arteries from the middle cerebral artery;
- the posteromedial and posterolateral choroidal arteries and the thalamoperforate arteries from the posterior cerebral artery;
- the peduncular and amygdaloid branches from the anterior choroidal artery.

This series of perforating vessels will be studied in relationship to their vascularization of the basal ganglia. They assure the supply of blood to the deep structures of the telencephalon and diencephalon.

In addition to the perforating branches, each of these groups of arteries (with the exception of the anterior choroidal arteries, which penetrate the temporal horns) provide branches to the surface of the brain whose fine terminal ramifications supply either the cerebral cortex or white matter. The size of the area of cortical vascularization of each of these branches varies according to its size and distribution:

- The anterior cerebral arteries supply the anterior two-thirds of the internal surfaces of the hemispheres, the corpus callosum, a parasagittal segment of the external surfaces of the hemispheres, and the internal part of the orbital surfaces of the frontal lobes.
- The middle cerebral arteries supply the majority of the convexities of both hemispheres from the frontal to the occipital poles (except for the parasagittal fringe previously mentioned).
- The anterior choroidal arteries supply the anterior segment of the hippocampus.
- The posterior cerebral arteries supply the posterior thirds of the internal surfaces of the hemispheres (cuneus), the occipitotemporal junctions, and a part of the hippocampus.

It is in this order that we shall approach the study of each of these vessels.
The early proposition of Foix and Hillemand (1925) has turned out to be a very important consideration in the topographic study of the cerebral vessels: regardless of the variations in course and division of the cortical branches, the analysis of large numbers of dissected brains reveals a fixed territory of distribution for each of the major cerebral arteries. Whether they branch early or late, or whether they are composed of one principal trunk or of several accessory divisions, all specimens contain the same cerebral arteries (which emphasizes the importance of a precise nomenclature).
The relatively fixed distribution of these arteries in man permits the recognition of essentially constant relationships between these vessels and certain sulci and fissures. These relationships are as apparent during angiography as during dissection. Consequently, at the level of the

hemispheres there is not only a fixed arterial distribution, but also an indirect method for the precise localization of the cerebral convolutions.

A. Anterior Cerebral Artery

I. Anatomic Study of the Anterior Cerebral Artery

The medial terminal branch of the internal carotid artery, the anterior cerebral artery, passes medially and anteriorly, above the optic chiasm and optic nerves. The anterior communicating artery connects both anterior cerebral arteries in the interhemispheric fissure. The anterior cerebral artery then describes a wide curve in the sagittal plane in contact with the corpus callosum. This explains the name "pericallosal artery" chosen by certain authors. It terminates as the artery of the splenium of the corpus callosum (LAZORTHES, 1956).

The anatomic and radiologic study of the anterior cerebral artery has been the subject of many works by DURET (1874), HEUBNER (1872), CRITCHLEY (1930) and more recently by LAZORTHES (1956), BAPTISTA (1963), RING (1963), MOSCOW, MICHOTEY and SALAMON (1974). Several anomalies of the anterior cerebral artery have been described. These occur particularly at the level of the circle of Willis, but may involve the trunk as well (e.g. a supernumerary anterior cerebral artery or a hypoplastic trunk with supply from the opposite anterior cerebral artery).

The cortical branches of the anterior cerebral artery may arise individually, as isolated arteries, or from a common trunk which runs in the cingulate sulcus. Most often a single major branch serves each territory; however, any territory may contain more than one branch. Although the origins and branching patterns of these cortical arteries are quite variable, the territories they supply are constant and these branches can be classified according to their territory of vascularization. Furthermore, certain constant relationships exist between these arteries and the principal sulci and fissures of the internal surface of the cerebral hemisphere. These relationships permit the localization of these sulci, by careful identification of the branches of the anterior cerebral artery.

Branches of the Anterior Cerebral Artery

Branch to the orbital surface of the frontal lobe
Branches to the internal surface of the frontal lobe
Branch to the paracentral lobule
Branches to the internal aspect of the parietal lobe
Branches to the corpus callosum

The anterior cerebral artery supplies an extensive territory which includes the internal surface of the superior frontal gyrus, the internal two-thirds of the orbital surface of the frontal lobe, the cingulate gyrus, the paracentral lobule, the precuneus and the corpus callosum. On the external surface of the cerebral hemisphere it supplies the superior portion of the cerebral convexity where its branches anastomose with cortical branches of the middle cerebral artery. The anterior cerebral artery also helps to vascularize the hypothalamus and the basal ganglia. (See arteries of the basal ganglia.)

a) Branch to the Orbital Surface of the Frontal Lobe (Figs. 42–49)

The orbitofrontal artery is the first cortical branch of the anterior cerebral artery and is analogous to the orbitofrontal branch of the middle cerebral artery. It can arise independently from the anterior cerebral artery or from a common trunk with the frontopolar artery. Less commonly, it may occur as a branch of the callosomarginal trunk. Generally, there is a single orbitofrontal artery which supplies the gyrus rectus and the orbital surface of the middle frontal gyrus. In the region of the external aspect of the orbital sulci, or H-shaped sulcus, it anastomoses with the orbitofrontal branches of the middle cerebral artery.

b) Branches to the Internal Surface of the Frontal Lobe (Figs. 42–49)

Frontopolar artery
Anterior internal frontal artery
Middle internal frontal artery
Posterior internal frontal artery

The frontopolar artery generally arises directly as a single branch from the anterior cerebral artery, but may share a common origin with the orbitofrontal artery. Less frequently, it may be part of a callosomarginal trunk, together with other branches to the medial surface of the frontal lobe. It arises in the region of the genu of the corpus callosum and runs anteriorly, most often in the subfrontal sulcus. This relationship permits the recognition of this sulcus. The frontopolar artery supplies the edge of the subfrontal sulcus, the inferior part of the cingulate gyrus and, anteriorly to it, the most anterior part of the internal surface of the superior frontal gyrus.

The anterior internal frontal artery most often appears as a single artery, which arises independently from the anterior cerebral artery. On occasions it shares a common origin with either the frontopolar or middle internal frontal artery. It also may be one of the branches of the callosomarginal trunk, which runs in the cingulate sulcus.

The position of the callosomarginal trunk permits the recognition of this sulcus at angiography. This latter situation is, however, not very common.
The anterior internal frontal artery often divides early into two or more branches. Rarely, two separate anterior internal frontal arteries are present. The distribution of this artery is to the anterior third of the internal surface of the superior frontal gyrus and the anterior part of the cingulate gyrus.

The middle internal frontal artery, like the anterior internal frontal artery, most commonly arises directly from the trunk of the anterior cerebral artery. Less frequently, it arises from a common origin with the other internal frontal arteries, or as a branch of the callosomarginal trunk together with the other branches to the internal aspect of the frontal lobe and paracentral lobule. However, in no case does it share a common origin with the internal parietal arteries.
The middle internal frontal artery is usually single and divides into two or more branches. Rarely, there are two separate middle internal frontal arteries. Its territory corresponds to the midportions of the cingulate gyrus and the internal surface of the superior frontal gyrus.

The posterior internal frontal artery, as with the other internal frontal arteries, arises either directly from the anterior cerebral artery, together with other neighboring cortical branches, or as a division of a callosomarginal trunk. Very often, a branch of the posterior internal frontal artery follows the course of the paracentral sulcus and serves to indicate the anterior margin of the paracentral lobule. The territory supplied by the posterior internal frontal artery is the posterior third of the internal surface of the superior frontal gyrus and the adjacent part of the cingulate gyrus.
Together, the internal frontal arteries provide the vascular supply to the internal aspect of the superior frontal gyrus. All of the internal frontal branches, as well as the paracentral and internal parietal arteries have characteristic reflections at the superior margin of the brain. Each artery runs a short course on the external surface of the hemisphere and contributes to the vascularization of the corresponding gyri. At this level anastomoses between the cortical branches of the anterior and middle cerebral arteries occur, as described by VAN DER ECKEN (1953, 1959).

c) Branch to the Paracentral Lobule
(Figs. 42–49)

The artery to the paracentral lobule or the paracentral artery arises from the anterior cerebral artery alone, in combination with neighboring vessels, or as a branch of the callosomarginal trunk. In approximately half of the paracentral arteries a branch runs in the marginal limb of the cingulate sulcus, thus marking the posterior limit of the paracentral lobule. At times, in addition, another branch of this artery courses in the paracentral sulcus. The territory of the paracentral artery, on the internal surface of the brain, is the paracentral lobule and the subjacent cingulate gyrus. On the external surface it supplies the superior part of the precentral and postcentral gyri.

d) Branches to the Internal Aspect of the Parietal Lobe
(Figs. 42–49)

Superior internal parietal artery
Inferior internal parietal artery

The internal aspect of the parietal lobe derives its blood supply from two internal parietal arteries. The larger of these, and often the largest branch of the anterior cerebral artery, is the ***superior internal parietal artery.*** The smaller is the ***inferior internal parietal artery.*** After the origin of the superior branch, the anterior cerebral artery is markedly reduced in caliber.
As with other branches of the anterior cerebral artery, several variations in the origin and branching patterns of these arteries are noted. However, in no instance do the parietal arteries share a common trunk with the internal frontal branches. It would, therefore, seem that an embryologic division in the distribution of the anterior cerebral artery occurs in the region of the paracentral lobule. Rarely, the internal parietal arteries can arise from the opposite anterior cerebral artery. A major branch of the superior internal parietal artery is usually found in the marginal limb of the cingulate sulcus, which is the posterior boundary of the paracentral lobule.
The inferior internal parietal arteries are often small and multiple. They most often arise from the narrowed anterior cerebral artery distal to the origin of the superior internal parietal artery and just before the artery passes around the splenium of the corpus callosum.
The territory of supply of the internal parietal arteries is the adjacent portion of the cingulate gyrus and the precuneus, with the exception of its most posterior part, which is supplied by occipitoparietal branches of the posterior cerebral artery.

e) Branches to the Corpus Callosum
(Figs. 42, 46, 47)

Pericallosal artery
Anterior artery to the corpus callosum
Posterior pericallosal artery

The principal artery to the corpus callosum is the anterior cerebral artery itself, which is known as the pericallosal artery. This artery is attached to the corpus callosum by multiple perforating branches which enter it. Also, an area beneath the genu of the corpus callosum is supplied by a branch of the anterior cerebral artery, the anterior artery to the corpus callosum. In addition, in the region of the corpus callosum, a branch of the anterior cerebral artery reaches the free margin of the falx to supply its inferior portion. The splenium is supplied by the terminal branch of the anterior cerebral artery, the artery of the splenium or posterior pericallosal artery. Its terminal branches anastomose with analogous branches of the posterior cerebral artery. It also anastomoses, in the region of the choroidal fissure, with the posteromedial branches of the posterior choroidal arteries.

II. Radiologic Study of the Anterior Cerebral Artery

The radiologic anatomy of the anterior cerebral artery was studied by FISHER in 1938. He proposed a division of this artery into a single precommunicant segment (A1) and 4 postcommunicant segments: 2 ascending segments (A2 and A3), and 2 horizontal segments (A4 and A5).

The division of this artery into pre- and postcommunicant segments gives rise to the falacious notion that the anterior cerebral artery terminates at the origin of the anterior communicating artery, with the postcommunicant segment being called the pericallosal artery.

LINDGREN (1957) also described the pre- and postcommunicant segments of the anterior cerebral artery. DILENGE and CONSTANS (1963) suggested the possibility that the anterior cerebral artery meanders from the midline in normal patients.

KRAYENBUHL and YASARGIL (1968) studied the variations in course and caliber of the first segment of the anterior cerebral artery. In the frontal projection especially, the number of possible variations is large. Seven principal categories were used to describe these normal variations of the precommunicant segment: (1) horizontal; (2) convex superiorly; (3) convex inferiorly; (4) inclined upwards; (5) inclined downwards; (6) angular, and (7) looped. The first three variations make up more than 50% of all age groups; the last two have only been reported in people from 51 to 74 years of age.

The diameters of the first segments of the anterior cerebral arteries are unequal in 58% of the cases reported by KRAYENBUHL and YASARGIL (1968). Hypoplasia or atresia was noted with a frequency of 5.3%. BAPTISTA (1963) and LAZORTHES (1956) studied the congenital variations which occur in the anterior cerebral artery, especially the supernumerary or median anterior cerebral artery, which may vary in length.

During angiography, opacification of the anterior cerebral artery on the side of injection seldom fails unless there is atresia of the first segment (provided, of course, that spasm has not been caused by a subintimal needle tip). Contrast medium opacifies the complete anterior cerebral artery in 65 to 80% of cases. Contralateral opacification depends exclusively on the hemodynamics of the circle of Willis.

RING and WADDINGTON (1968) performed a detailed study of the vascularization of the internal surface of the brain by the anterior cerebral artery, especially the internal frontal and parietal regions. Similar work has also been performed in our laboratory by MOSCOW, MICHOTEY and SALAMON (1974), and FARNARIER (1974). Their dissections and sectional radiographs permit the proposition of a classification of the branches of the anterior cerebral artery (Figs. 57, 58).

Carotid angiography (especially when normal) usually demonstrates the same major branches of the cerebral arteries seen during dissection. Each branch of the anterior cerebral artery can be described by the same anatomic terminology, whether demonstrated at dissection or angiography. We consequently deplore the modification or alteration of the existing nomenclature (as proposed in certain treatises).

With the exception of the first segment (Fig. 55), the anterior cerebral artery and the majority of its branches are best seen in the lateral projection. HUANG (1973), however, has proposed a method of localizing the sulci on the orbital surface of the frontal lobe by analysis of the course of the orbitofrontal artery in the frontal projection.

In the lateral projection it is easy to identify the orbitofrontal artery close to the roof of the orbit. This is followed by the frontopolar artery, the anterior, middle and posterior internal frontal arteries, the artery to the paracentral lobule, and finally the two internal parietal arteries (Figs. 52–54, 58). In general the caliber of the anterior cerebral artery is markedly reduced after the origin of the superior internal parietal artery. The artery to the splenium of the corpus callosum is not always discernible.

The anterior cerebral artery follows the superior aspect of the corpus callosum and is visible throughout its course. On the other hand, the callosomarginal artery is extremely variable. It may be a short trunk, which gives rise to only two internal frontal arteries, or a long arcade supplying the internal branches from the frontopolar artery to the artery of the paracentral lobule.

The courses of these branches, as seen angiographically, offer the possibility of tracing indirectly the contours of the major fissures and sulci of the internal surface of the brain (Fig. 59). The course of the anterior cerebral artery outlines the corpus callosum to the splenium, and the callosomarginal sulcus is defined by the internal frontal arteries. The margins of the paracentral lobule are shown by the posterior internal frontal artery and the artery of the paracentral lobule.

Completing their course on the internal surface of the brain, these arteries arrive at the superior aspect and continue out onto the external surface of the brain. The characteristic angiographic appearance at this point resembles a hairpin and this permits recognition of the external surface, especially in the region of the precentral and postcentral gyri.

The constancy of these branches, despite the variation of their origins, permits the use of a reference template for studying each branch (SALAMON *et al.*, 1975). This permits detailed study of each artery on the internal surface of the brain, and also any expansive processes in this region. It also allows the study of the modifications in the courses of these vessels caused by intracerebral and extracerebral masses. In a similar manner, it makes occluded vessels easier to identify and helps define the vascular pedicles of tumors or angiomas.

The study of the anterior cerebral artery not only provides one of the most important angiographic references, the cerebral midline, but also provides a reliable method for studying the gyri of the internal surface of the cerebral hemisphere. This is by reference to the branches that supply the orbital and internal surfaces of the frontal lobe, and the internal surfaces of the parietal lobe and paracentral lobule.

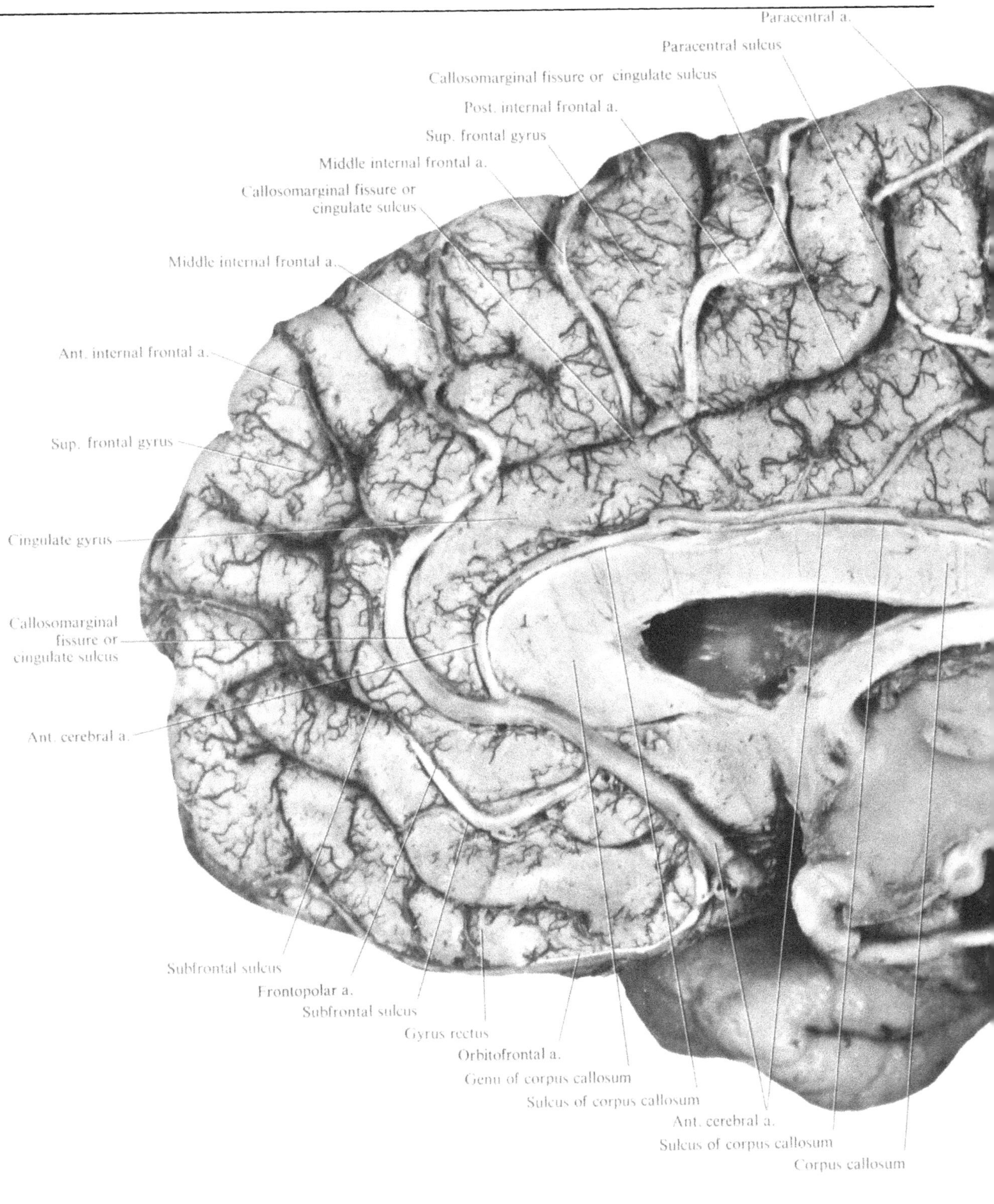

Fig. 42. Dissection of the right cerebral hemisphere after selective injection of the anterior cerebral artery, medial view

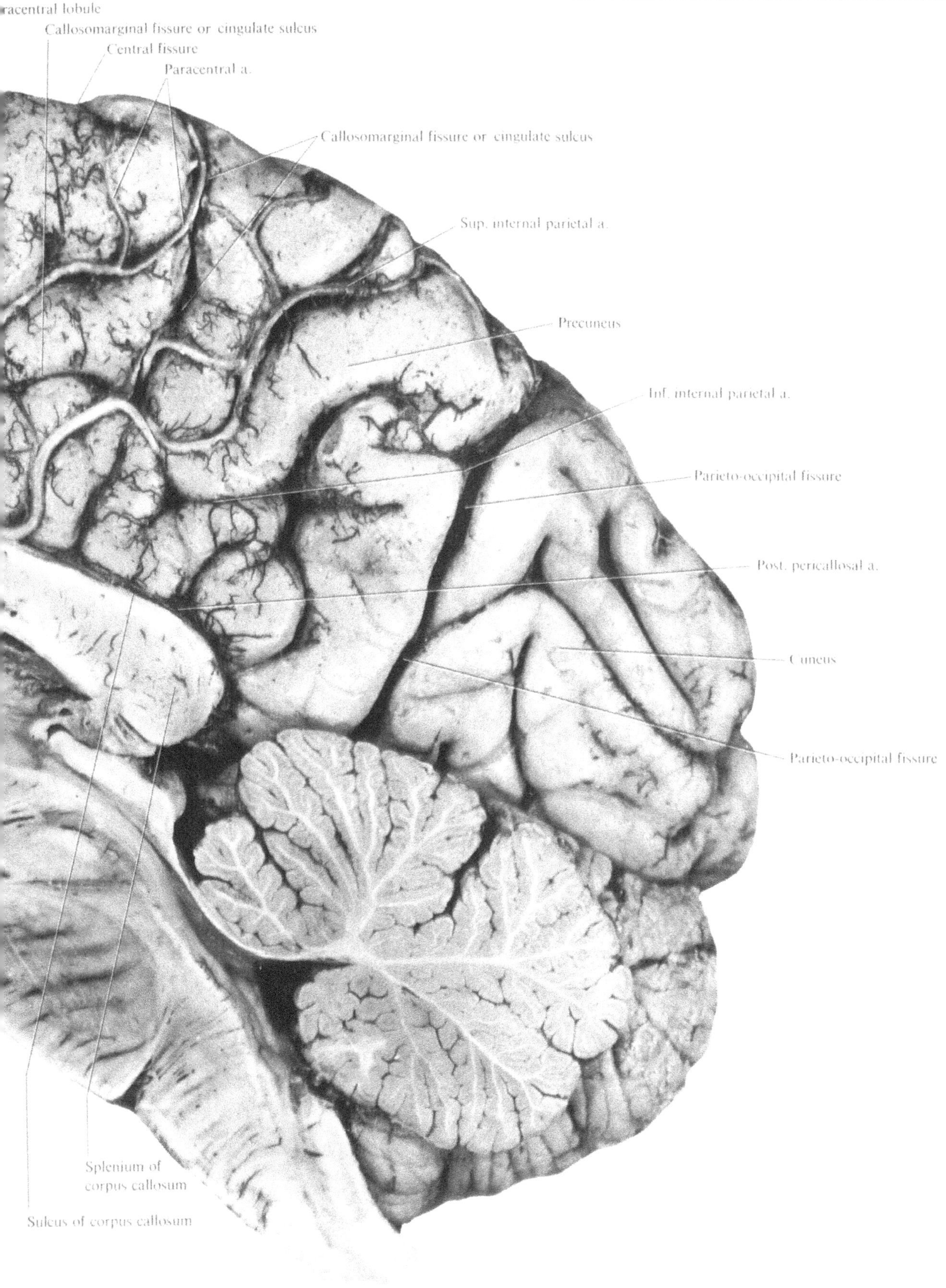

racentral lobule
Callosomarginal fissure or cingulate sulcus
Central fissure
Paracentral a.
Callosomarginal fissure or cingulate sulcus
Sup. internal parietal a.
Precuneus
Inf. internal parietal a.
Parieto-occipital fissure
Post. pericallosal a.
Cuneus
Parieto-occipital fissure
Splenium of
corpus callosum
Sulcus of corpus callosum

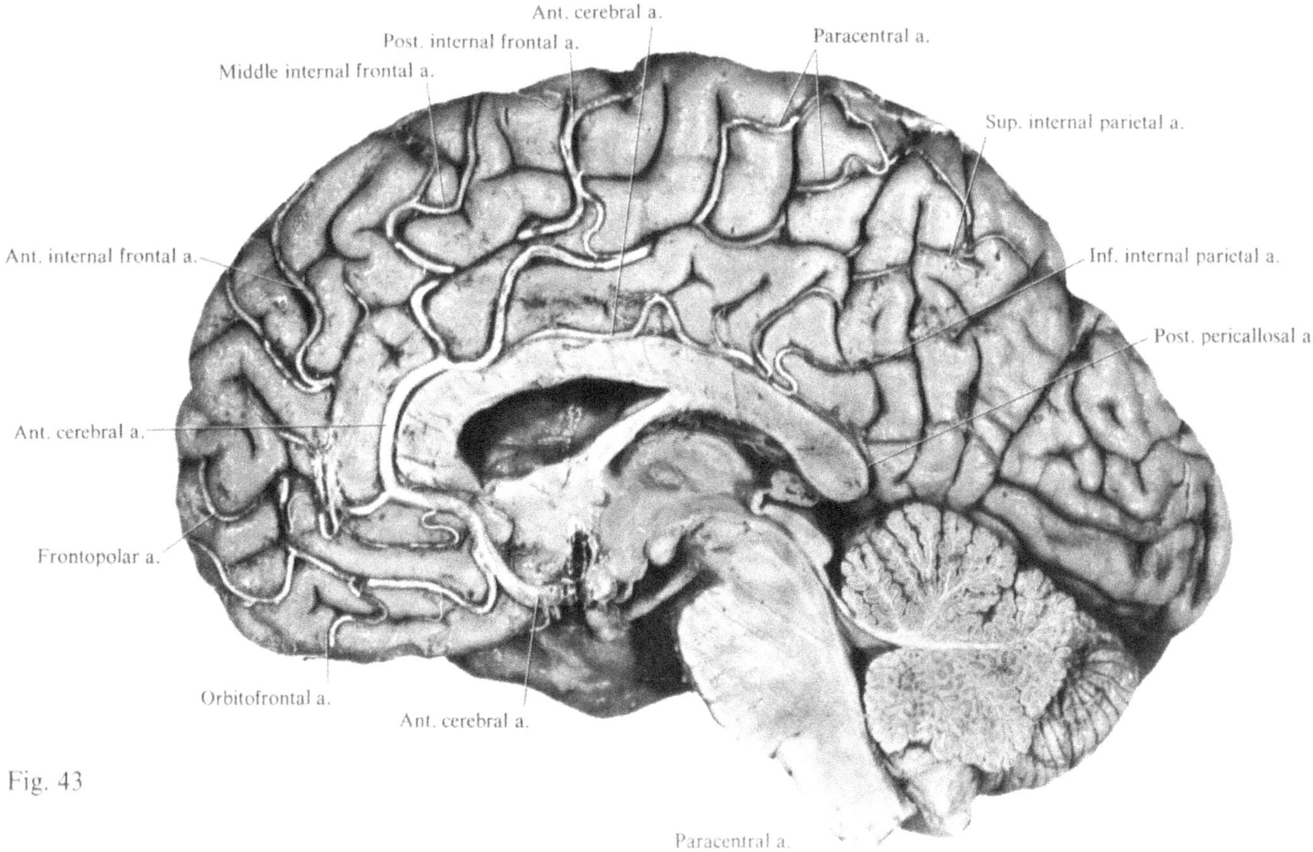
Ant. cerebral a.
Post. internal frontal a.
Middle internal frontal a.
Paracentral a.
Sup. internal parietal a.
Ant. internal frontal a.
Inf. internal parietal a.
Post. pericallosal a.
Ant. cerebral a.
Frontopolar a.
Orbitofrontal a.
Ant. cerebral a.

Fig. 43

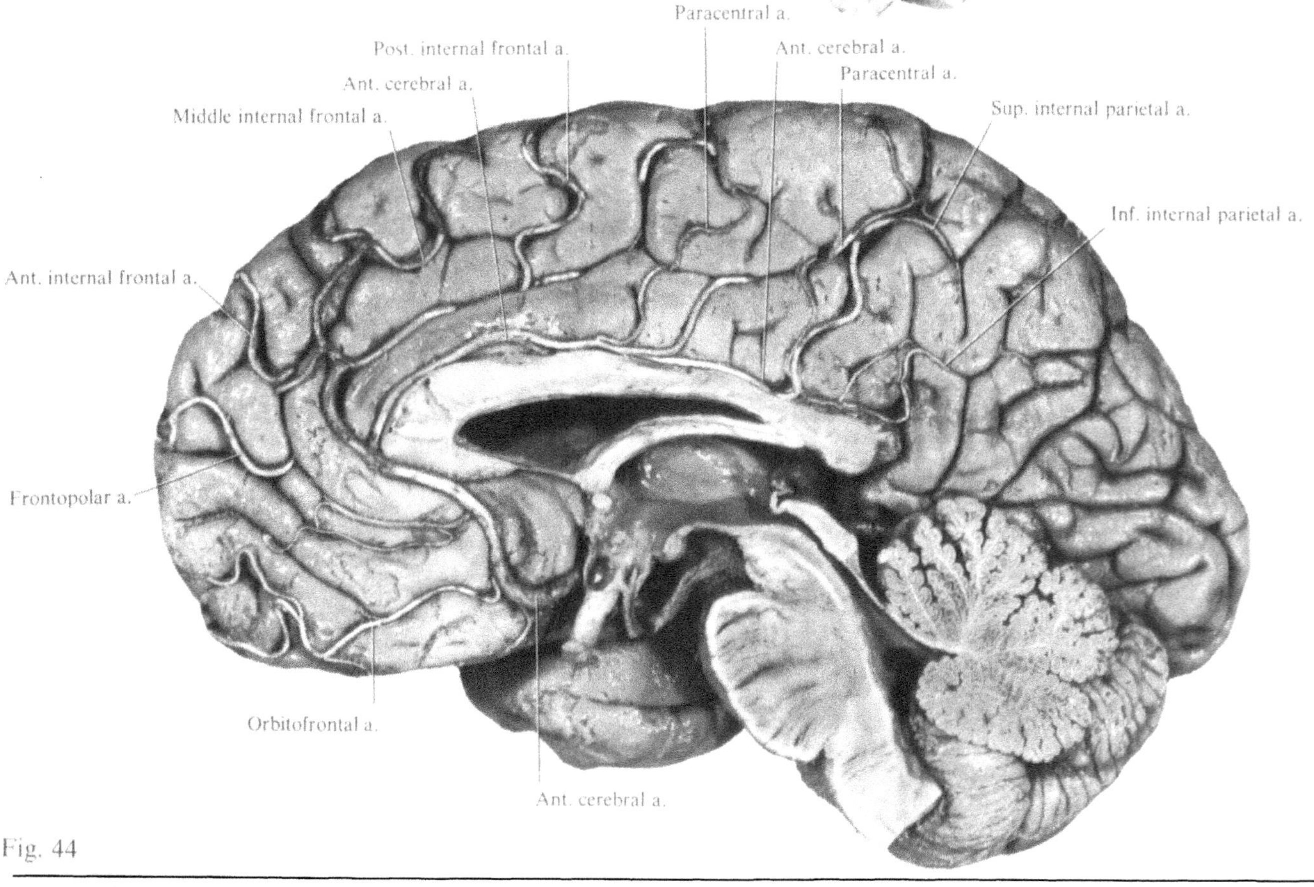
Paracentral a.
Post. internal frontal a.
Ant. cerebral a.
Ant. cerebral a.
Paracentral a.
Middle internal frontal a.
Sup. internal parietal a.
Inf. internal parietal a.
Ant. internal frontal a.
Frontopolar a.
Orbitofrontal a.
Ant. cerebral a.

Fig. 44

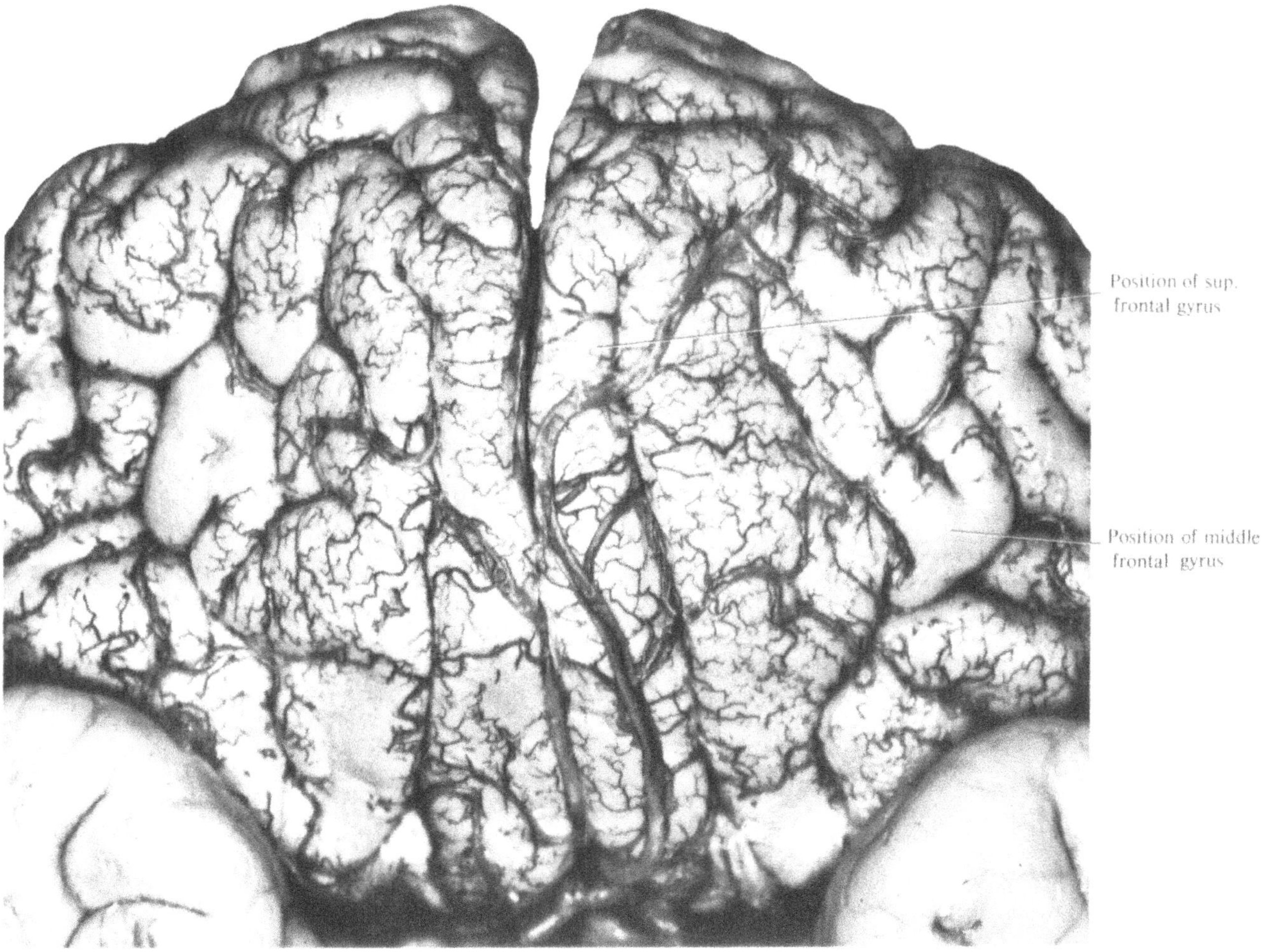

Fig. 45. Dissection of the cerebral hemispheres after selective injection of the anterior cerebral arteries, inferior view

◁

Fig. 43. Dissection of the right cerebral hemisphere after selective injection of the anterior cerebral artery, medial view

Fig. 44. Dissection of the right cerebral hemisphere after selective injection of the anterior cerebral artery, medial view

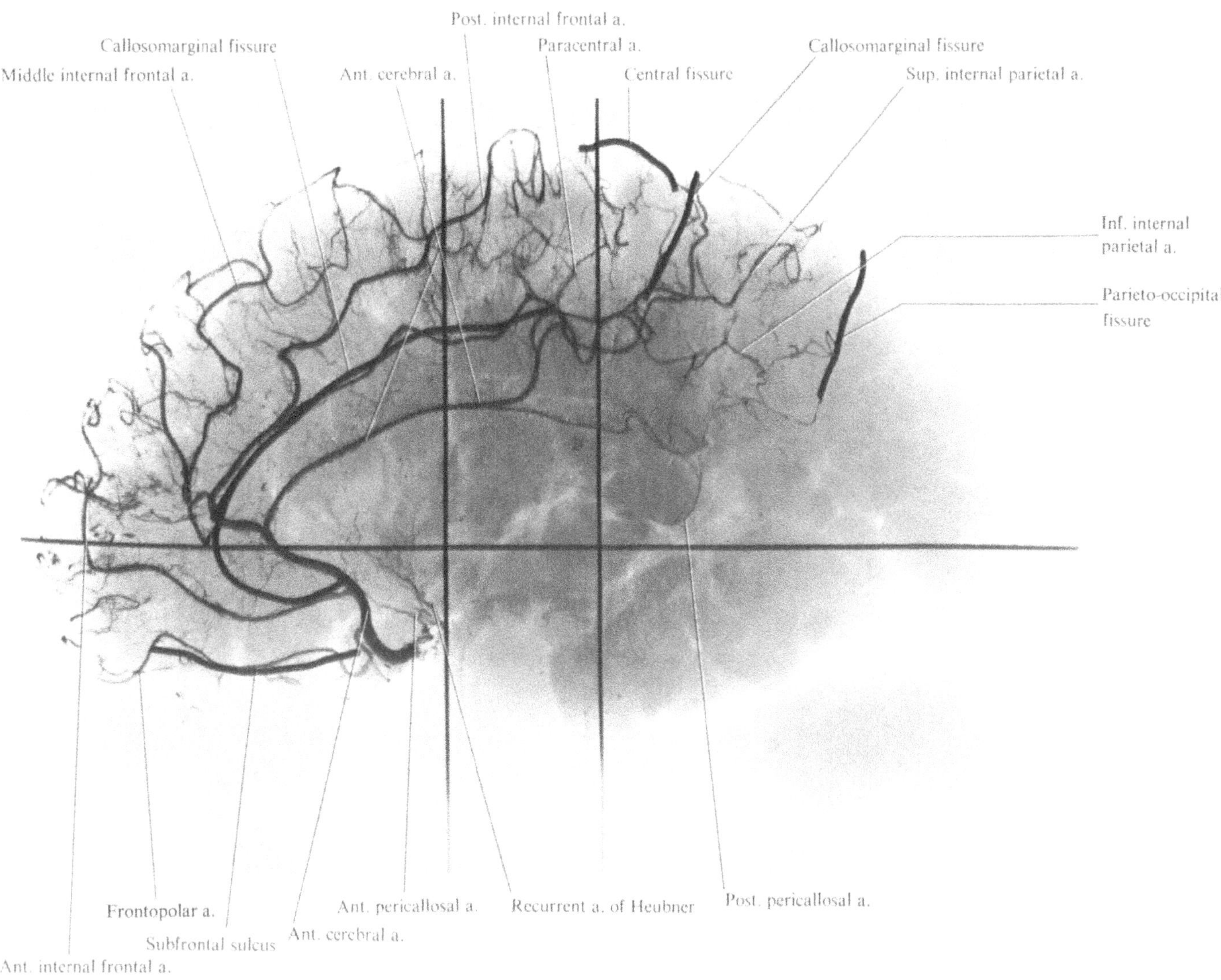

Fig. 46. Radiograph after selective injection of the right anterior cerebral artery, lateral view
Note that metallic wires have been placed in the parieto-occipital fissure, central fissure, cingulate sulcus, and subfrontal sulcus. Other vertical and horizontal wires pass through the anterior and posterior commissures

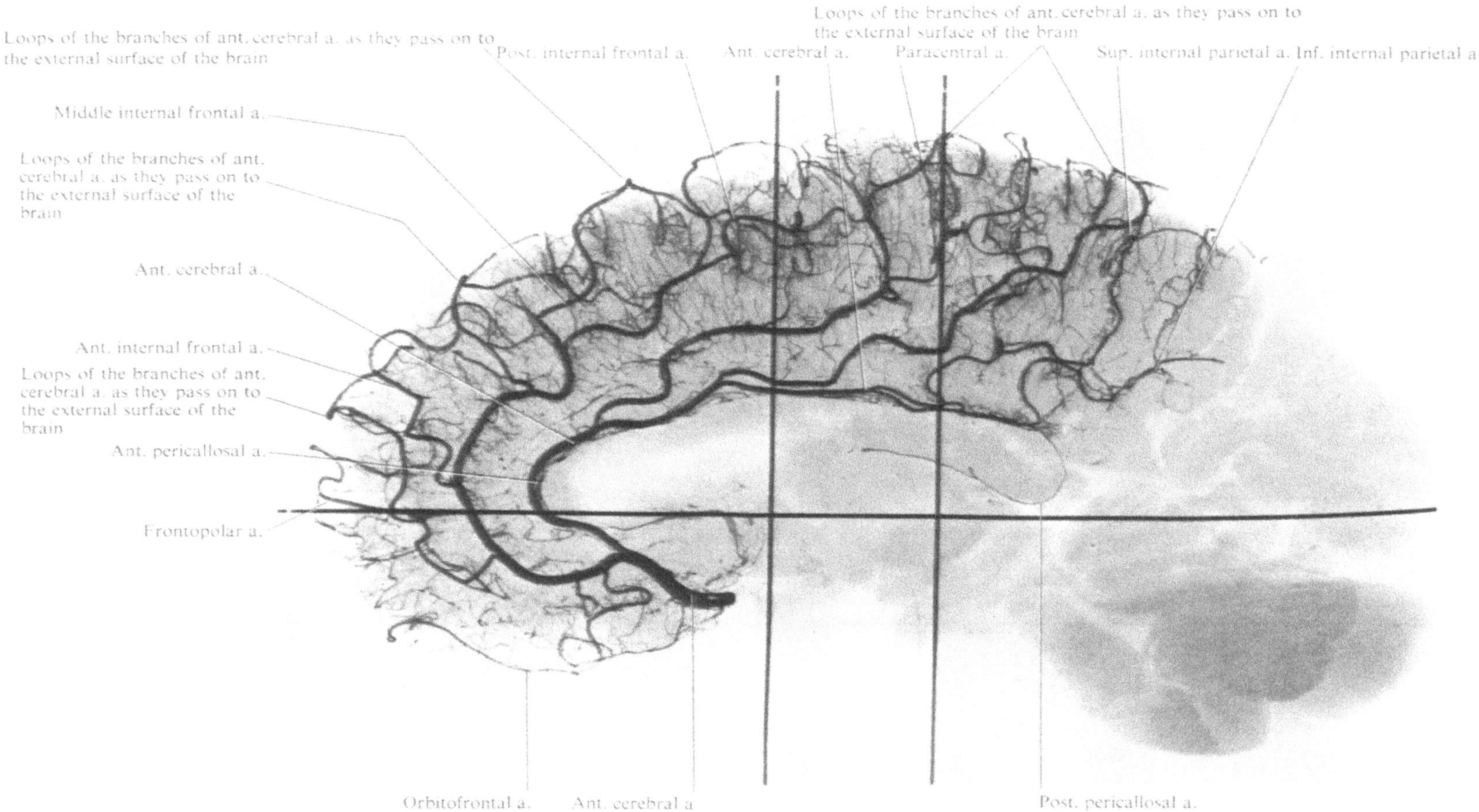

Fig. 47. Radiograph after selective injection of the right anterior cerebral artery, lateral view
Note that vertical metallic wires pass through the anterior and posterior commissures. A horizontal wire passes through both commissures

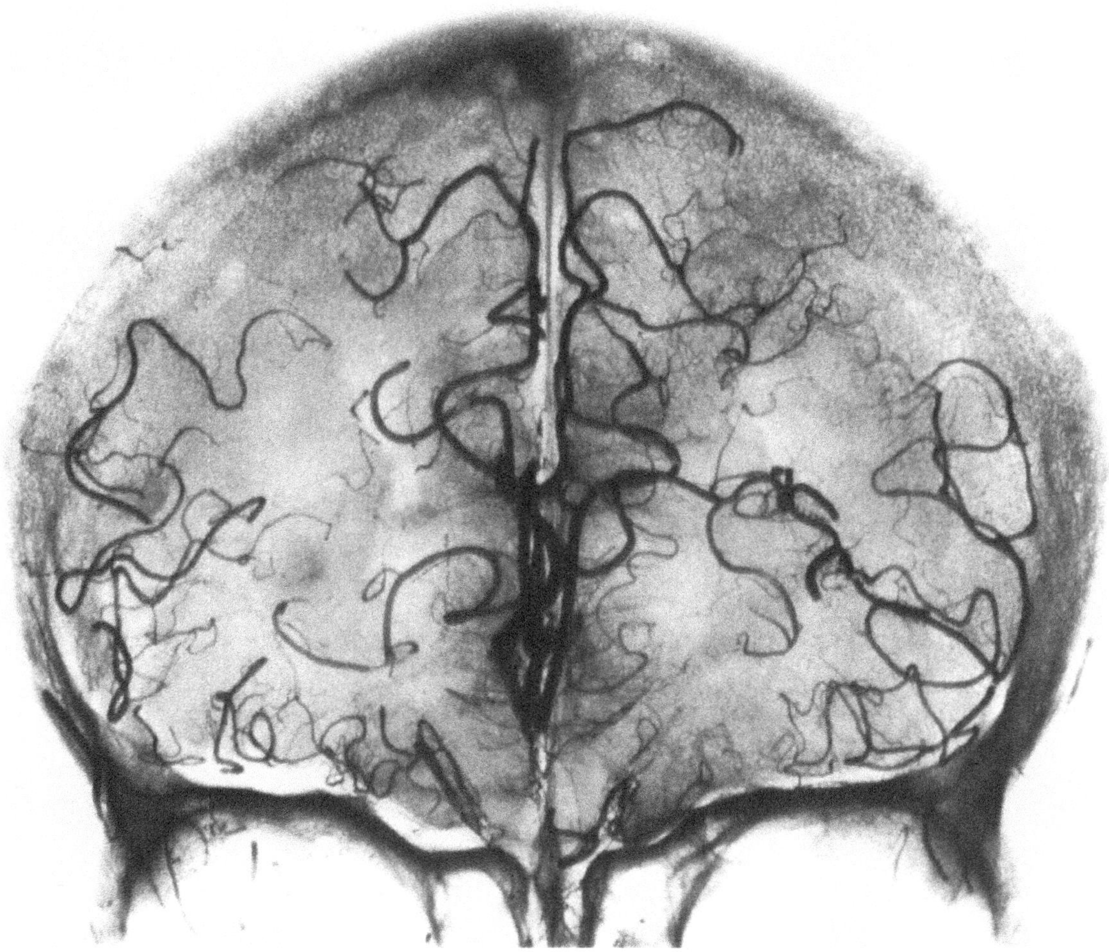

Fig. 48. Frontal section of the head after selective injection of the carotid artery, showing the territory of the anterior cerebral artery

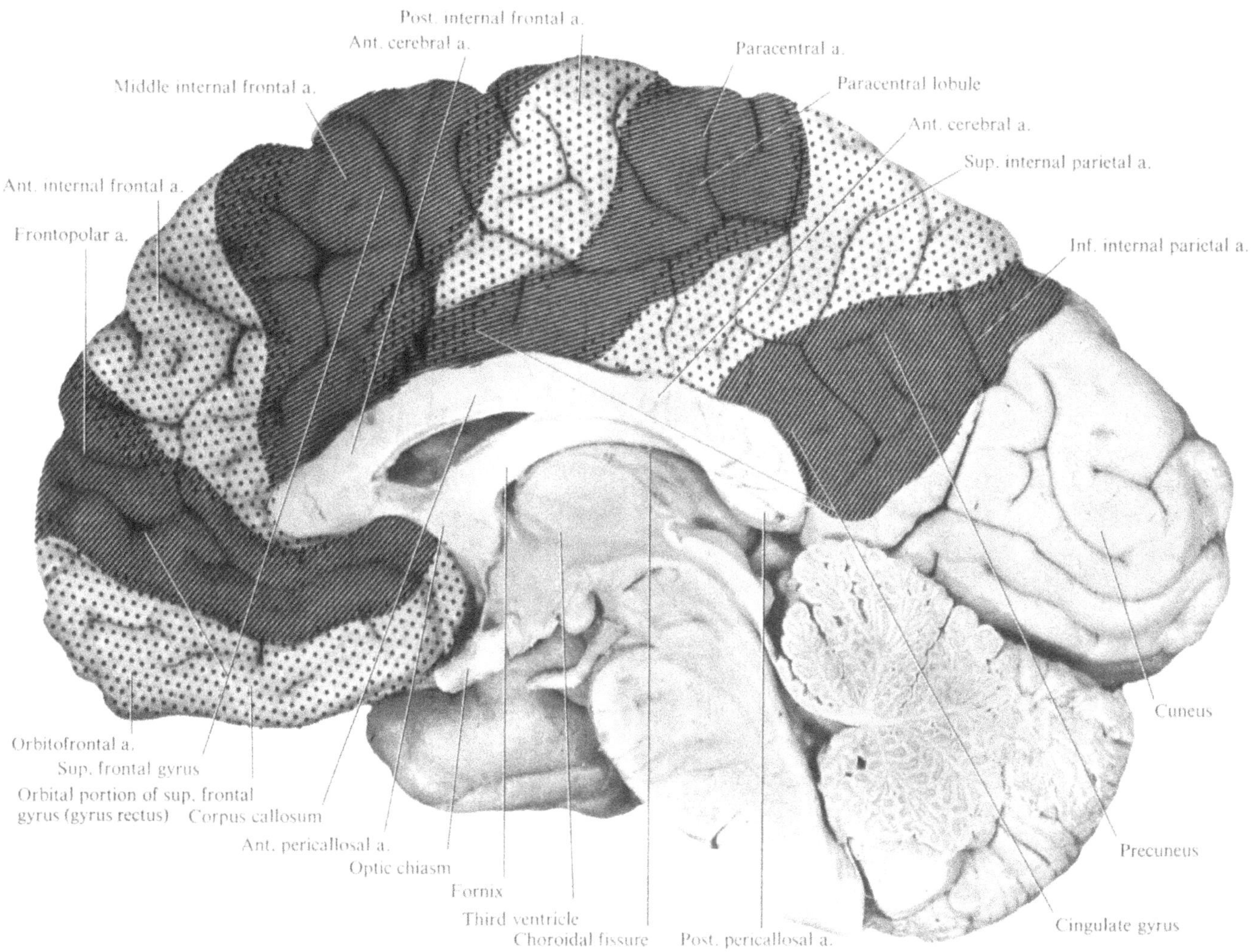

Fig. 49. Schematic representation of the territories of the anterior cerebral artery, on the internal surface of the cerebral hemisphere

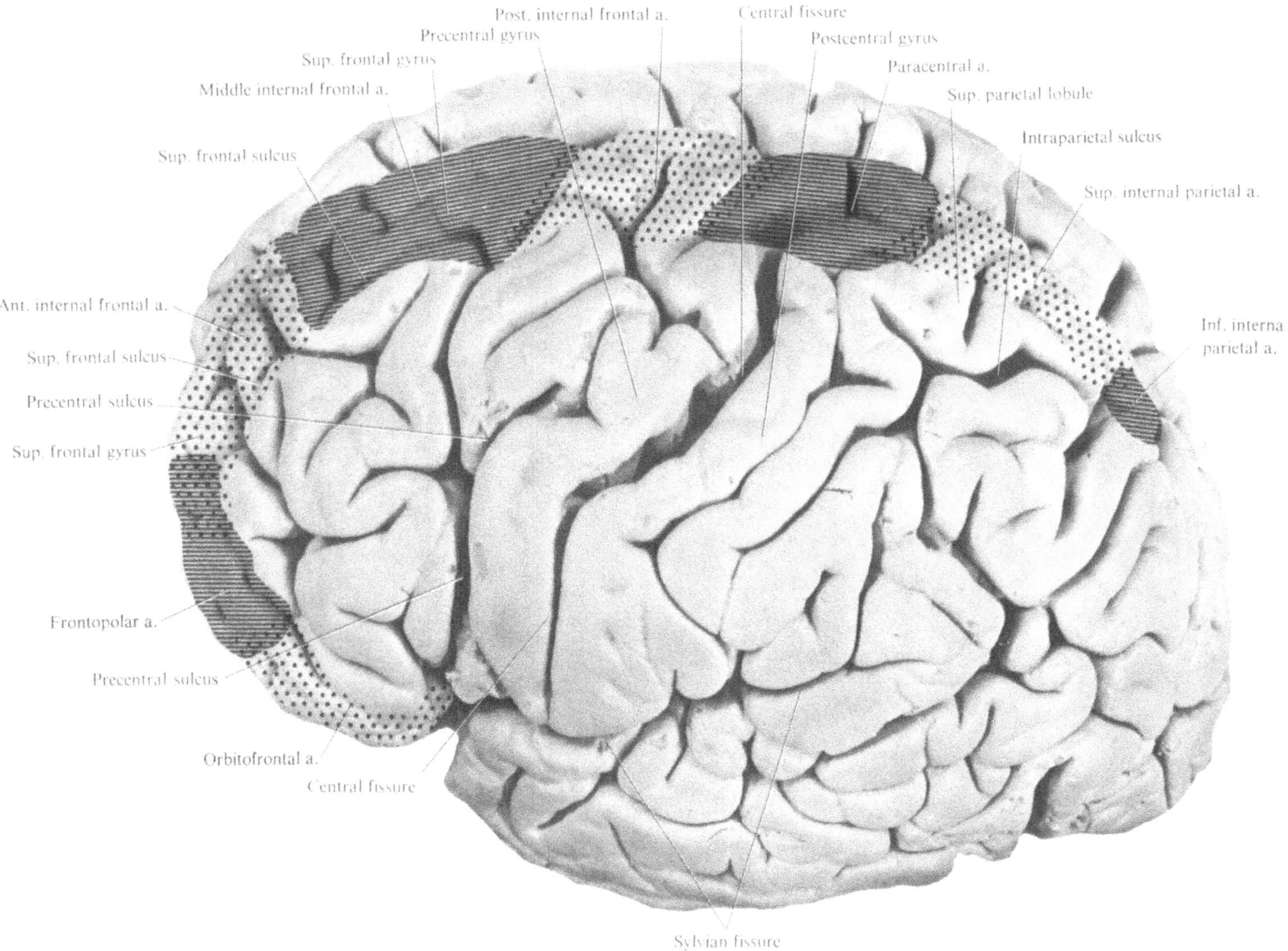

Fig. 50. Schematic representation of the territories of the anterior cerebral on the external surface of the cerebral hemisphere

▷

Fig. 51. Schematic representation of the territories of the anterior cerebral artery on the inferior surface of the frontal lobe. (*OF* orbitofrontal a., *FP* frontopolar a.)

Fig. 52. Carotid angiogram, lateral view

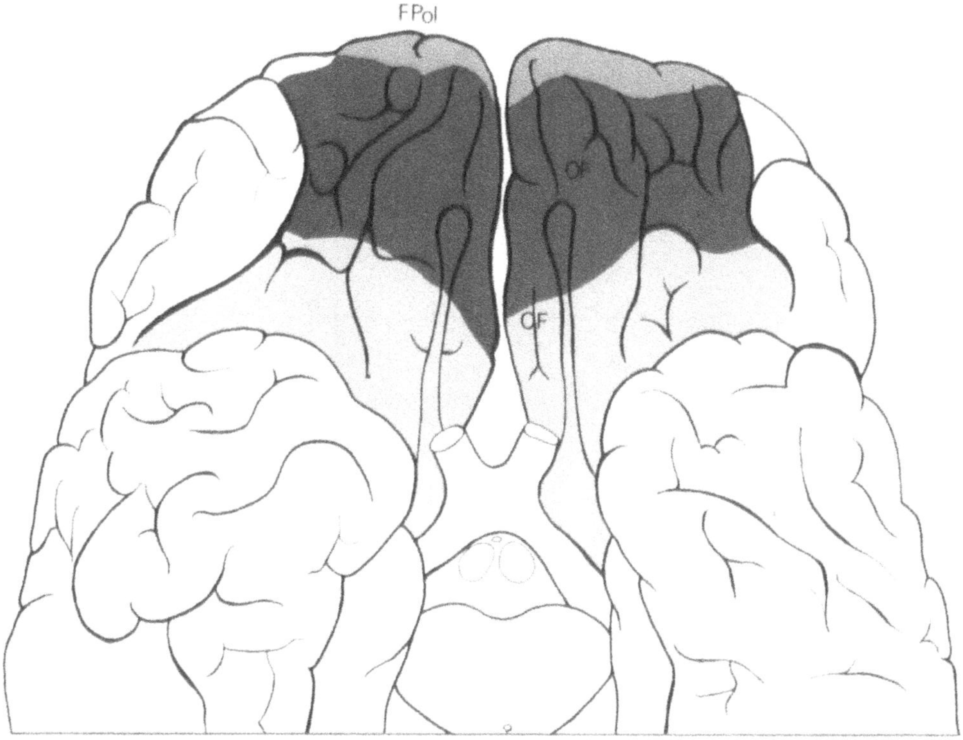
FPol
OF
OF

Fig. 51

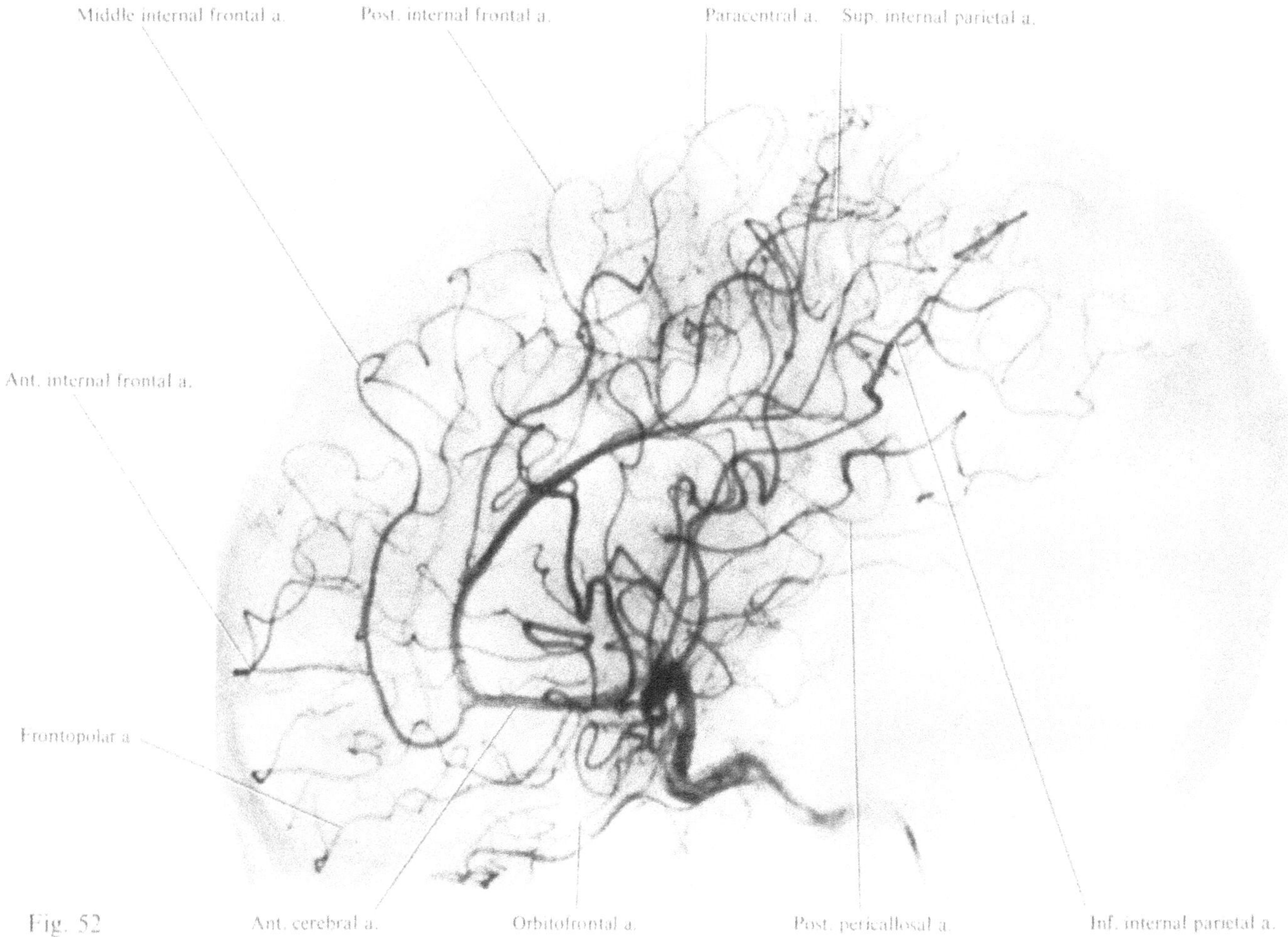
Middle internal frontal a.
Post. internal frontal a.
Paracentral a.
Sup. internal parietal a.
Ant. internal frontal a.
Frontopolar a.
Ant. cerebral a.
Orbitofrontal a.
Post. pericallosal a.
Inf. internal parietal a.

Fig. 52

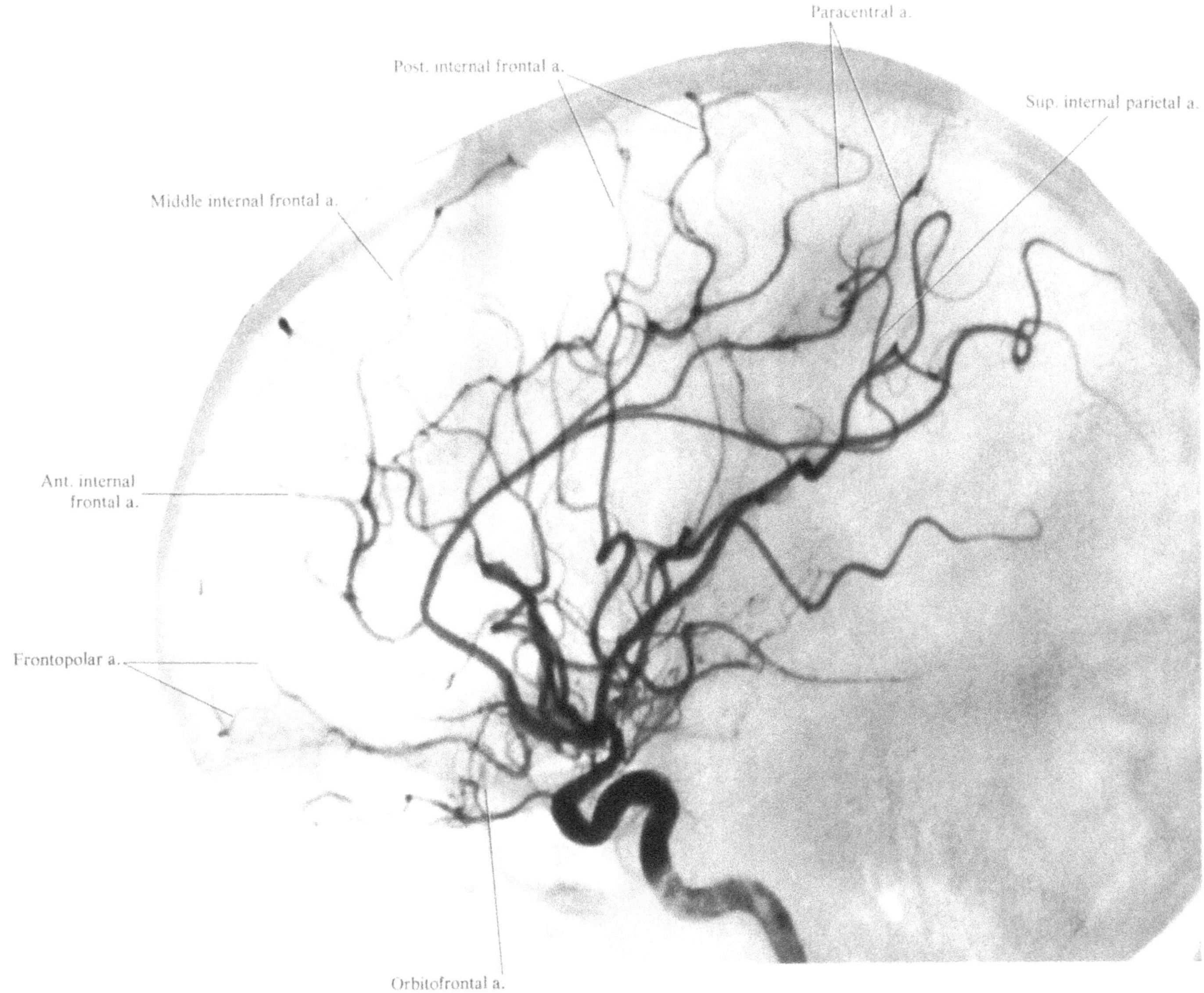

Fig. 53. Carotid angiogram, lateral view

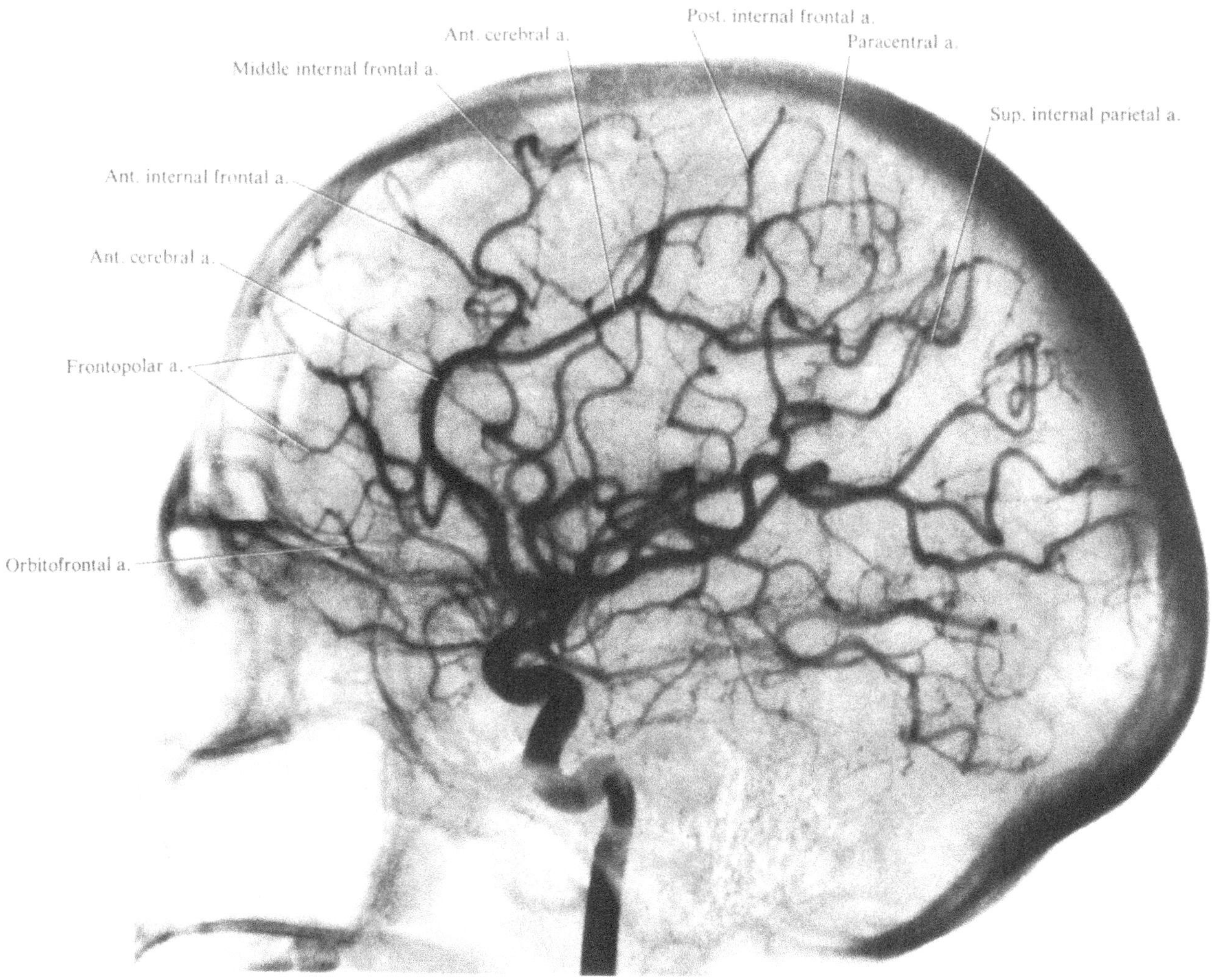

Fig. 54. Carotid angiogram, lateral view

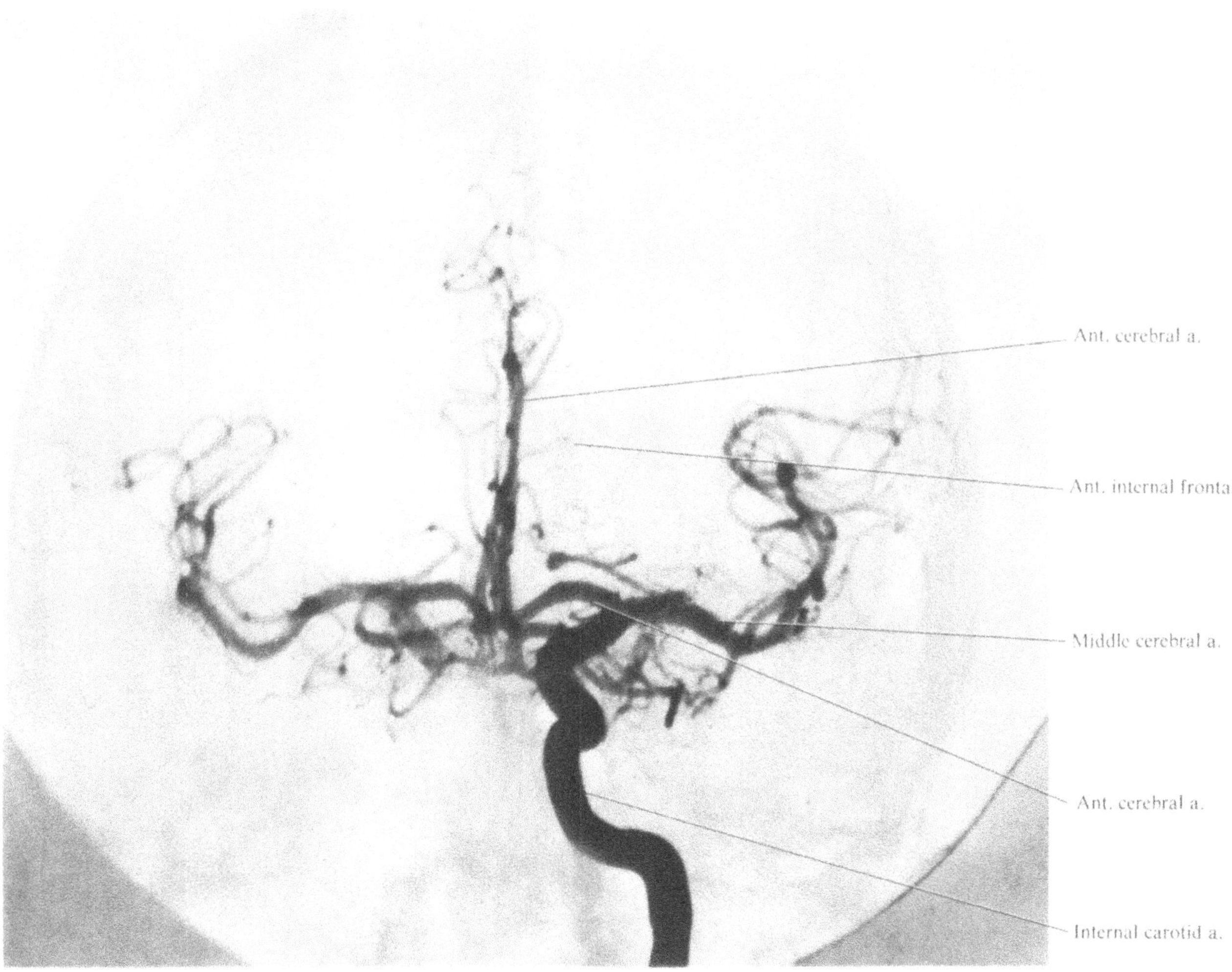

Fig. 55. Left carotid angiogram, frontal projection, with right carotid compression

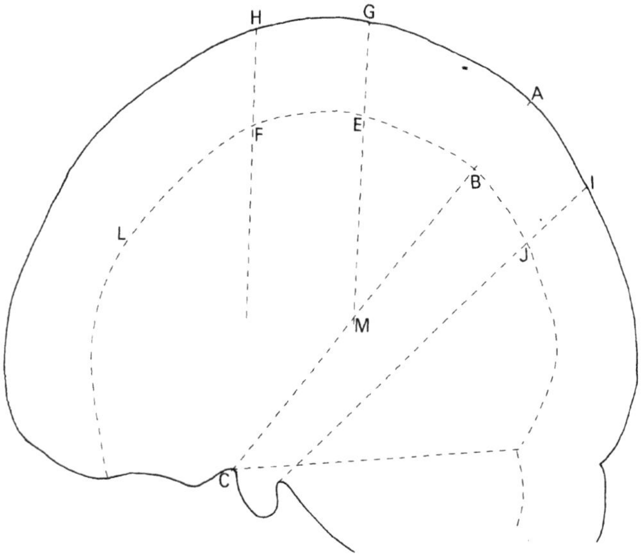

Fig. 56. Procedure of RING and WADDINGTON (1968) for the determination of the vascular territories of the anterior cerebral artery in the lateral projection

(1) A line (L) is constructed, 2.5 cm inside the inner table and parallel to it
(2) The clinoparietal line of TAVERAS and WOOD (1964) is drawn from the anterior clinoid process (C) to a point (A), situated 9 cm above the internal occipital protuberance
(3) The intersection of lines (L) and CA defines point (B)
(4) The midpoint of line CB is defined as point (M)
(5) From point (M), a vertical line is drawn, parallel to the coronal suture. This line defines point (E) where it crosses line (L) and point (G), where it intersects the inner table

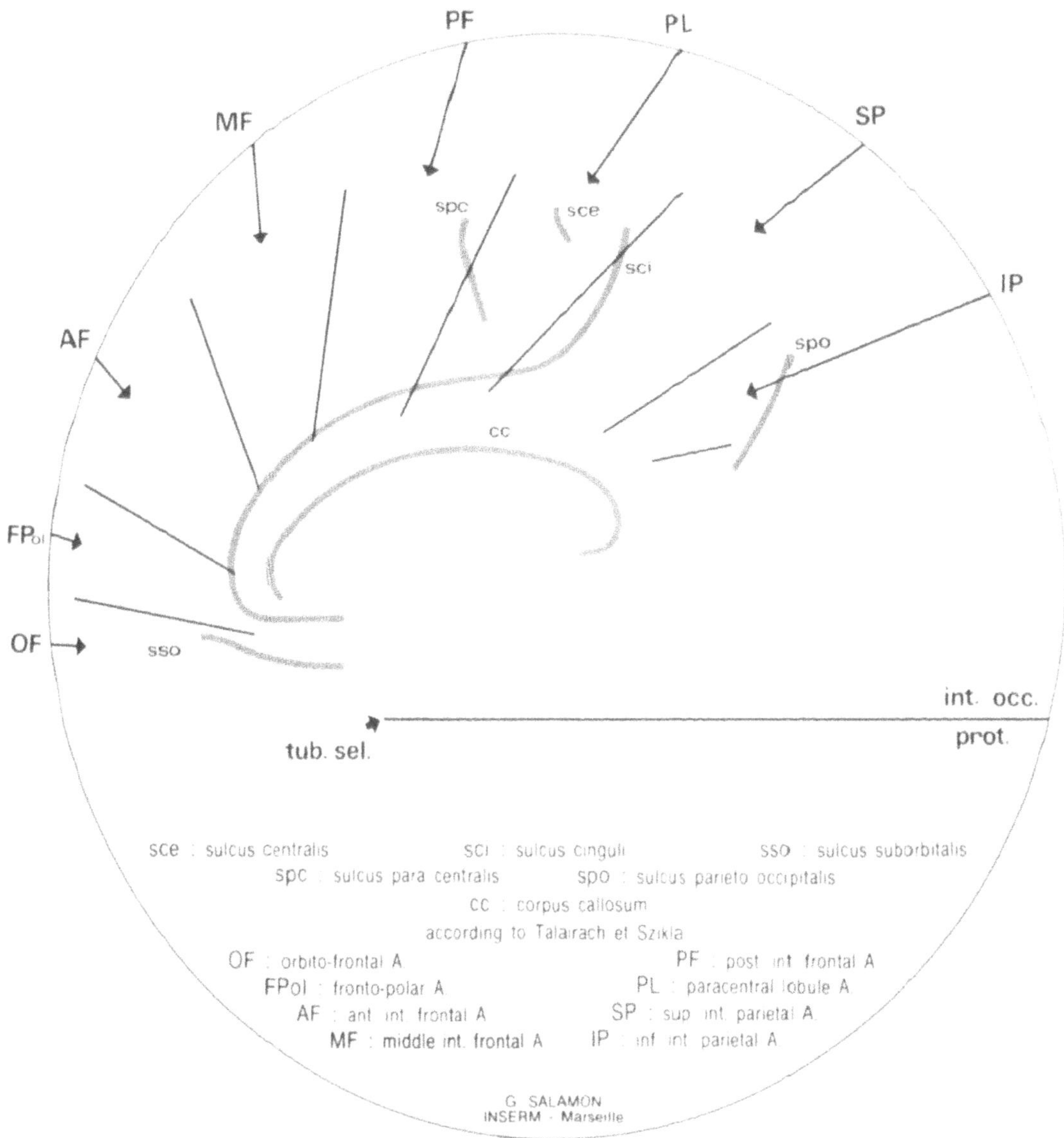

Fig. 57. Localization of the branches of the anterior cerebral artery (author's method). The transparent plastic disc indicates the course and territory of each branch of the anterior cerebral artery

◁

Fig. 56 (continued)

(6) A vertical line HF is drawn through the coronal suture parallel to line GEM. Point (H) is at the inner table and point (F) is on line (L)

(7) Point (I) is located at the midpoint of the inner table between point (G) and the internal occipital protuberance

(8) Point (J) is located on line (L) where it intersects a line connecting point (I) with the posterior clinoid process

Space EFGH corresponds to the paracentral lobule

Space EGIJ corresponds to the precuneus

In front of the plane HF is the vascular territory of the internal frontal arteries

The paracentral lobule (EFGH) is supplied by the artery of the paracentral lobule

The precuneus (EGIJ) is vascularized by the internal parietal arteries

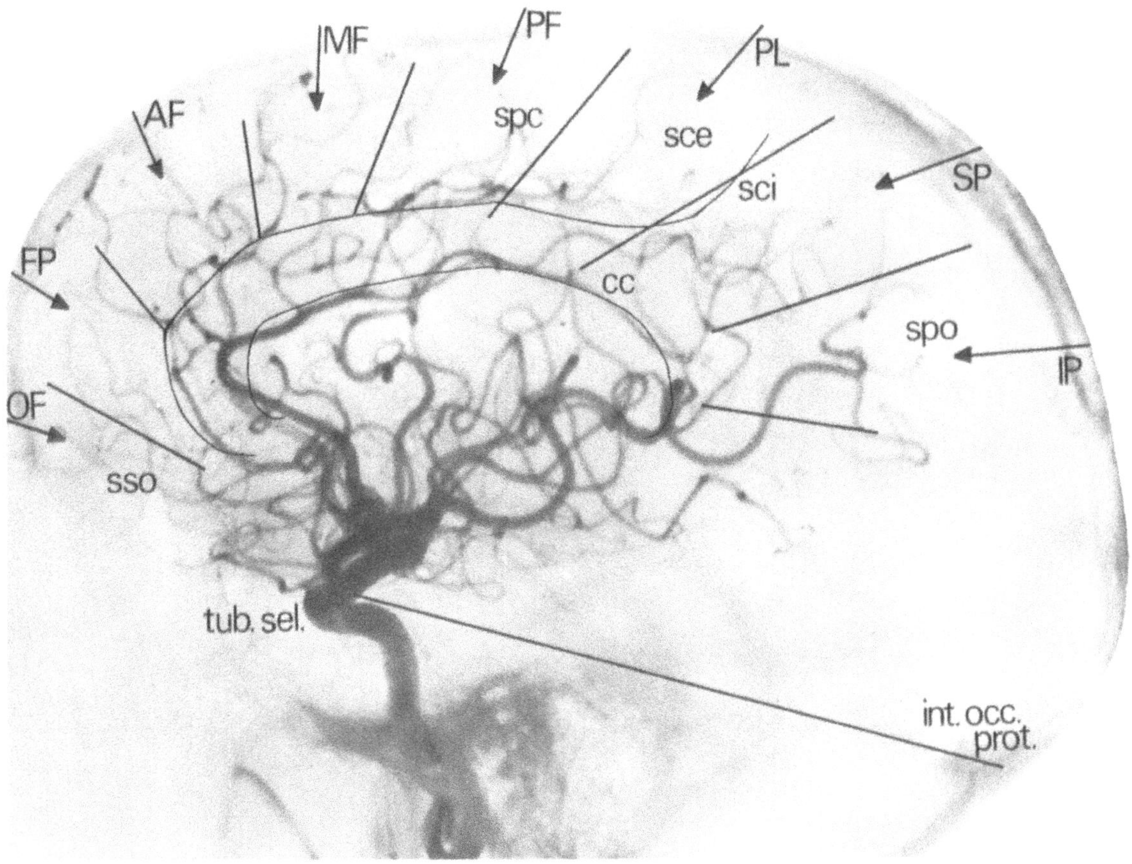

Fig. 58. Left carotid angiogram, lateral projection with superimposition of the disc described in Fig. 57

▷

Fig. 59 A–B. Localization of the sulci on the internal surface of the cerebral hemisphere, using the cortical branches of the anterior cerebral artery

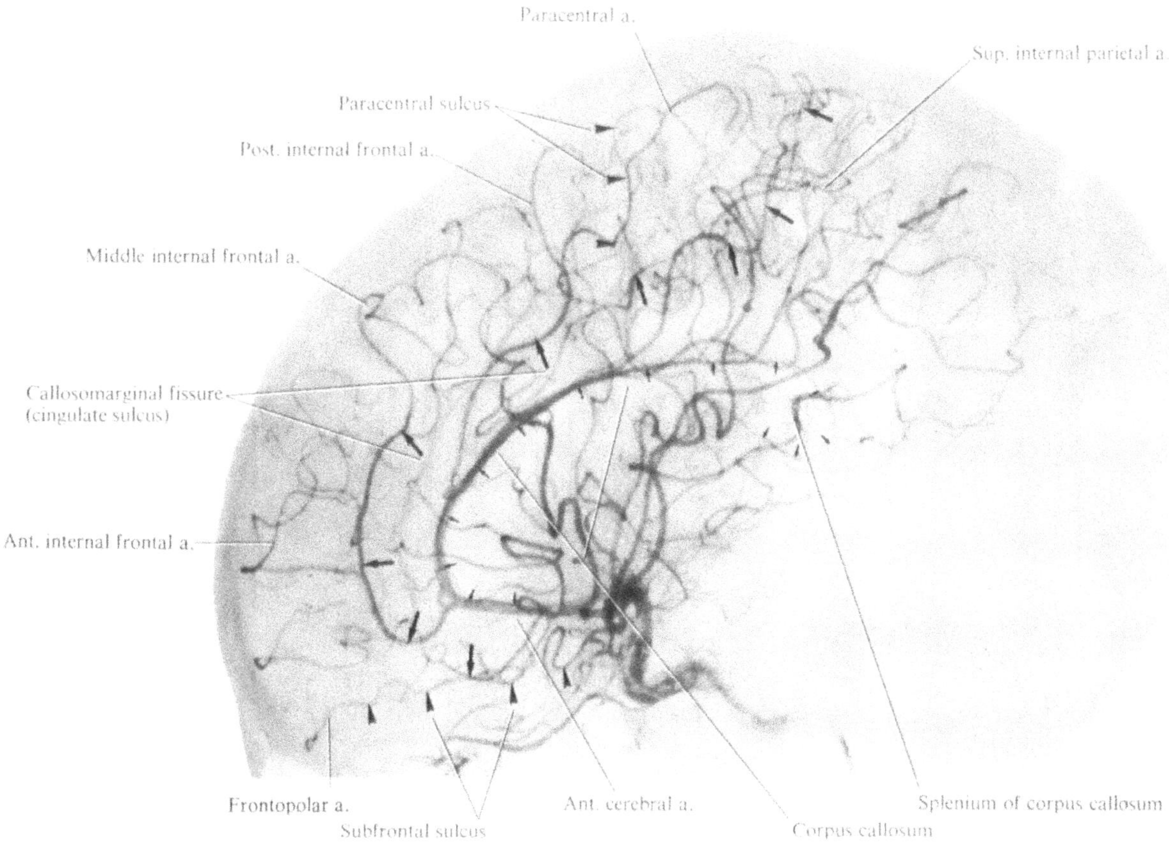

Fig. 59 A

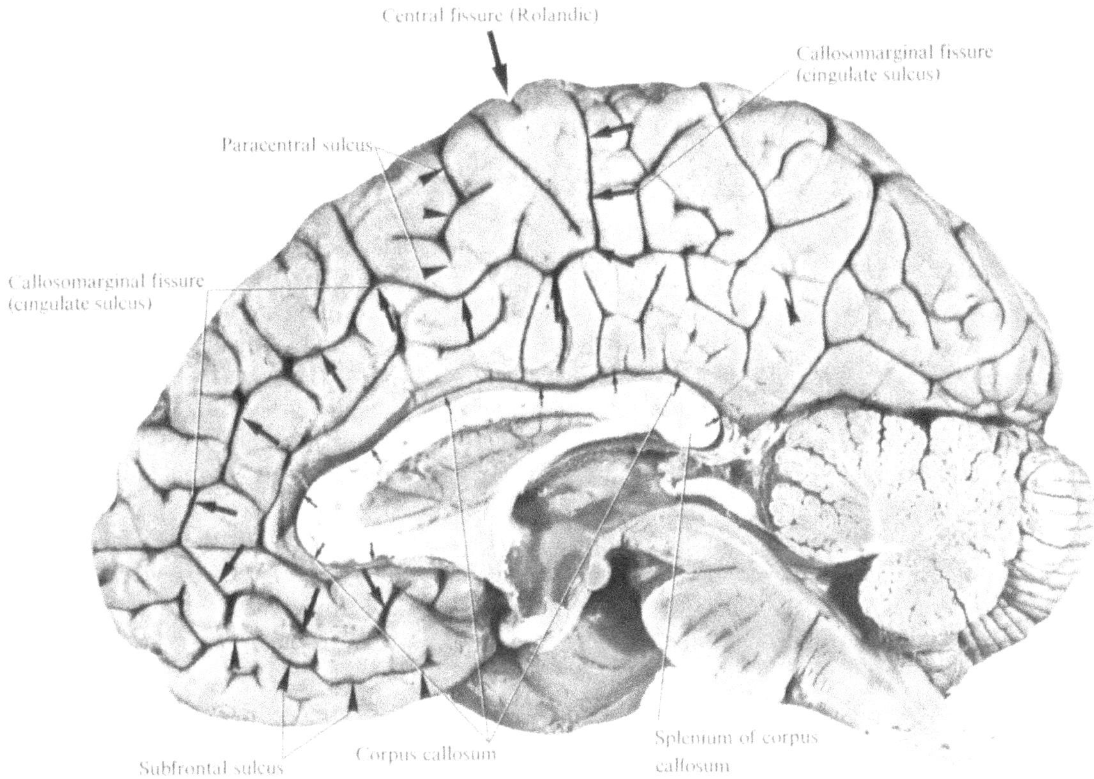

Fig. 59 B

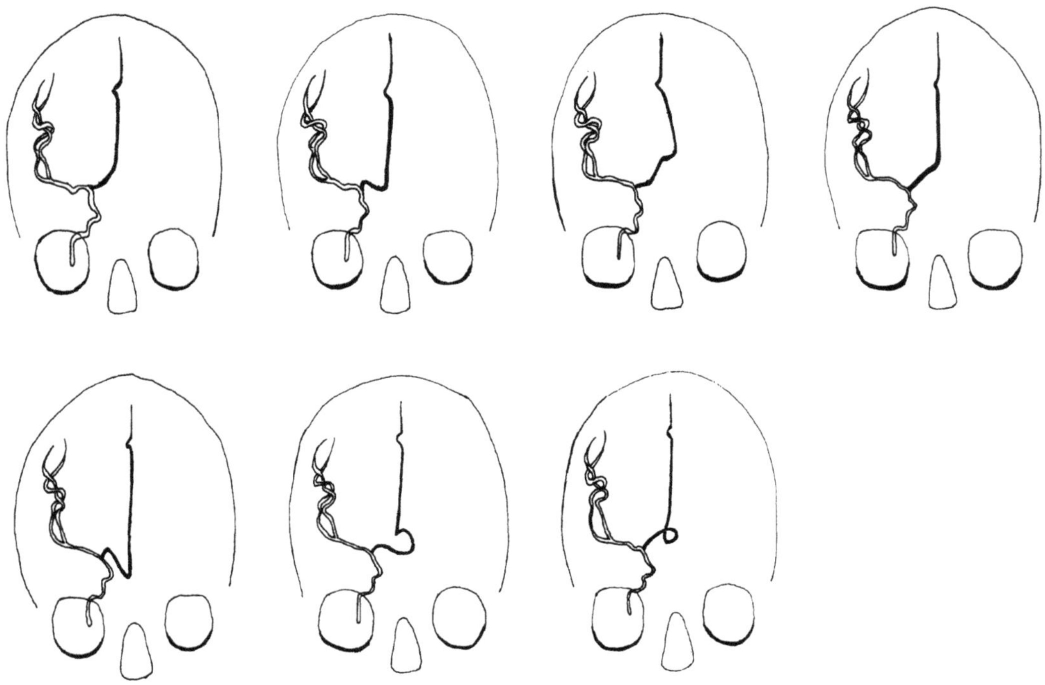

Fig. 60. Schematic representation (KRAYENBUHL and YASARGIL (1968)) of the different types of first segments of the anterior cerebral artery

B. Middle Cerebral Artery

I. Anatomic Study of the Middle Cerebral Artery

The middle cerebral artery is the largest division of the internal carotid artery. It measures 4.5 mm in diameter at its origin from the supracavernous portion of the internal carotid artery. The course of the middle cerebral artery is rather complex. It passes laterally and superiorly in its first segment, running between the uncus of the hippocampus and the olfactory stalk. In the region of the anterior perforated substance it gives rise to the lenticulostriate arteries which vascularize the basal ganglia (see p. 195) via the perforating arteries.

In its second segment, the middle cerebral artery turns 90° and enters the depths of the Sylvian fissure to reach the insula. At this level it divides into its major branches. These branches, as they pass out of the Sylvian fissure and around the frontal, parietal, or temporal opercula, constitute the last segment of the middle cerebral artery. They follow a sinuous course, ascending or descending, depending upon their territory of distribution.

The study of the middle cerebral artery has been the subject of many anatomic and radiologic studies: DURET (1874), TESTUT (1906), MOUTIER (1908), TIXIER (1912), FOIX and LEVY (1927), GABRIELLE, LATARJET *et al.* (1949), LAZORTHES (1961), and more recently RING and WADDINGTON (1967), and SALAMON and MICHOTEY (1972). The anatomoses between the middle cerebral artery and other arteries of the brain have been studied by ADAMS and VAN DER ECKEN (1959), GOUAZE *et al.* (1972).

By its branches, the middle cerebral artery supplies the major portion of the external surface of the cerebral hemisphere. In this chapter the patterns of division of the middle cerebral artery within the Sylvian fissure and the course and territory of each branch will be presented.

In a general way, these arteries have characteristic courses running either on the surface or deep within the sulci. When they cross the sulci they present characteristic loops. By anatomic analysis of the sulci, each of the major branches of the middle cerebral artery can be found. Conversely, analysis of the course of each vessel permits recognition of the principal fissures and sulci of the brain. Consequently the boundaries of the cerebral gyri can be located by identifying these arteries.

1. Patterns of Division of the Middle Cerebral Artery within the Sylvian Fissure

(Fig. 70)

Schematically, the middle cerebral artery presents two principal patterns of division: bifurcation or trifurcation. In the bifurcation pattern, there is an anterior and a posterior trunk. The orbitofrontal, prefrontal, precentral and central arteries arise from the anterior trunk. The remaining branches usually take their origin from the posterior trunk. However, some variation is seen in the origin of the parietal arteries, which may arise from either the anterior or posterior trunk.

In the second type of division there are three principal trunks of equal size, which arise within a few millimeters of each other. The orbitofrontal, prefrontal and precentral arteries are branches of the anterior trunk. (The last of these branches may arise from the middle trunk as well.) The middle trunk gives rise to the central arteries, the anterior and posterior parietal arteries, and the angular gyrus artery. The temporo-occipital artery may come from either the middle or posterior trunk. All of the temporal arteries arise from the posterior trunk.

Other patterns of division are less common. A single trunk may be present, terminating as the angular gyrus artery. Conversely, multiple branches may fan out within the Sylvian fissure, without a true common trunk.

2. Frontal Branches of the Middle Cerebral Artery

(Figs. 61–68)

Orbitofrontal artery
Prefrontal artery
Precentral artery
Central artery

The orbitofrontal artery is quite variable in its origin but in general it emerges from the Sylvian fissure at the level of the pars orbitalis of the inferior frontal gyrus. It is directed towards the orbital surface of the inferior frontal gyrus and supplies this portion of the frontal lobe.

The prefrontal artery leaves the Sylvian fissure at the level of the pars triangularis of the inferior frontal gyrus, or just anterior or just posterior to it. It divides into two or three principal branches on the external surface of the frontal lobe. These branches follow an ascending course and present characteristic loops as they cross the inferior frontal sulcus.

The territory of supply of the prefrontal artery is the pars orbitalis, the pars triangularis and a part of the pars opercularis of the inferior frontal gyrus, and most of the middle frontal gyrus. Distally, its branches anastomose with corresponding branches of the anterior cerebral artery in the region of the superior frontal gyrus. The diploidal branching pattern of the prefrontal arteries is peculiar to these vessels and they have been referred to as the "candelabra arteries".

The precentral artery reaches the precentral sulcus after emerging from the Sylvian fissure at the base of the precentral gyrus. One or two major branches are present at its origin. Anteriorly to the precentral sulcus, the precentral artery supplies the posterior part of the middle frontal gyrus. Posteriorly to the precentral sulcus, it supplies the inferior half of the precentral gyrus.

The central artery leaves the Sylvian fissure by passing over the frontoparietal operculum or the base of the postcentral gyrus. Two branches are usually present at the frontoparietal operculum. The anterior branch enters the inferior part of the central fissure while the posterior branch reaches the central fissure higher up. These two arteries often have a long course in the depths of the central fissure. The relationship between the central artery and the central fissure is rather characteristic and permits the identification of this fissure at angiography.

The territory of the central artery lies anteriorly and posteriorly to the central fissure. Anteriorly, it supplies the upper part of the precentral gyrus, with the exception of the most superior part which derives its blood supply from the anterior cerebral artery. Posteriorly, it serves the inferior third or half of the postcentral gyrus.

3. Parietal Branches of the Middle Cerebral Artery

(Figs. 61–68, 71)

Anterior parietal artery
Posterior parietal artery
Angular gyrus artery

The anterior parietal artery can arise as an isolated branch or in common with either the posterior parietal artery or posterior branch of the central artery. In general, it is a single artery and has a characteristic course. It follows the intraparietal sulcus in its inferior portion and when the intraparietal sulcus changes its direction, this artery generally follows the postcentral sulcus. Its territory of vascularization includes the superior half or two-thirds of the postcentral gyrus and the anterior part of the inferior parietal lobule.

The posterior parietal artery appears on the surface of the brain at the posterior extremity of the Sylvian fissure. It has an ascending course at the level of the posterior part of the inferior parietal lobule. Unlike the other ascending branches of the middle cerebral artery, which run deeply within the sulci, its course is superficial. Near its origin, the posterior parietal artery gives rise to a major branch, the artery to the supramarginal gyrus.
The territory of the posterior parietal artery corresponds to the posterior part of the inferior parietal lobule, the inferior part of the superior parietal lobule, and the supramarginal gyrus. The superior parietal lobule is supplied equally by branches of the anterior cerebral artery, while the supramarginal gyrus receives contributions from the angular gyrus artery.

The angular gyrus artery has been considered by certain authors as the trunk of the middle cerebral artery or at least its terminal branch. It emerges from the Sylvian fissure in various ways. It may appear on the external surface anywhere from the parietal operculum to the posterior extremity of the Sylvian fissure. If it leaves at the level of the parietal operculum, it crosses the superior temporal gyrus, and enters the superior temporal sulcus. It then reaches the angular gyrus,which it supplies. If it emerges more posteriorly, it follows the direction of the Sylvian fissure. During its course it gives rise to branches to the supramarginal gyrus. In the majority of cases it divides into two branches; the superior one serves the angular gyrus, while the inferior branch is directed towards the occipital lobe to vascularize the superior and middle occipital gyri.
The territory of the angular gyrus artery is very large and includes the posterior part of the superior temporal gyrus, the supramarginal gyrus, the angular gyrus, and the upper halves of the superior and middle occipital gyri. In the region of the superior temporal gyrus the territory of the angular gyrus artery overlaps the territory of the temporo-occipital artery. At the level of the supramarginal gyrus it overlaps the territory of the posterior parietal artery. Lastly, it also shares a common territory with the occipitotemporal branch of the posterior cerebral artery.

4. Temporal and Temporo-Occipital Branches of the Middle Cerebral Artery
(Figs. 61–68, 71)

Temporo-occipital artery
Posterior temporal artery
Middle temporal artery
Inferior temporal artery
Temporal polar artery

The temporo-occipital artery is single and emerges quickly from the Sylvian fissure, often at the level of the fronto-parietal operculum. It can, however, emerge more posteriorly. The temporo-occipital artery crosses the superior temporal gyrus and follows the superior temporal sulcus. In the temporo-occipital region it divides into two terminal branches, which supply the middle and inferior occipital gyri. When the temporo-occipital artery is well developed, the posterior temporal artery is small and the reverse is true when the posterior temporal artery is large. Apart from branches to the posterior part of the middle and inferior temporal gyri, the territory of the temporo-occipital artery corresponds to the inferior occipital gyrus. At the occipital pole the temporo-occipital artery anastomoses with analogous branches of the posterior cerebral artery.

The posterior temporal artery leaves the Sylvian fissure at the level of the frontoparietal operculum. It has a step-like course, following first the superior temporal sulcus and later the inferior temporal sulcus, after having crossed both the superior and middle temporal gyri. It supplies the middle and posterior parts of the superior temporal gyrus, the posterior third of the middle temporal gyrus, and the posterior extremity of the inferior temporal gyrus.

The middle temporal artery leaves the Sylvian fissure more anteriorly, in the region of the pars opercularis. It crosses the superior and middle temporal gyri before finally entering the inferior temporal sulcus. Its course is analogous to that of the preceding artery, but it is located anteriorly to it. Its territory is the middle portion of the superior and middle temporal gyri, and the middle and posterior portions of the inferior temporal gyrus.

The anterior temporal artery shares the supply of the anterior portion of the external surface of the temporal lobe with the temporal polar artery. It leaves the Sylvian fissures anteriorly to the middle temporal artery and presents a characteristic step-like course similar to the other temporal arteries.

The temporal polar artery is often neglected in anatomical work (Wickbom, 1948). Its existence is constant and it should not be considered a branch of the anterior temporal artery. It arises very early on from the trunk of the middle cerebral artery. The temporal polar artery has an undulating course on the internal aspect of the temporal lobe before arriving on the external surface. Here it crosses the superior and middle temporal gyri. Its territory of distribution corresponds to the temporal pole.

5. Insular Branches

The insular branches are composed of many small vessels which arise from the middle cerebral trunk or its branches. It is not possible to distinguish or name these branches to the insula individually. They arise exclusively from the trunks that pass through the Sylvian fissure.

II. Radiologic Study of the Middle Cerebral Artery

In 1938, FISHER studied the radiologic anatomy of the middle cerebral artery and proposed his personal subdivision of this artery into M1, M2 and M3 segments, depending on its horizontal, insular or cortical location.
Numerous methods have been proposed for studying the axis of the Sylvian triangle. WORINGER and GERNEZ (1948) related the Sylvian axis to a line connecting the anterior clinoid process with the external occipital protuberance; these two lines normally form an angle of 40° (Fig. 82). KRAYENBUHL and YASARGIL (1968) observed that a line passing through the roots of the upper incisors and the carotid siphon also passed through the Sylvian axis (Fig. 82).
TAVERAS and WOOD (1964) related the axis of the Sylvian triangle to the clinoparietal line (Fig. 82). This line extends from the anterior clinoid process to a point 9 cm above the internal occipital protuberance.
The angiographic anatomy of the middle cerebral artery was the subject of a detailed monograph by DILENGE. Other important radiologic descriptions include those of WICKBOM (1948), GREITZ and LINDGREN (1948), ABRAMS(1961), KRAYENBUHL and YASARGIL (1968), and TAVERAS and WOOD (1964).
KRAYENBUHL and YASARGIL (1968) described important normal variations of the horizontal segment of the middle cerebral artery (Fig. 88).
A very precise study is the treatise of RING and WADDINGTON (1967), based upon the works of FOIX and LEVY (1927), which proposed an original method for studying the cortical branches of the middle cerebral artery (Fig. 79).
In our own laboratory, MICHOTEY (1972) performed a series of important dissections of each branch of the middle cerebral artery and its territory of cortical vascularization (Fig. 71). These dissections form the basis of our system for localizing the cortical branches of the middle cerebral artery. Localization of the gyrus of Heschl, by branches of the parietal arteries, was performed by SZIKLA and TALAIRACH (1976) during unique dissections under stereotactic control.
The configuration of the insular branches was also the subject of works by TAVERAS and WOOD (1964), SCHLESINGER (1953), VLAHOVITCH *et al.* (1964, 1968, 1970, 1973) (Figs. 83, 84).
TAVERAS and WOOD (1964) studied the reflections of the insular branches in the frontal projection. Two important Sylvian points were described. The superficial point corresponds to the arterial segment closest to the inner table from which it is separated by 20 to 32 mm (Fig. 84). The deep point corresponds to the deepest arterial segment just as it leaves the insula and is separated from the inner table by 30 to 43 mm.
VLAHOVITCH (1964, 1968, 1970, 1973) was especially interested in the localization of the insula on lateral radiographs (Fig. 83). He described the Sylvian triangle in detail, defining its limits. The upper limit of this triangle, which is called its base, is the superior insular line. (He also described a supra-insular line, parallel to the previous one and situated at the level of the frontoparietal cortex.)
According to the results of VLAHOVITCH (1964, 1968, 1970, 1973), the superior insular line runs parallel to the orbitomeatal line, midway between the external auditory canal and the inner table of the skull, on a perpendicular to the orbitomeatal line. The anterior insular point is on the superior insular line, 4 to 5 mm in front of or behind a point perpendicularly above the midpoint of the orbitomeatal line. The posterior insular point is also on the same line, and is up to 17 mm behind the perpendicular from the external auditory canal.
GUYOT and PHILIPPON (1969) described a method for using the opercular points to localize the Sylvian fissure.
Personally, we use the bicommissural line and the method of TALAIRACH and SZIKLA (1967) for localization of the insula. The insular branches of the middle cerebral artery fit well into this system of localization, especially in the normal patient.
Without detailing the course and possible variations of the middle cerebral artery at this time, it is important to realize that its branches are best visualized in the lateral projection (Figs. 72–76).
The most anterior branch, the *orbitofrontal artery*, runs parallel to the roof the orbit. It participates in the vascularization of the inferior surface of the frontal lobe with an analogous branch from the anterior cerebral artery, the orbitofrontal artery.

The second branch or *prefrontal artery* has been called the "candelabra artery" since its original description by MONIZ (1927, 1934). This name arises from the diploidal branching pattern exhibited by this artery, which supplies the middle part of the inferior and middle frontal gyri. Its characteristic branching pattern allows localization of the inferior and superior frontal sulci (Fig. 85).
The *precentral or pre-Rolandic artery* usually ascends parallel to the precentral sulcus.
The presence of two separate *central arteries* is practically constant. After their opercular origin, both are directed towards the central fissure (of Roland), which they penetrate deeply. Two characteristic loops identify this change of direction and consequently localize the central fissure and the adjacent motor and sensory areas (Fig. 85).
The anterior and posterior parietal arteries vascularize most of the parietal lobe with contributions from the angular gyrus artery (Fig. 86). A characteristic right-angle bend identifies the point at which the anterior parietal artery passes from the intraparietal sulcus into the postcentral sulcus.
The *angular gyrus artery* is the largest branch of the middle cerebral artery. It continues along the direction of the Sylvian fissure to the region of the angular gyrus. The terminal segment of this artery curves over the top of the angular gyrus, presenting a characteristic curve concave inferiorly. This curve, the general direction and the length serve to identify the angular gyrus artery.
The other long branch of the middle cerebral artery, the *temporo-occipital artery,* also distinguishes itself by its length and characteristic curve in the region of the occipital pole. Its degree of development is inversely related to that of the posterior temporal artery.
The posterior, middle and anterior temporal arteries identify themselves by their typical bayonette-like courses. Each branch crosses the superior temporal gyrus to enter the superior temporal sulcus. They then follow a short posterior course in this sulcus, before leaving and then crossing the middle temporal gyrus. Finally they enter the inferior temporal sulcus, where they again have a posterior course. These paths readily identify the superior temporal sulcus as it parallels the Sylvian fissure, and this helps to define the supramarginal and angular gyri (Fig. 87).
The temporal polar artery is less frequently identified angiographically than the other branches of the middle cerebral artery. It runs at the level of the uncus to reach its most anterior part.
Thus it is possible to distinguish angiographically the various branches of the middle cerebral artery, with sufficient detail to provide anatomic correlation comparable to that obtained during dissection or radiography of injected specimens. Careful analysis of the branches of the middle cerebral artery will localize the majority of the sulci on the external surface of the brain (Figs. 85–87). This close angiographic and anatomic correlation makes the study of these important arteries an unsurpassed morphologic and functional exploration of the brain.

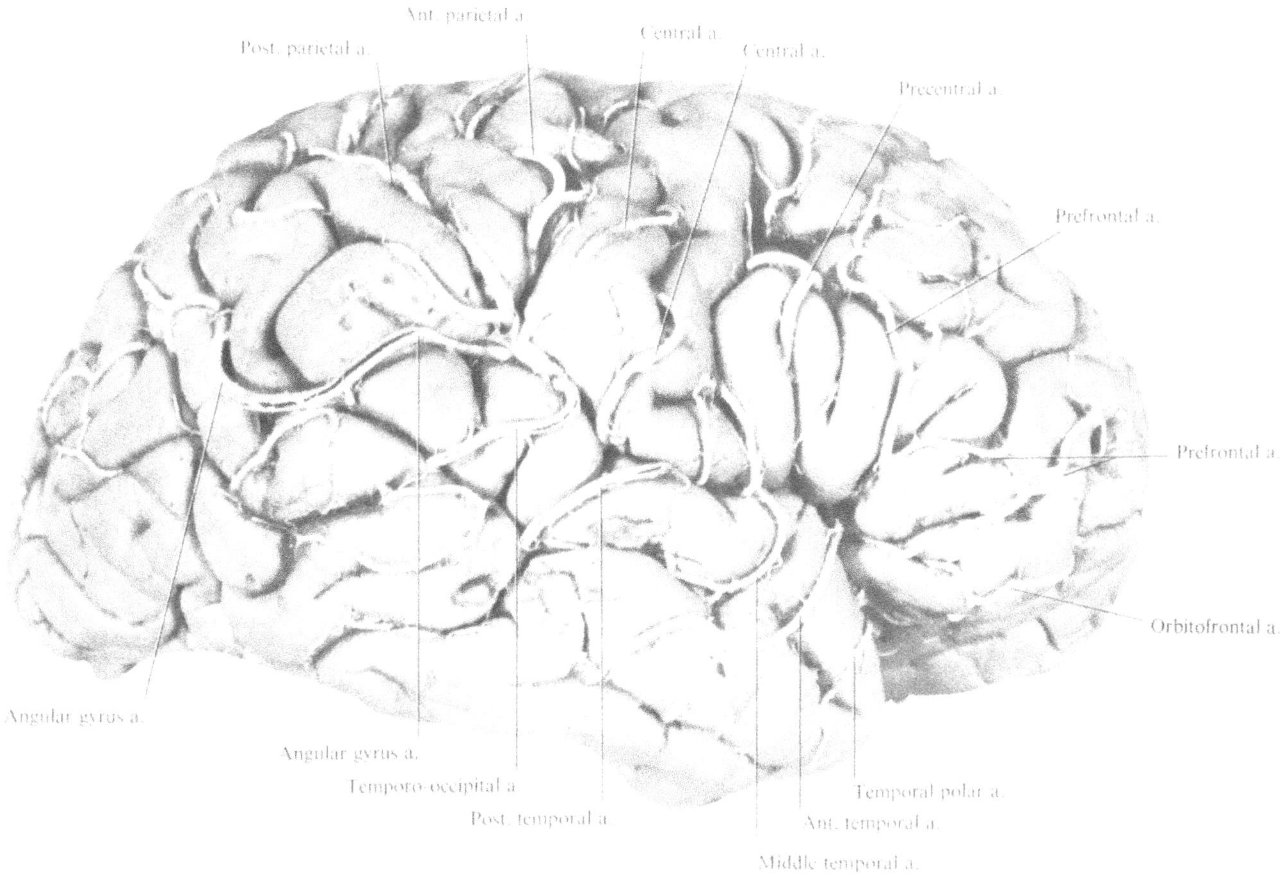

Fig. 61. Dissection of the right cerebral hemisphere after selective injection of the middle cerebral artery, lateral view

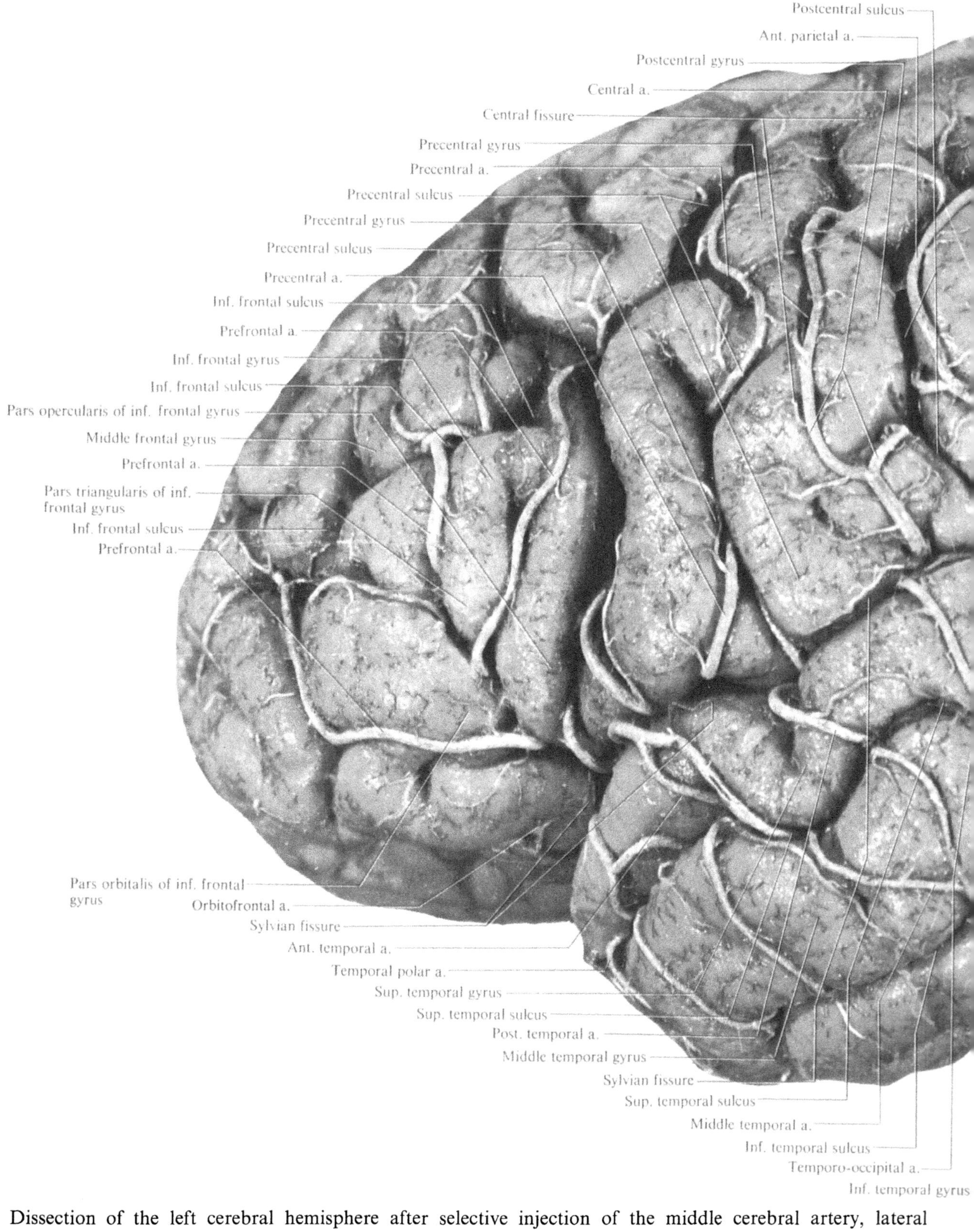

Fig. 62. Dissection of the left cerebral hemisphere after selective injection of the middle cerebral artery, lateral view

Note on this specimen the relationships between the inferior frontal sulcus and the loops of the prefrontal artery and the superior temporal sulcus and the curves of the temporal lobe arteries. Note also the characteristic course of the anterior parietal artery which permits the recognition of the intraparietal sulcus

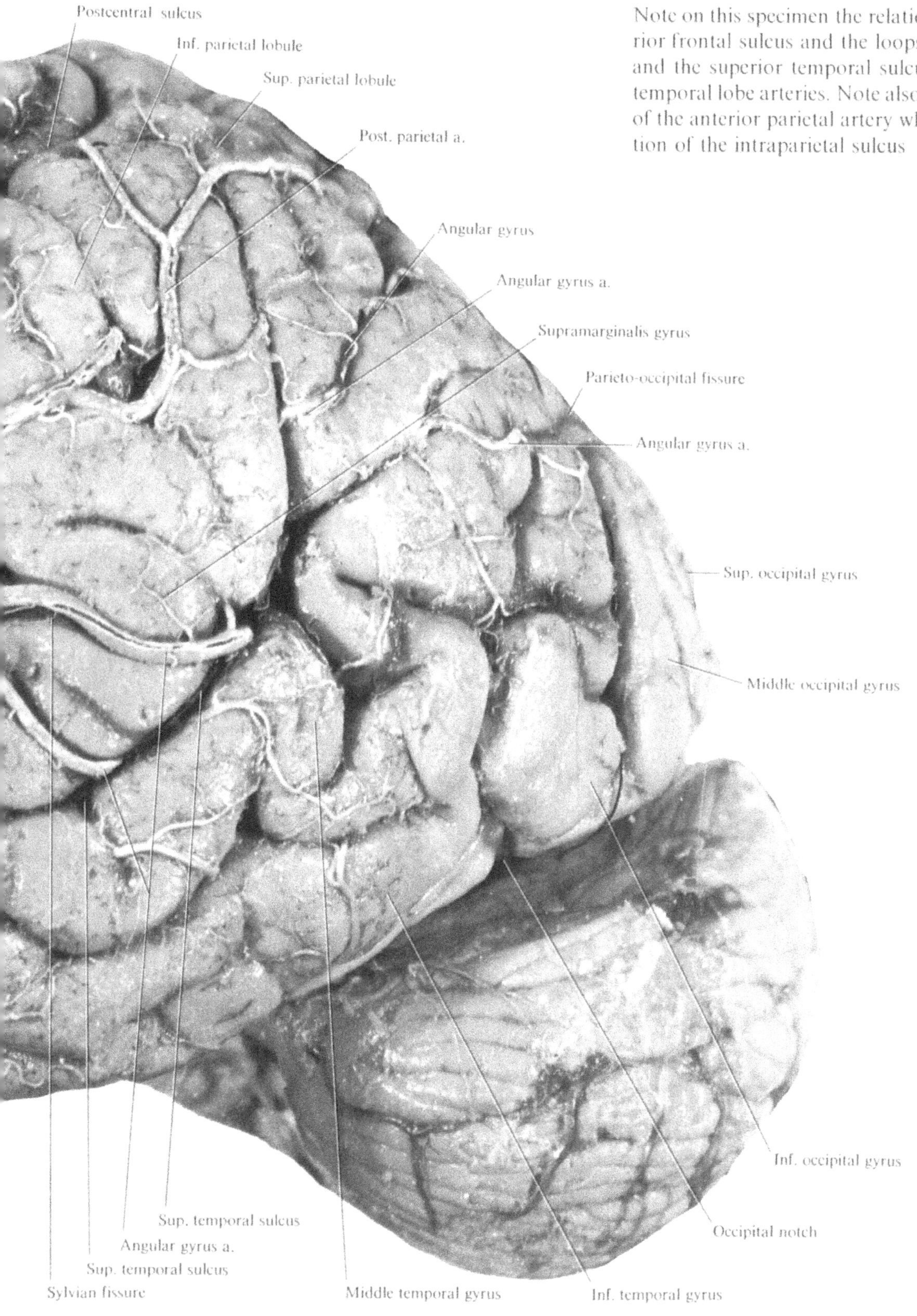

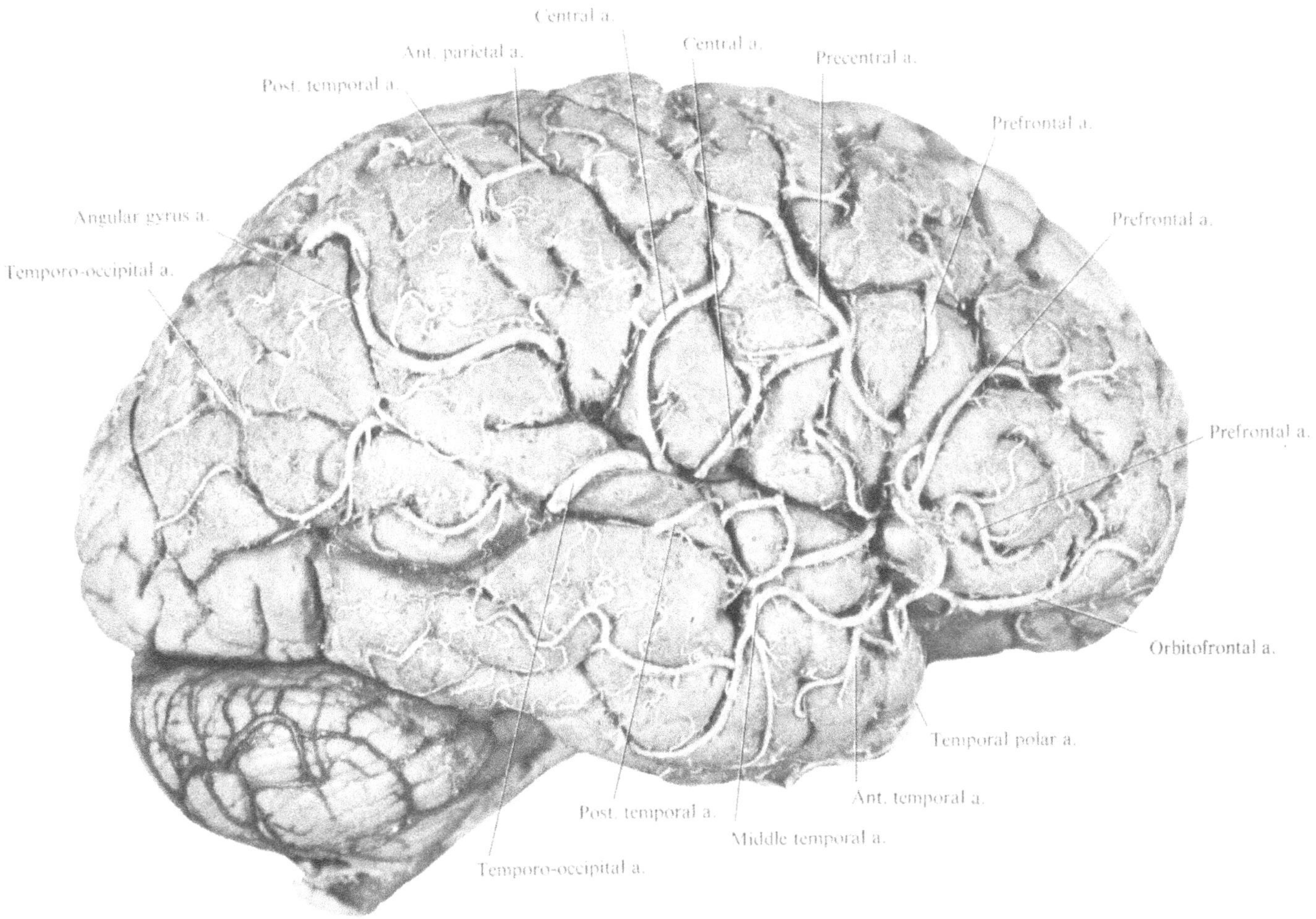

Fig. 63. Dissection of the right cerebral hemisphere after selective injection of the middle cerebral artery, lateral view

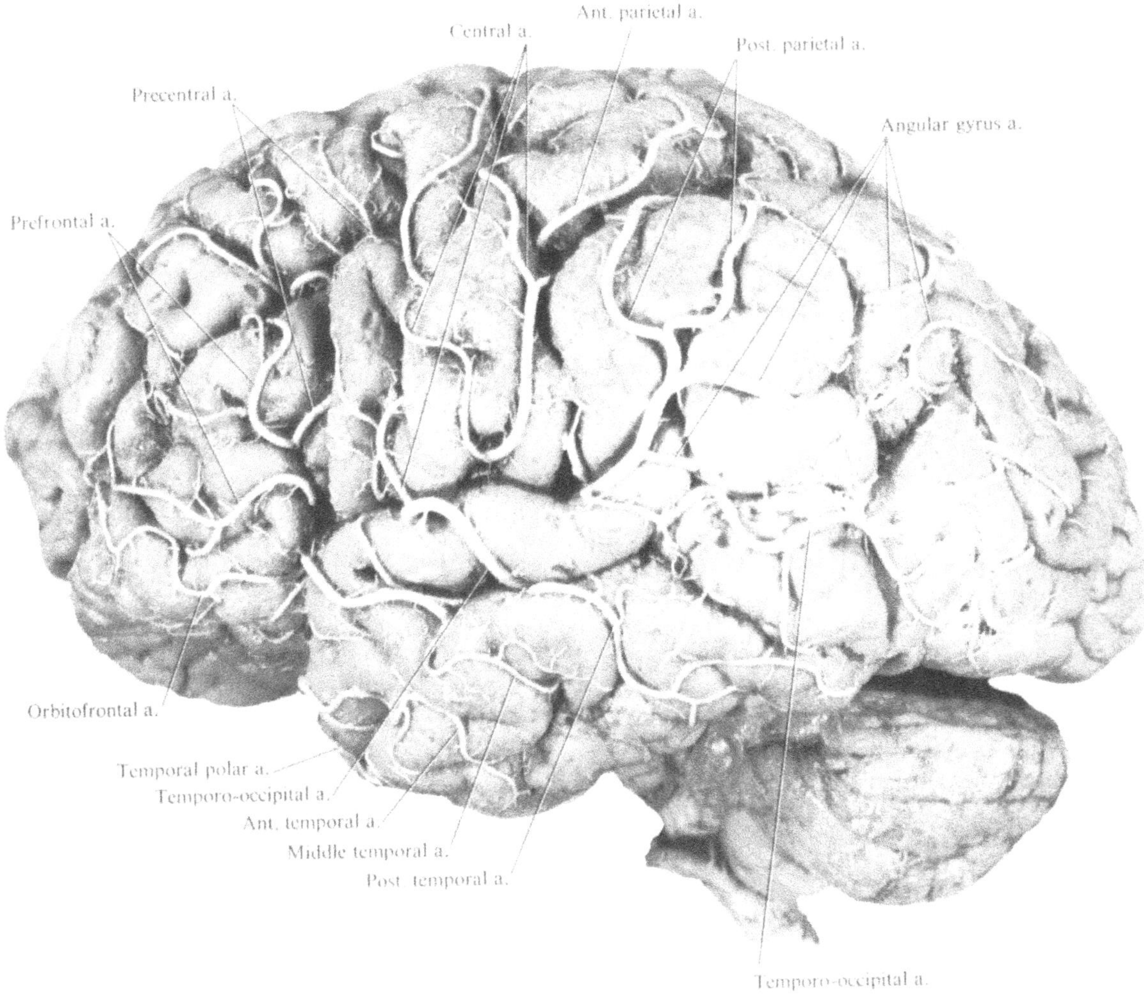

Fig. 64. Dissection of the left cerebral hemisphere after selective injection of the middle cerebral artery, lateral view

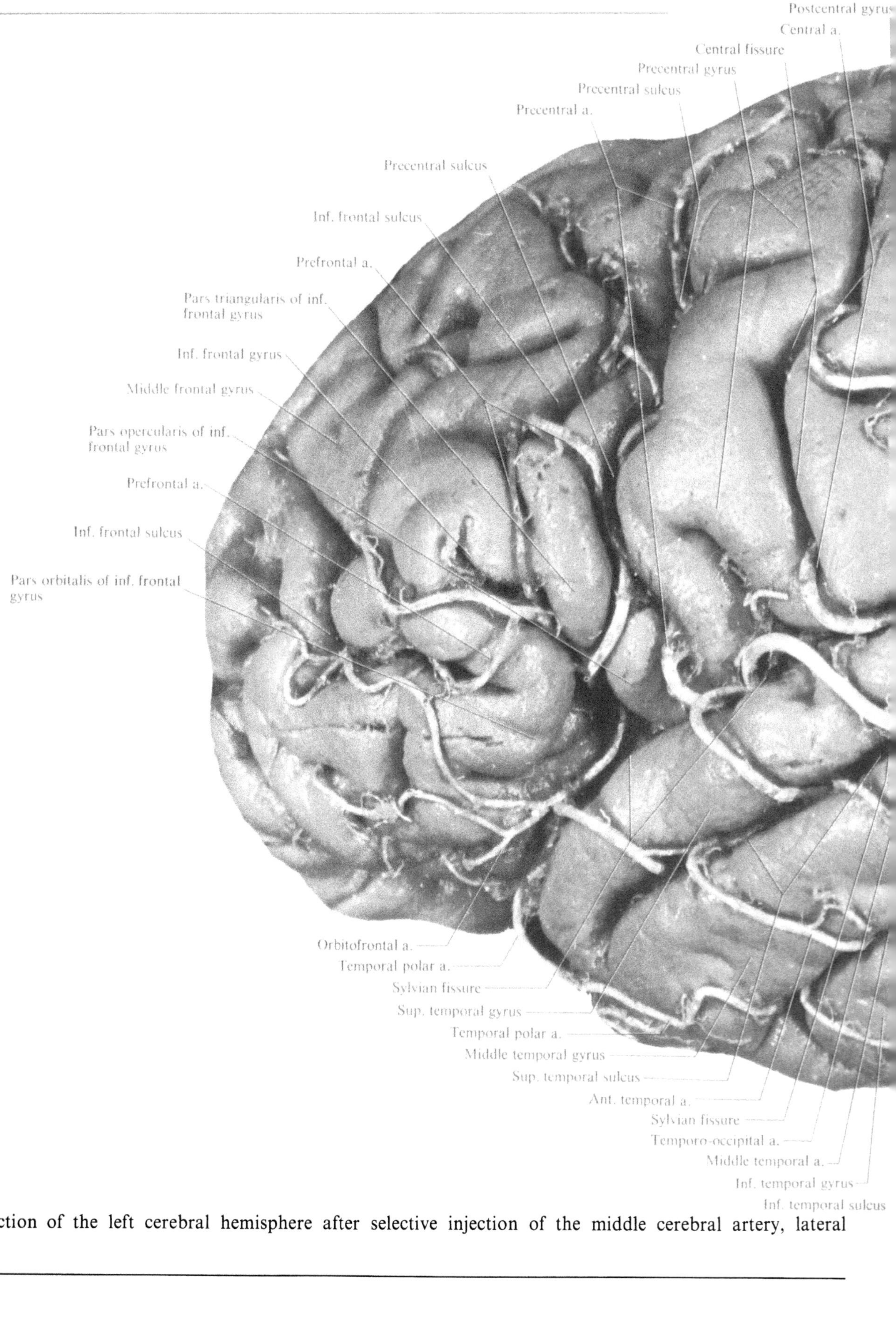

Fig. 65. Dissection of the left cerebral hemisphere after selective injection of the middle cerebral artery, lateral view

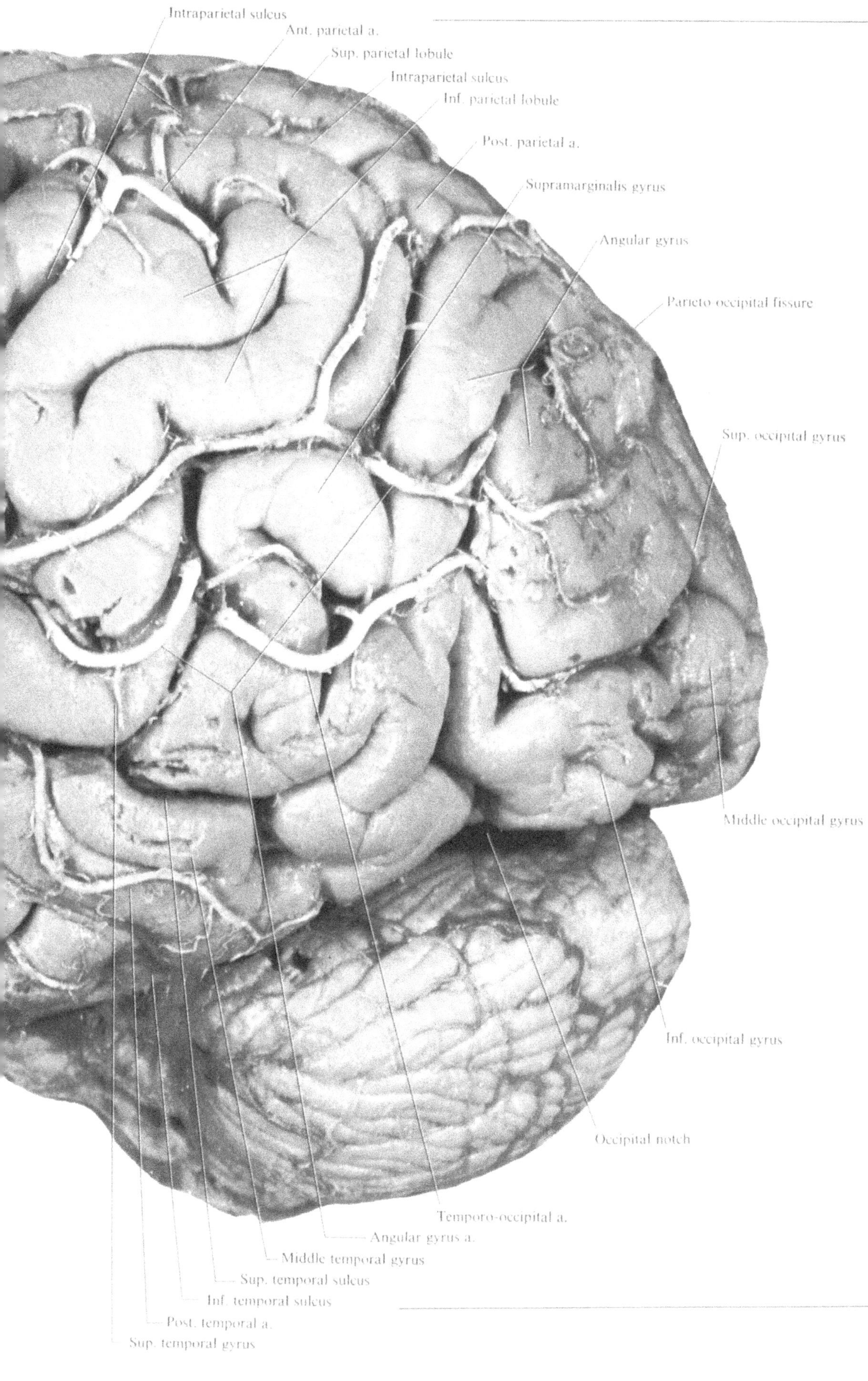

Intraparietal sulcus
Ant. parietal a.
Sup. parietal lobule
Intraparietal sulcus
Inf. parietal lobule
Post. parietal a.
Supramarginalis gyrus
Angular gyrus
Parieto occipital fissure
Sup. occipital gyrus
Middle occipital gyrus
Inf. occipital gyrus
Occipital notch
Temporo-occipital a.
Angular gyrus a.
Middle temporal gyrus
Sup. temporal sulcus
Inf. temporal sulcus
Post. temporal a.
Sup. temporal gyrus

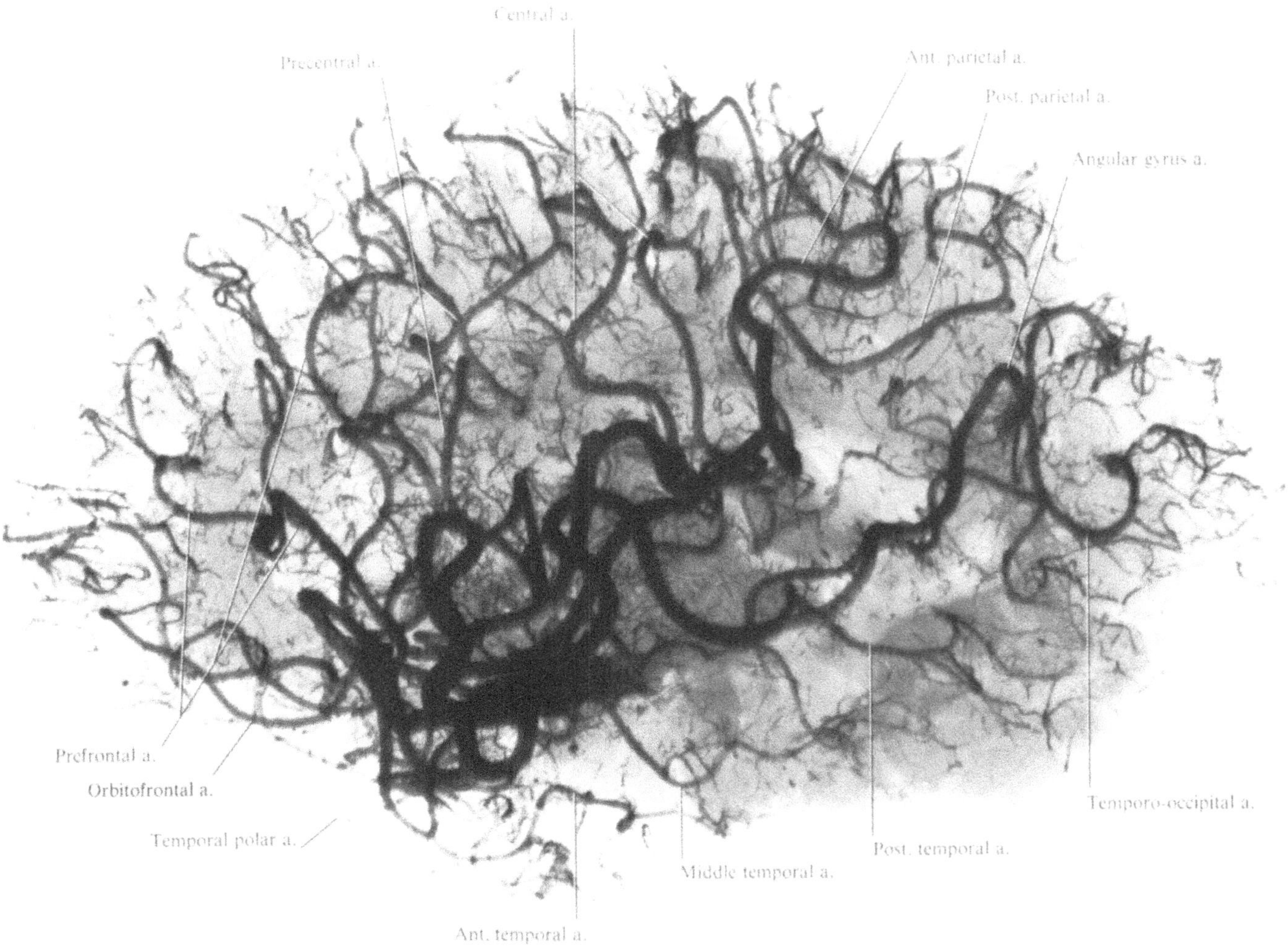

Fig. 66. Radiograph after selective injection of the left middle cerebral artery, lateral view

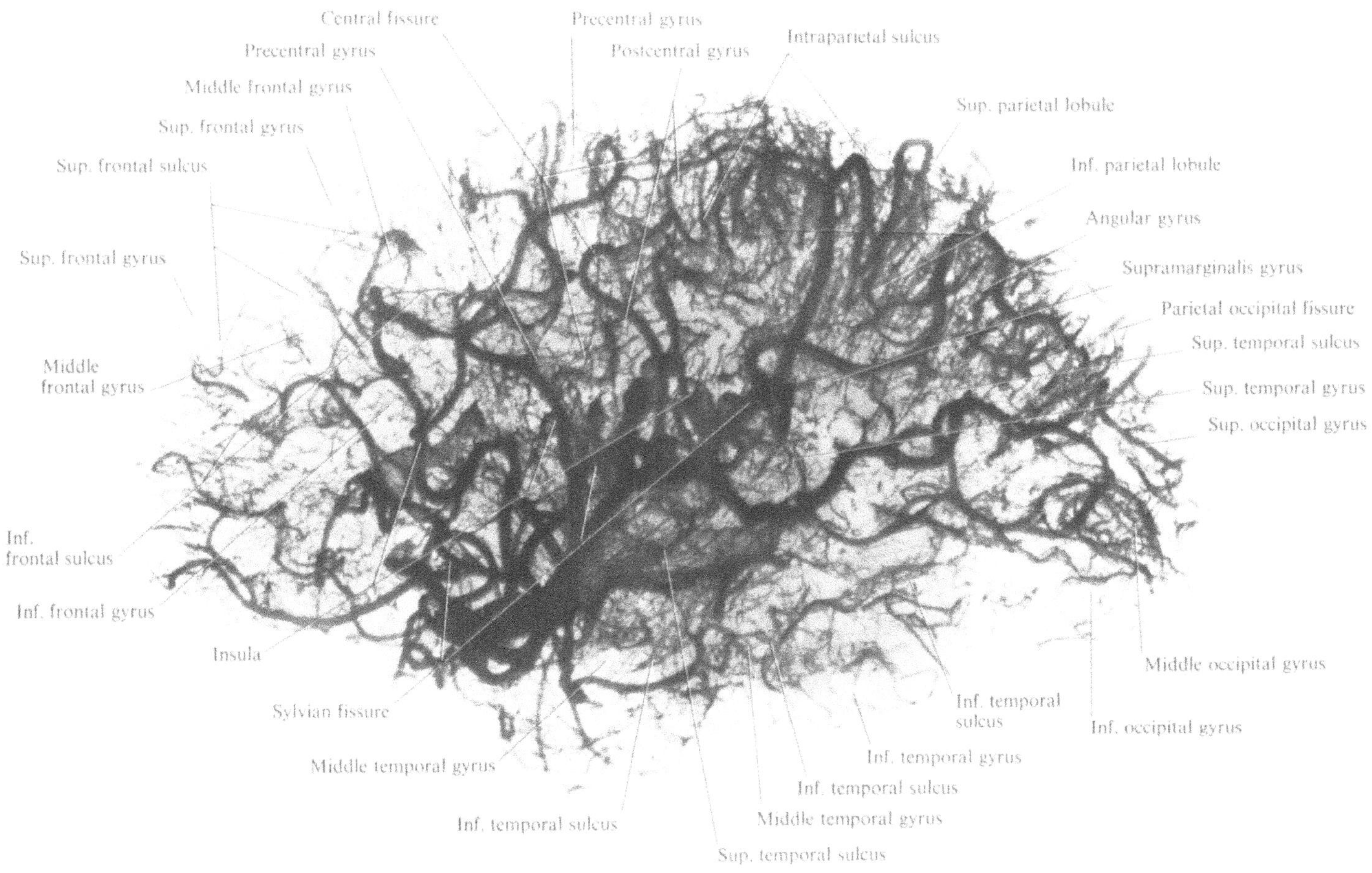

Fig. 67. Radiograph after selective injection of the left middle cerebral artery, lateral view
In this specimen, metallic wires have been placed in the major fissures and sulci of the convexity. The close relationships between the sulci and the loops of the cortical branches of the middle cerebral artery can be readily seen.
It is therefore possible to recognize the topography of the convolutions of the external surface of the cerebral hemisphere

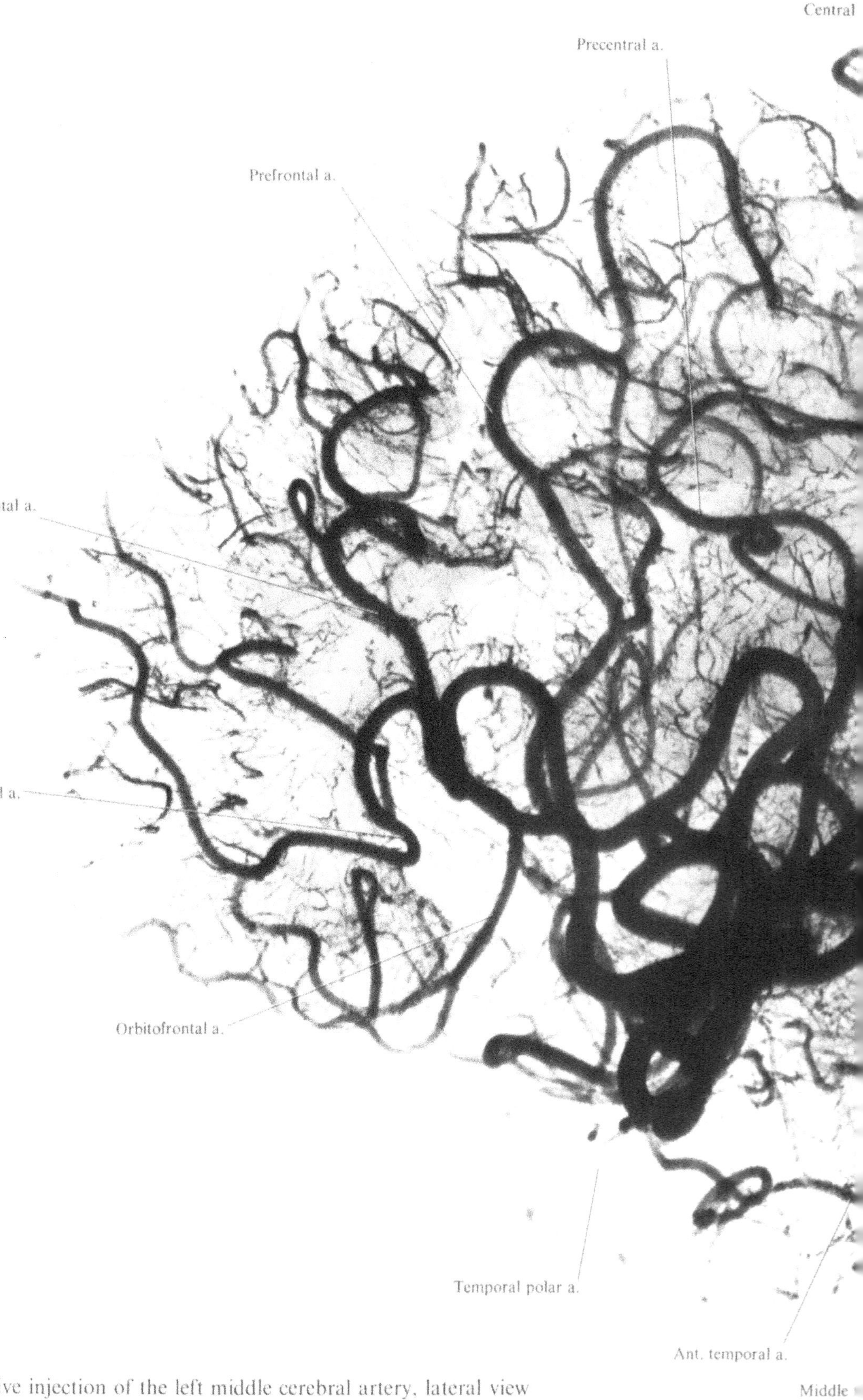

Fig. 68. Radiograph after selective injection of the left middle cerebral artery, lateral view

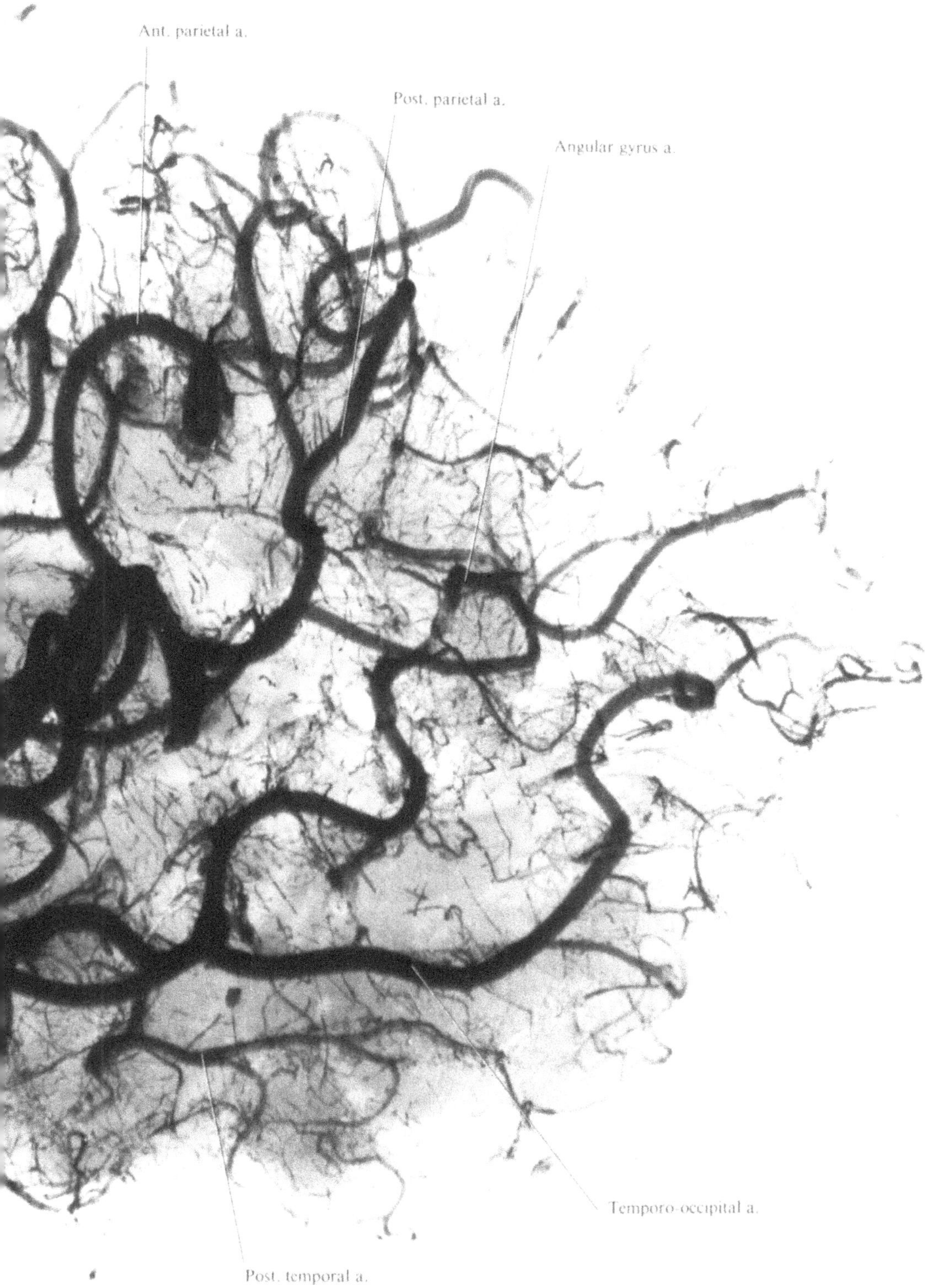
Ant. parietal a.
Post. parietal a.
Angular gyrus a.
Temporo-occipital a.
Post. temporal a.

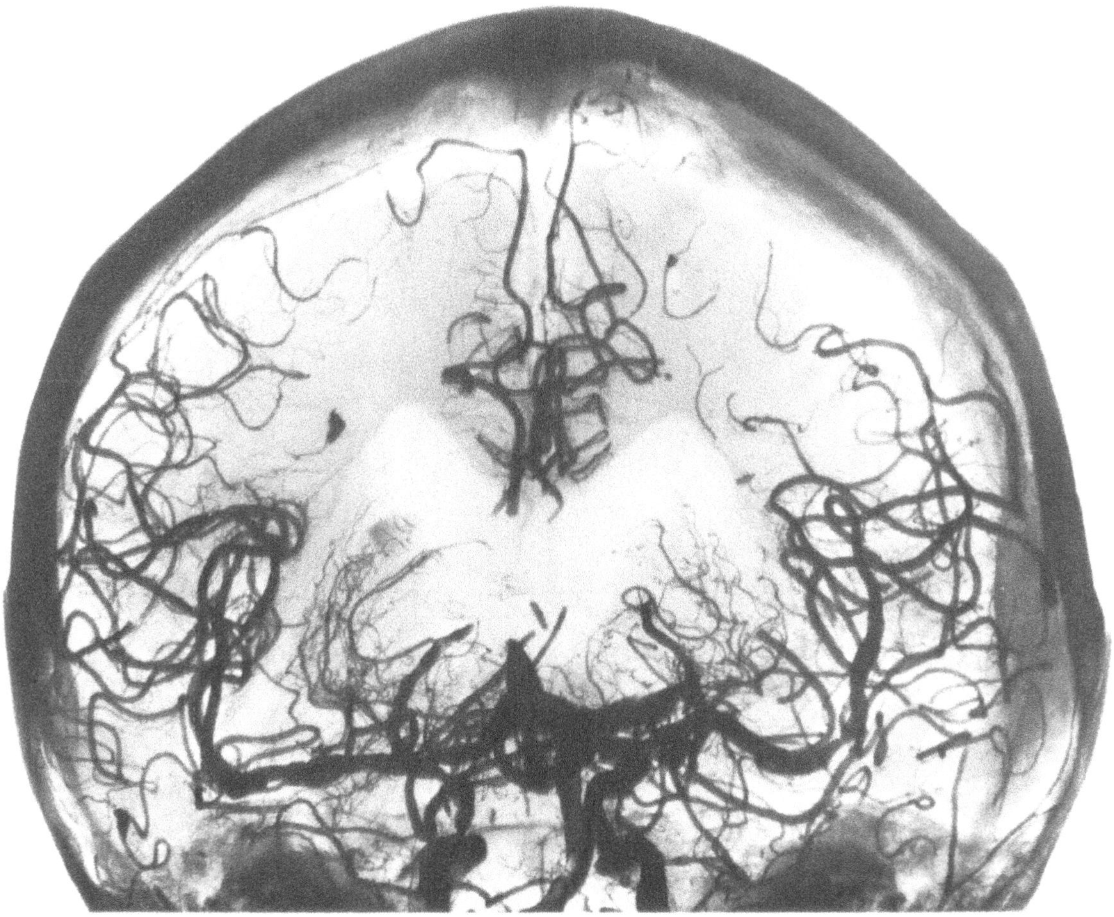

Fig. 69. Frontal section of the head after selective injection of the carotid artery, showing the territory of the middle cerebral artery

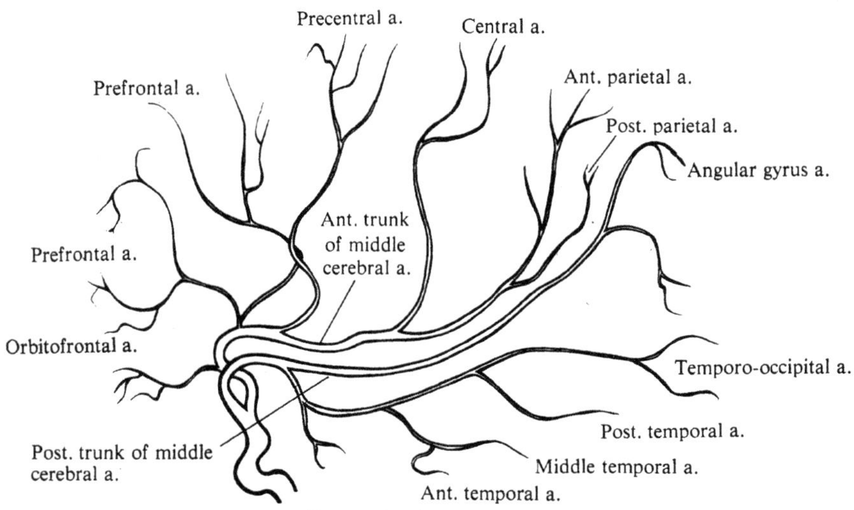

Fig. 70 A. Bifurcation pattern of division

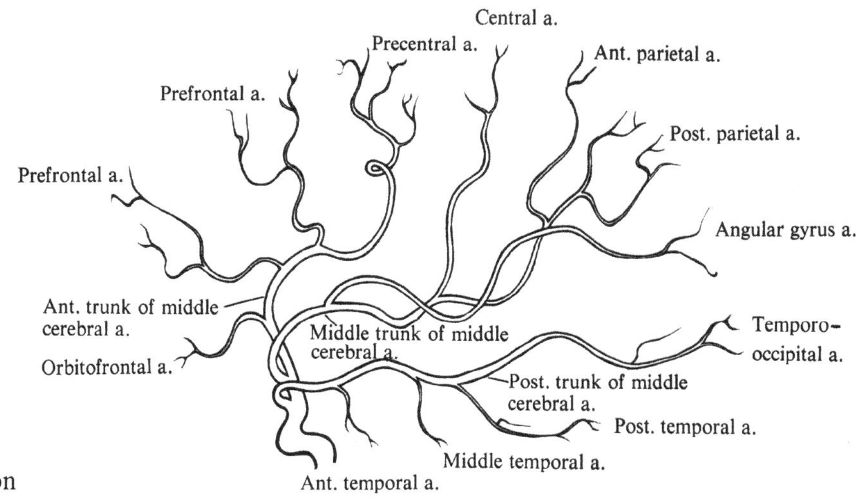

Fig. 70B. Trifurcation pattern of division

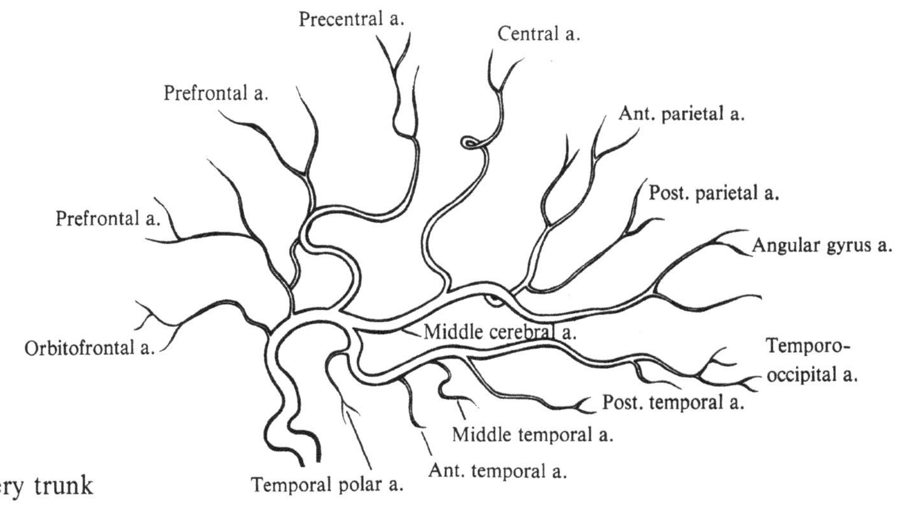

Fig. 70C. Single middle cerebral artery trunk

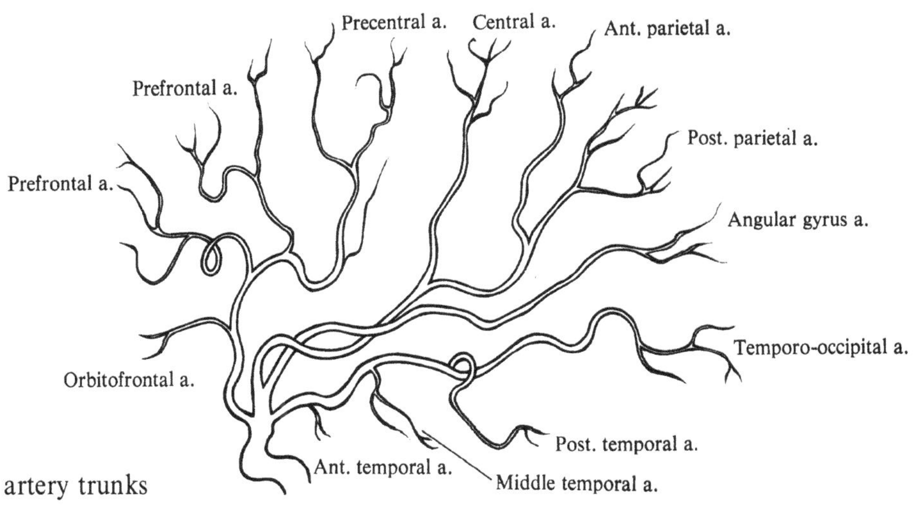

Fig. 70D. Multiple middle cerebral artery trunks

Fig. 70A–D. Division patterns of the middle cerebral artery

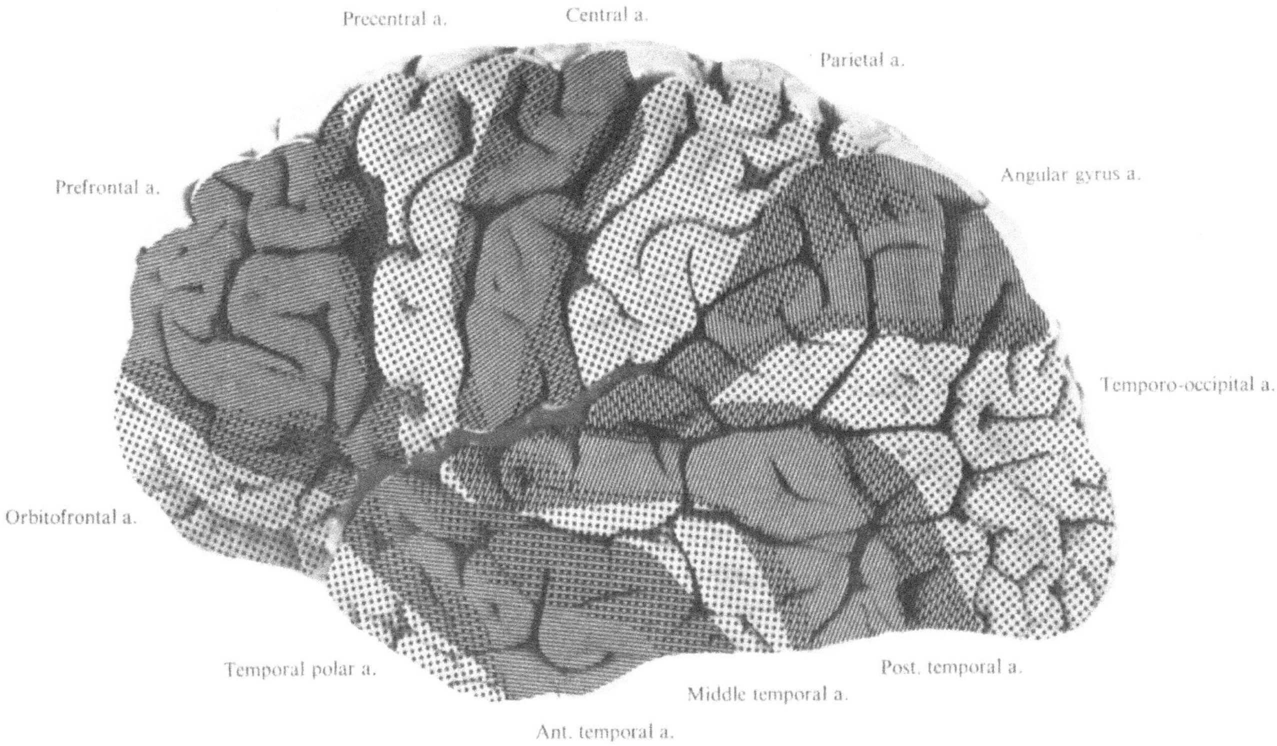

Fig. 71. Schematic representation of the territories of the middle cerebral artery on the external surface of the cerebral hemisphere

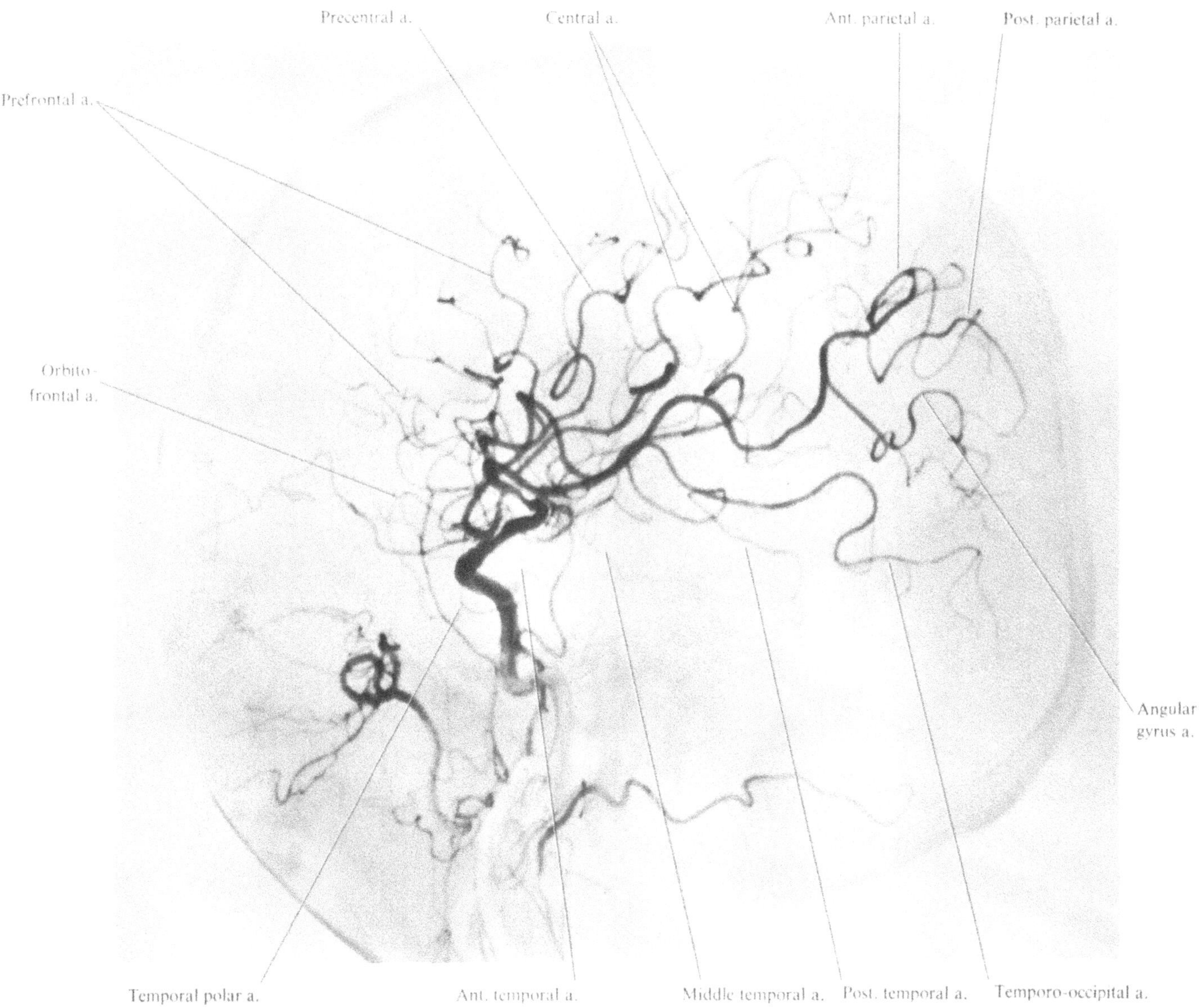

Fig. 72. Carotid angiogram, lateral projection. Only the middle cerebral artery has been filled

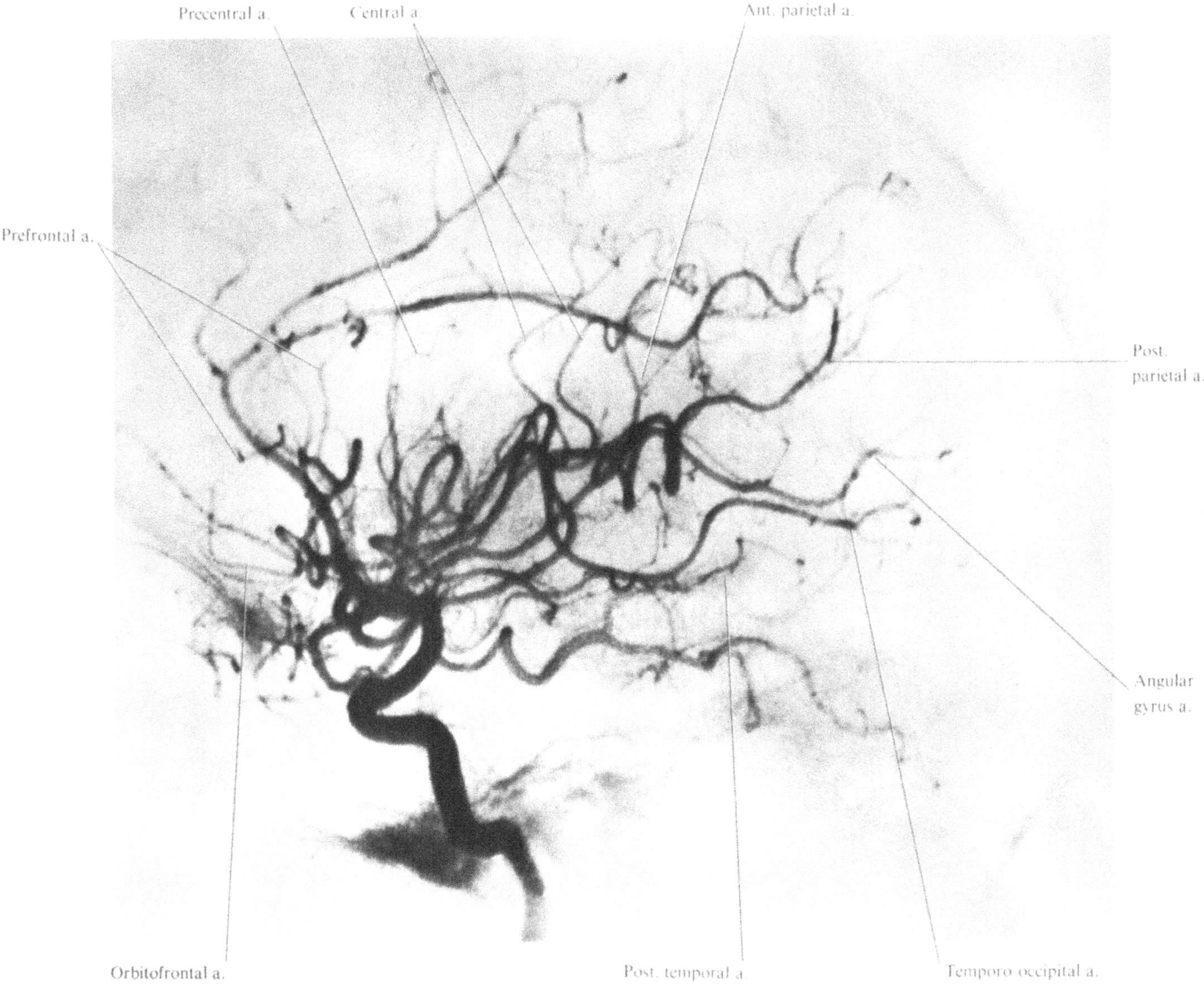

Fig. 73. Carotid angiogram, lateral projection. Due to filling of the posterior cerebral artery, it is difficult to identify the branches to the anterior temporal lobe

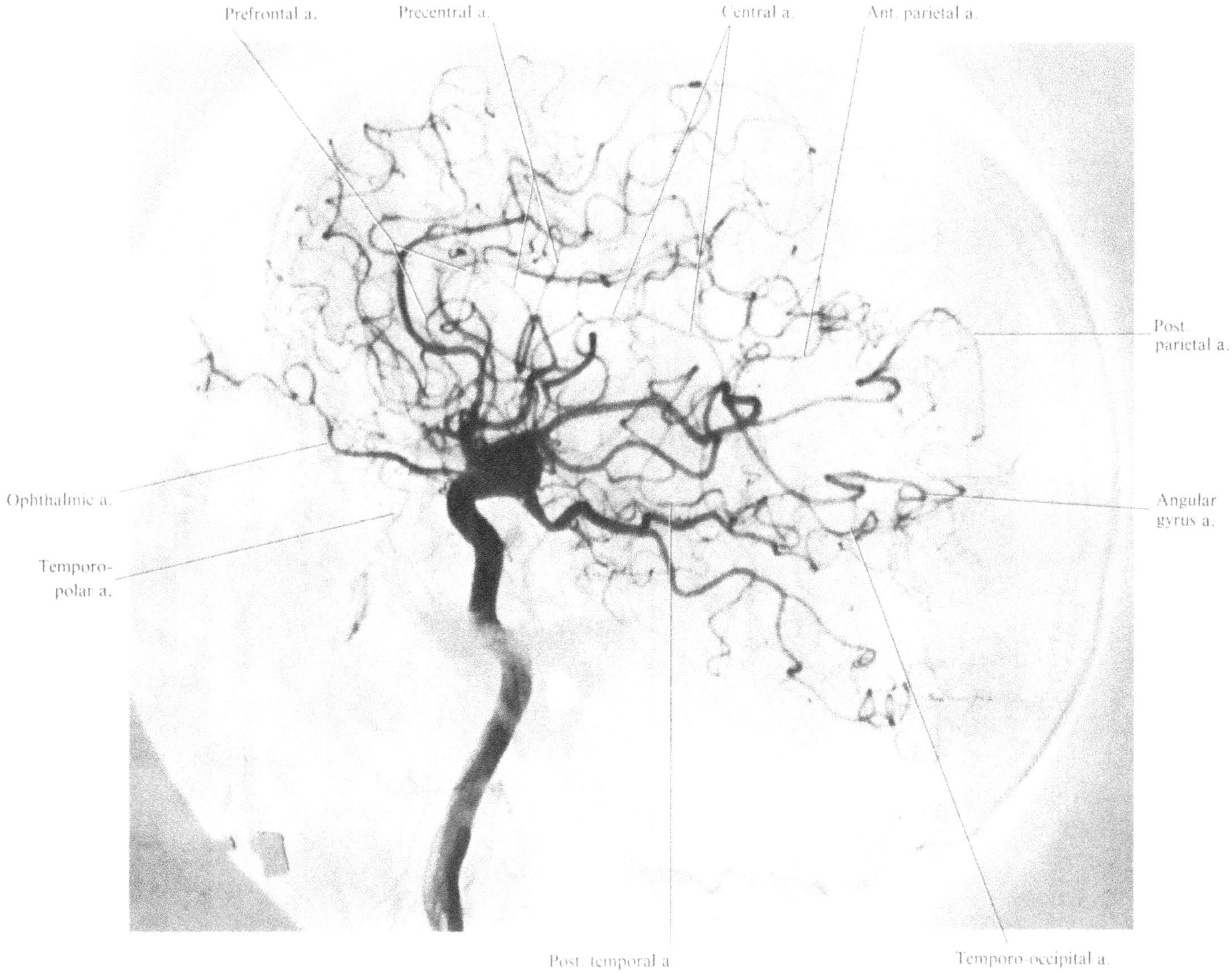

Fig. 74. Carotid angiogram, lateral projection. The orbitofrontal branch of the middle cerebral artery cannot be identified because the ophthalmic artery is so large

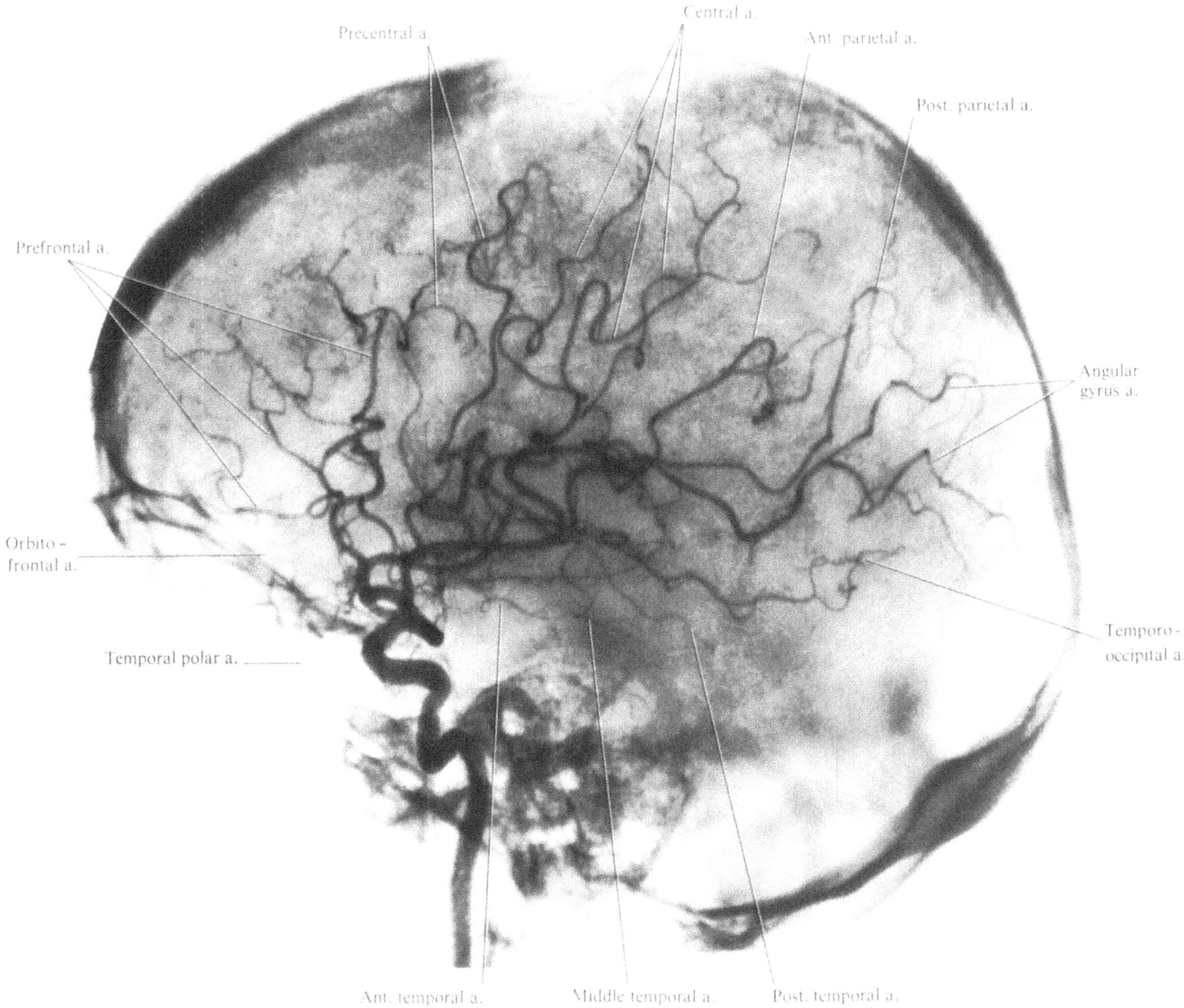

Fig. 75. Carotid angiogram, lateral view

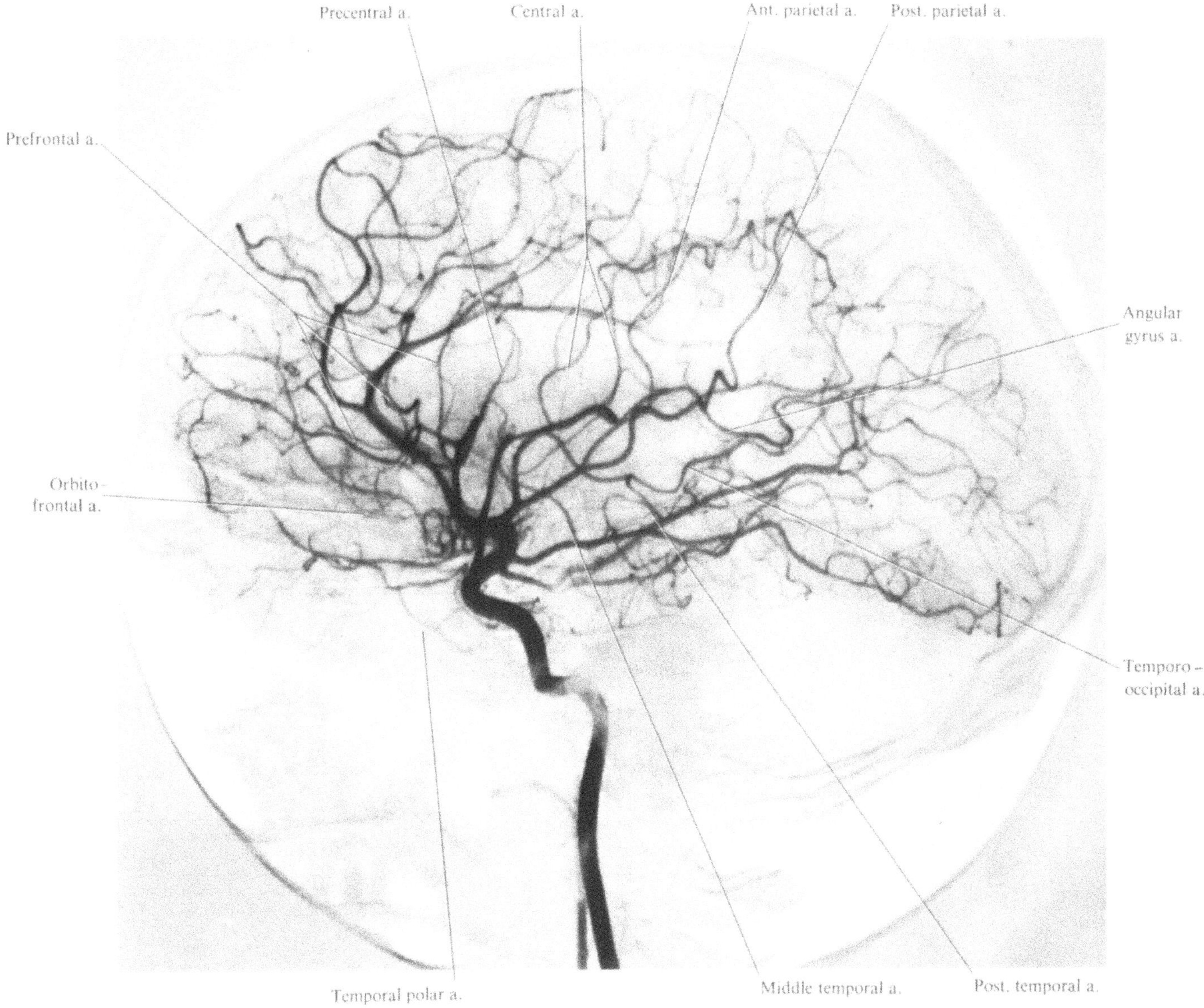

Fig. 76. Carotid angiogram, lateral view

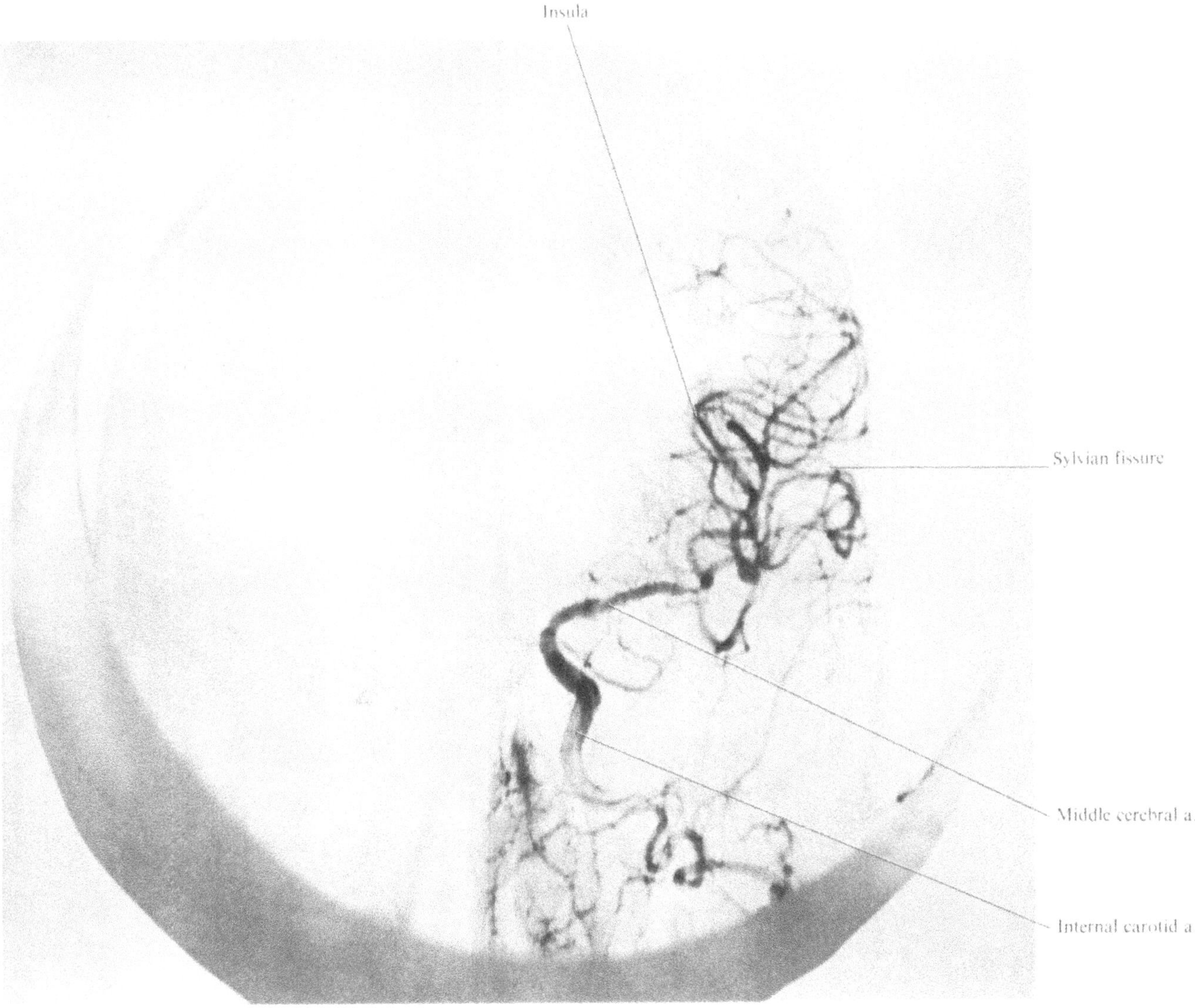

Fig. 77. Left carotid angiogram, frontal projection. Only the middle cerebral artery has been filled

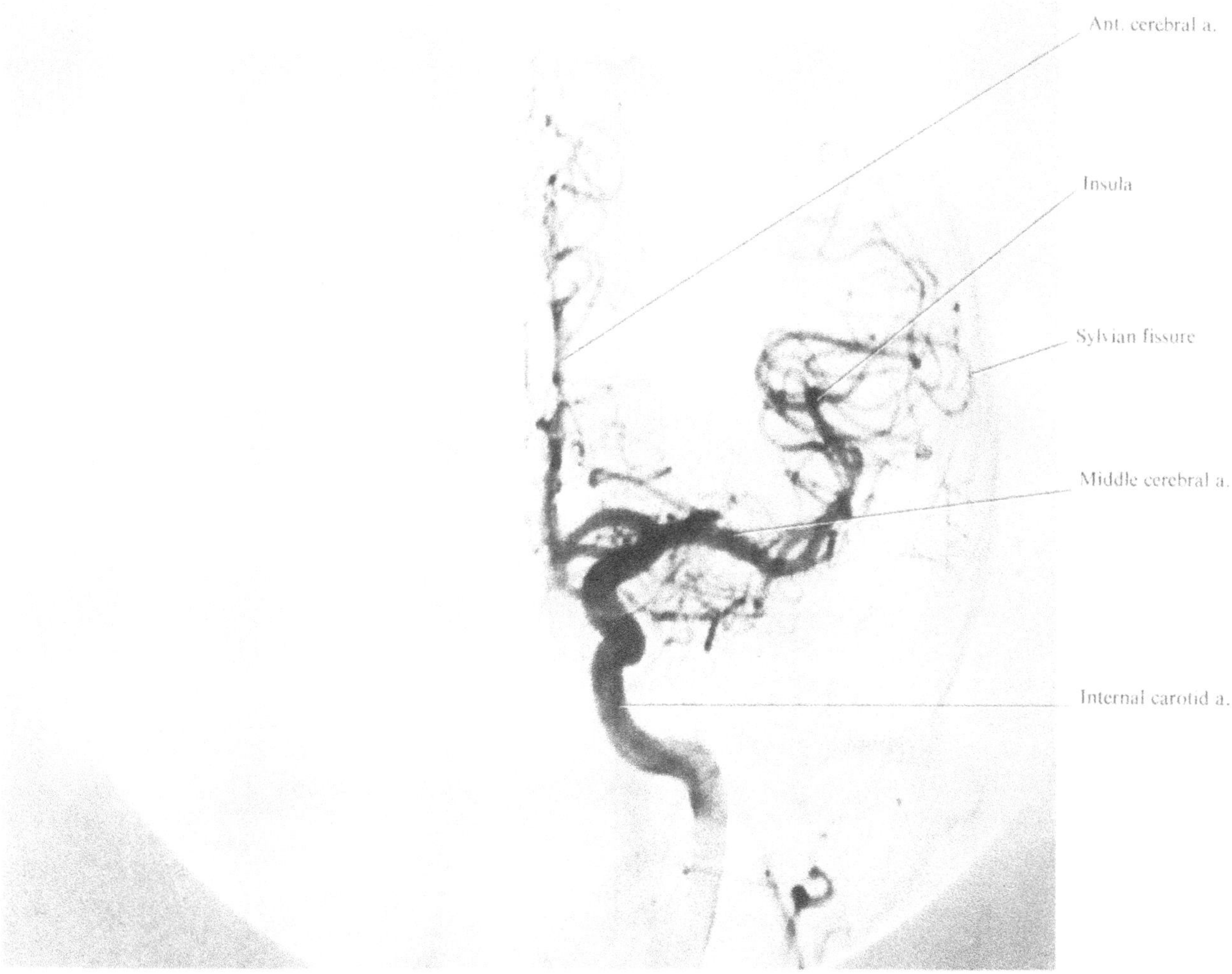

Fig. 78. Left carotid angiogram, frontal projection

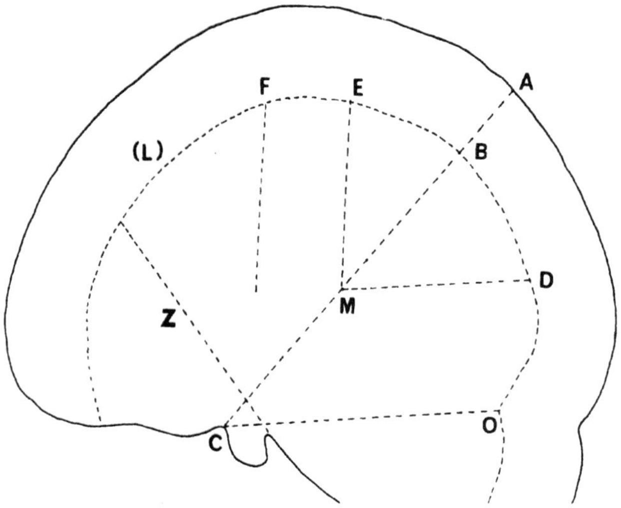

Fig. 79. Schematic representation of the method of RING and WADDINGTON (1967) for determining the vascular territories of the branches of the middle cerebral artery.

(1) Construct a line (L), 2.5 cm within the inner table and parallel to it, to a point (O), anterior to the internal occipital protuberance.

(2) Construct the clinoparietal line (of TAVERAS and WOOD, 1964) from the anterior clinoid process (C), to a point (A), situated on the inner table 9 cm above the internal occipital protuberance. This line defines point (B) where it crosses line (L).

(3) From the midpoint (M) of line BC, construct a line parallel to line CO. This defines point (D) where the line crosses line (L).

(4) Construct a line parallel to the coronal suture and passing through point (M). This line crosses line (L) at point (E).

(5) Construct another vertical line (F), 2.5 cm in front of and parallel to line ME.

(6) Construct a line (Z), connecting the midpoint of the anterior arc of line (L), i.e. anterior to point (F), with the dorsum sellae.

The clinoparietal line CA represents the axis of the middle cerebral artery in adults.

Space OCMD corresponds to the vascular territory of the posterior temporal artery, DMB to that of the angular gyrus artery, and BME to that of the posterior parietal artery.

The open-ended quadrilateral EMF corresponds to the vascular territory of the central artery (or arteries) and permits the identification of the motor area anteriorly and the sensory area posteriorly.

In front of and beneath the anterior line (Z) is the vascular territory of the orbitofrontal artery; above and behind is that of the prefrontal or candelabra artery.

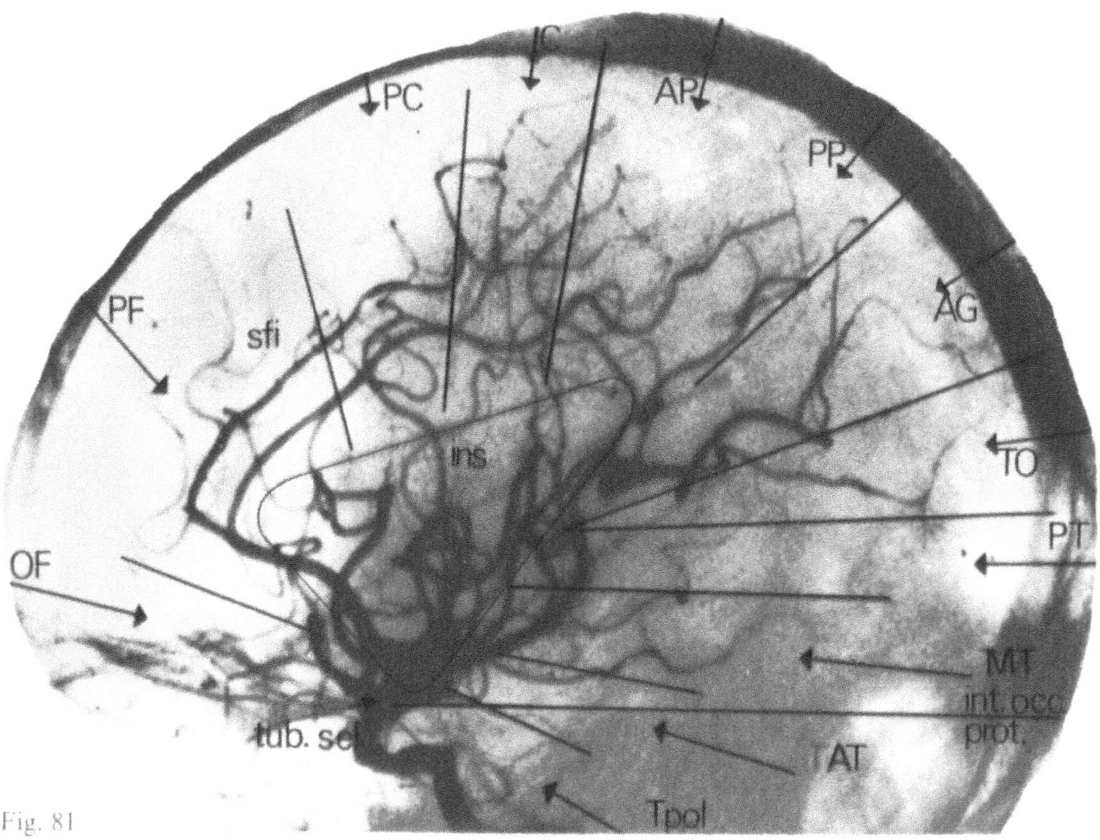

Fig. 81

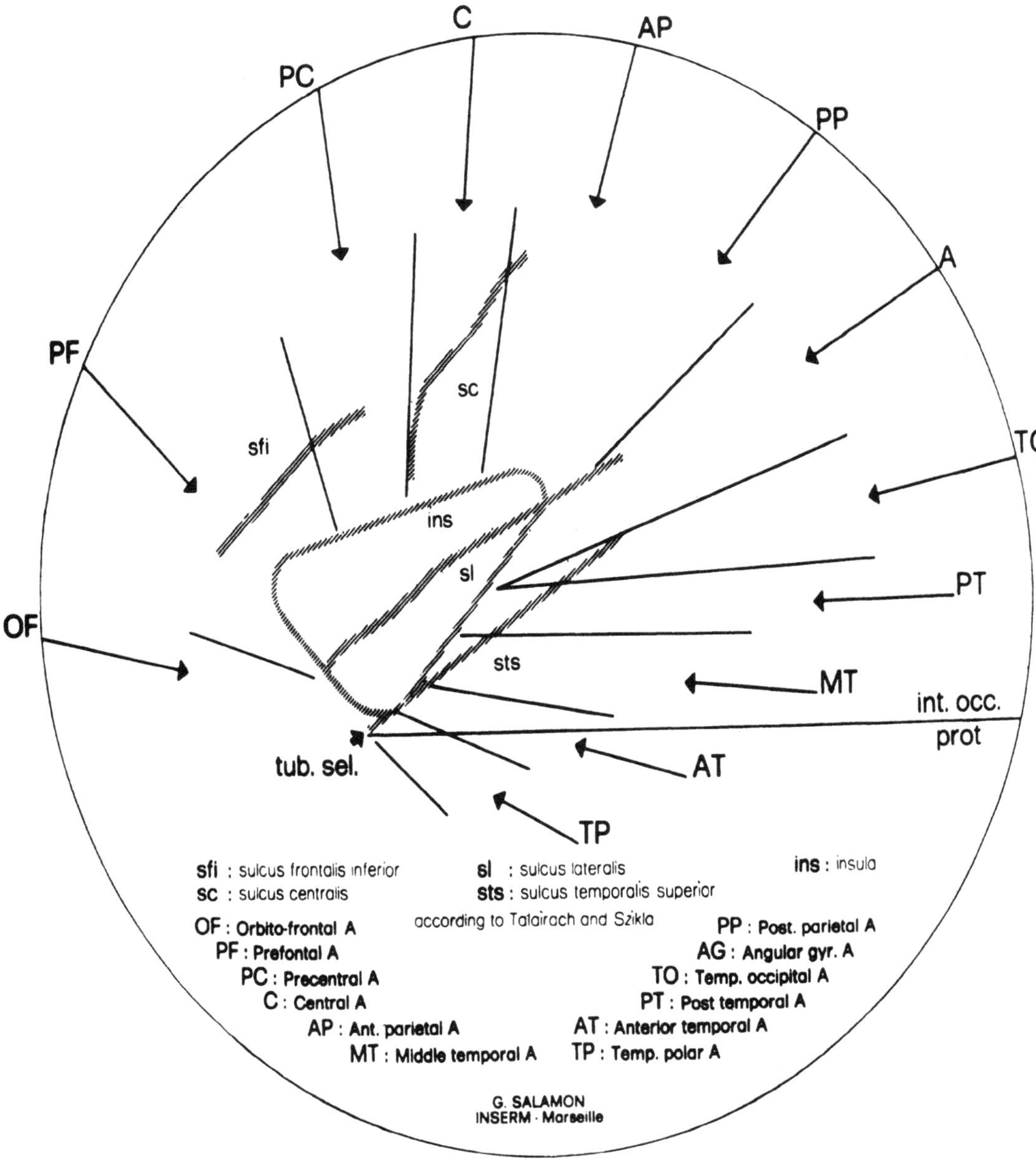

Fig. 80. Photograph of the transparent plastic template, used by the author to localize the cortical branches of the middle cerebral artery. This disc is used by superimpose upon any lateral carotid angiogram

◁

Fig. 81. Identification of the cortical branches of the middle cerebral artery using the disc illustrated in Fig. 80

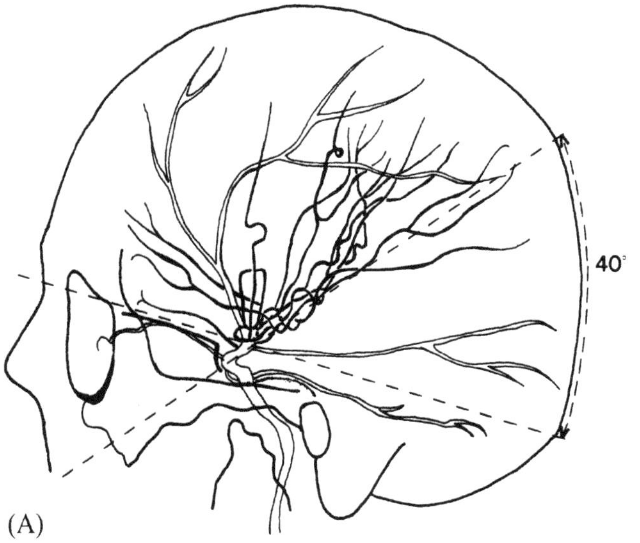

(A)

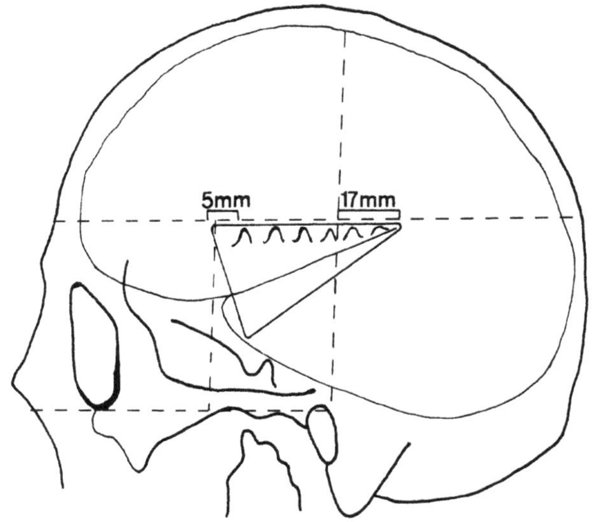

Fig. 83. Representation of the method of VLAHOVITCH *et al.* (1964, 1968, 1970, 1973) for localizing the insula. The superior insular line is parallel to the orbitomeatal line and it bisects a perpendicular to the latter line which extends from the external auditory canal to the inner table. The numbers on the figure indicate the normal variation in the location of the anterior and posterior insular points

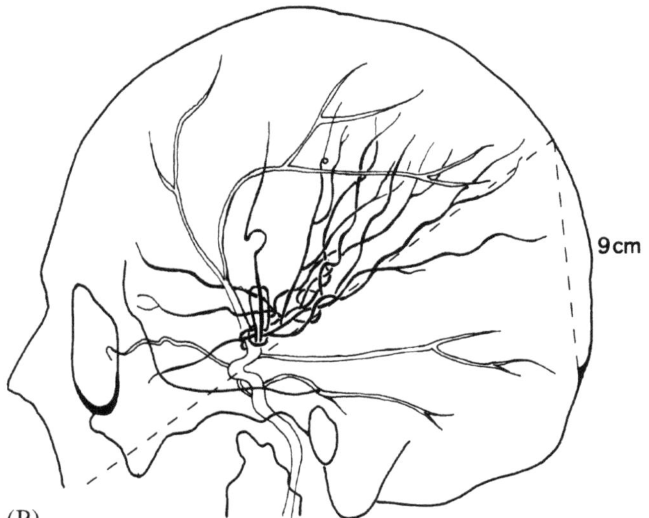

(B)

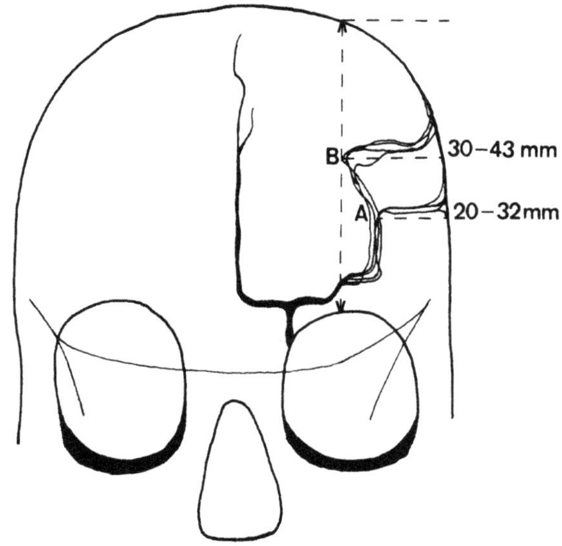

Fig. 84. Schematic representation of the superficial and deep Sylvian points of TAVERAS and WOOD (1964) as seen in the frontal projection

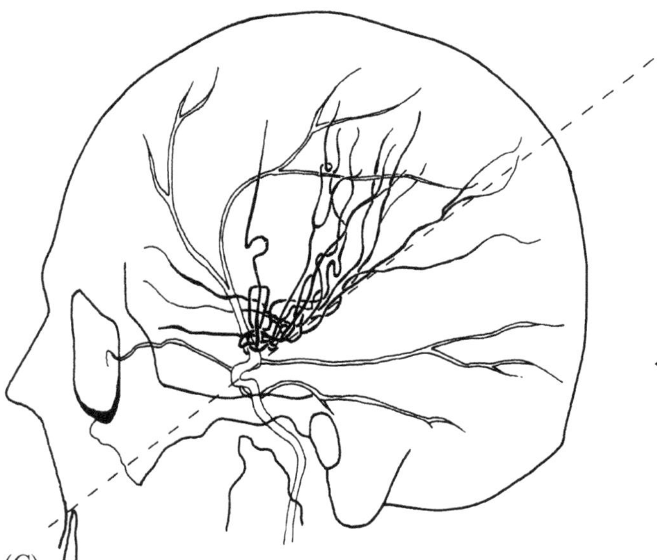

(C)

◁ Fig. 82A–C. Methods of localization of the axis of the Sylvian triangle
A. Method of WORINGER and GERNEZ (1948)
B. Method of TAVERAS and WOOD (1964): the clinoparietal line
C. Method of KRAYENBUHL and YASARGIL (1968): the incisive-siphon line

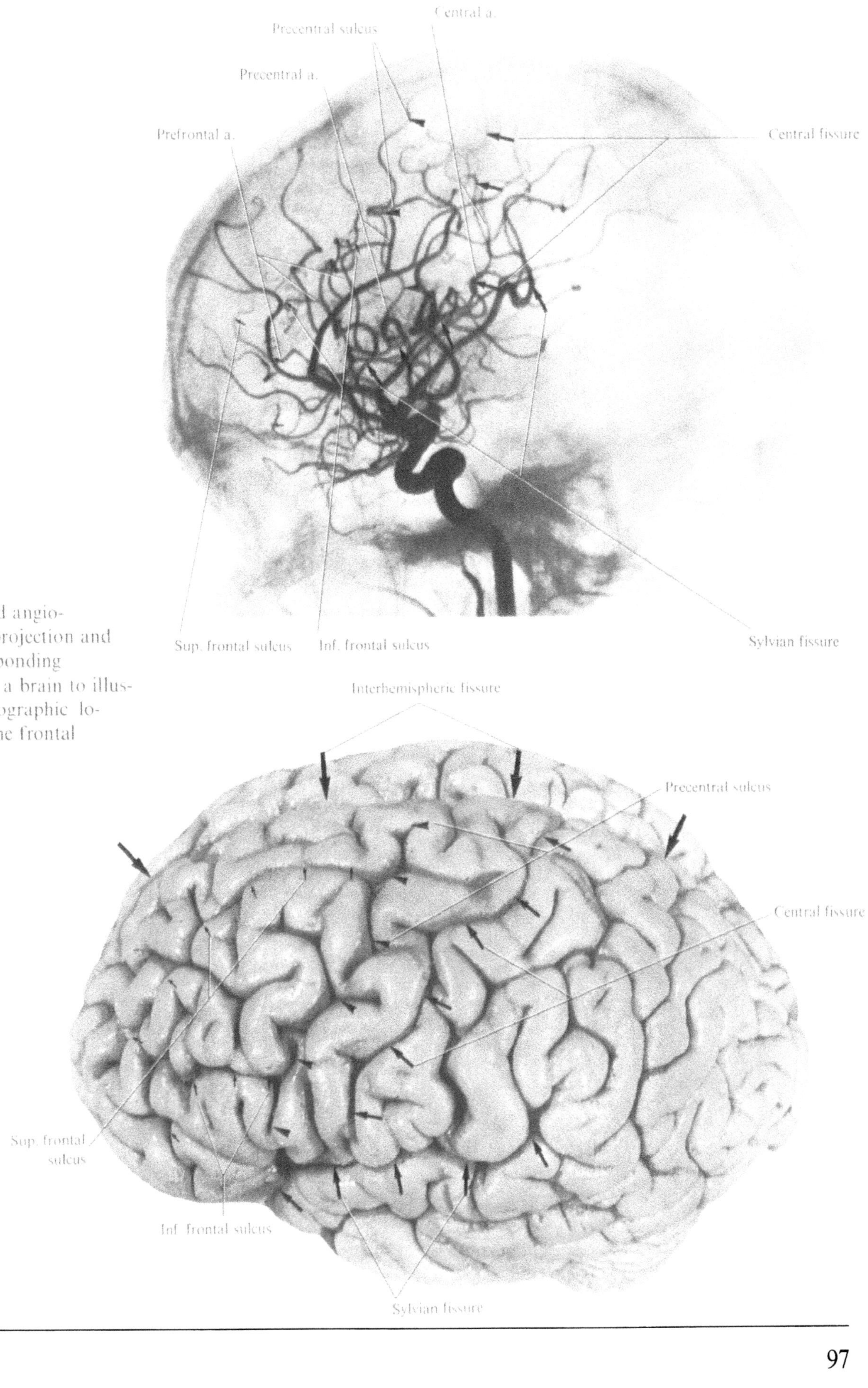

Fig. 85
Upper: Carotid angiogram, lateral projection and *Lower:* corresponding lateral view of a brain to illustrate the angiographic localization of the frontal sulci

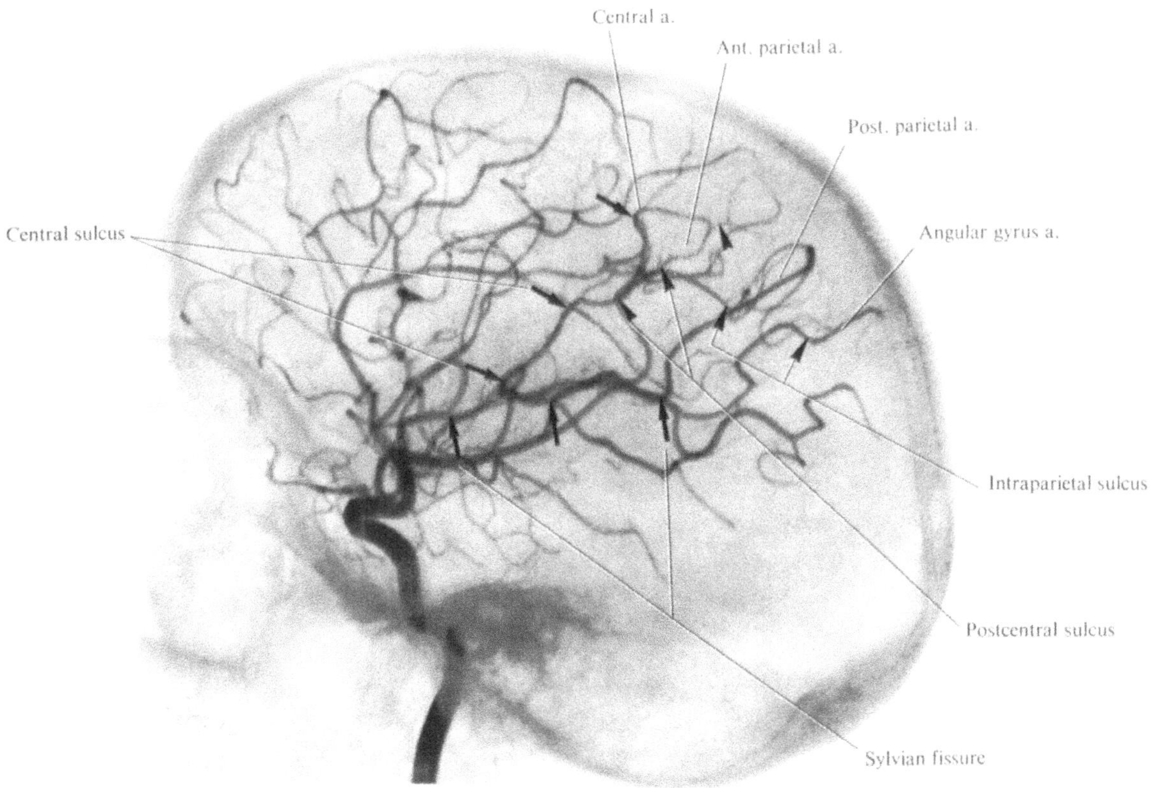

Fig. 86 A. Carotid angiogram, lateral projection and

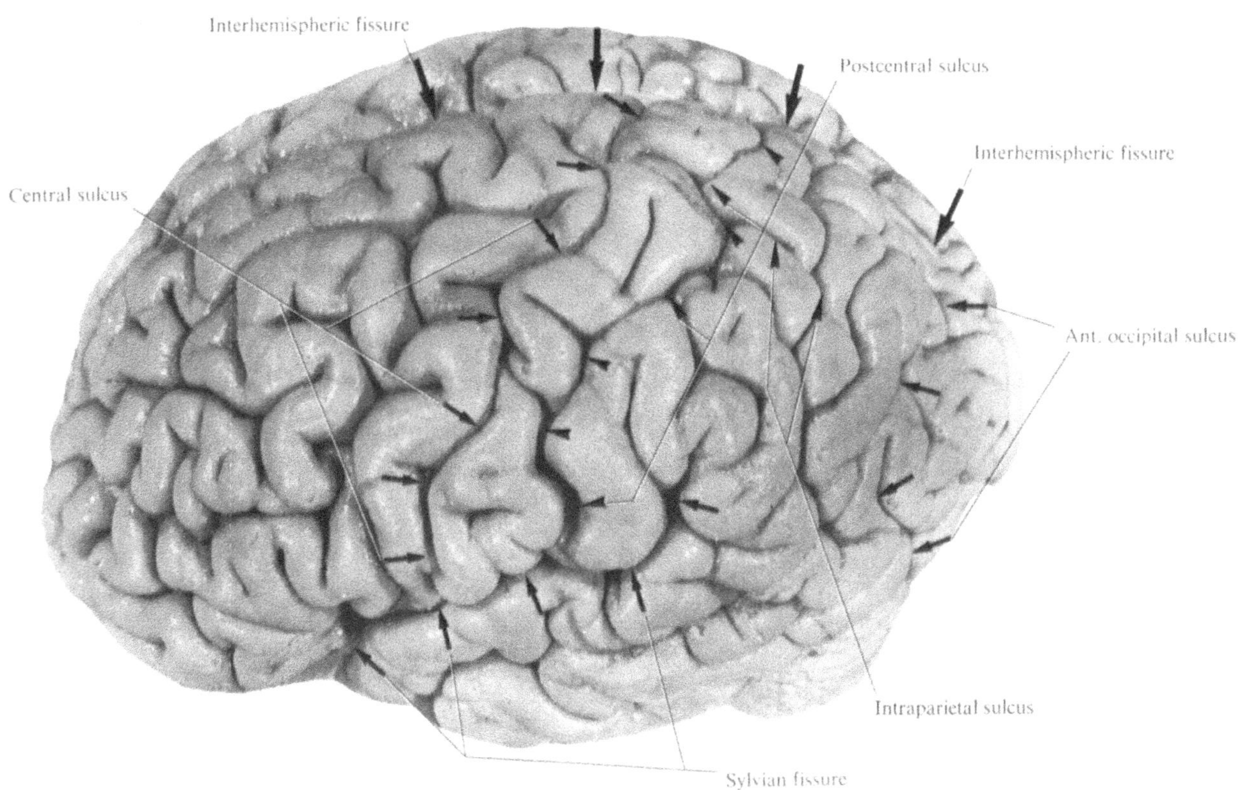

Fig. 86 B. corresponding lateral view of a brain to illustrate the angiographic localization of the parietal sulci

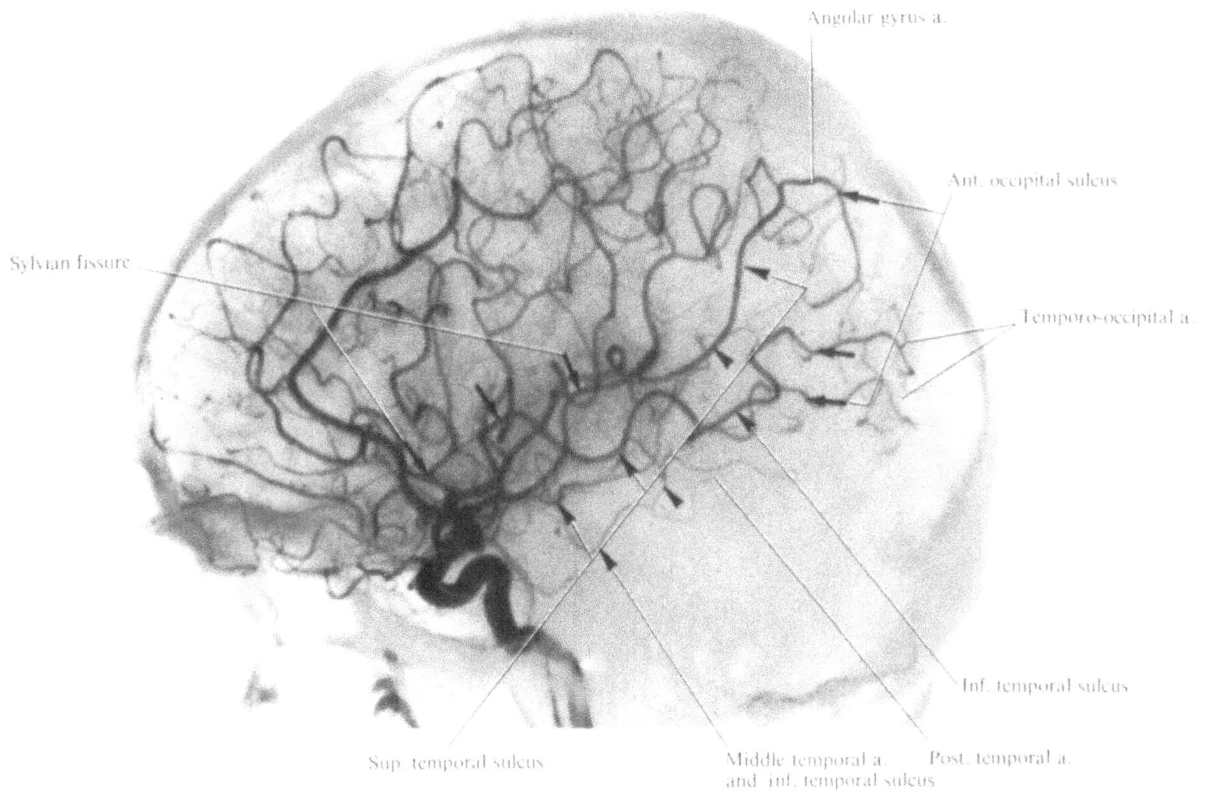

Fig. 87 A. Carotid angiogram, lateral projection and

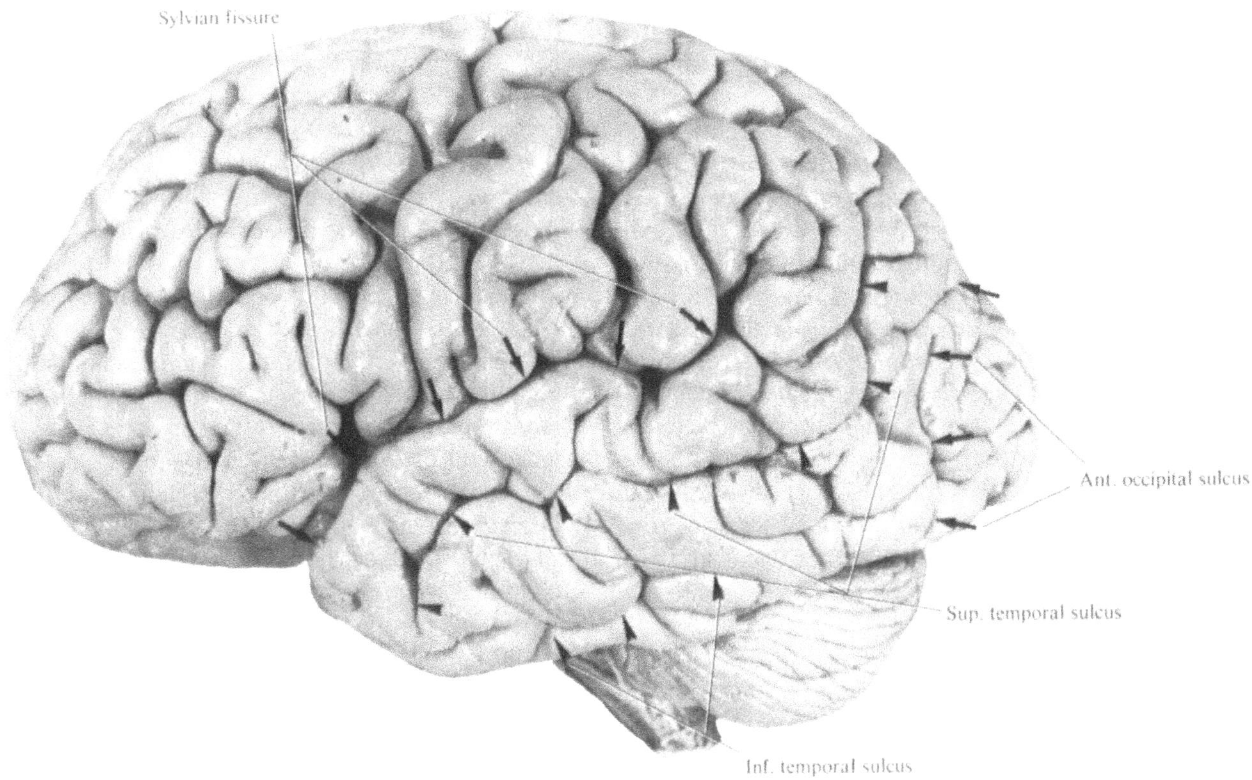

Fig. 87B. corresponding lateral view of a brain illustrate the angiographic localization of the temporal sulci

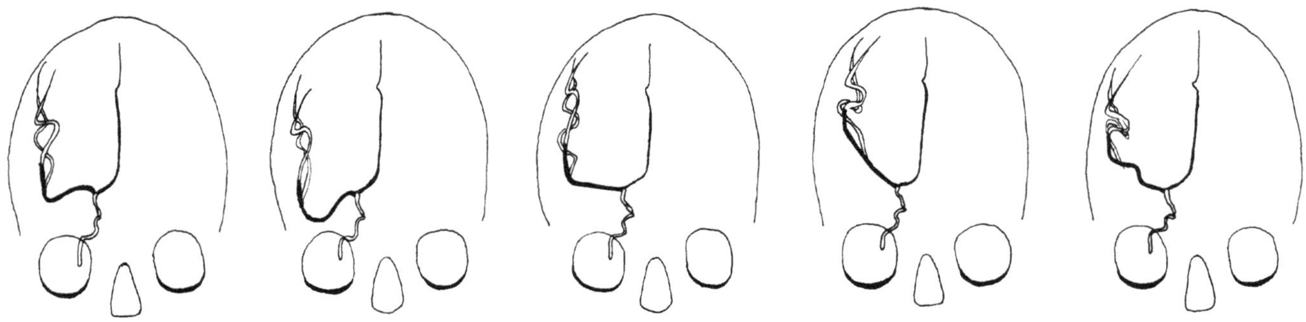

Fig. 88. Schematic representation, in frontal projection, of the normal variations in the horizontal segment of the middle cerebral artery (after KRAYENBUHL and YASARGIL, 1968)

C. Anterior Choroidal Artery

I. Anatomic Study of the Anterior Choroidal Artery

Previously studied by DURET (1874), HEUBNER (1872), FOIX and NICOLESCO (1925), ABBIE (1933), BEEVOR (1907, 1909), ALEXANDER (1942) and KOLISKO (1891), the anterior choroidal artery has stimulated recent investigation because of the surgical interest attached to its ligation in the treatment of Parkinson's disease (COOPER, 1954) and the radiologic interest resulting from its angiographic study. These recent works are those of CARPENTER, NOBACK and MOSS (1954), MOUNIER, BOUCHET and COSTAZ (1955), OTOMO (1965), SJOGREN (1956), THERON (1976).

The anterior choroidal artery arises from the posterolateral aspect of the internal carotid artery after it leaves the cavernous sinus. Classically its origin is found approximately 2 mm proximal to the origin of the anterior cerebral artery. This occurred in 76% of the cases studied by CARPENTER *et al.* (1954). In 11.7% of their cases it arose from the middle cerebral artery, in 6.7% it arose from the posterior communicating artery, and in 3.3% its origin was at the point of bifurcation into anterior and middle cerebral arteries.

The posterior communicating artery, which is larger, always arises from the posteromedial aspect of the internal carotid artery, usually 2 to 3 mm proximal to the anterior choroidal artery.

The average diameter of the anterior choroidal artery, at its origin, is about 0.5 mm. Despite its small diameter, it is a long artery and may terminate near the foramen of Monro or in the choroid plexus of the frontal horn.

The anterior choroidal artery presents two different segments during its course. In its first segment it crosses the chiasmatic cistern in its lateral and posterior portion (Figs. 89, 90), and then it follows the optic tract running between the cerebral peduncle and the medial surface of the hippocampus. In this segment the artery has an oblique course directed laterally and superiorly (Figs. 89, 90). In its second segment, the anterior choroidal artery passes through the choroidal fissure to enter the temporal horn of the lateral ventricle. It then follows the choroid plexus of the temporal horn around the atrium and terminates near the foramen of Monro (Figs. 91, 92).

The collateral supply of the anterior choroidal artery was of particular interest to ABBIE (1933). His study demonstrated connections between this artery and the posterolateral choroidal artery in the region of the lateral geniculate body and within the choroid plexus of the lateral ventricle.

The importance of the regions supplied by the anterior choroidal artery is striking. It participates in the vascularization of the optic tracts and the external part of the lateral geniculate body. It supplies branches to Ammon's horn, the pyriform cortex, the uncus and the amygdaloid body. It contributes to the supply of the anterior third of the base of the cerebral peduncle, the substantia nigra and the red nucleus. Intracerebral branches go to the thalamus, the tail of the caudate nucleus, the retrolenticu-

lar portion of the internal capsule and the lateral portion of the anterior commissure. All these branches are in addition to its more obvious joint supply to the choroid plexus of the lateral ventricle, together with the postero-lateral choroidal artery.
The richness of this vast anastomotic network explains the rarity of the classical clinical picture of occlusion of the anterior choroidal artery: hemiplegia, hemianesthesia, and hemianopsia.

II. Radiologic Study of the Anterior Choroidal Artery

The angiographic anatomy of the anterior choroidal artery was initially described by SJOGREN (1956), more recently by THERON (1976). According to KRAYENBUHL and YASARGIL (1968), and DILENGE (1962), it is visible on 85% of all carotid angiograms.
In the lateral projection, the anterior choroidal artery appears to be the second branch of the internal carotid artery after the latter emerges from the cavernous sinus (Figs. 94, 95). Situated 2 to 3 mm above the posterior communicating artery, its first segment passes obliquely upwards and posteriorly, in the ambient cistern, with a slight curve concave superiorly. In this segment its path lies adjacent to the optic tracts.
In the frontal projection the origin of the anterior choroidal artery is masked by the internal carotid artery. It is first seen in this projection as it passes above the horizontal segment of the middle cerebral artery and then appears to cross the origins of the lenticulostriate arteries (Fig. 93).
SJOGREN (1956) identified the close relationship between the anterior choroidal artery, the posterior cerebral artery, and the basal vein of Rosenthal as they traverse the ambient cistern (Fig. 96). THERON (1976) proposed a method for detecting displacements of this artery on lateral angiograms.
At the end of its first segment, the anterior choroidal artery dives abruptly through the choroidal fissure to enter the temporal horn of the lateral ventricle. A characteristic right-angle kink identifies this landmark. A subsequent reduction in caliber usually impairs precise definition of this artery, as it continues its course along the surface of the choroid plexus of the lateral ventricle. However, the frequently visualized blush of the choroid plexus (or the artery itself if seen) displays the characteristic curve of the temporal horn of the lateral ventricle.
The identification of collateral branches of the anterior choroidal artery is exceptional. On the other hand, anastomotic channels occasionally opacify the terminal segment of this artery during selective vertebral angiography.

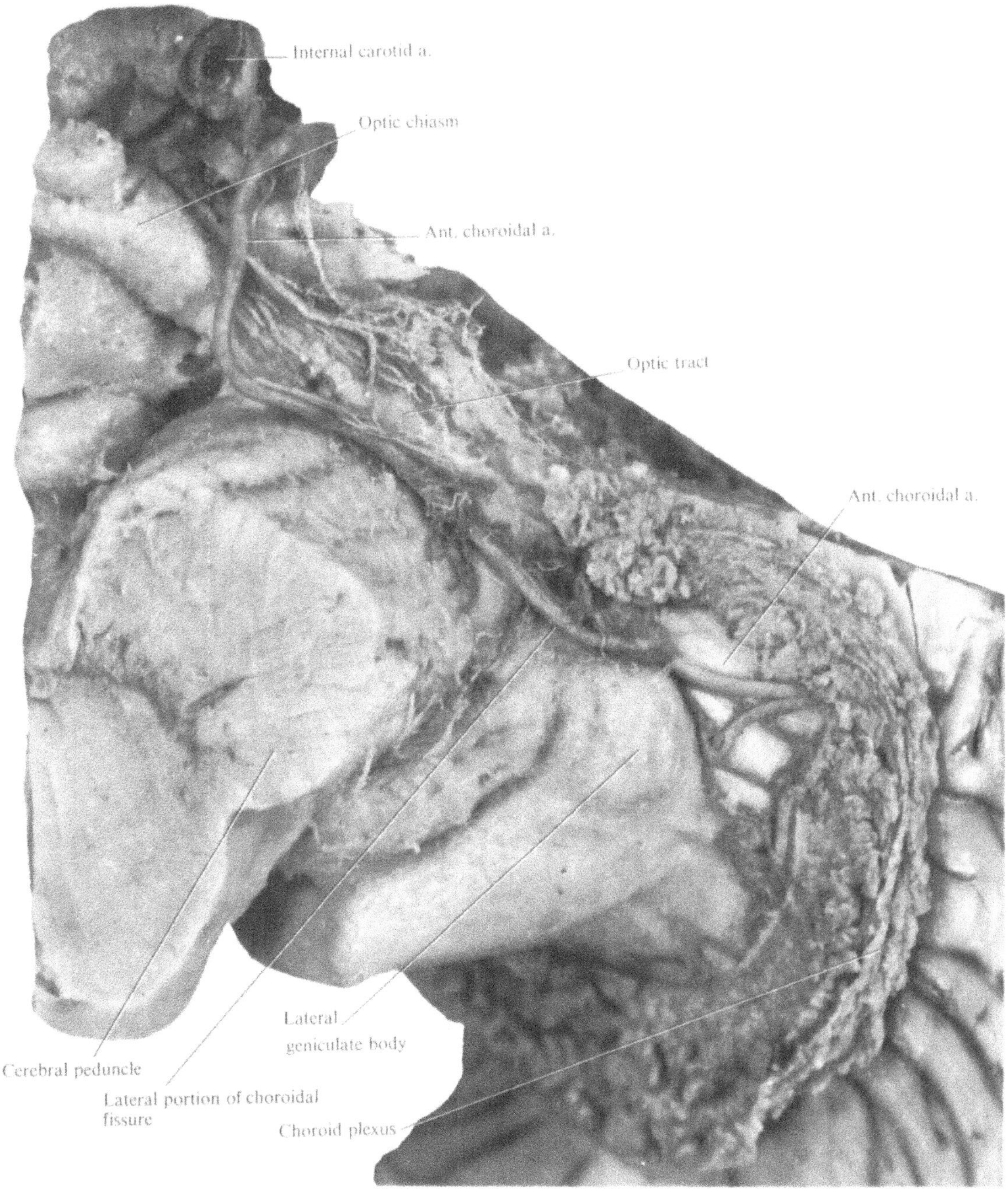

Fig. 89. Dissection after selective injection of the anterior choroidal artery, inferior view

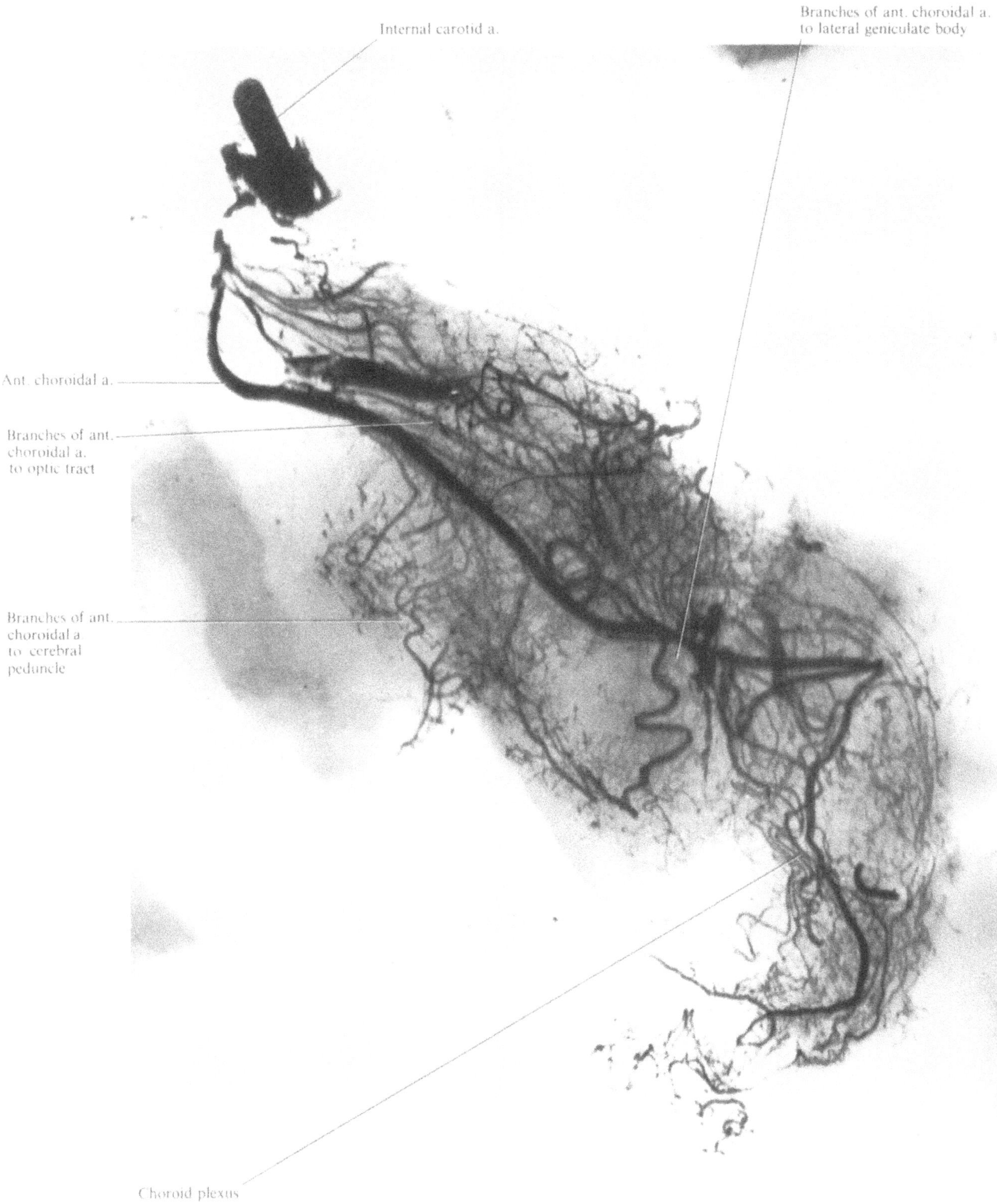

Fig. 90. Radiograph after selective injection of the anterior choroidal artery, inferior view

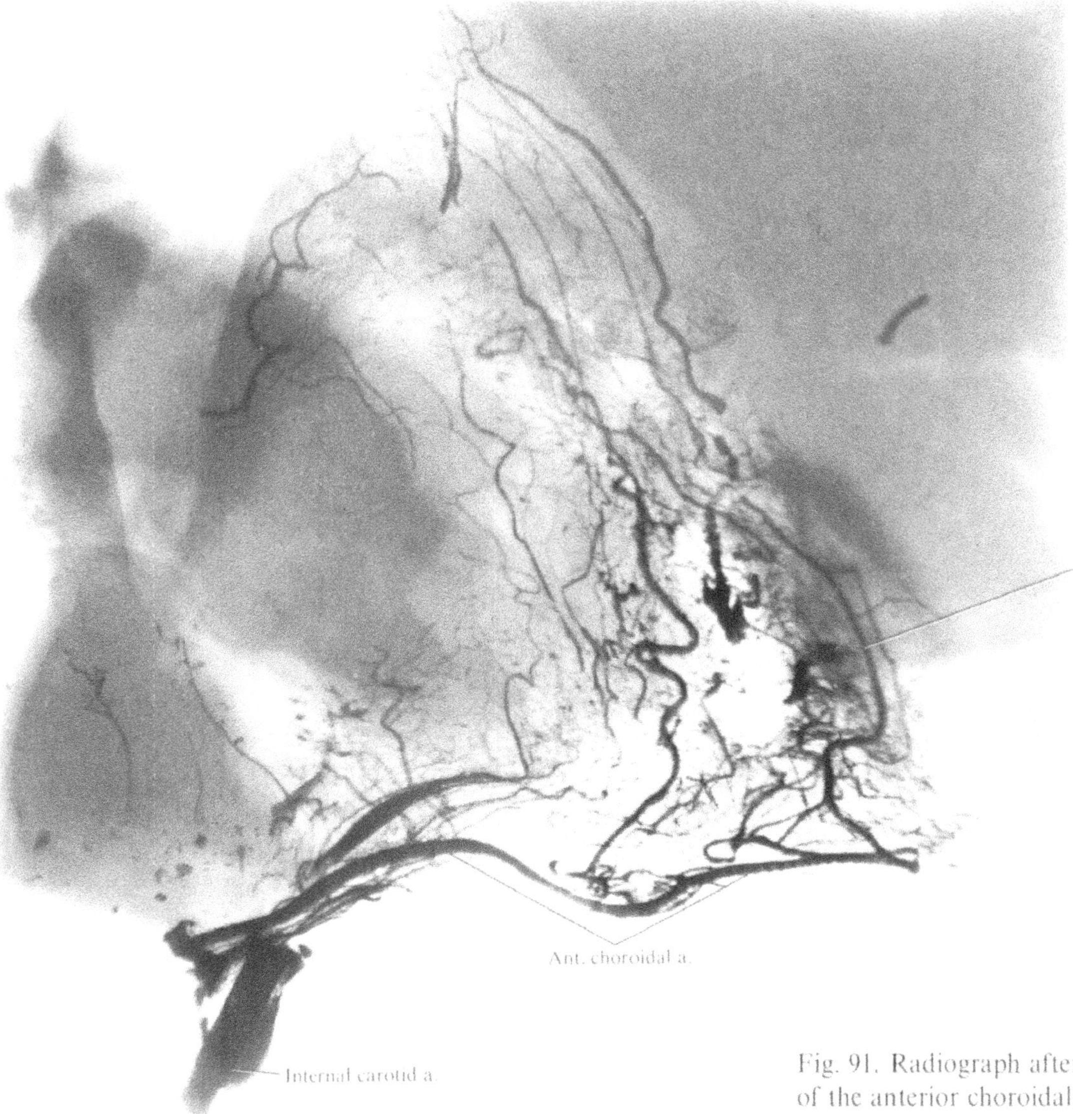

Fig. 91. Radiograph after selective injection of the anterior choroidal artery, lateral view

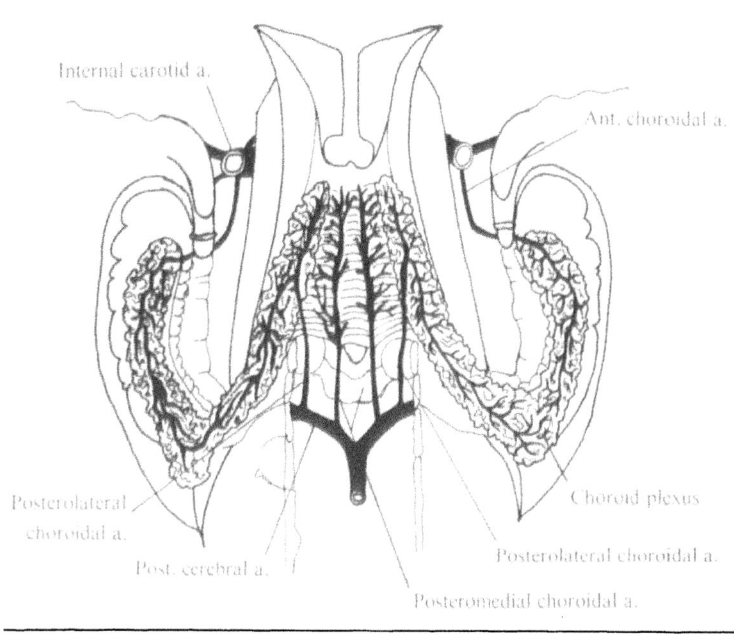

Fig. 92. Schematic representation of the choroidal arteries (after the work of TESTUT, 1948)

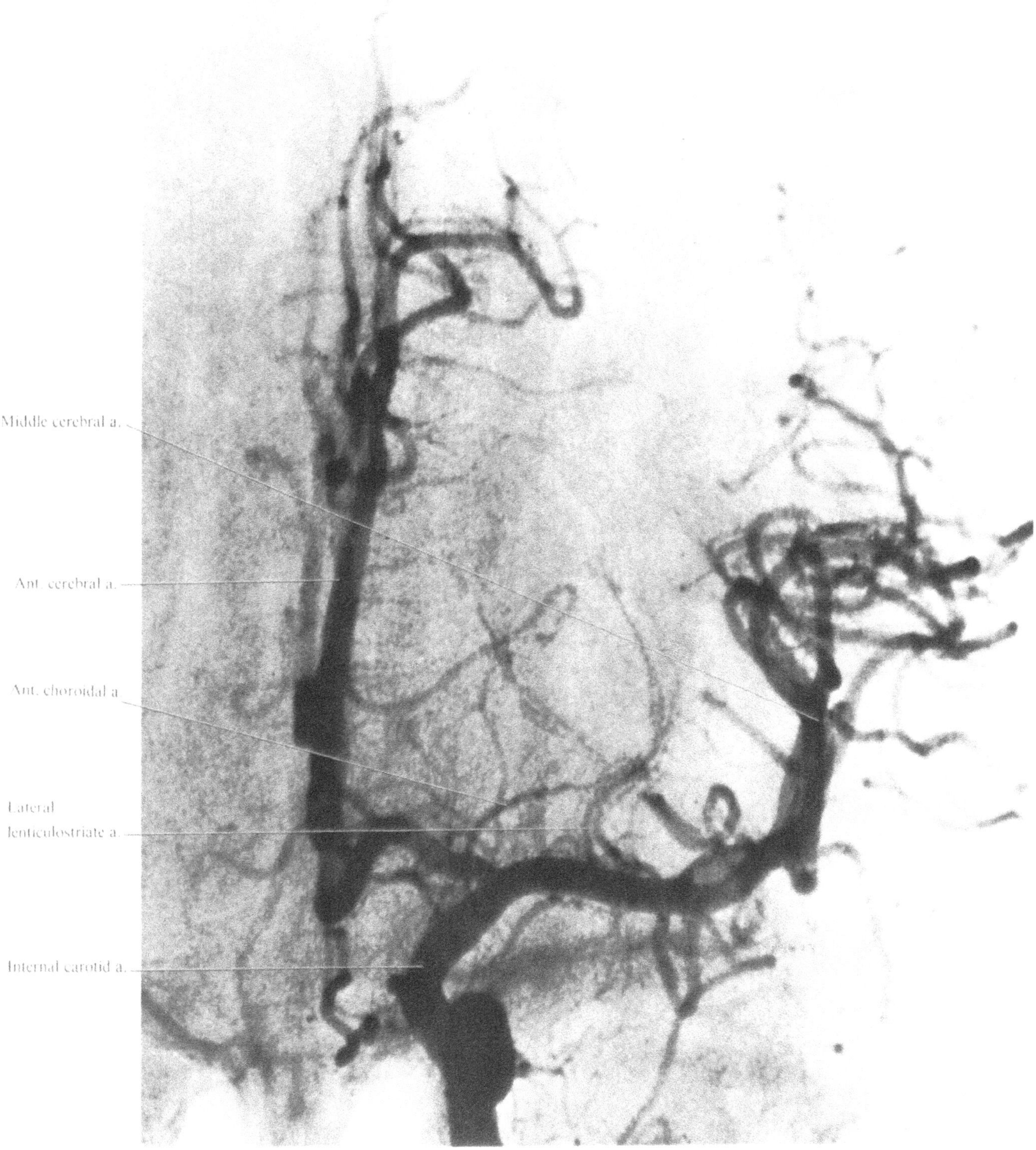

Fig. 93. Left carotid angiogram, frontal projection (× 2.5 magnification)

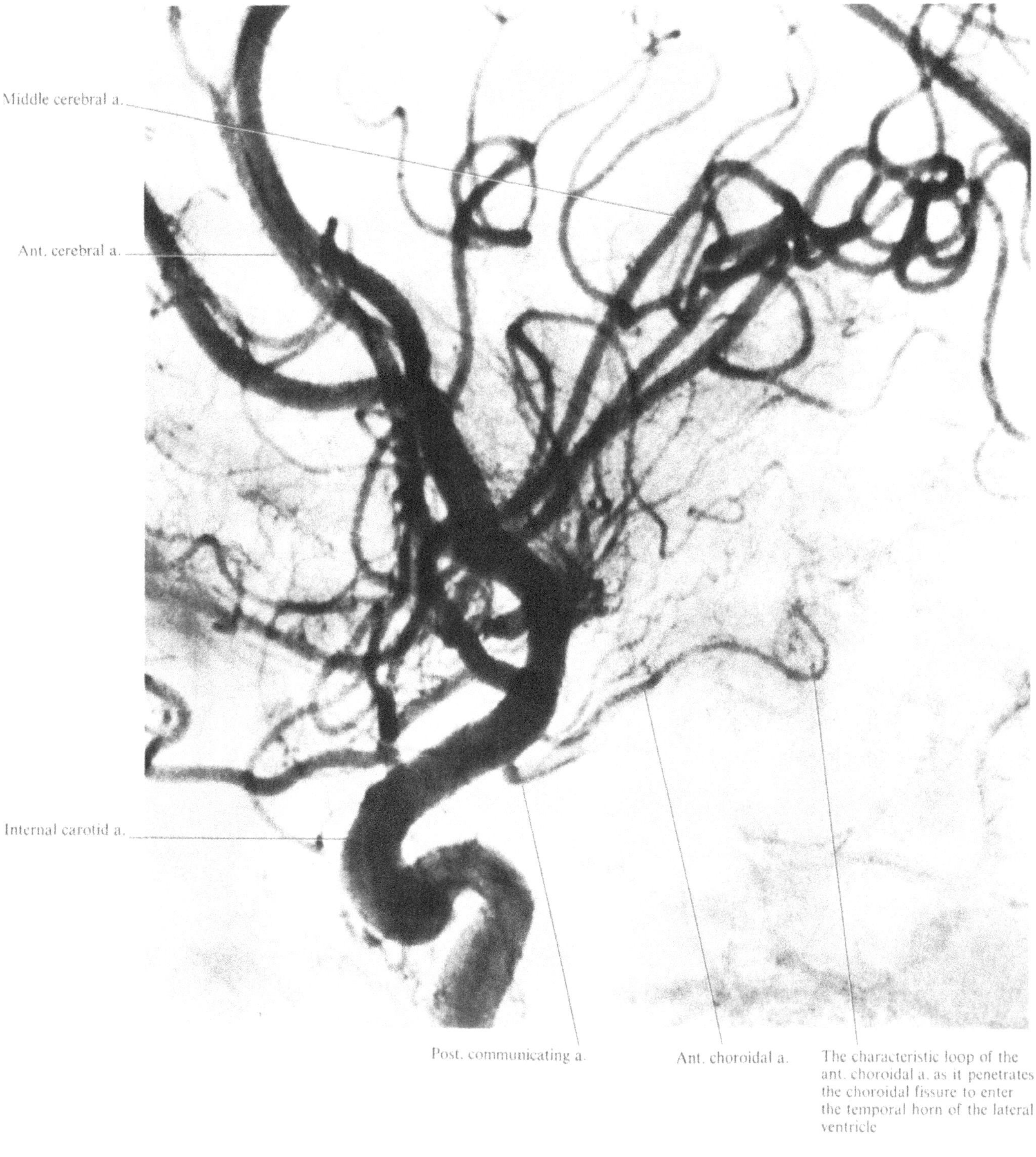

Fig. 94. Left carotid angiogram, lateral projection (× 2.5 magnification)

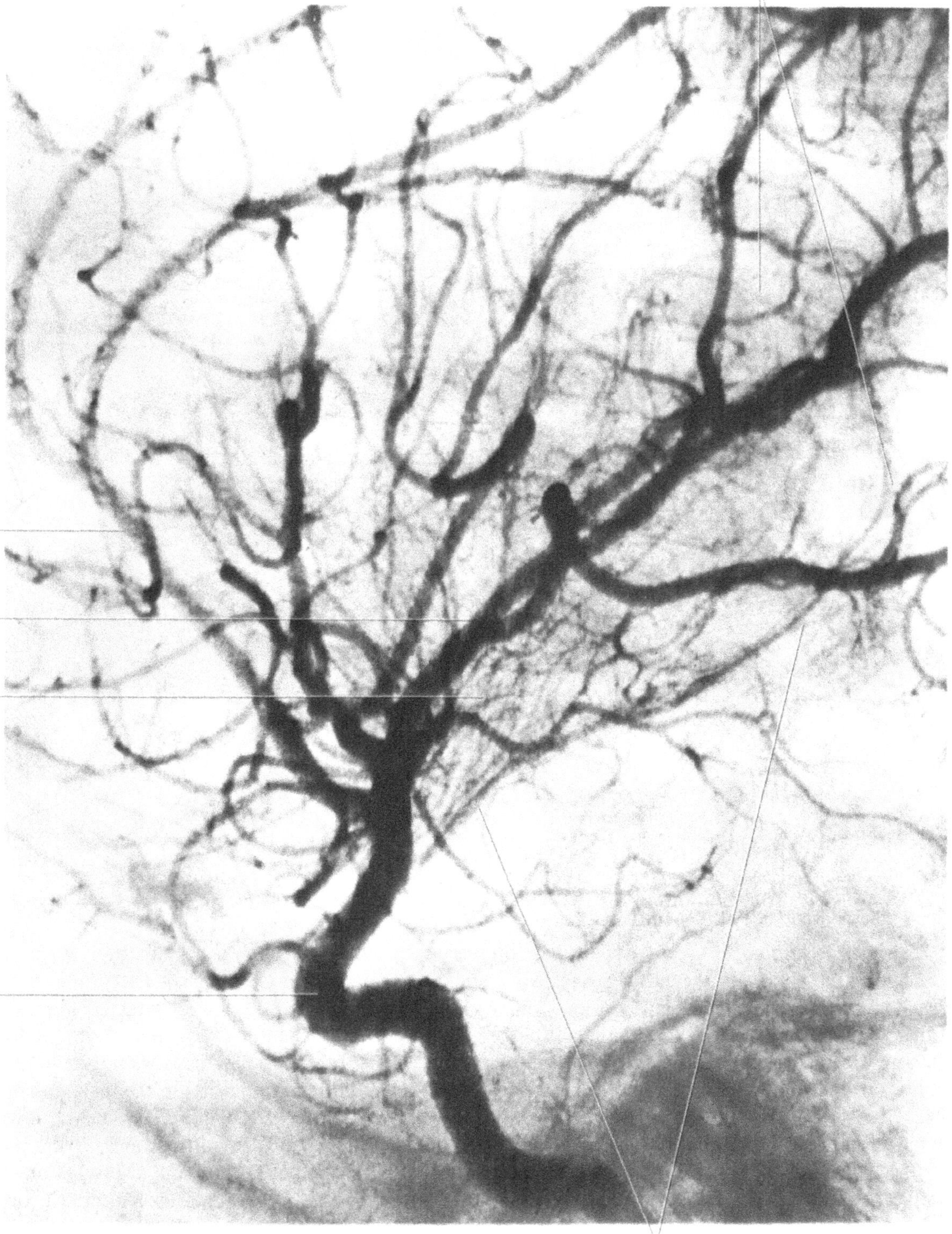

Fig. 95. Left carotid angiogram, lateral projection

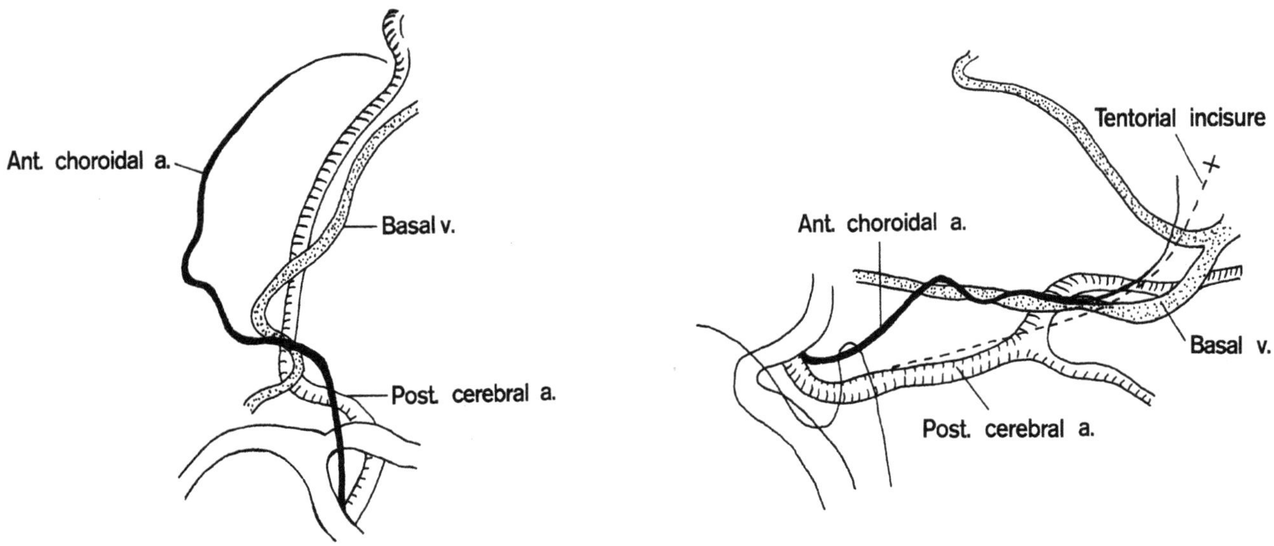

Fig. 96. Schematic representation of the course of the anterior choroidal artery in frontal and lateral projections (after Sjogren, 1956). The course of this artery is related to that of the basal vein of Rosenthal and the posterior cerebral artery

D. Posterior Cerebral Artery

I. Anatomic Study of the Posterior Cerebral Artery

The posterior cerebral arteries, despite their origins as the terminal branches of the basilar artery, have an embryology and territory of vascularization similar to the other arteries that supply the cerebral hemispheres. They link up with the latter vessels via the posterior communicating arteries, which connect them with the internal carotid arteries.

Each posterior cerebral artery supplies a deep portion of the brain and also provides hemispheric vascularization to the internal surface of the occipital lobe, a portion of the internal surface of the parietal lobe, and most of the fusiform, lingual and hippocampal gyri. Its temporal territory extends to the temporal pole.

The anatomic studies of the posterior cerebral artery include the early works of Duret (1874), Foix and Hillemand (1925), and the more recent studies of Lazorthes (1961), Kaplan and Ford (1966), Margolis and Newton (1970), Salamon, Michotey and Bank (1976).

From its origin, at the bifurcation of the basilar artery (Figs. 102, 103), the posterior cerebral artery passes along the anterior and then lateral surface of the cerebral peduncle, presenting a curve convex medially (Figs. 97–99). In this region the oculomotor nerve separates it from the superior cerebellar artery (or arteries) which arises from the distal basilar artery. The posterior cerebral artery continues to the region of the quadrigeminal plate.

After its origin, the posterior cerebral artery provides perforating branches to the thalamus, the thalamoperforate arteries. Other deep branches, arising from its circumpeduncular portion, include the posteromedial and posterolateral choroidal arteries, along with the quadrigeminal arteries and the posterior group of perforating thalamic branches, the thalamogeniculate arteries. The terminal deep branch of the posterior cerebral artery is the posterior pericallosal or splenial artery.

A certain amount of confusion exists with regard to the nomenclature of the hemispheric branches of the posterior cerebral artery. If these branches vascularize the occipitotemporal region, and the hippocampal, lingual and fusiform gyri, they merit the term occipitotemporal arteries. If, however, the most anterior branches supply only the inferior surface of the temporal lobe, then these branches merit the distinction of more precise nomenclature. Since our dissections reveal the latter situation, we prefer to classify the hemispheric branches of the posterior cerebral artery as the inferior temporal arteries and the occipitotemporal arteries (Figs. 97–103).

Despite a wide range of variation, it is possible to distinguish two principal branches of the inferior temporal artery, one anterior and the other posterior (Figs. 98, 99, 102, 103). The anterior inferior temporal artery courses anteriorly and laterally from its origin, while the posterior inferior temporal artery is directed laterally.

The occipitotemporal artery is generally single and presents various patterns of division (Figs. 98, 99, 102, 103). The posterolateral course of its branches continues the posterior end of the fan-like distribution of the inferior temporal arteries. Characteristic loops occur whenever any of these branches cross the collateral or occipitotemporal fissures.

The continuation of the posterior cerebral artery, the calcarine artery, passes along the internal surface of the occipital lobe to enter the calcarine fissure (Figs. 97–103). It usually provides one or two collateral branches to the internal surface of the cuneus and the adjacent parietal lobe (the occipitoparietal artery).

In summary, the hemispheric territory of the posterior cerebral artery is supplied as follows:

The anterior and posterior inferior temporal arteries vascularize the inferior and internal surfaces of the temporal lobe up to its anterior end.

The occipitotemporal artery supplies the posterior portion of the fusiform and lingual gyri.

The calcarine artery vascularizes the internal surface of the occipital lobe and, via its occipitoparietal branch, the posterior part of the precuneus.

Anastomoses connect the terminal ramifications of the hemispheric branches of the posterior cerebral artery, with similar ramifications of the anterior and middle cerebral arteries.

II. Radiologic Study of the Posterior Cerebral Artery

Vertebral angiography, particularly the angiographic study of the posterior cerebral arteries, has been the subject of numerous recent works. DECKER (1953) has shown that the vascular territory of the posterior cerebral artery is relatively fixed. DILENGE (1962), and later SALTZMANN (1959), studied the conditions required for filling these arteries via the carotid arteries. YASARGIL (1962) described an axis from the tuberculum sellae to the lambda, which defines the course of the posterior cerebral artery, as viewed in the lateral projection. Recently, HUANG (1974) pointed out the relationship between the branches of the posterior cerebral artery and the collateral sulcus. Numerous works have also detailed the perforating branches which arise from the posterior cerebral artery [GALLOWAY and GREITZ (1960), LAZORTHES and SALAMON (1971), GEORGE, SALAMON and KRICHEFF (1975), HARA and FUJINO (1966)].

In the lateral projection, the initial segment of the posterior cerebral artery extends from the basilar tip to the region of the quadrigeminal plate (Figs. 104–107). In front of the basilar artery, opacification of the posterior communicating artery is frequently seen.

This circumpeduncular segment of the posterior cerebral artery usually presents a slightly curved course, concave superiorly. It is in this segment that the thalamoperforate and thalamogeniculate arteries arise, along with the posteromedial and posterolateral choroidal arteries.

In the region of the quadrigeminal plate, the posterior cerebral artery gives rise to its important hemispheric branches. The most anterior are the inferior temporal arteries and, more posteriorly is the occipitotemporal artery.

The trunk of the posterior cerebral artery continues posteriorly as the calcarine artery. Asymmetry is frequently present between the two calcarine arteries, especially in their relationship to the midline, but these arteries usually present a characteristic curve corresponding to the calcarine fissure. They also give rise to one or two occipitoparietal arteries which supply the precuneus, together with parietal branches from the anterior cerebral artery.

In the frontal view the branches of the posterior cerebral artery are best visualized in the half-axial projection (Figs. 109, 110). The circumpeduncular segments of each side are relatively characteristic. Although superimposed upon one another, the hemispheric branches of the posterior cerebral artery are distinguished from the cerebellar hemispheric branches of the superior cerebellar artery by their course, their greater degree of tortuosity, and their slightly greater caliber.

The loops of the inferior temporal and occipitotemporal arteries frequently outline the courses of the collateral and occipitotemporal sulci. The course of the calcarine artery usually localizes the calcarine fissure (Figs. 112, 113).

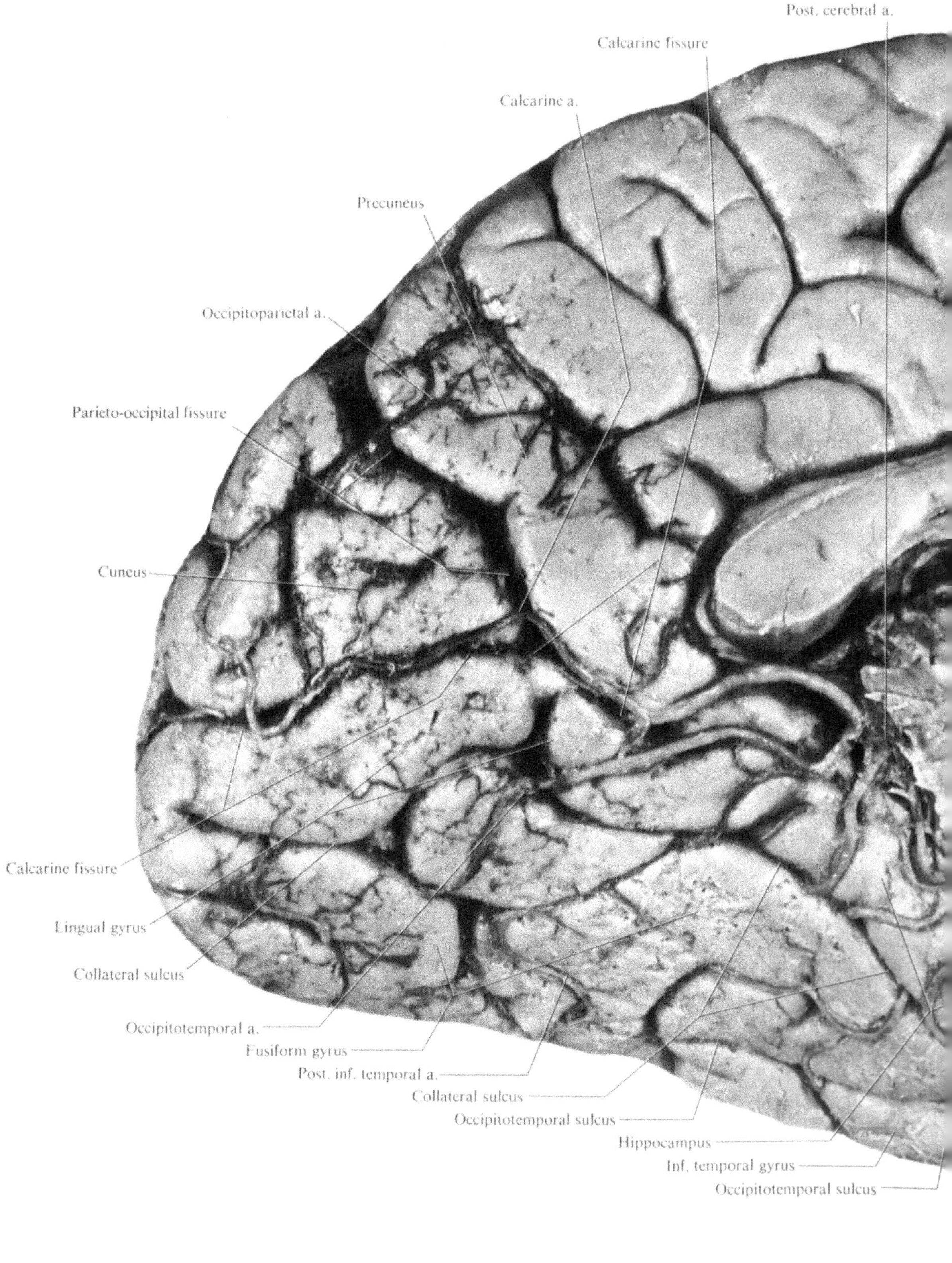

Fig. 97. Dissection of the left cerebral hemisphere after selective injection of the posterior cerebral artery, inferomedial view

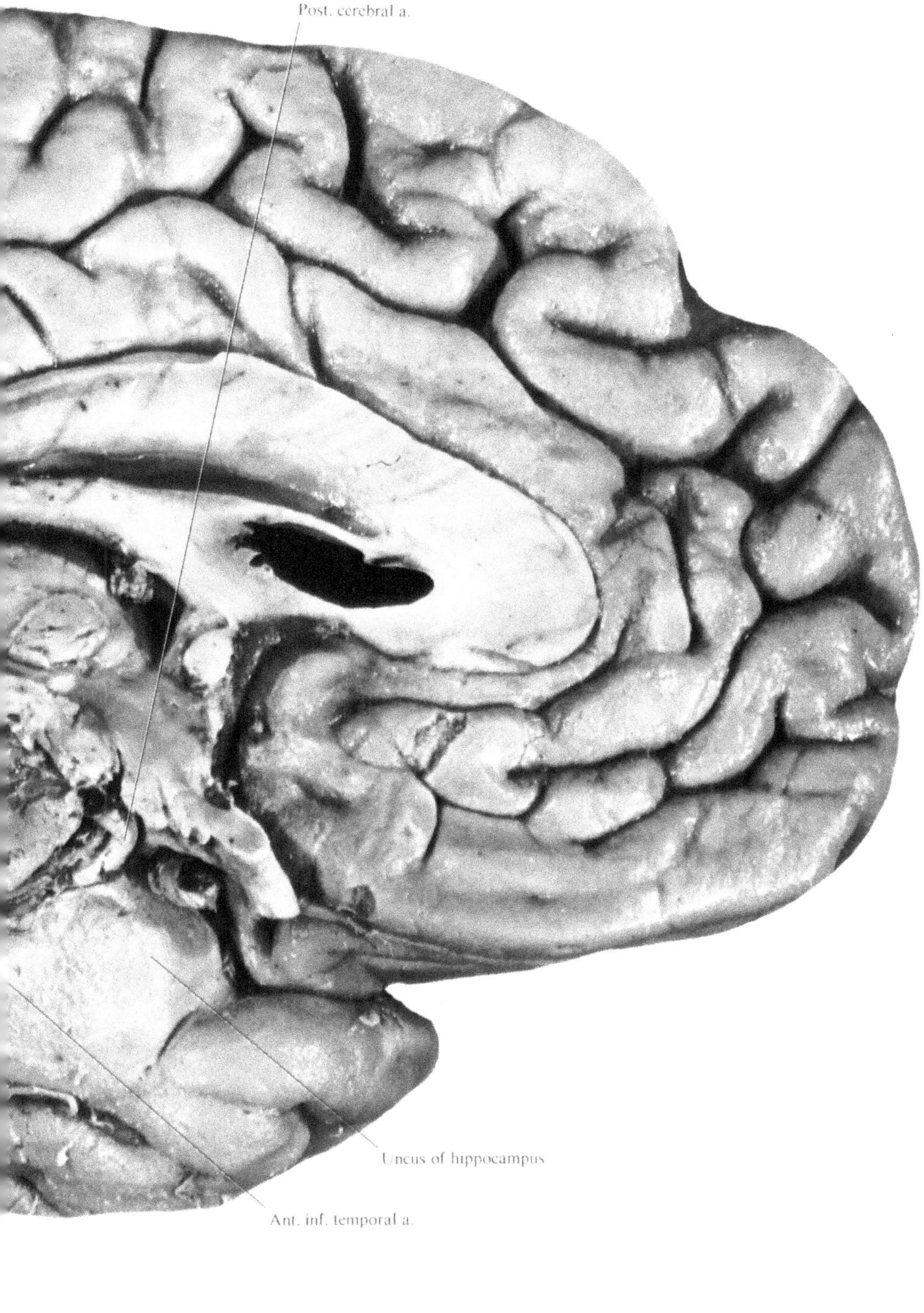
Post. cerebral a.
Uncus of hippocampus
Ant. inf. temporal a.

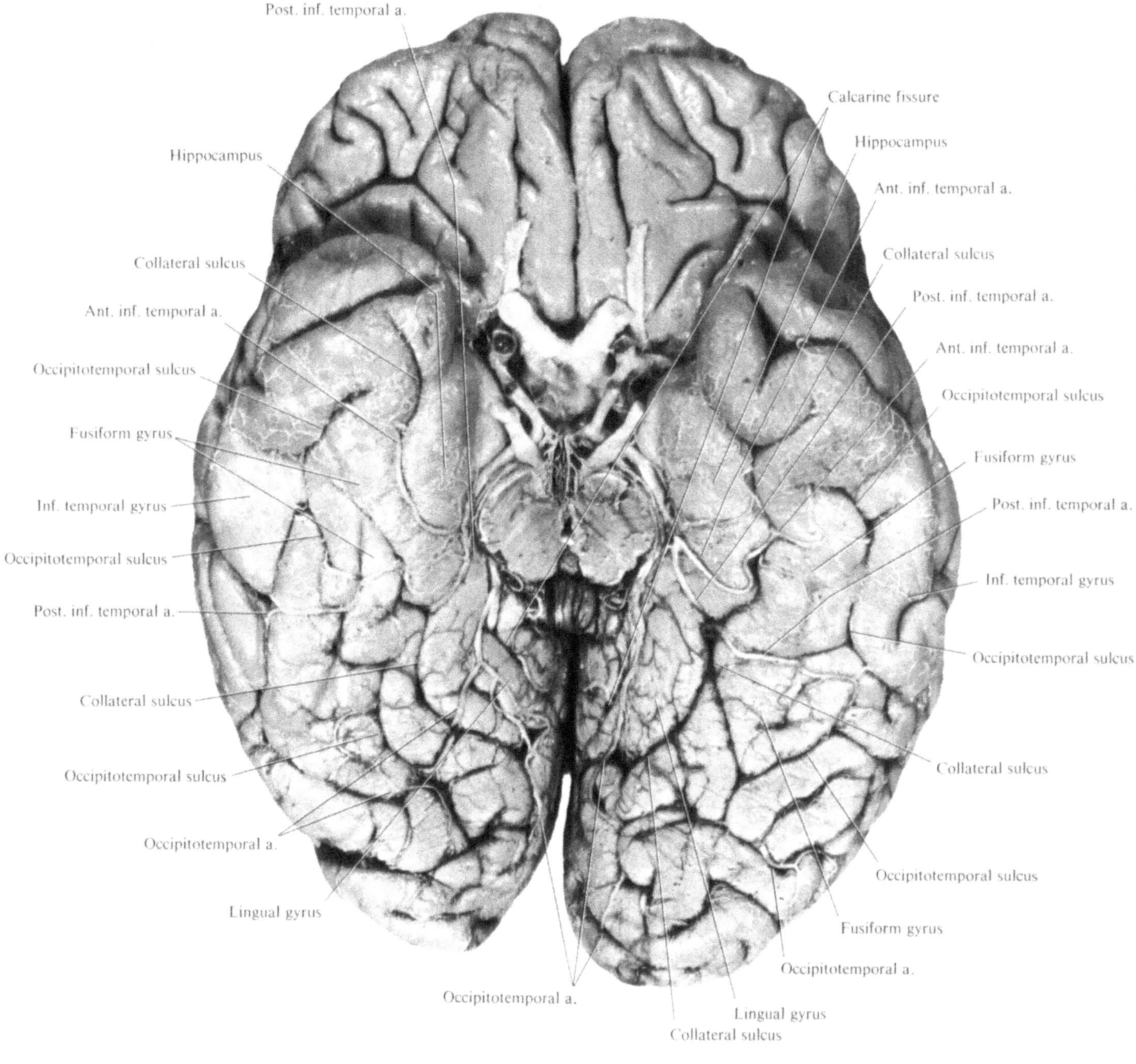

Fig. 98. Dissection of the cerebral hemisphere after selective injection of the posterior cerebral arteries, inferior view. Note that the calcarine artery is not visible in this projection

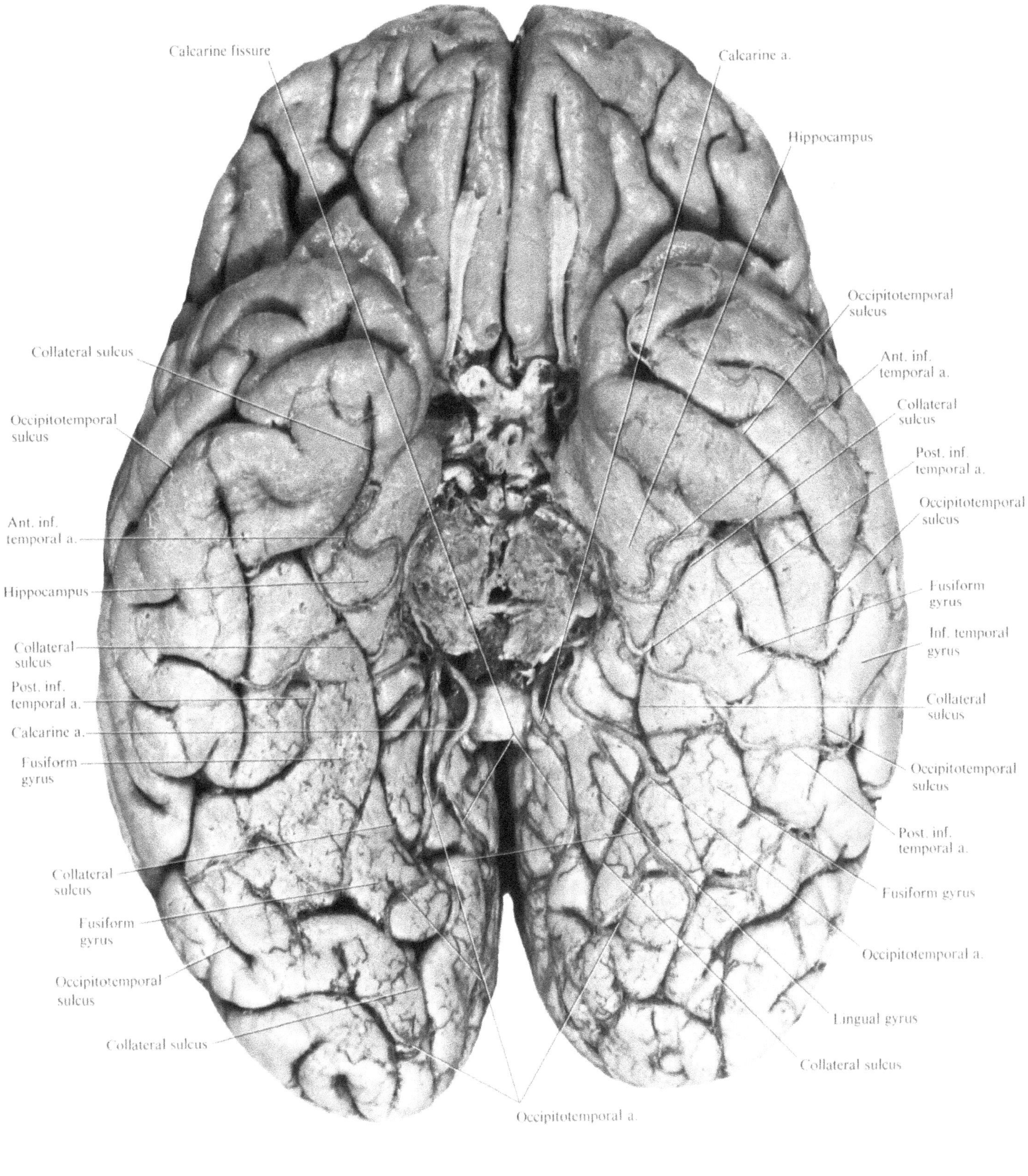

Fig. 99. Dissection of the cerebral hemisphere after selective injection of the posterior cerebral arteries, inferior view

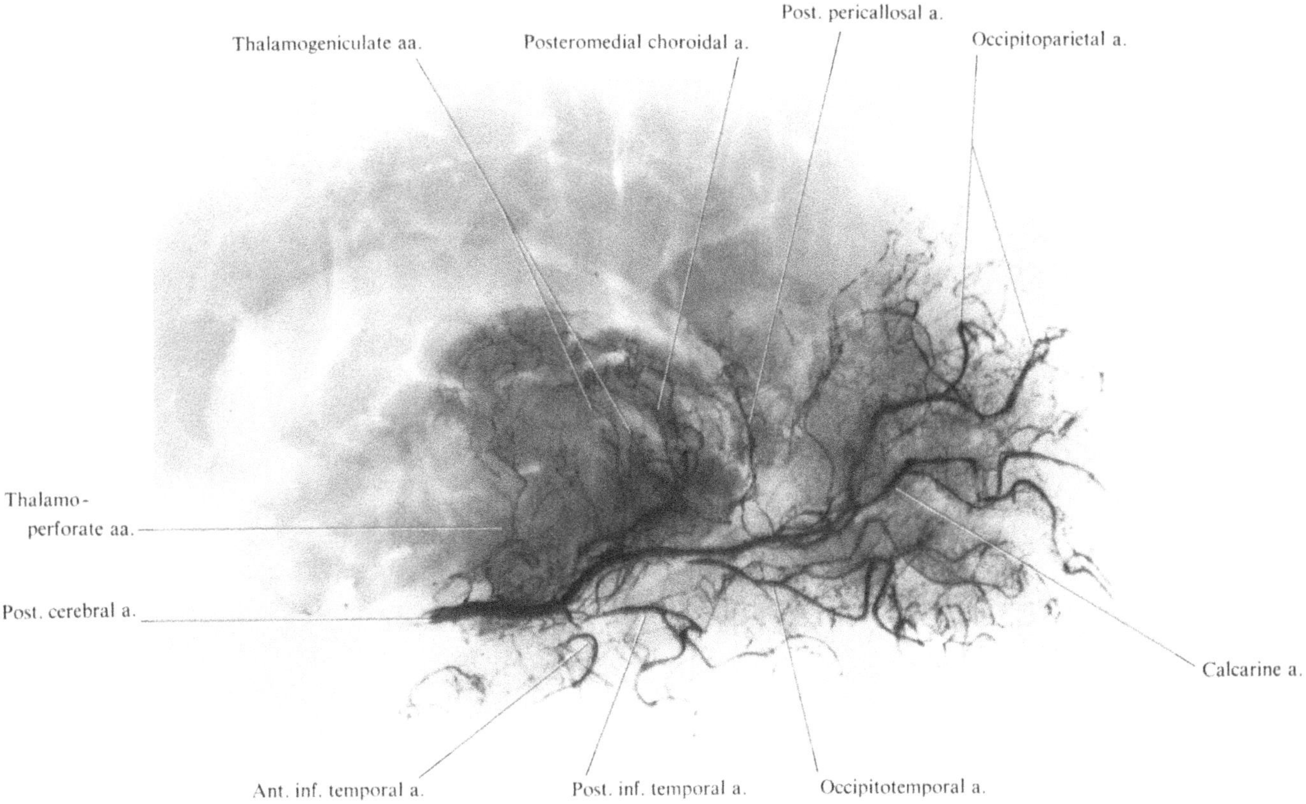

Fig. 100. Radiograph after selective injection of the left posterior cerebral artery, lateral view

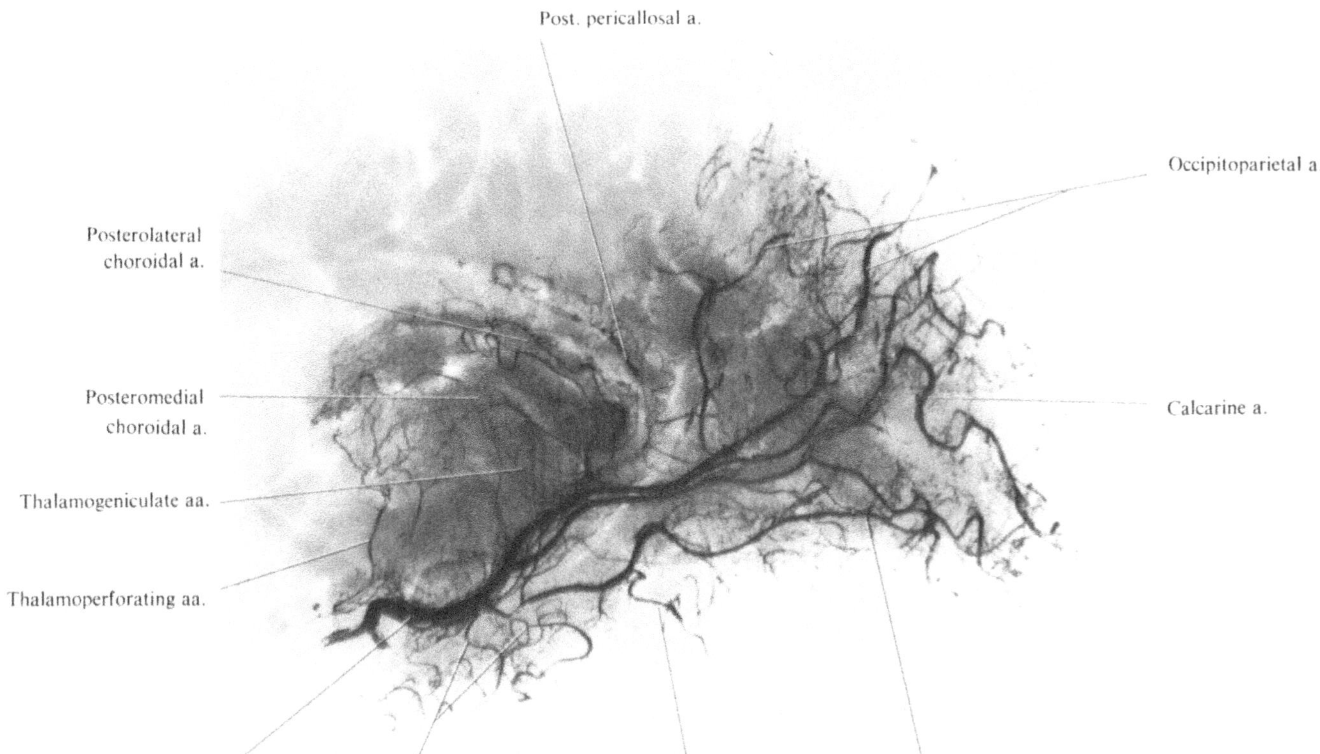

Fig. 101

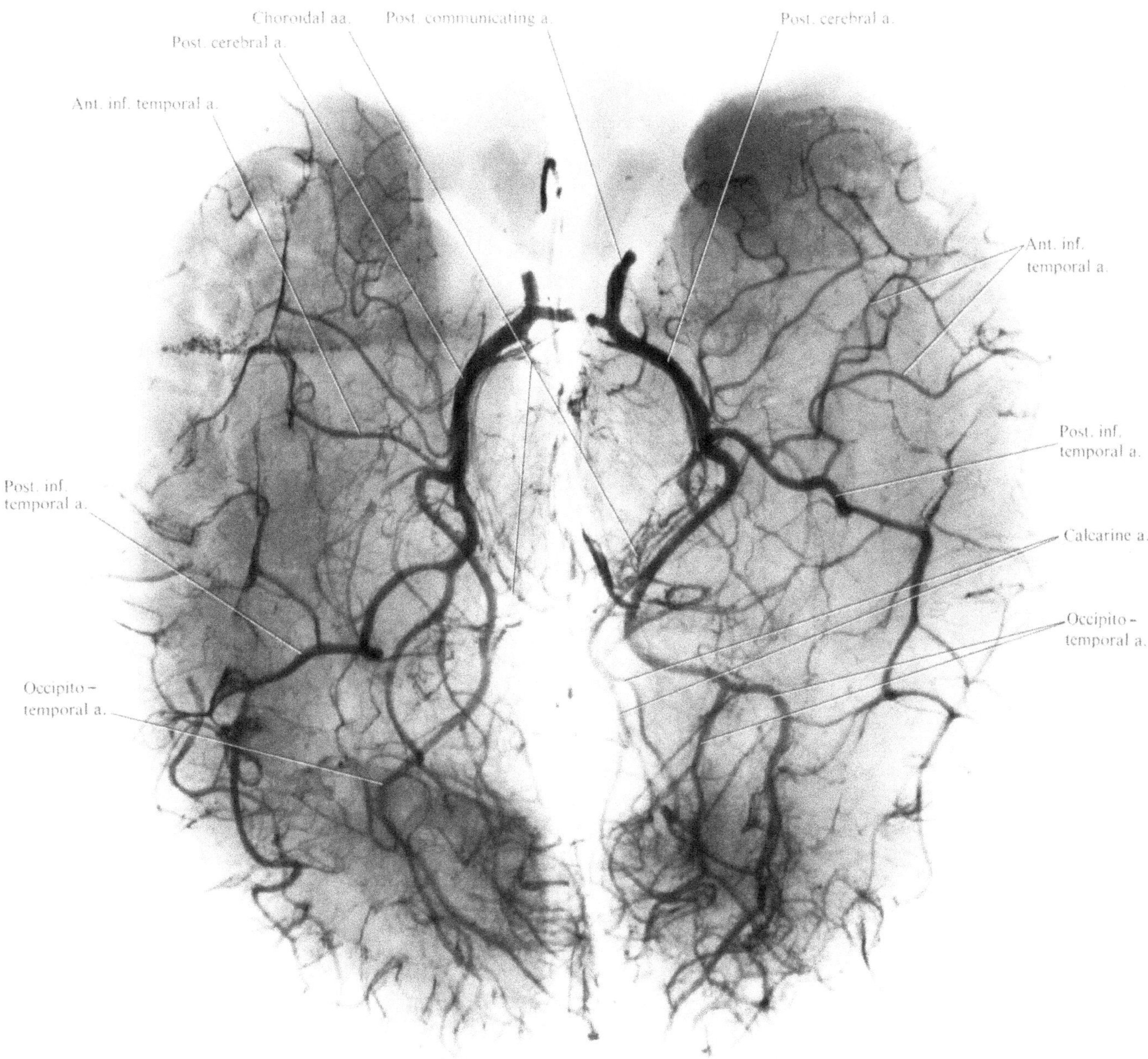

Fig. 102. Radiograph after selective injections of the posterior cerebral arteries, inferior view

◁

Fig. 101. Radiograph after selective injection of the left posterior cerebral artery, lateral view

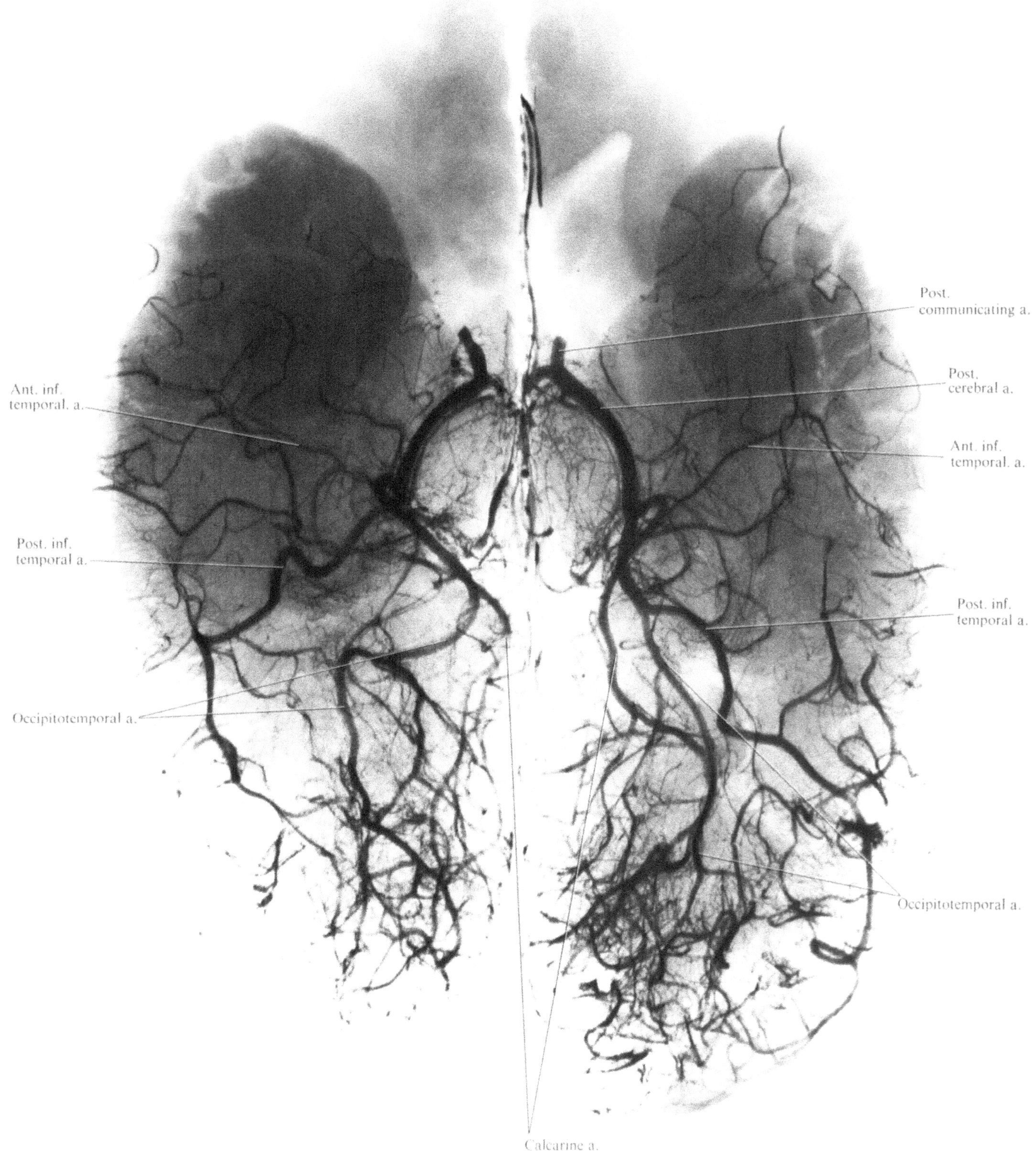

Fig. 103. Radiograph after selective injections of the posterior cerebral arteries, inferior view

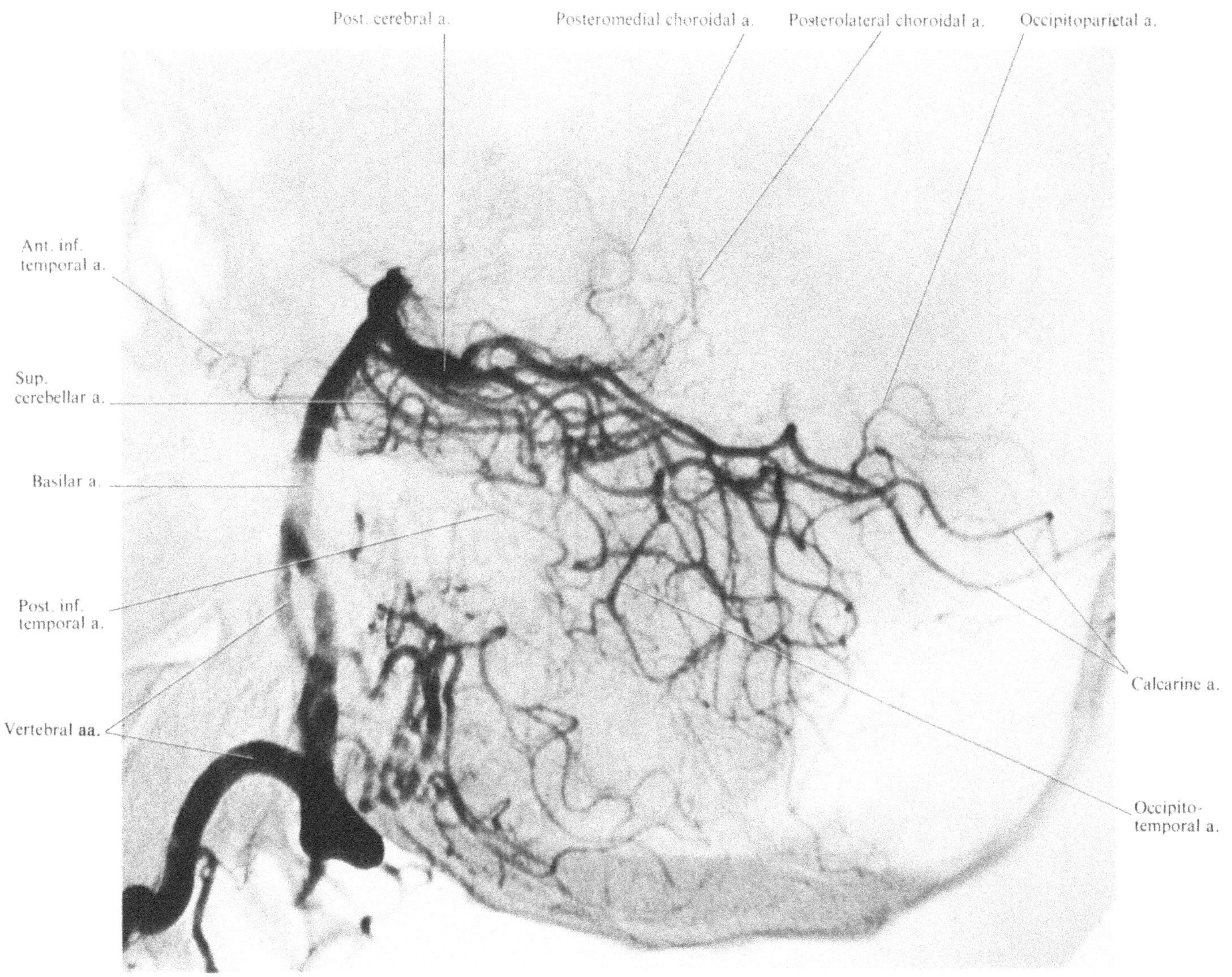

Fig. 104. Vertebral angiogram, lateral projection

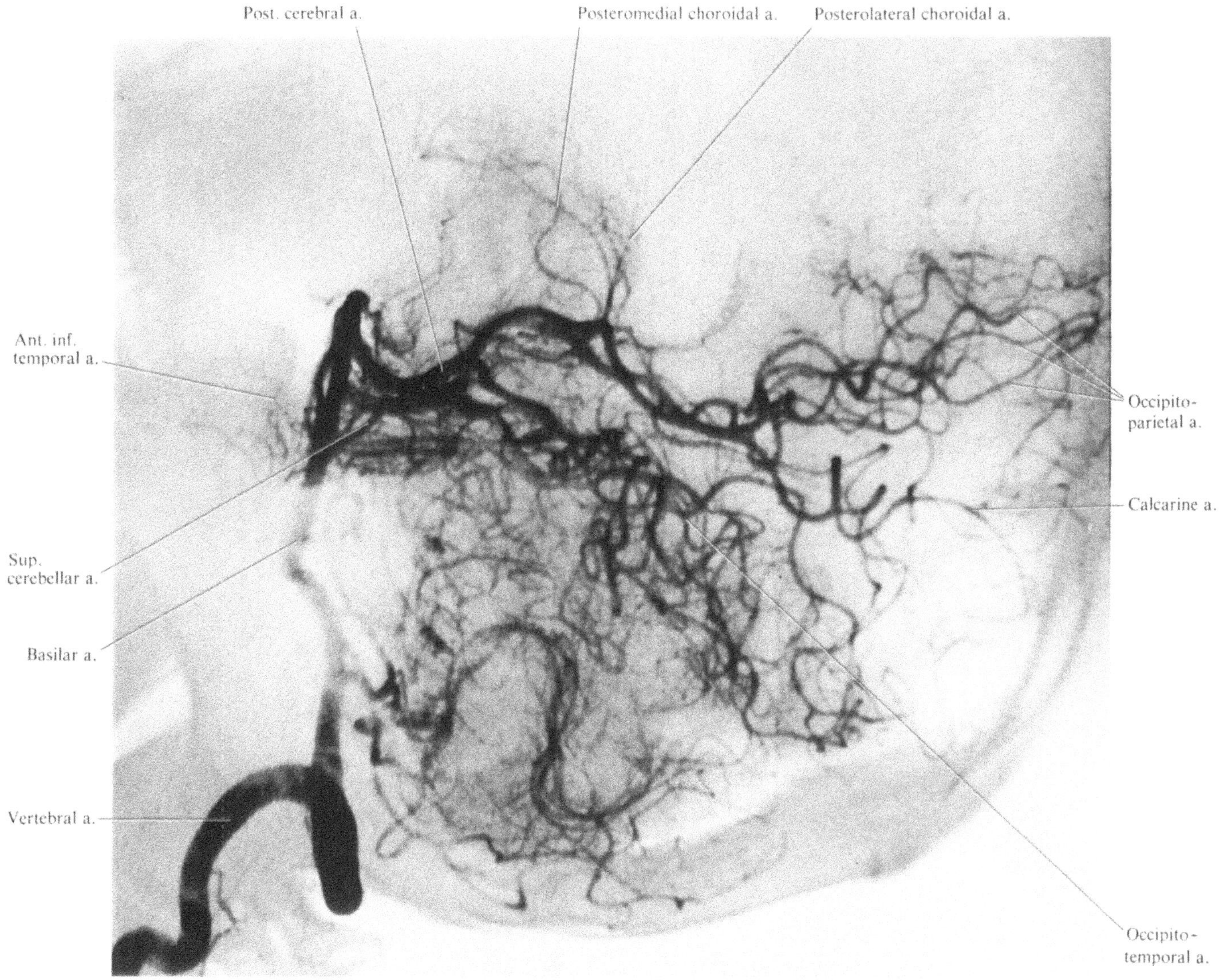

Fig. 105. Vertebral angiogram, lateral projection

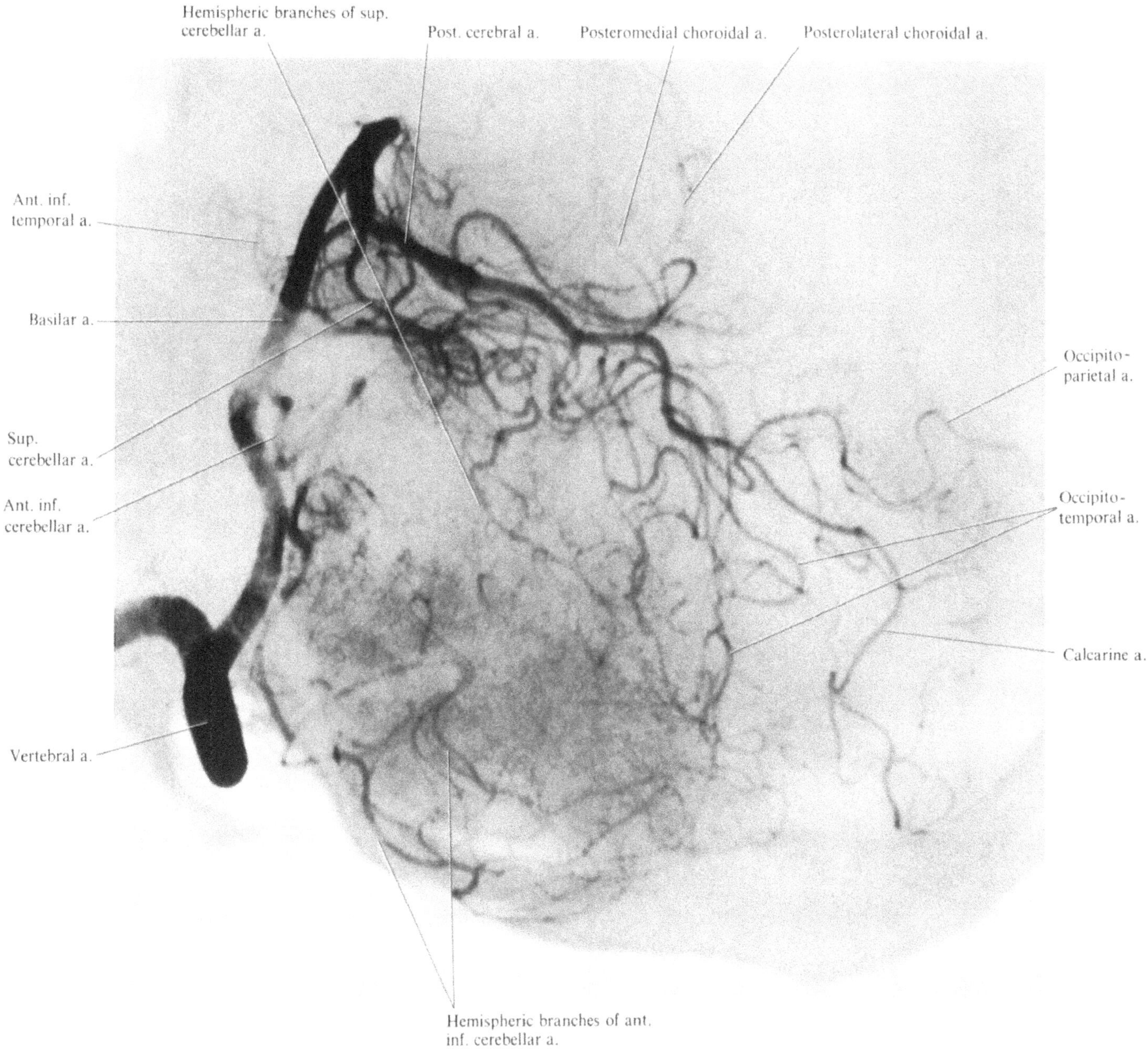

Fig. 106. Vertebral angiogram, lateral projection

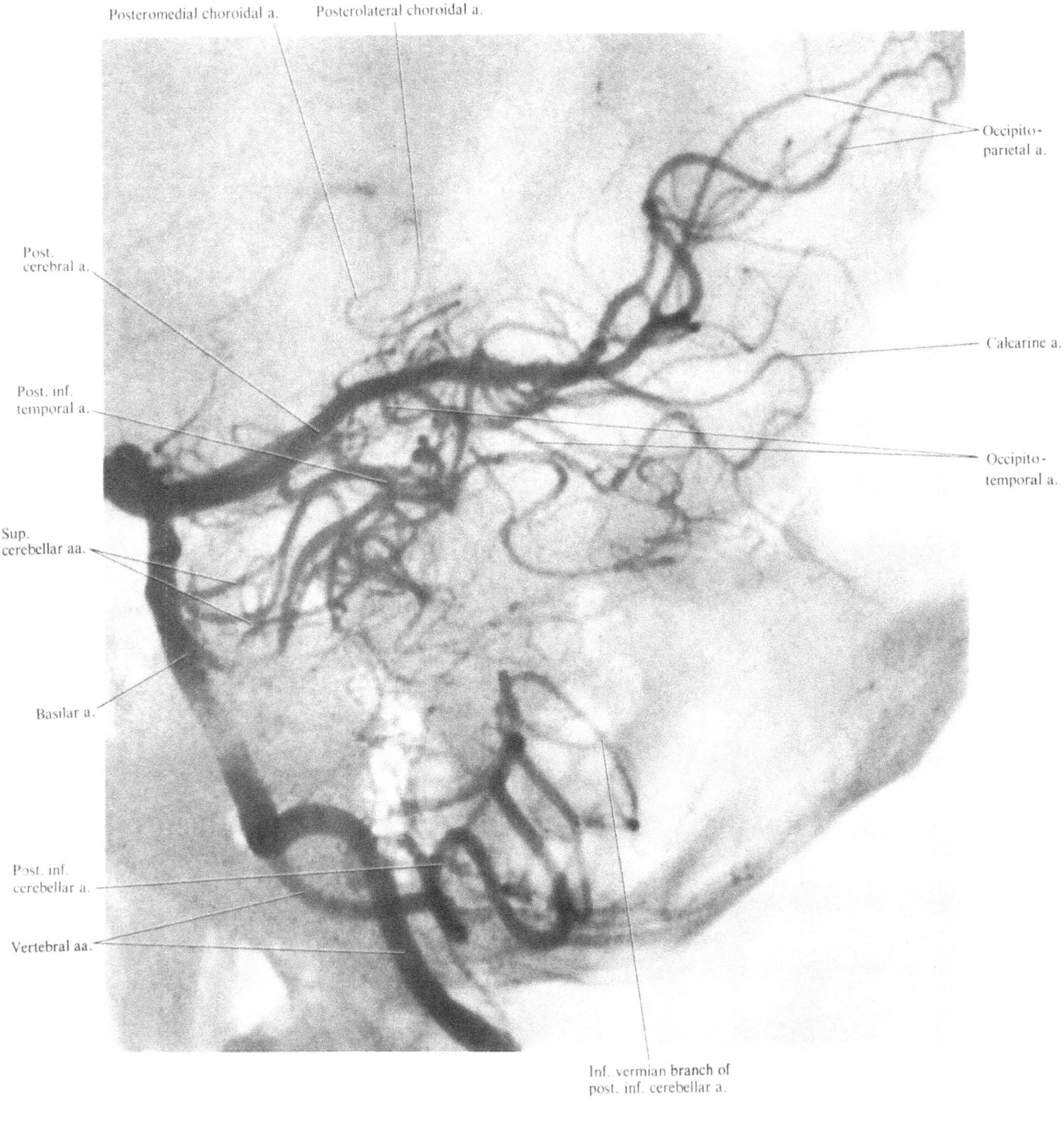

Fig. 107. Vertebral angiogram, lateral projection

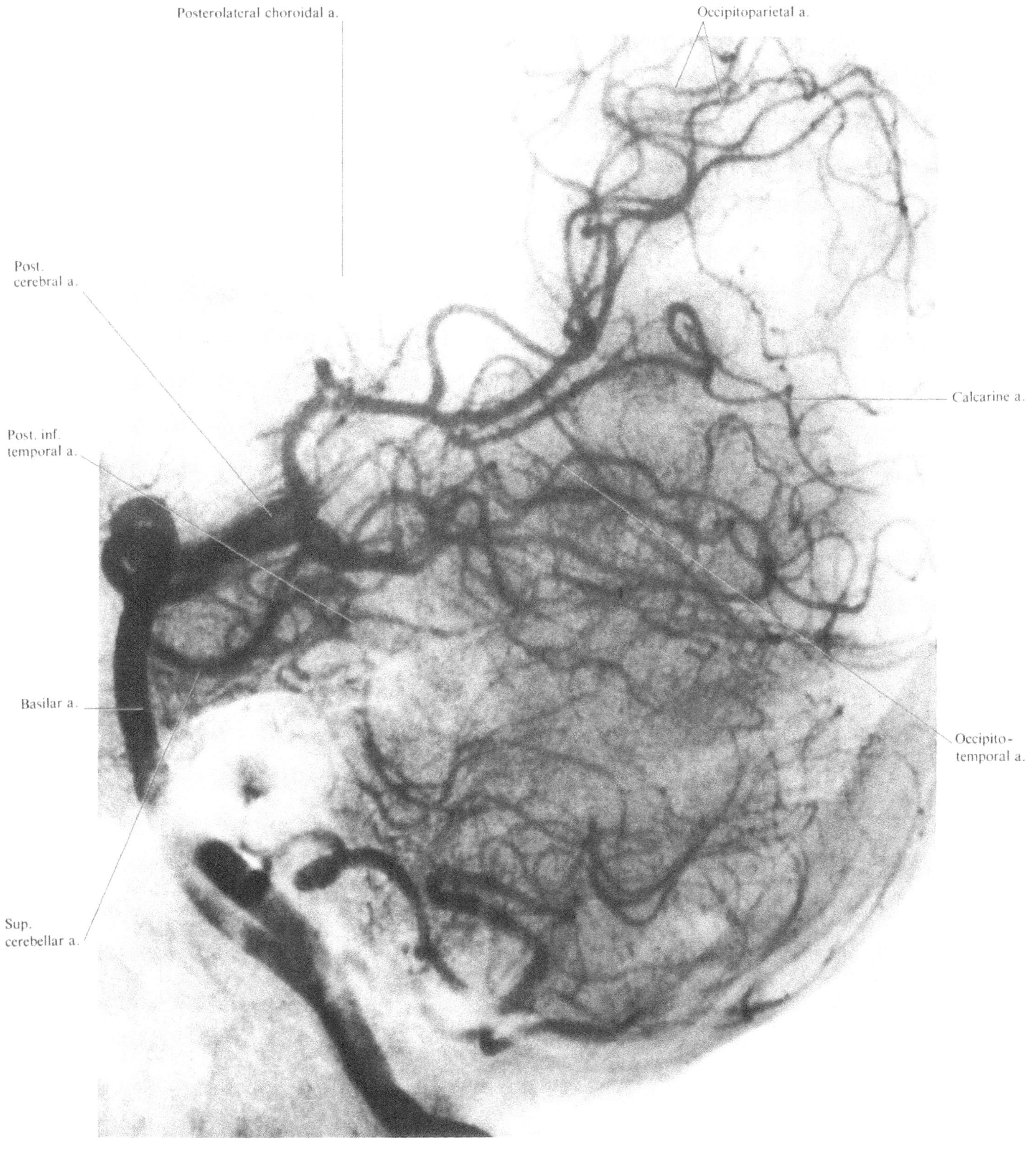

Fig. 108. Vertebral angiogram, lateral projection

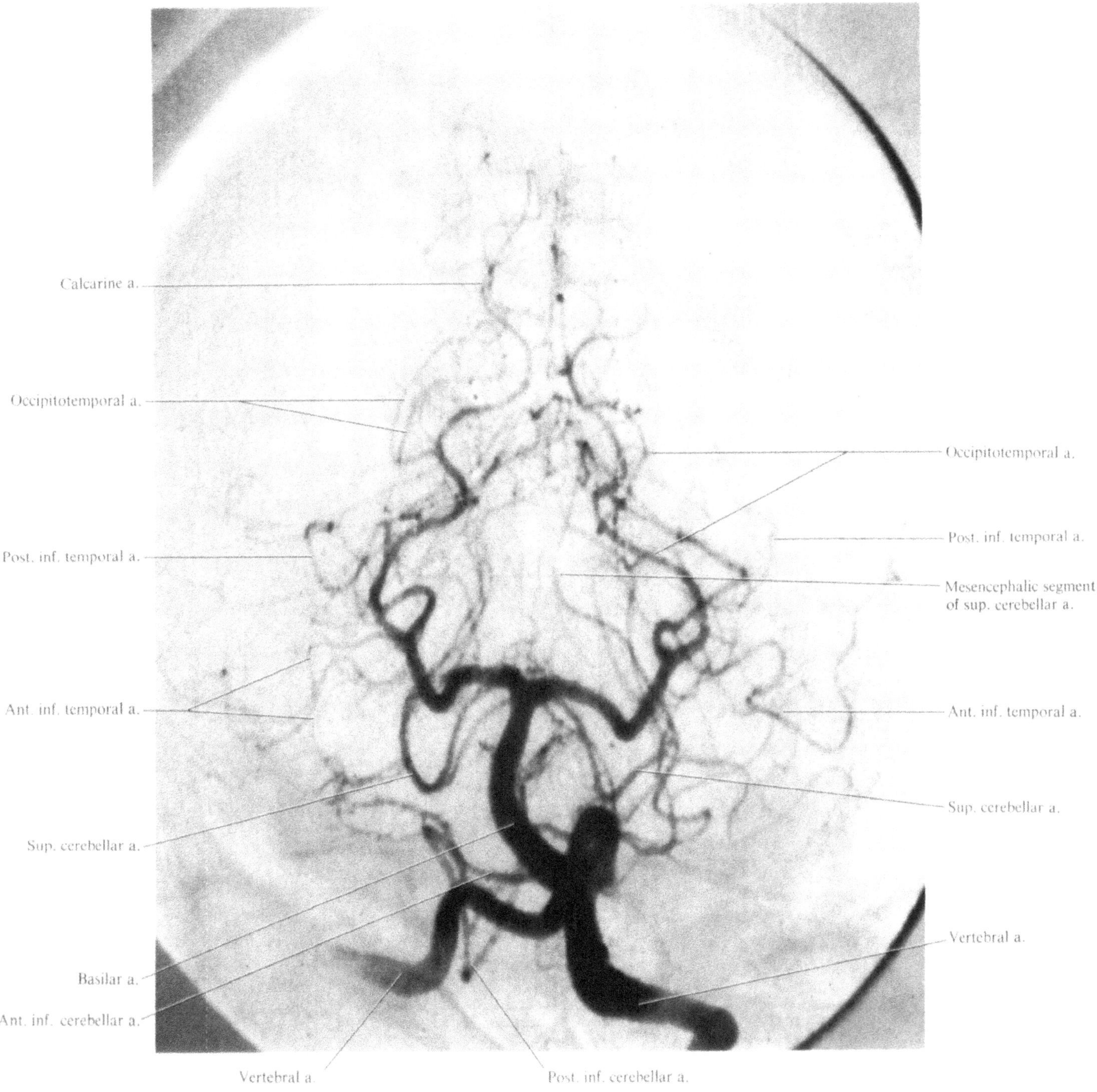

Fig. 109. Vertebral angiogram, showing distribution of the posterior cerebral arteries, frontal projection

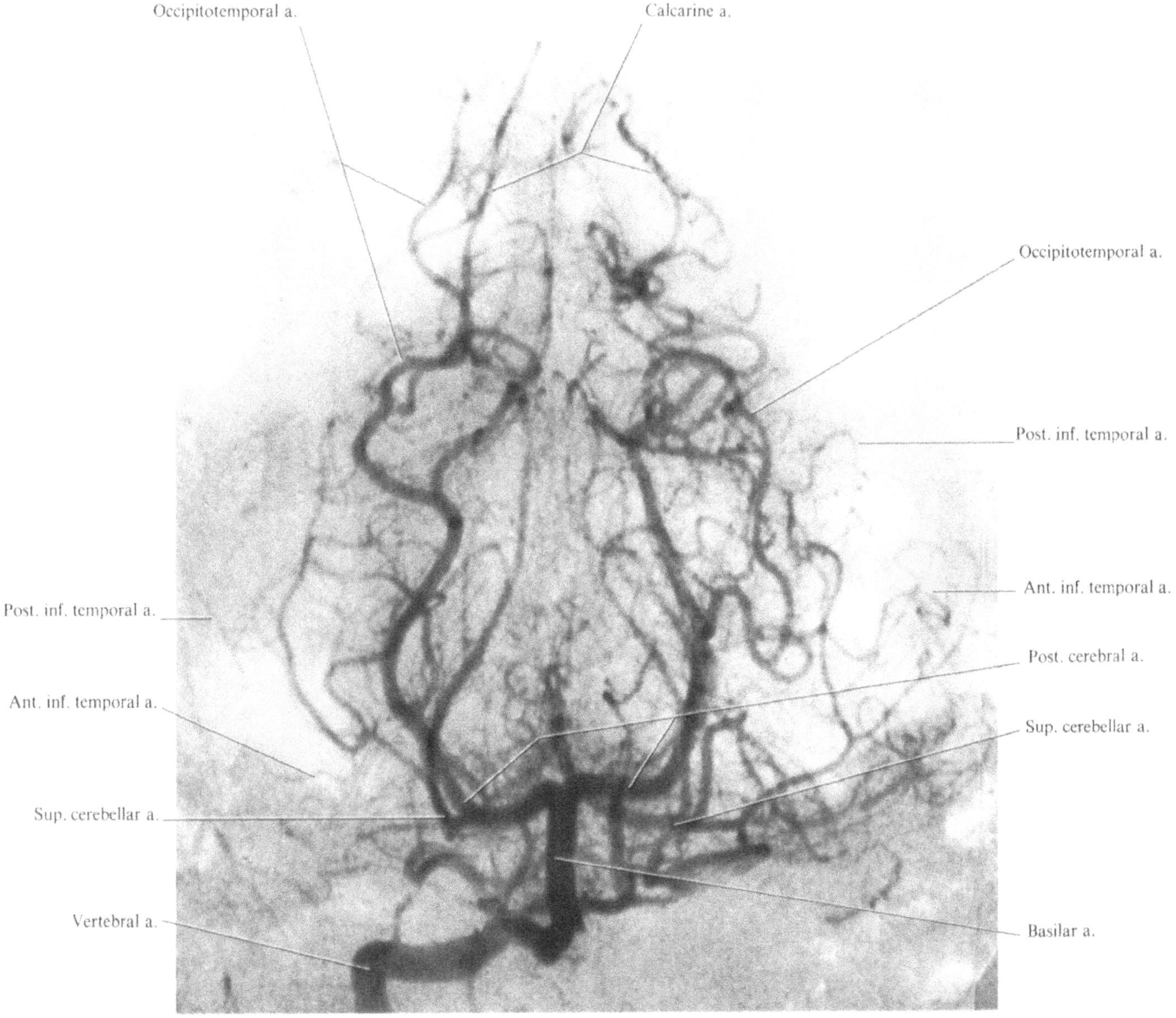

Fig. 110. Vertebral angiogram, half axial projection

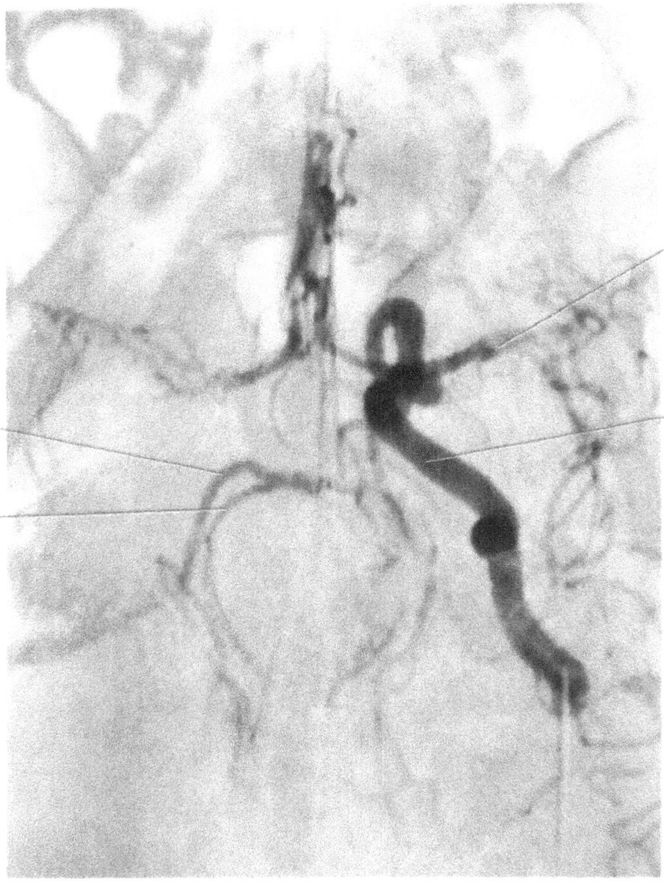

Fig. 111. Carotid angiogram, axial projection, showing filling of the posterior cerebral and superior cerebellar arteries, via the posterior communicating artery

▷

Fig. 112 A–B. Vertebral angiogram, lateral projection (A), and corresponding photograph of the medial surface of the cerebral hemisphere (B), showing the localization of the important fissures and sulci

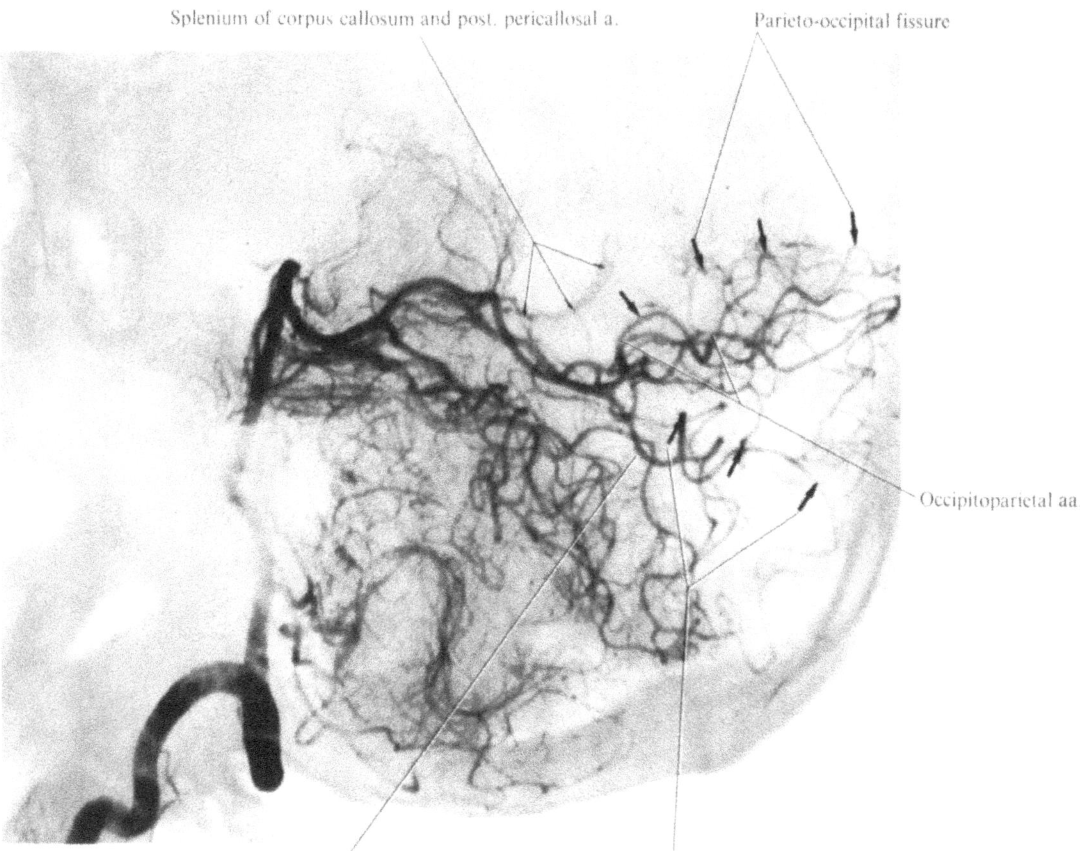

Fig. 112A

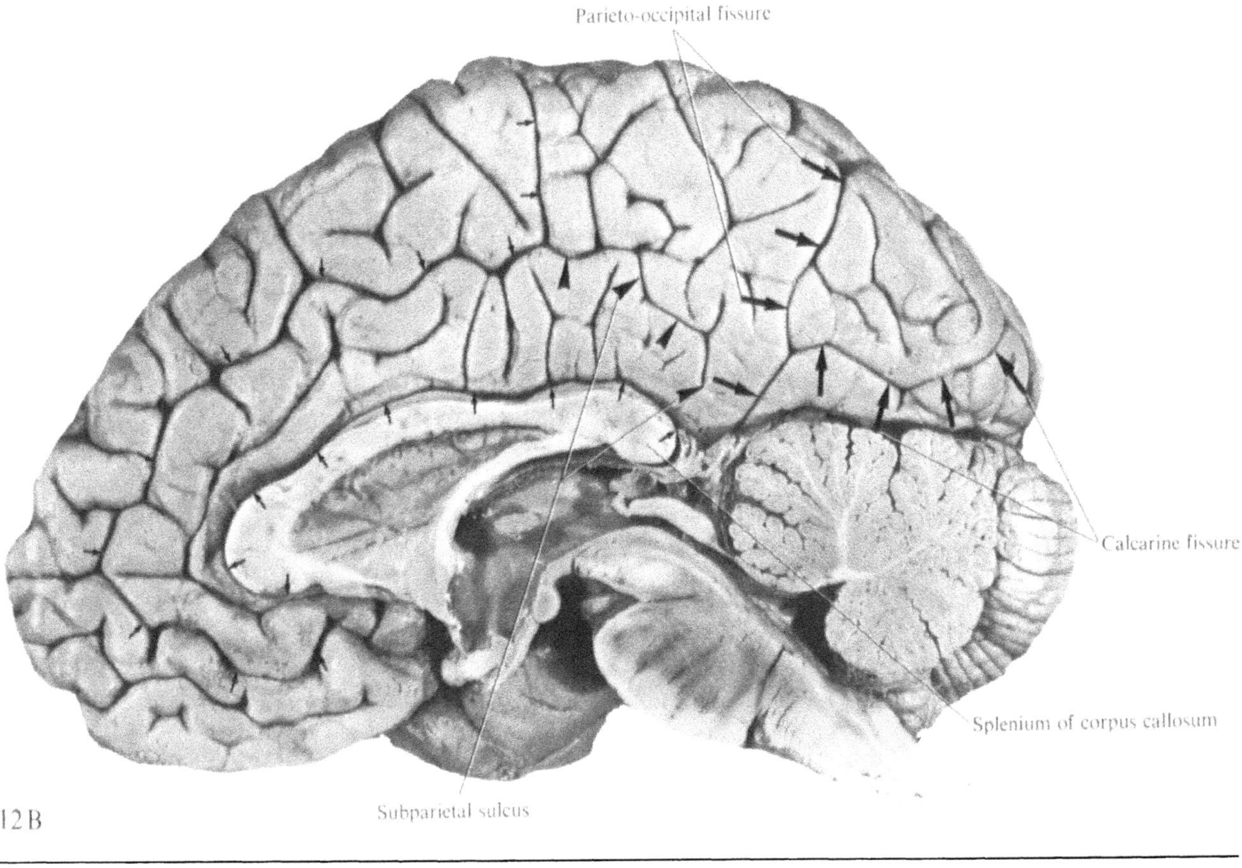

Fig. 112B

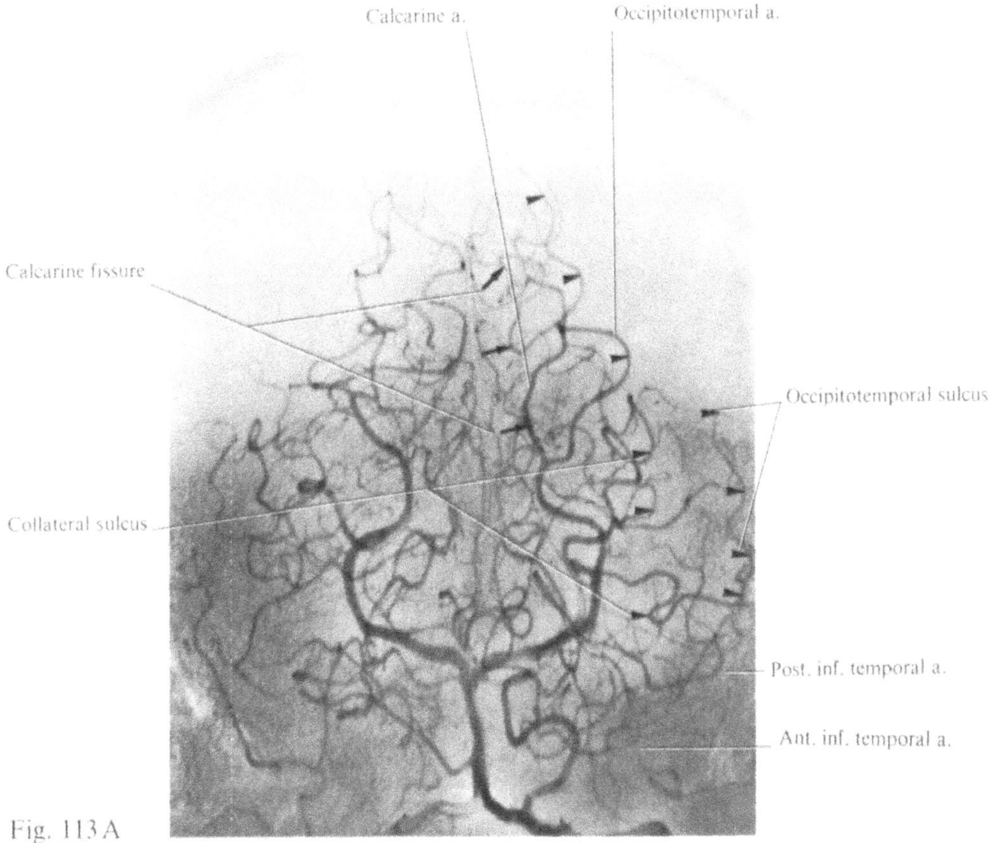

Fig. 113A

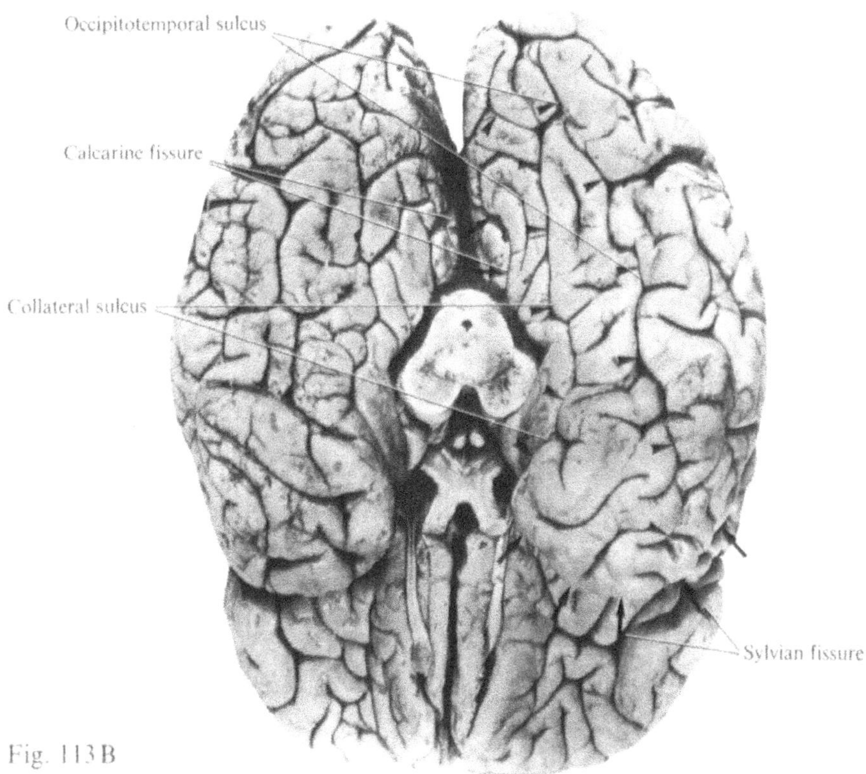

Fig. 113B

Fig. 113A–B. Vertebral angiogram, frontal projection (A), with corresponding view of the inferior surface of the cerebral hemispheres (B), showing the localization of the important fissures and sulci

Chapter 4
Basal Cerebral Vein

A. Normal Anatomy

The basal cerebral vein described by ROSENTHAL in 1824 has been the subject of many investigations.

The vein is formed by the union of the anterior cerebral, deep middle cerebral and inferior striate veins, on the undersurface of the anterior perforated substance. The combined trunk, the basal cerebral vein, then passes posteromedially above the uncus to reach the anterior part of the cerebral peduncle, where it receives the peduncular vein. The basal cerebral vein then runs posterolaterally, receiving the inferior ventricular vein and its tributaries, at the level of the most lateral portion of the cerebral peduncle. The vein then turns posteromedially and is joined by the lateral mesencephalic tributary, at the level of the lateral mesencephalic sulcus. Medial temporal and posterior thalamic tributaries join the basal cerebral vein as the latter runs further posteromedially and superiorly, to finally join the great cerebral vein or the posterior portion of the internal cerebral vein.

For descriptive purposes, the basal cerebral vein may be divided into three segments: (I) the first, anterior, or striate segment; (II) the second, middle or peduncular segment; and (III) the third, posterior or posterior mesencephalic segment. The junction between the first and second segments is located at the most medial point in the course of the vein, anteriorly to the cerebral peduncle. The junction between the second and third segments lies at the level of the lateral mesencephalic sulcus, immediately anteriorly to the lateral mesencephalic vein (Figs. 114, 115). Tributaries of each segment are as follows:

I. First Segment

1. Deep middle cerebral vein and its insular tributaries
2. Inferior striate veins
3. Olfactory vein
4. Fronto-orbital veins
5. Anterior cerebral and pericallosal veins
6. Veinlets from the optic chiasm, optic tract and adjacent structures

II. Second Segment

1. Peduncular vein and its inferior thalamic tributaries
2. Inferior ventricular vein and its tributaries
3. Uncal cortical or other medial temporal cortical veins
4. Veinlets from the optic tract and adjacent structures

III. Third Segment

1. Lateral mesencephalic vein
2. Lateral atrial vein
3. Medial temporal and occipitotemporal cortical veins
4. Posterior longitudinal hippocampal vein
5. Posterior thalamic veins

These relationships are shown in diagrammatic form in Fig. 114.

I. First Segment of the Basal Cerebral Vein and Its Tributaries (Figs. 114–118, 122–126)

The first segment of the basal cerebral vein is formed by the union of the deep middle cerebral vein and the inferior striate veins on the undersurface of the anterior perforated substance. It runs medially, posteriorly and somewhat inferiorly, receiving the fronto-orbital, olfactory and anterior cerebral veins and also veinlets from the optic tract and adjacent structures. It runs above the uncus to reach the area where the optic tract, the anterior border of the cerebral peduncle and the superolateral margin of the recurved uncus are approximated. This is the most medial point in the course of the basal cerebral vein, where it is lying anteriorly to the cerebral peduncle. Beyond this point, the second segment of the vein begins by turning posterolaterally to pass around the brain stem.

1. Deep Middle Cerebral Vein

(WOLF and HUANG, 1963) (Figs. 114, 115, 124, 125, 128, 129)

Typically, the *precentral insular*, *central insular* and *posterior insular veins*, lying respectively in the precentral sulcus, central sulcus and posterior limiting sulcus of the insula, run downwards and forwards towards the pole of the insula, where they unite to form the deep middle cerebral vein. Unlike the other insular veins, the *anterior insular vein* takes a somewhat meandering course downwards in the anterior limiting sulcus, between the corrugated anterior surface of the insula and the opposing frontal operculum. At the level of the limen insulae, this anterior insular vein turns medially and posteriorly, to join the deep middle cerebral vein, medial to the point of union of the other insular veins. The posterior insular vein, which is usually the most prominent and constant of all the insular veins, takes a straight antero-inferior course in the lateral view. The exception is at its origin, where it takes a slightly curved course, convex postero-inferiorly.

A straight line extending posterosuperiorly from the straight portion of the posterior insular vein, intersects the internal cerebral vein at a point averaging 7 mm behind its midpoint. The origin of the posterior insular vein, however, is usually level with the midportion of the internal cerebral vein. The line extending upwards from the central insular vein intersects the internal cerebral vein about 1 cm behind the venous angle, which is located at the foramen of Monro. The precentral insular vein, on the other hand, when extended upwards, lies a short distance anteriorly to the venous angle (Figs. 124A, 129A).

In some cases, these insular veins may lie, not deep within the sulci, but on the surface of the long or short gyri of the insula (Fig. 115B). Furthermore, any or all of these veins may be replaced by laterally running veins that drain into the superficial middle cerebral, ascending cortical or descending cortical veins (Figs. 124A, 125B, 128).

2. Inferior Striate Veins

(ROSA and BORZONE, 1973; SCHLESINGER, 1939; STEPHENS and STILLWELL, 1969; WOLF *et al.*, 1955) (Figs. 114, 115, 122–124, 125B, 129–130, 131A, 132B)

The inferior striate veins, which drain the inferior part of the corpus striatum, converge towards the anterior perforated substance, where they join the deep middle cerebral vein. These veins, therefore, have, in the lateral view, a fan-shaped appearance with the apex pointing to the anterior perforated substance. In the anteroposterior view the central part of the fan, formed by the inferior striate veins, is convex laterally. Among them, one or two veins may be especially prominent. They originate from the anterior pole of the putamen and run postero-inferiorly in a somewhat arcuate fashion, convex laterally, to join the deep middle cerebral vein at the anterior perforated substance. In the lateral view, however, these long curved veins appear straight and course postero-inferiorly towards the anterior perforated substance. These veins belong to the anterocentral (or anteromedial) group of the inferior striate veins (WOLF and HUANG, 1963) (Figs. 125B, 130A). Although division of the superior striate veins into external and internal groups can be made with ease, division of the inferior striate veins is more difficult, since the former spread anteroposteriorly over a wide area, whereas the latter converge toward, a small area, the anterior perforated substance. Unlike their arterial counterparts (the lenticulostriate arteries), the inferior striate veins usually have no appreciable cisternal segments, between the point of emergence from the brain substance and the point of entry into the deep middle cerebral vein. Even when prominent, the cisternal segments may easily escape detection on angiograms, since, like the first segment of the basal cerebral vein, they are intimately attached to the undersurface of the anterior perforated substance. In these cases, the parenchymal segments of the inferior striate veins appear to join directly the deep middle cerebral vein in both lateral and anteroposterior views, on the angiogram.

3. Olfactory Vein

(BROWNING, 1884; HUANG and WOLF, 1974)
(Figs. 114, 116, 117, 118, 120, 125A, 126, 129, 131A, 132A)

The olfactory vein originates in the olfactory sulcus above the olfactory bulb, and runs backwards and upwards in the depths of the sulcus (first or ascending fissural segment). It then runs backwards and downwards, leaving the olfactory sulcus either medially or laterally to the olfactory trigone (second or descending fissural segment). After emerging from the sulcus and running around the inferior aspect of the olfactory stria, which is located a short distance above the tuberculum sellae, the vein passes upwards on the postero-inferior aspect of the frontal lobe, to reach the anterior perforated substance, where it joins the deep middle cerebral, the fronto-orbital or the anterior cerebral vein (third or retrofissural segment) (Figs. 126, 131A). Although the olfactory vein usually runs backwards to join the first segment of the basal cerebral vein, in some cases a vein in the olfactory sulcus may drain anteriorly to join a frontopolar or an ascending frontal cortical vein.

4. Fronto-Orbital Veins
(BEKOV, 1965; WOLF *et al.*, 1963) (Figs. 114, 115, 117, 124, 128, 131A, 132A)

The fronto-orbital veins begin on the orbital surface of the frontal lobe, usually in or adjacent to the H-shaped sulci and most frequently from the medial orbital sulcus (medial orbital vein). They pass backwards, around the inferior and posterior borders of the postorbital lobule, to reach the anterior perforated substance, where they join the deep middle cerebral vein, the olfactory vein or the sphenoparietal sinus.

5. Anterior Cerebral and Pericallosal Veins
(BEAU and RABISCHONG, 1959; BEKOV, 1965; BEN AMOR and WACKENHEIM, 1973; WOLF and HUANG, 1963) (Figs. 114, 116A, 117, 118, 120, 122–125A, 126, 128, 131A, 133A)

Anteriorly, the pericallosal vein lies in the sulcus of the corpus callosum, adjacent to the anterior cerebral artery and joins the inferior sagittal sinus directly or the superior sagittal sinus indirectly, through a medial cortical vein or veins (supracallosal segment). Likewise, the portion of the pericallosal vein running around the genu of the corpus callosum (genual segment) may travel upwards or forwards to open into one of the sagittal sinuses. It may, however, pass postero-inferiorly on the medial aspect of the subcallosal gyrus, anterior to the lamina terminalis (terminal segment).
Not infrequently, tributaries originating from the rostral and inferior rostral sulci (horizontal sulci lying immediately anteriorly to the paraterminal body or the parolfactory area), converge posteriorly and form a single trunk, the *paraterminal vein.* This vein continues backwards and joins the distal end of the anterior cerebral vein, or the terminal segment of the pericallosal vein usually at the level of the lower border of the subcallosal gyrus. Before turning laterally onto the inferior aspect of the cerebral hemisphere, behind the medial olfactory stria, the terminal segment of the pericallosal vein communicates with its fellow of the opposite side, through the *anterior communicating vein.* The vein beyond this point is known as the anterior cerebral vein. It runs laterally to reach the anterior perforated substance and joins the deep middle cerebral vein or the olfactory vein.

6. Veinlets from the Optic Chiasm, Optic Tract and Adjacent Structures
(BEKOV, 1965)

As it runs posteromedially, the basal cerebral vein receives tributaries from the optic tract, the mammillary body, the infundibulum and adjacent structures. Because of their small size, these veins are, in general, useful only rarely in pathologic cases.
The *premammillary veins* drain the antero-inferior part of the thalamus and the hypothalamus. These veins emerge from the area lateral and anterior to the mammillary body, medial to the optic tract (Figs. 117, 118, 120). Although these veins most frequently join the posterior part of the first segment of the basal cerebral vein, not infrequently they open into the beginning of the second segment or its peduncular tributary (Figs. 122C, 122D, 125B).

II. Second Segment of the Basal Cerebral Vein and Its Tributaries
(Figs. 114–118, 120, 121, 124, 125, 127, 128)

The second segment of the basal cerebral vein begins above the recurved uncus, immediately anteriorly to the cerebral peduncle. There it receives the peduncular vein and then runs posterolaterally, between the anterolateral aspect of the cerebral peduncle and the posteromedial aspect of the recurved uncus. Immediately behind the uncus, the inferior ventricular vein joins the second segment, at the most lateral point in the course of the basal cerebral vein around the brainstem. The second segment then turns posteromedially and superiorly to reach the lateral mesencephalic sulcus, where it becomes continuous with the third segment.

1. Peduncular Vein
(BEKOV, 1965; HUANG and WOLF, 1974)
(Figs. 114–118, 122, 124B, 125B, 129B, 130, 134A)

The peduncular vein, also called the interpeduncular vein, receives numerous inferior thalamic tributaries. After emerging from the interpeduncular fossa, the vein runs laterally around the anterior aspect of the cerebral peduncle, to open into the beginning of the second segment of the basal cerebral vein. The peduncular vein frequently communicates with that of the opposite side through the *posterior communicating vein* (Figs. 115, 116, 130B). In contrast to the anterior communicating vein, the posterior communicating vein may be quite large and often communicates inferiorly with the anterior pontomesencephalic vein, in the interpeduncular fossa (Fig. 130).

2. Inferior Ventricular Vein
(WOLF and HUANG, 1964) (Figs. 114, 119, 121, 122, 127)

The inferior ventricular vein is formed by the union of the inferior ventricular subependymal, temporal tip subependymal, anterior hippocampal, anterior longitudinal hippocampal, and uncal cortical or other medial temporal cortical veins.

The *inferior ventricular subependymal vein* originates in the region of the lateral wall of the body or the anterior wall of the atrium of the lateral ventricle. It takes an arcuate course downwards and forwards running on the anterior aspect of the atrium and in the roof of the temporal horn, usually lying laterally to the tail of the caudate nucleus (the transverse caudate tributary). At the level of the inferior end of the choroid fissure, the inferior ventricular subependymal vein turns medially. After receiving the temporal tip subependymal vein, it crosses, medially, the tail of the caudate nucleus and again receives a vein running adjacent to the stria terminalis (the *terminal vein*) (Fig. 122A). These transverse caudate and terminal tributaries of the inferior ventricular subependymal vein correspond to the lateral and medial tributaries of the temporal horn described by WACKENHEIM and his coworkers (BEN AMOR and WACKENHEIM, 1973). The inferior ventricular subependymal vein then passes above (or deep to) the stria terminalis, lamina affixa and tenia choroidea and is joined by a small inferior choroidal vein before leaving the temporal horn.

The combined venous trunk, the inferior ventricular vein, continues medially, receiving the *anterior longitudinal hippocampal* and *anterior hippocampal veins*, before opening into the basal cerebral vein, usually at the most lateral point in its course around the cerebral peduncle.

The venous drainage of the midportion of the hippocampal formation is by the *transverse hippocampal subependymal veins*, emerging from the fimbrio-dentate sulcus, and transverse hippocampal pial veins, arising from the depths of the hippocampal sulcus (WOLF and HUANG, 1964). These veins join, at right angles, the anterior longitudinal hippocampal vein which runs forwards along the medial aspect of the corrugated dentate gyrus, to open into the stem of the inferior ventricular vein, often together with the anterior hippocampal vein (Figs. 114, 122A–B, 128).

The anterior part of the hippocampal formation (pes hippocampi) is drained by the *anterior hippocampal vein* (HUANG and WOLF, 1974). This vein, which originates from the depths of the digitations and pes of the hippocampus, runs posterosuperiorly and medially in the anterior hippocampal sulcus, below the recurved uncus (the uncal portion of the hippocampal sulcus). It joins either the stem of the inferior ventricular vein or, in some cases, the basal cerebral vein near its junction with the inferior ventricular vein. Not infrequently, one or more *uncal cortical veins* join the basal cerebral vein or the inferior ventricular vein in this region. One should not, however, confuse these uncal cortical veins, which ramify on the surface of the uncal cortex, with the usually designated uncal vein (WOLF *et al.*, 1963), which is always located anteriorly to the uncus. The location of the stem of the inferior ventricular vein and the course of its anterior hippocampal tributary are important angiographically, since they determine respectively, the site of the inferior end of the choroid fissure (the inferior choroidal point) and the location of the anterior hippocampal sulcus. The latter marks the postero-inferior border of the recurved uncus (Figs. 117, 122, 124A, 125A, 128, 131A).

III. Third Segment of the Basal Cerebral Vein and Its Tributaries
(Figs. 114, 115, 117, 120–122, 130, 131)

The third segment begins in the region of the lateral mesencephalic sulcus where it receives the lateral mesencephalic vein (HOCHSTETTER, 1938; LAINE *et al.*, 1956; WACKENHEIM and BRAUN, 1970) (Figs. 114, 115, 117, 121, 122, 130, 131). The vein runs posteromedially and superiorly, receiving numerous fine posterior thalamic tributaries and the medial temporal or occipitotemporal cortical veins, to join the great cerebral vein or the posterior part of the internal cerebral vein. The lateral atrial vein and the posterior longitudinal hippocampal vein may join this segment.

Other veins which may open into the third segment are the medial atrial, internal occipital, splenial and rarely the precentral cerebellar, superior vermian, medial posterior thalamic, superior thalamic and pineal veins.

1. Lateral Mesencephalic Vein
(HOCHSTETTER, 1938; LAINE *et al.*, 1956; WACKENHEIM and BRAUN, 1970)
(Figs. 114, 115, 117, 121, 122, 130, 131)

The lateral mesencephalic vein, running in the lateral mesencephalic sulcus, may drain either upwards to join the basal cerebral or posterior mesencephalic vein (*ascending lateral mesencephalic vein*), or downwards to open into the brachial tributary of the petrosal vein (*de-*

scending lateral mesencephalic vein). More often, however, it serves as an anastomosis between a supratentorial vein (the basal cerebral vein) and an infratentorial vein (the petrosal vein). This *anastomotic lateral mesencephalic vein*, observed for the first time in cerebral angiograms by WOLF, HUANG and NEWMAN in 1963, may be divided into three segments: (1) a supratentorial segment, running transversely below the medial geniculate body and above the parahippocampal gyrus to join the basal cerebral vein; (2) a mesencephalic segment, located in or adjacent to the lateral mesencephalic sulcus; and (3) an infratentorial segment, running forwards on the superior and anterior aspects of the brachium pontis. This last segment is the brachial tributary of the petrosal vein (Figs. 114, 131).

2. Lateral Atrial Vein

(LAINE *et al.*, 1956; PATURET, 1964; WOLF and HUANG, 1964) (Figs. 114, 122A)

The lateral atrial vein is a variant of the inferior ventricular vein. It originates on the lateral wall of the atrium and runs forwards in the roof of the temporal horn. At some distance behind the inferior choroidal point, the vein turns medially, crossing the undersurface of the tail of the caudate nucleus and passing deep to or above the stria terminalis, lamina affixa and tenia choroidea and it joins the third segment of the basal cerebral vein.

3. Medial Temporal and Occipitotemporal Cortical Veins

(Figs. 114, 120, 122, 128)

The medial temporal cortical vein begins on the undersurface of the midtemporal lobe, frequently from the region of the collateral or occipitotemporal sulcus, and runs medially and superiorly, to join the basal cerebral vein. The occipitotemporal cortical vein originates more posteriorly from the lingual or occipitotemporal gyrus or from the adjacent sulcus. It runs anteriorly and medially to open into the posterior part of the basal cerebral vein, directly or indirectly, through the stem of the medial atrial or internal occipital veins.

4. Posterior Longitudinal Hippocampal Vein

(HUANG and WOLF, 1974; WOLF and HUANG, 1964) (Figs. 114, 122)

The posterior longitudinal hippocampal vein receives, at right angles, the short, fine tributaries emerging from the posterior part of the hippocampal sulcus. It runs posteromedially and superiorly, along the medial aspect of the dentate gyrus, to open into the stem of the medial atrial vein or, in rare instances, directly into the posterior part of the basal cerebral vein.

5. Posterior Thalamic Veins

(GIUDICELLI and SALAMON, 1970) (Figs. 114B, 121A, 122C, 268C)

The posterior thalamic veins are fine short veins which drain the postero-inferior part of the thalamus and adjacent structures. They enter the posterior part of the basal cerebral or posterior mesencephalic vein. The medial aspect of the pulvinar is, however, usually drained by the superior thalamic vein or the medial posterior thalamic (or superior pineal) vein, which open into the internal cerebral, the great cerebral or, in rare instances, the basal cerebral vein.

B. Anatomic Variations

According to PADGET (1957), the primitive telencephalic, diencephalic and mesencephalic veins drain posterolaterally into a tentorial sinus in the early stages of embryonic life. With elongation and attenuation of this tentorial sinus, due to posterior expansion of the cerebral hemisphere, a shorter, more direct venous channel is formed by secondary longitudinal anastomoses of the deep telencephalic vein, the ventral diencephalic vein, the mesencephalic vein and also the dorsal diencephalic tributary of the internal cerebral vein or the superior mesencephalic tributary of the great cerebral vein. The basal cerebral vein, thus formed, drains posteromedially and superiorly to join the Galenic venous system. The posterolateral drainage of these veins into the lateral sinus, seen in the chicken, cat, horse and dog, is therefore phylogenetically a less advanced form of venous drainage, than the posteromedial drainage into the Galenic venous system seen in the human (PADGET, 1957).

Because of the complicated processes involved in the development of the basal cerebral vein, it is not surprising to see numerous anatomic variations of this vein (BABIN, 1971; HUANG and WOLF, 1974; STEPHENS and STILWELL, 1969; WOLF *et al.*, 1963). These are frequently encountered in cerebral angiograms and are to be expected (Figs. 129–137). The basal cerebral vein may drain into the posterior portion of the internal cerebral vein, instead of the more usual opening into the great cerebral vein (Fig. 133A). It may join the anterior, middle, or posterior portion of the straight sinus, either directly or indirectly through a tentorial sinus (Figs. 114D, 132A). Not infrequently, a combination of posteromedial drainage on one side and posterolateral drainage on the other side may be observed. When the primitive metencephalic vein is involved in the formation of the basal cerebral vein, the latter vein may communicate with posterior fossa veins through the anastomotic lateral mesencephalic vein and/or the anterior pontomesencephalic vein (HUANG *et al.*, 1968; HUANG and WOLF, 1974) (Figs. 114, 130, 131, 133A, 134B–C). In rare cases in which the primitive myelencephalic vein is also involved, the anterior pontomesencephalic vein may connect further inferiorly with the anterior medullary vein and drain into the inferior end of the inferior petrosal sinus or into the circular sinus, around the foramen magnum (Fig. 118). [DUVERNOY (1975), STEPHENS and STILLWELL (1969).]

The previously described posterior mesencephalic vein (HUANG and WOLF, 1965), which originates from the mesencephalon and runs posteriorly to join the posterior part of the internal cerebral or great cerebral vein, is a variant of the second and third segments, or of only the third segment, of the basal cerebral vein. This posterior mesencephalic vein may replace the basal cerebral vein or may be present in addition to a complete form of this vein. In the latter case, the posterior mesencephalic vein may be more appropriately called the *accessory basal cerebral vein.* In rare instances, several accessory posterior mesencephalic veins may be observed (Fig. 131A).

Failure of anastomosis between the first and second segments of the basal cerebral vein may result in formation of a prominent uncal vein (BEKOV, 1965; WOLF *et al.*, 1963). The *uncal vein,* which may also be called the medial vallecular vein (HUANG *et al.*, 1975) or, more precisely, the preuncal vein, drains forwards and downwards to open into the cavernous or paracavernous sinus, anteriorly to the rhinal sulcus (Figs. 114, 129, 133). When part of the third segment fails to participate in the development of the basal cerebral vein, the first and second segments may drain infratentorially into the petrosal vein, through the anastomotic lateral mesencephalic vein (Fig. 131A). The anastomotic lateral mesencephalic vein may also connect the third segment of the basal cerebral vein with the petrosal venous system (Fig. 131B). The inferior ventricular vein, with or without the first segment of the basal cerebral vein, may drain via the anastomotic lateral mesencephalic vein into the straight sinus, the lateral sinus, or the superior petrosal sinus (Figs. 130, 131A, 132A, 133). In rare instances, in which the stem of the petrosal vein is absent, its tributaries may drain upwards and backwards into the Galenic system via the brachial, anastomotic lateral mesencephalic and posterior mesencephalic veins (Fig. 134B). In some cases, the first segment of the basal cerebral vein may drain into the second and third segments of the basal cerebral vein of the opposite side, via the posterior communicating vein (Fig. 134A). Through the latter vein, the anterior part of the basal cerebral vein may, in some instances, open into the uncal vein of the opposite side. Rarely observed is a prominent longitudinal hippocampal vein, replacing the usual basal cerebral vein (WOLF and HUANG, 1964). The former vein usually runs posteromedially and superiorly to join the stem of the medial atrial vein and open into the posterior portion of the internal cerebral vein. An unusual connection between the basal cerebral vein and the sphenoparietal sinus (WOLF *et al.*, 1963), and a rare form of drainage of the superior thalamic vein into the basal cerebral vein or into the posterior fossa venous system through the anastomotic lateral mesencephalic vein, have also been observed (Fig. 134C).

A communication between the dorsal pharyngeal tributary of the pro-otic sinus and a facial tributary of the primitive maxillary vein, at the level of the foramen ovale or the accessory sphenoidal foramen, becomes the sphenoidal or accessory sphenoidal emissary vein, allowing anastomosis between the cavernous sinus and the extracranial pterygoid plexus (PADGET, 1957). The anterior part of the basal cerebral vein or the uncal vein, therefore, may drain extracranially through these foramina of the middle fossa (HUANG and WOLF, 1974; WOLF *et al.*, 1963).

Major anatomic variations of the basal cerebral vein are diagramatically illustrated in Figs. 135–137.

Fig. 114A. Normal anatomy and variations of the basal cerebral vein and its tributaries, submentovertical view
Covered portions are indicated by dashed lines.
On the left (reader's right), the major part of the temporal lobe has been removed to show the undersurface of the insula and the temporal horn of the lateral ventricle, to illustrate a complete form of the basal cerebral vein. On the right (reader's left), a fragmented form of basal cerebral vein, with each venous stem draining independently, is shown. The first (1), second (2) and third segments (3) of the basal cerebral vein, the anterocentral group of the inferior striate veins (arrow), and the premammillary veins (arrowhead) are indicated. (Courtesy of HUANG and WOLF, 1974. C.V. MOSBY Co)

Fig. 114B. Normal anatomy of the basal cerebral vein and its tributaries, lateral view
The drawing, showing a parasagital section of the cerebral hemisphere at the level of the anterior perforated substance, illustrates the relationships of the Sylvian vallecula to the midline chiasmatic, interpeduncular and pontine cisterns. The dural sinuses are shaded. The anterior portion of the basal cerebral vein drains forwards and downwards as the uncal (or medial vallecular) vein. The anterior cerebral vein (arrow) receives the terminal segment of the anterior pericallosal vein and the paraterminal vein. A rather typical obtuse angle is formed between the stem of the paraterminal vein and the anterior cerebral vein. The anterior communicating vein is often located in this area – usually 1 or 2 mm behind the apex of this obtuse angle. From the practical point of view, the apex of this angle may therefore be considered the site of the anterior communicating vein. More posteriorly, the basal cerebral vein communicates with the veins of the posterior fossa through the anterior pontomesencephalic and anastomotic lateral mesencephalic veins. The first (1), second (2) and third segments (3) of the basal cerebral vein, anterior hippocampal vein (a), anterior longitudinal hippocampal vein (b), anterior cerebral vein (arrow) and posterior thalamic veins (arrowhead) are indicated

Figs. 114A and 114B see pp. 134–135

Fig. 114C. Normal anatomy and variations of the basal cerebral vein and its tributaries, semiaxial view
On the right (reader's left), a complete form of the basal cerebral vein is illustrated. On the left (reader's right), the first segment of the basal cerebral vein drains forwards and downwards as the uncal (or medial vallecular) vein, whereas the second and third segments of the vein drain posteromedially and superiorly to join the great cerebral vein. 1, 2, and 3 indicate the first, second and third segments of the basal cerebral vein

Fig. 114D. Variations in the course of the basal cerebral vein within the tentorium (tentorial sinuses)
On the left (reader's right), part of the tentorium and temporal lobe have been removed to illustrate the course of the anterior portion of the basal cerebral vein and its tributaries. Posteriorly, it runs within the tentorium and joins the straight sinus or lateral sinus at variable points. The first (1), second (2) and third segments (3) of the basal cerebral vein and the premammillary veins (↨) are labelled.
On the right (reader's left), the superficial Sylvian vein runs posteriorly and opens into a tentorial sinus, which in turn joins either the lateral or straight sinus. The first segment (1) of the basal cerebral vein drains antero-inferiorly, as the uncal vein. The second segment (2), receiving the peduncular, inferior ventricular and lateral atrial veins, drains infratentorially into the superior petrosal sinus via the anastomotic lateral mesencephalic vein. Two posterior mesencephalic veins, derived from the third segment (3), form a common stem with the medial atrial vein and open into the posterior portion of the basal cerebral vein. The anterocentral group of the inferior striate veins is also labelled on the right (↑)

Figs. 114C and 114D see pp. 136–137 ▷

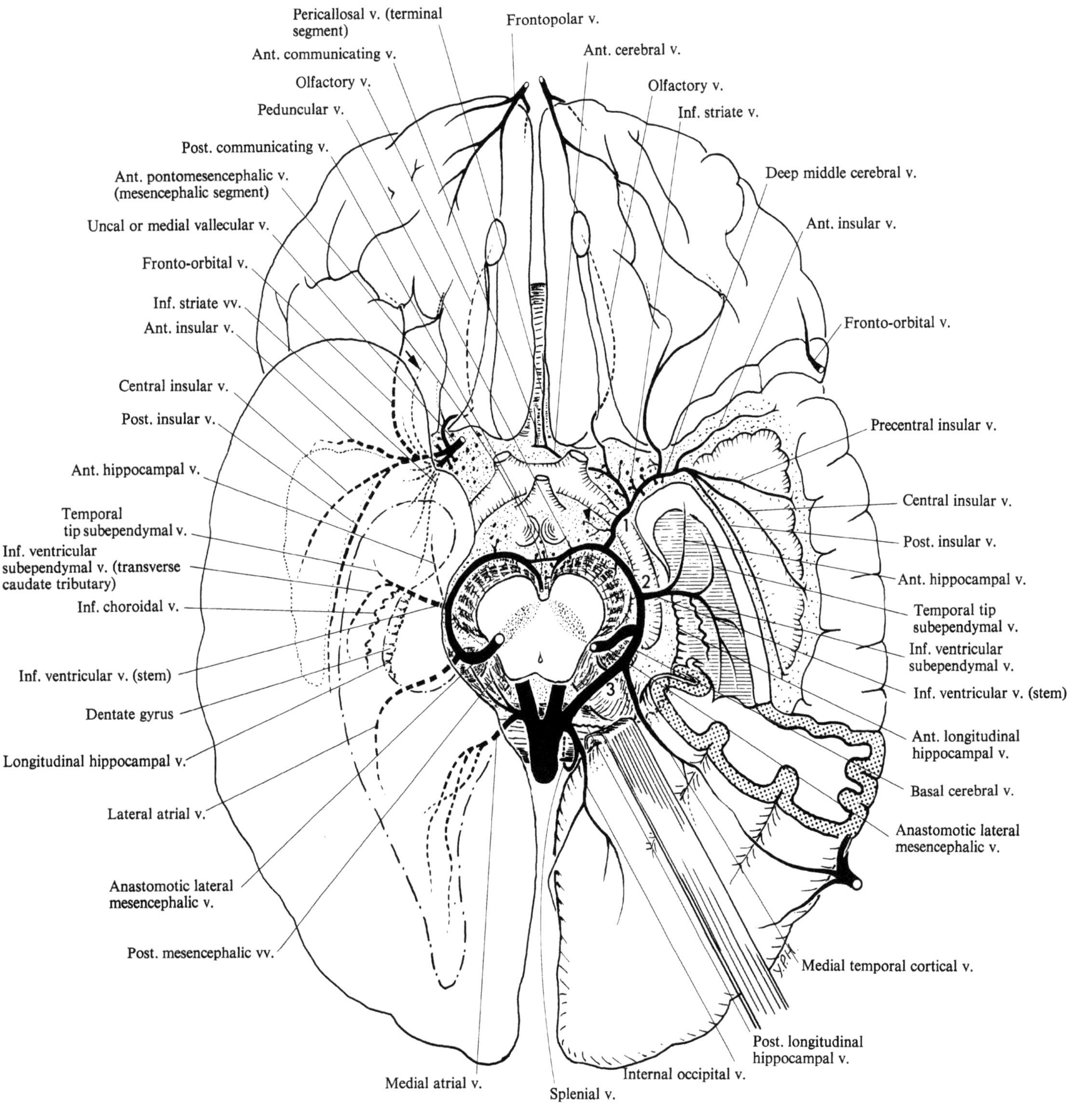

Pericallosal v. (terminal segment)
Frontopolar v.
Ant. communicating v.
Ant. cerebral v.
Olfactory v.
Olfactory v.
Peduncular v.
Inf. striate v.
Post. communicating v.
Ant. pontomesencephalic v. (mesencephalic segment)
Deep middle cerebral v.
Uncal or medial vallecular v.
Ant. insular v.
Fronto-orbital v.
Inf. striate vv.
Fronto-orbital v.
Ant. insular v.
Central insular v.
Precentral insular v.
Post. insular v.
Ant. hippocampal v.
Central insular v.
Temporal tip subependymal v.
Post. insular v.
Inf. ventricular subependymal v. (transverse caudate tributary)
Ant. hippocampal v.
Inf. choroidal v.
Temporal tip subependymal v.
Inf. ventricular subependymal v.
Inf. ventricular v. (stem)
Inf. ventricular v. (stem)
Dentate gyrus
Ant. longitudinal hippocampal v.
Longitudinal hippocampal v.
Basal cerebral v.
Lateral atrial v.
Anastomotic lateral mesencephalic v.
Anastomotic lateral mesencephalic v.
Post. mesencephalic vv.
Medial temporal cortical v.
Post. longitudinal hippocampal v.
Medial atrial v.
Internal occipital v.
Splenial v.
1
2
3
Y.P.H.

Fig. 114A

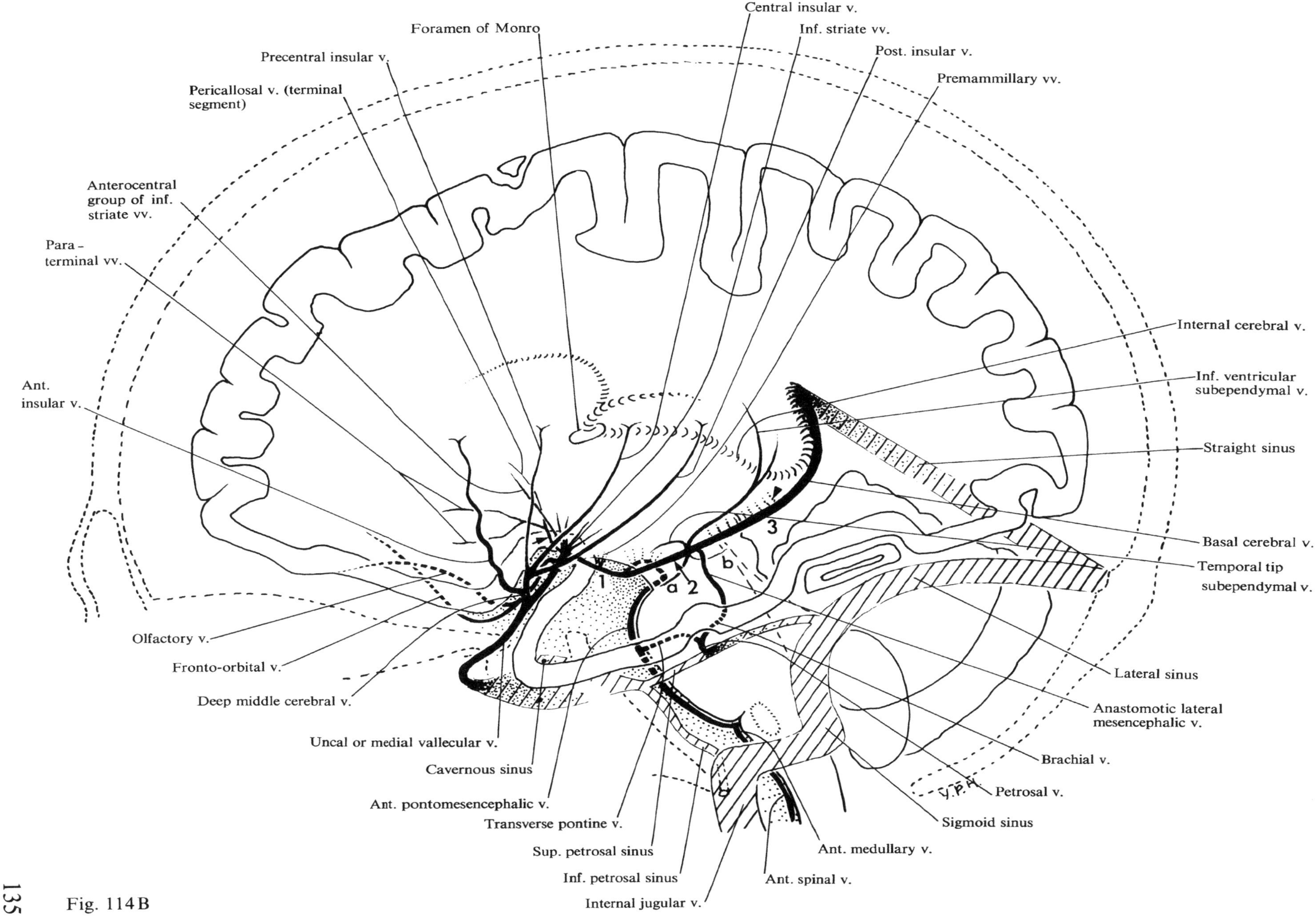
Foramen of Monro
Central insular v.
Inf. striate vv.
Post. insular v.
Premammillary vv.
Precentral insular v.
Pericallosal v. (terminal segment)
Anterocentral group of inf. striate vv.
Para-terminal vv.
Ant. insular v.
Internal cerebral v.
Inf. ventricular subependymal v.
Straight sinus
Basal cerebral v.
Temporal tip subependymal v.
Lateral sinus
Anastomotic lateral mesencephalic v.
Brachial v.
Petrosal v.
Sigmoid sinus
Ant. medullary v.
Ant. spinal v.
Internal jugular v.
Inf. petrosal sinus
Sup. petrosal sinus
Transverse pontine v.
Ant. pontomesencephalic v.
Cavernous sinus
Uncal or medial vallecular v.
Deep middle cerebral v.
Fronto-orbital v.
Olfactory v.
1
2
3
a
b

Fig. 114 B

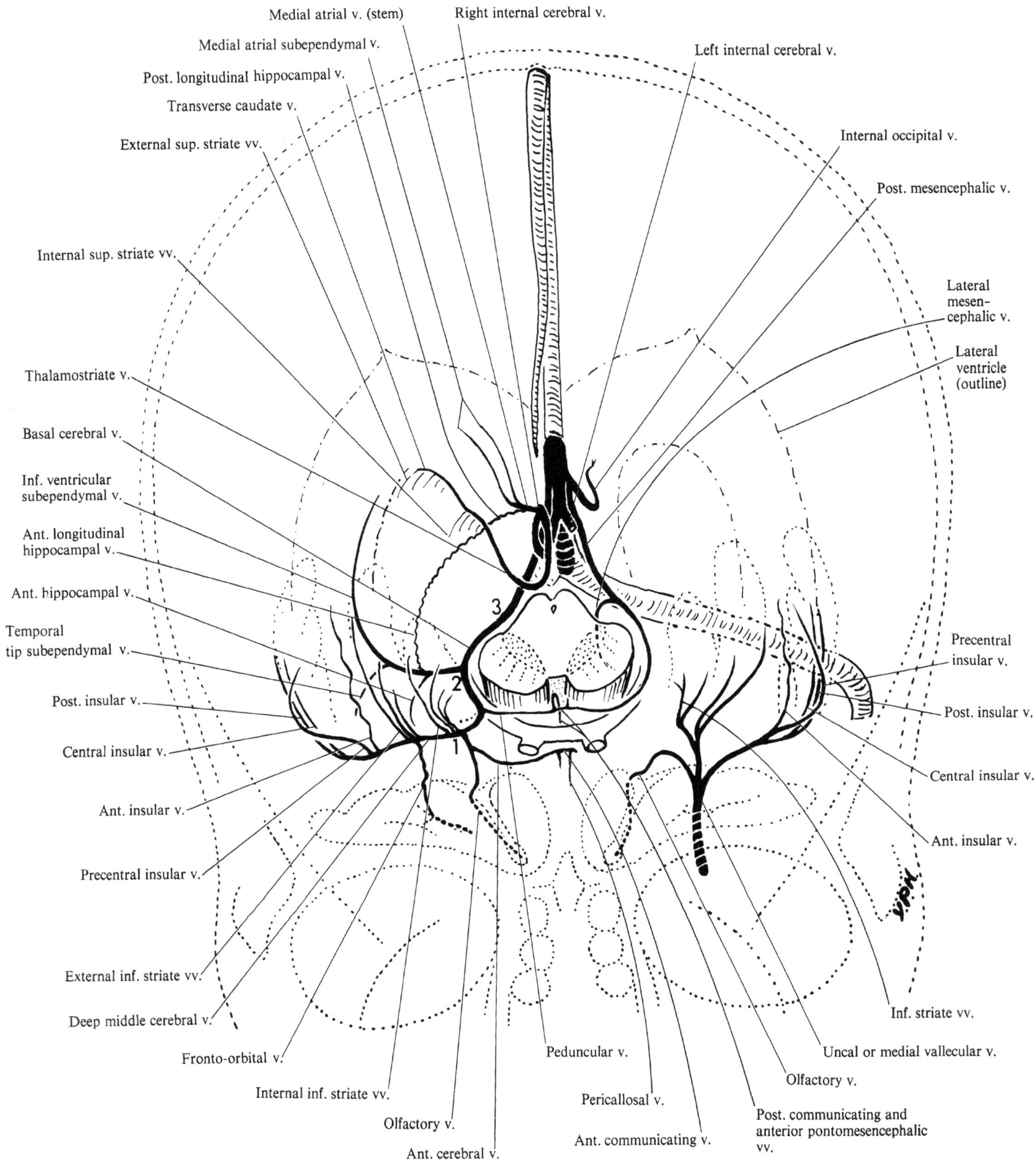

Medial atrial v. (stem)
Right internal cerebral v.
Medial atrial subependymal v.
Left internal cerebral v.
Post. longitudinal hippocampal v.
Transverse caudate v.
Internal occipital v.
External sup. striate vv.
Post. mesencephalic v.
Internal sup. striate vv.
Lateral mesen-cephalic v.
Lateral ventricle (outline)
Thalamostriate v.
Basal cerebral v.
Inf. ventricular subependymal v.
Ant. longitudinal hippocampal v.
Ant. hippocampal v.
Temporal tip subependymal v.
Precentral insular v.
Post. insular v.
Post. insular v.
Central insular v.
Central insular v.
Ant. insular v.
Ant. insular v.
Precentral insular v.
External inf. striate vv.
Deep middle cerebral v.
Inf. striate vv.
Fronto-orbital v.
Peduncular v.
Uncal or medial vallecular v.
Olfactory v.
Internal inf. striate vv.
Pericallosal v.
Olfactory v.
Post. communicating and anterior pontomesencephalic vv.
Ant. communicating v.
Ant. cerebral v.
1
2
3

Fig. 114C

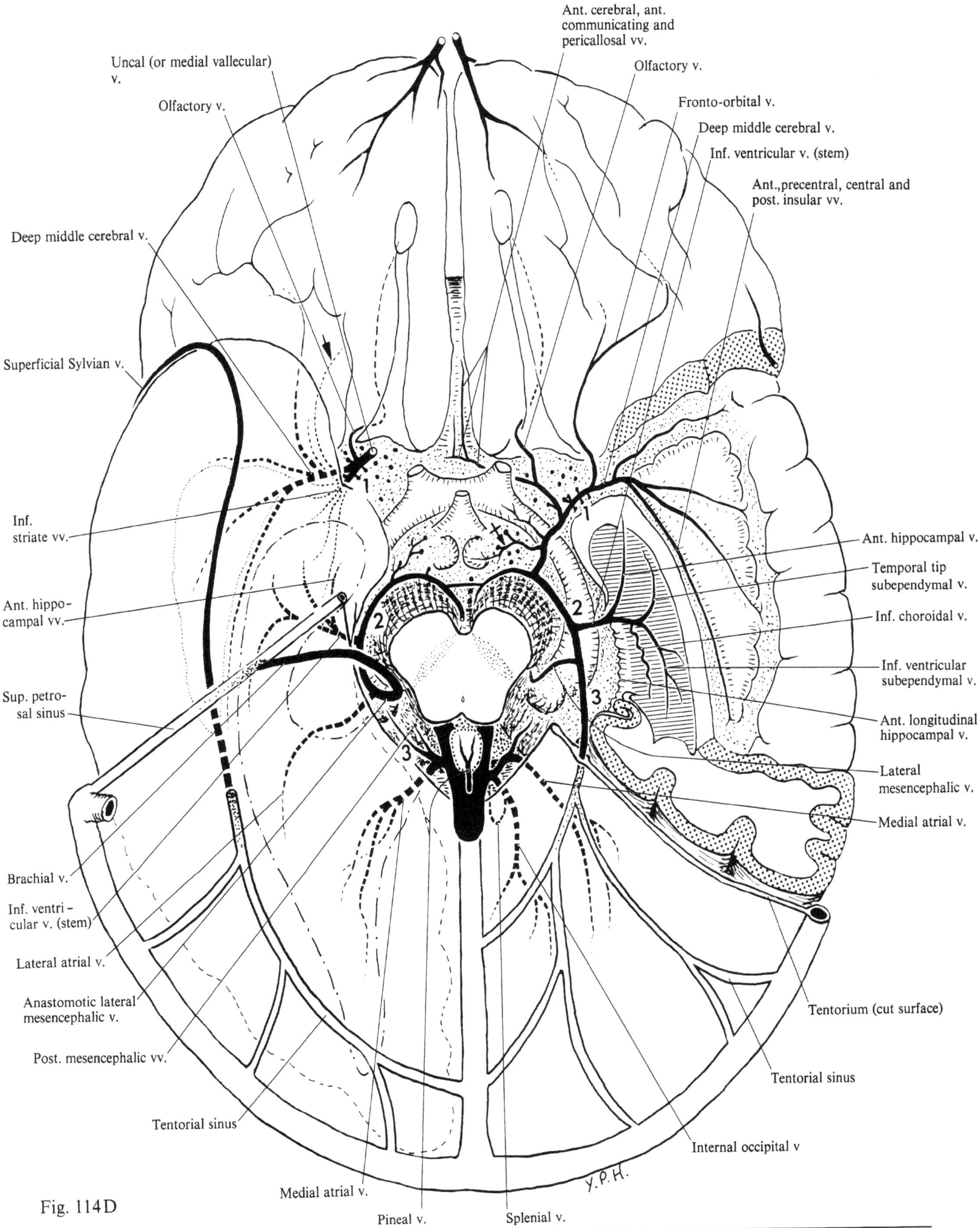
Ant. cerebral, ant. communicating and pericallosal vv.
Uncal (or medial vallecular) v.
Olfactory v.
Olfactory v.
Fronto-orbital v.
Deep middle cerebral v.
Inf. ventricular v. (stem)
Ant.,precentral, central and post. insular vv.
Deep middle cerebral v.
Superficial Sylvian v.
Inf. striate vv.
Ant. hippocampal v.
Temporal tip subependymal v.
Ant. hippo-campal vv.
Inf. choroidal v.
Inf. ventricular subependymal v.
Sup. petro-sal sinus
Ant. longitudinal hippocampal v.
Lateral mesencephalic v.
Medial atrial v.
Brachial v.
Inf. ventri-cular v. (stem)
Lateral atrial v.
Anastomotic lateral mesencephalic v.
Tentorium (cut surface)
Post. mesencephalic vv.
Tentorial sinus
Tentorial sinus
Internal occipital v
Medial atrial v.
Pineal v.
Splenial v.
1
1
2
2
3
3
3
Y.P.H.

Fig. 114D

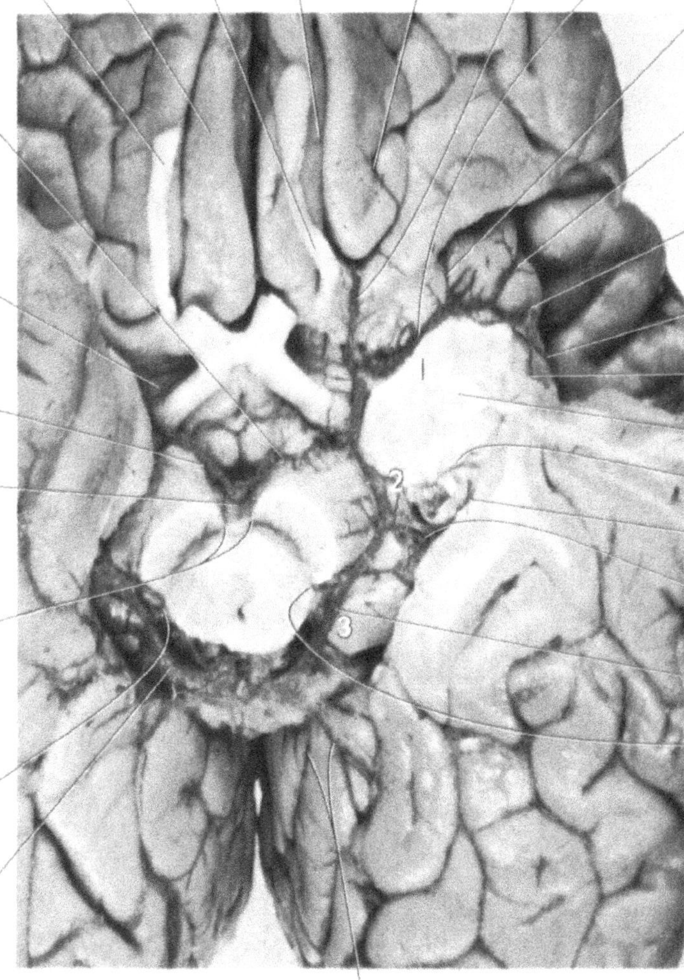

Fig. 115A. Anatomic specimen showing the course of the basal cerebral vein, view from below
On the left (reader's right), the anterior portion of the temporal lobe has been removed to show the entire course of the basal cerebral vein. The roof of the tip of the temporal horn of the lateral ventricle is also exposed

▷

Fig. 115B. Anatomic specimen showing the course of the basal cerebral vein. Same specimen as in Fig. 115A, view from below and from the left. The brain stem and cerebellum are, however, left intact

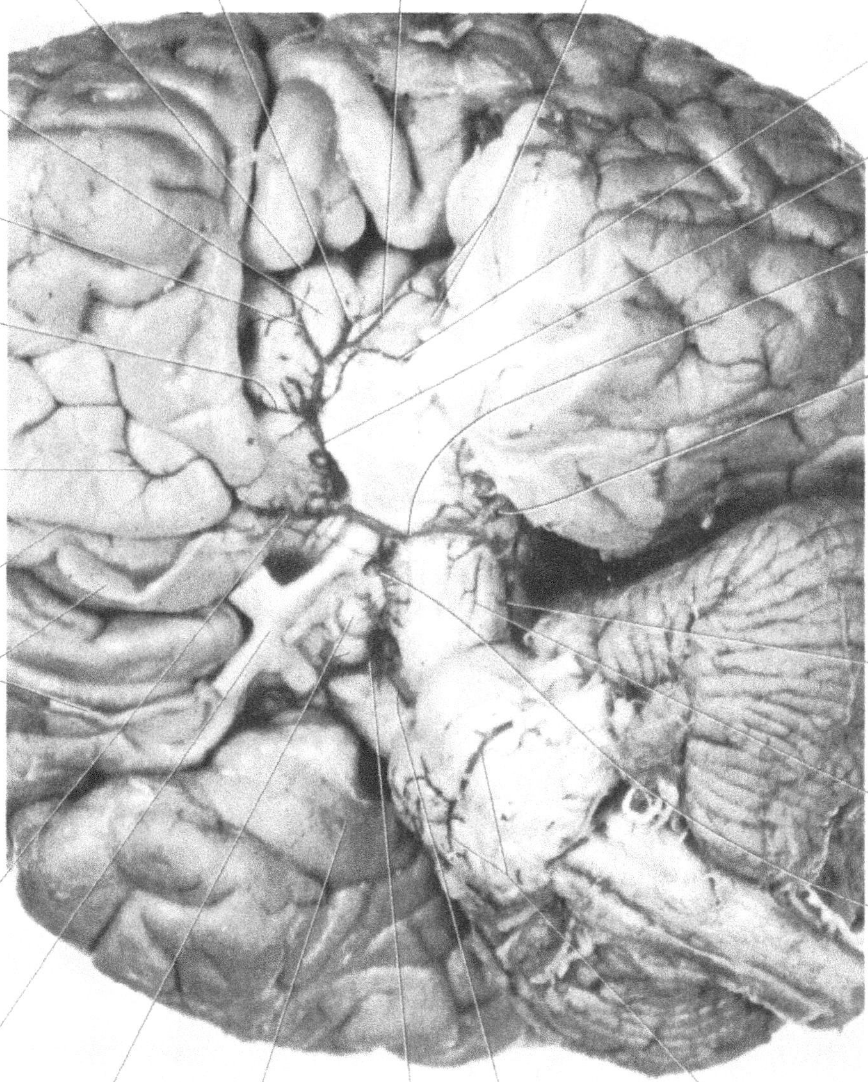

Fig. 115B

Fig. 116A. Anatomic specimen showing the course of the olfactory vein, view from below
Part of the medial orbital gyrus, or the lateral wall of the olfactory sulcus, has been removed to expose the olfactory vein on the left. The tip of the temporal lobe has been removed. The deep and superficial olfactory veins unite posteriorly to form a single trunk which in turn runs backwards to join the first segment of the basal cerebral vein (⇞). The major drainage of the olfactory vein is, however, into the sphenoparietal sinus through a prominent communicating vein (row of arrowheads)

Fig. 116B. Anatomic specimen showing the course of the olfactory vein. Same specimen as in Fig. 116A, view from below and from the left. The lateral wall of the olfactory sulcus and the tip of the temporal lobe have been removed, to expose the entire course of the olfactory vein.

Figs. 116A and 116B see pp. 140–141 ▷

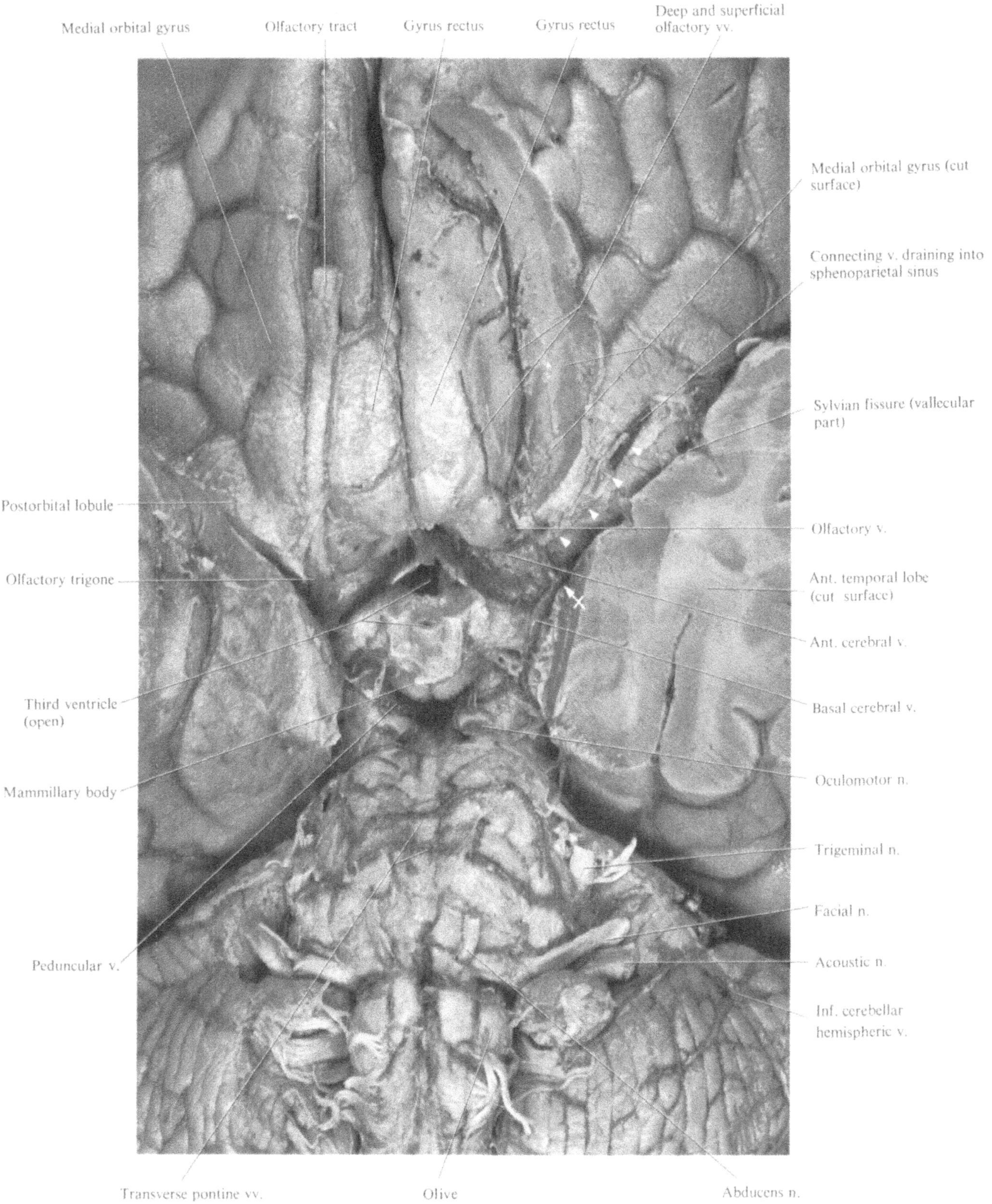
Medial orbital gyrus
Olfactory tract
Gyrus rectus
Gyrus rectus
Deep and superficial olfactory vv.
Medial orbital gyrus (cut surface)
Connecting v. draining into sphenoparietal sinus
Sylvian fissure (vallecular part)
Postorbital lobule
Olfactory v.
Olfactory trigone
Ant. temporal lobe (cut surface)
Ant. cerebral v.
Third ventricle (open)
Basal cerebral v.
Oculomotor n.
Mammillary body
Trigeminal n.
Facial n.
Peduncular v.
Acoustic n.
Inf. cerebellar hemispheric v.
Transverse pontine vv.
Olive
Abducens n.

Fig. 116A

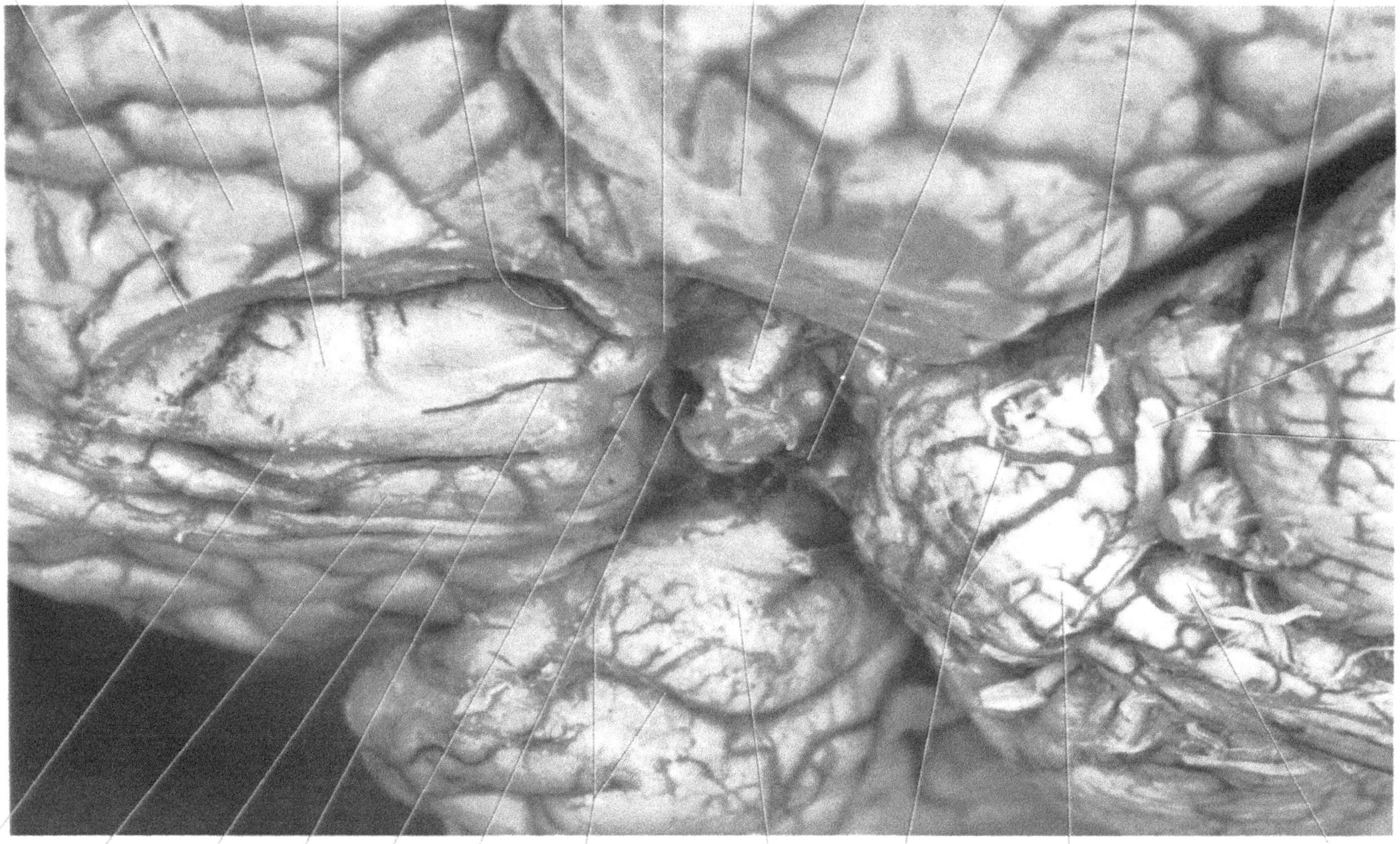
Medial wall of the olfactory sulcus
Medial orbital gyrus (cut surface)
Deep olfactory v. (second segment)
Connecting v. draining into sphenoparietal sinus
Ant. temporal lobe (cut surface)
Medial orbital gyrus
Deep olfactory v. (first segment)
Olfactory v. (third segment)
Optic tract
Peduncular vv.
Trigeminal n.
Inf. cerebellar hemispheric v.
Facial n.
Acoustic n.
Interhemi- spheric fissure
Gyrus rectus
Olfactory tract
Superficial olfactory v.
Post. wall of gyrus rectus
Third ventricle (open)
Vv. in the rhinal sulcus
Uncus
Transverse pontine vv.
Abducens n.
Olive

Fig. 116 B

Fig. 117. Anatomic specimen showing the course of the anterior cerebral, peduncular and posterior communicating veins, view from below
The optic chiasm and part of the optic tract have been removed, exposing the third ventricle at the level of the optic and infundibular recesses

Fig. 118. Anatomic specimen showing the anomalous anterior pontomesencephalic vein, draining the first segment of the basal cerebral vein into the posterior fossa, view from below
The anomalous anterior pontomesencephalic or lateral anterior pontomesencephalic vein, which runs not in the interpeduncular fossa but on the anterior aspect of the cerebral peduncle on the left, continues inferiorly to become the anterior medullary vein. The further course, into the vein of the first cervical root, is not shown. On the right, only the anterior part of the anastomotic lateral mesencephalic vein and its tributaries are seen

Figs. 117 and 118 see pp. 143–144.

Fig. 119. Lateral wall of the lateral ventricle showing the inferior ventricular tributary of the basal cerebral vein, view from the medial aspect (see Fig. 172B).
The cerebral hemisphere has been sectioned obliquely inferomedially, through the superolateral angle of the body of the lateral ventricle, obliquely inferolaterally through the thalamus, internal capsule and globus pallidus, and inferiorly through the collateral eminence of the temporal and occipital horns of the lateral ventricle (see insert). The lateral part of the hemisphere, containing the lateral wall of the lateral ventricle, is then viewed from its medial aspect. The subependymal veins belonging to the lateral group are therefore visible. The inferior ventricular subependymal vein begins by the union of the atrial subependymal tributaries, which converge on the anterior wall of the atrium (arrowhead). The combined trunk, the inferior ventricular subependymal vein, then runs downwards and forwards on the roof of the temporal horn and is joined by the temporal tip subependymal vein. Its further course towards the basal cerebral vein is not visible

Fig. 119 see p. 145 ▷

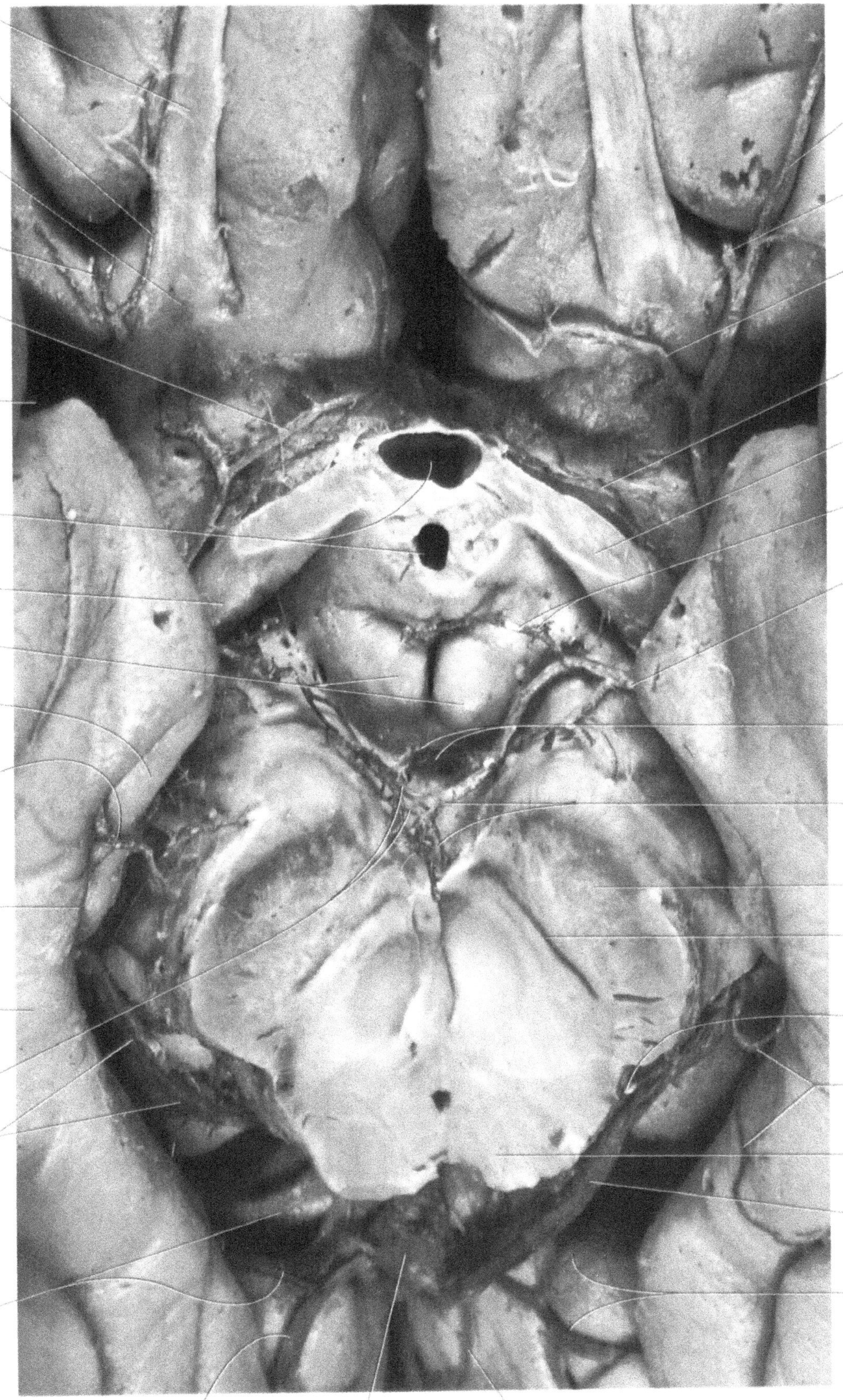

Olfactory tract
Superficial olfactory v.
Olfactory trigone
Deep olfactory v.
Ant. cerebral v.
Sylvian vallecula (medial part)
Third ventricle (optic and infundibular recesses)
Optic tract
Mammillary bodies
Recurved uncus
Ant. hippocampal v.
Ant. hippocampal fissure
Parahippocampal gyrus
Post. communicating vv.
Basal cerebral v.
Medial atrial vv.
Fronto-orbital (medial orbital) v.
Olfactory v.
Accessory ant. cerebral v.
Ant. cerebral v.
Optic tract (cut surface)
Premammillary vv.
Peduncular v.
Inf. thalamic vv.
Peduncular and ant. ponto mesencephalic vv.
Basis peduncli
Substantia nigra
Lateral mesencephalic v.
Medial temporal cortical vv.
Tectum
Basal cerebral v.
Medial atrial v.
Internal occipital v.
Great cerebral v.
Internal occipital v.

Fig. 117

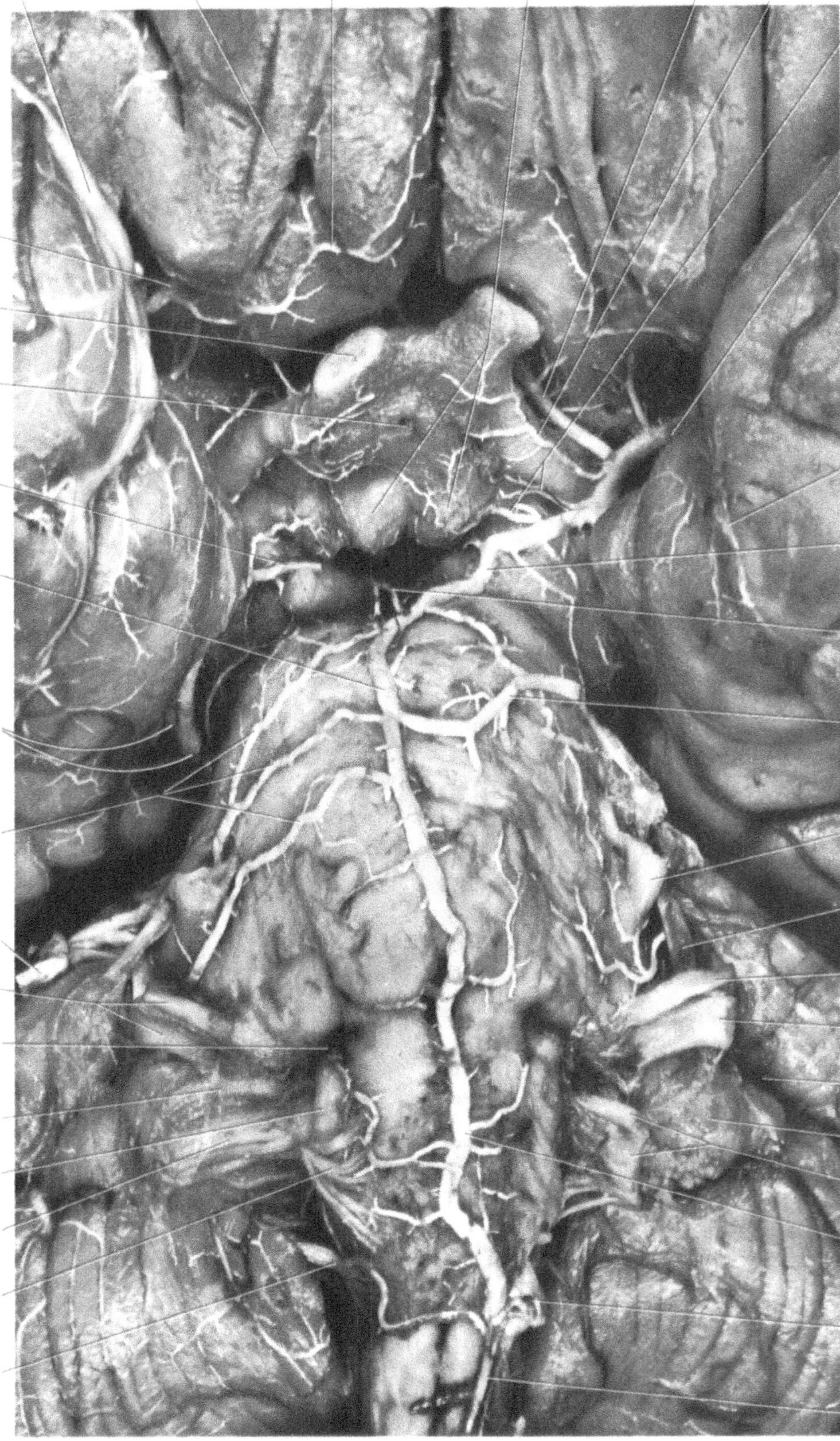
Superficial Sylvian v.
Olfactory tract
V. of gyrus rectus
Mammillary bodies
Ant. cerebral v.
Tributary from the optic tract
Mammillary and premammillary vv.
Deep middle cerebral v.
Olfactory v.
Optic n. (cut surface)
Infundibum
Peduncular v.
Anomalous ant. pontomesencephalic v. (pontine segment)
Anastomotic lateral mesencephalic v. and its inf. ventricular tributary
Transverse pontine vv.
Petrosal v.
Acoustic and facial nn.
Supraolivary fossette
Glossopharyngeal n.
Olive
Vagal n.
Hypoglossal n.
Accessory n.
V. of the rhinal sulcus
Anomalous ant. pontomesencephalic v.
Inf. thalamic v.
Transverse pontine v.
Trigeminal n.
V. of great horizontal fissure
Facial n.
Acoustic n.
Suprafloccular segment of great horizontal fissure
Flocculus
Glossopharyngeal and vagal nn.
Ant. medullary v.
Draining into v. of first cervical root
Ant. spinal v.

Fig. 118

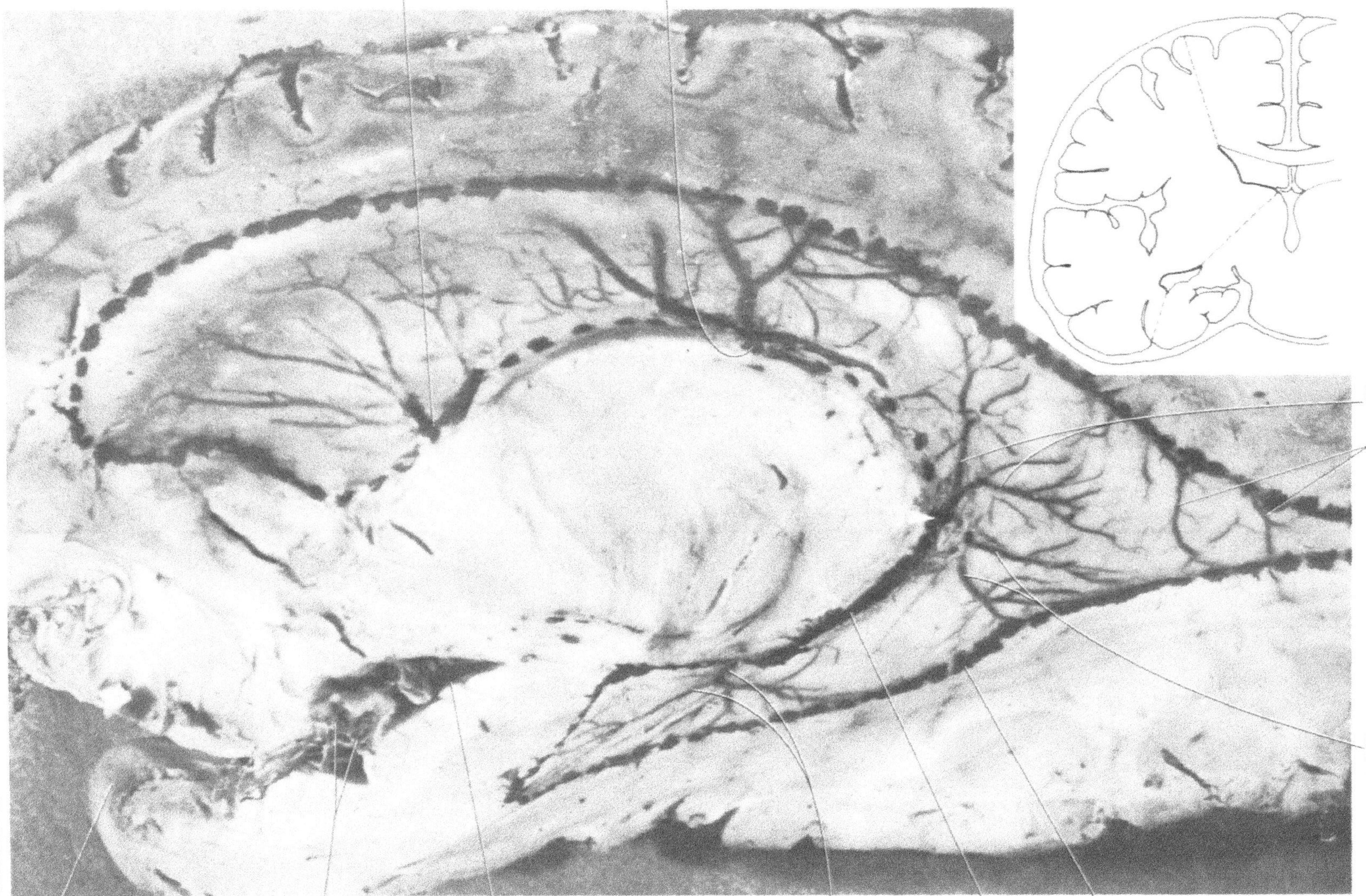
Thalamostriate v. (stem)
Direct lateral v.
Lateral atrial tributaries (inf. ventricular v.)
Medial atrial vv. on lateral wall of occipital horn
Lateral atrial tributaries (inf. ventricular v.)
Temporal pole
Branches of middle cerebral a.
Sylvian vallecula
Temporal tip subependymal v.
Inf. ventricular subependymal v.
Outline of the lateral ventricle (dotted line)

Fig. 119

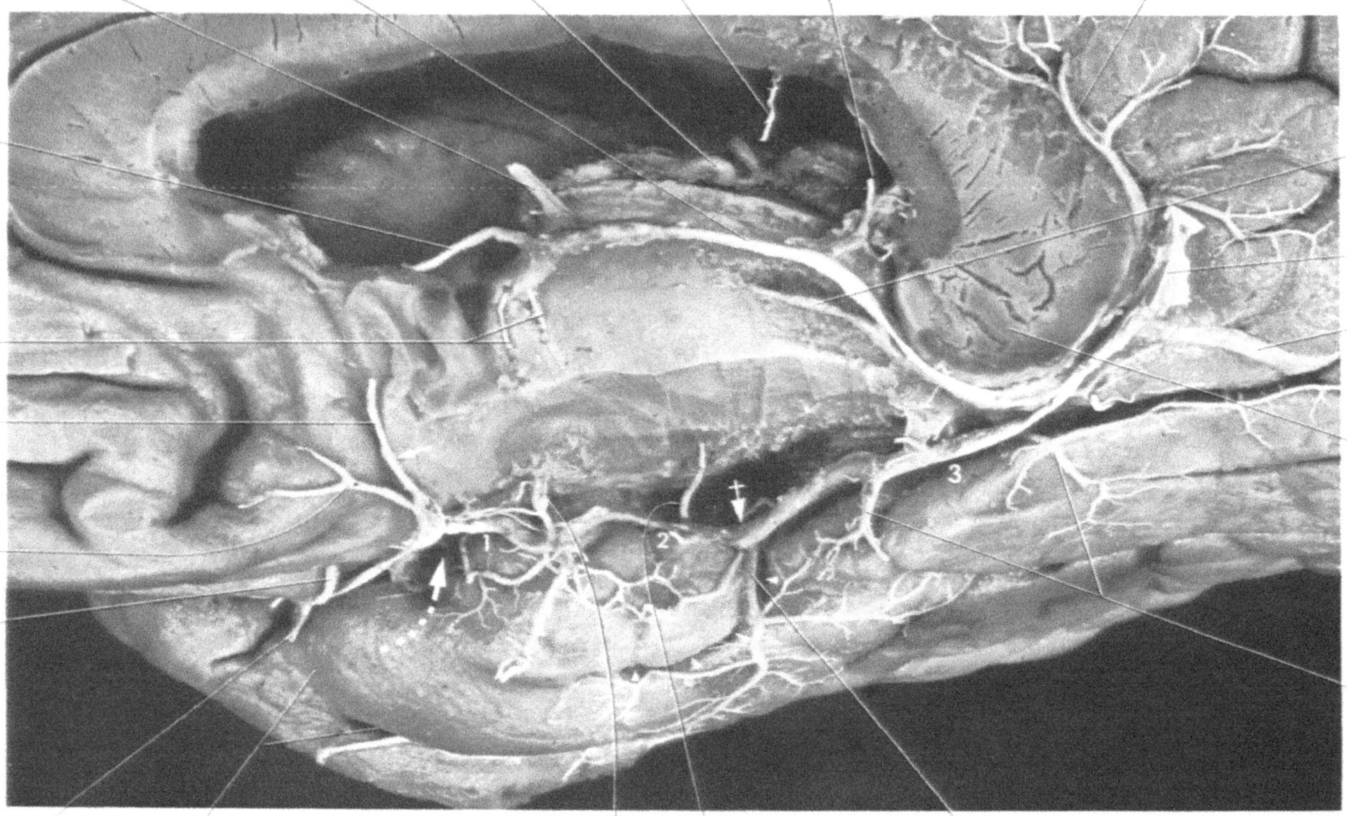

Fig. 120. Injected specimen showing the course of the basal cerebral vein and its tributaries, view from the medial aspect
The lower part of the thalamus, hypothalamus and upper brain stem have been removed. The locations of the anterior communicating vein (small arrow), anterior perforated substance (large arrow), inferior end of the choroid fissure (⍖) and anterior hippocampal sulcus (arrowheads) are labelled. The posterior part of the olfactory vein is anomalous and runs laterally, crossing the medial orbital gyrus, to join the uncal vein. The first (1), second (2) and third segments (3) of the basal cerebral vein are also labelled

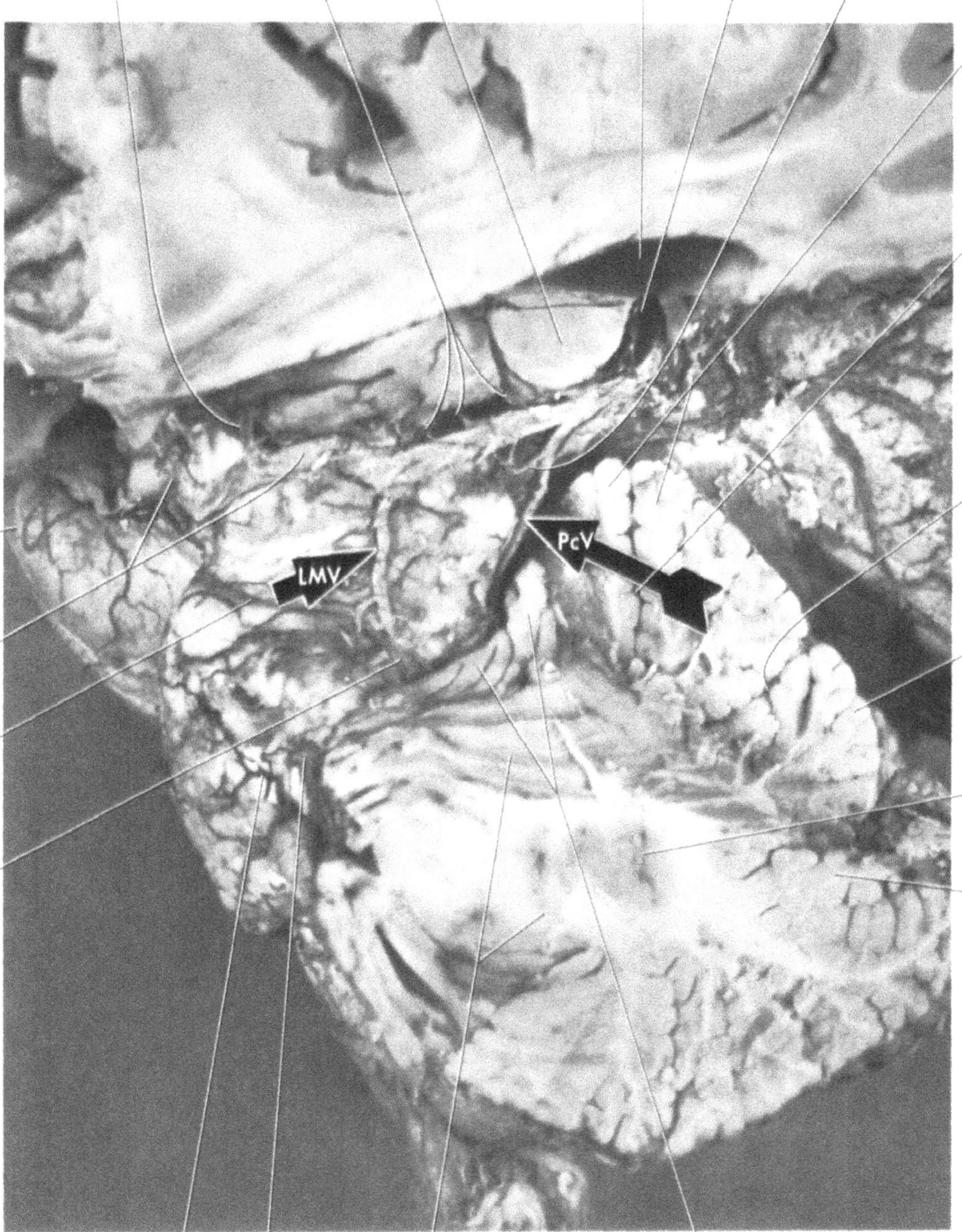

Fig. 121 A. Injected specimen showing the course of the second and third segments of the basal cerebral vein, view from the lateral aspect
On the left, the occipital lobe, the inferior part of the temporal lobe and the lateral portion of the cerebellum have been removed, exposing the temporal horn and the lateral aspect of the mesencephalon. The precentral cerebellar (PcV) and lateral mesencephalic veins (LMV) are labelled (large arrows)

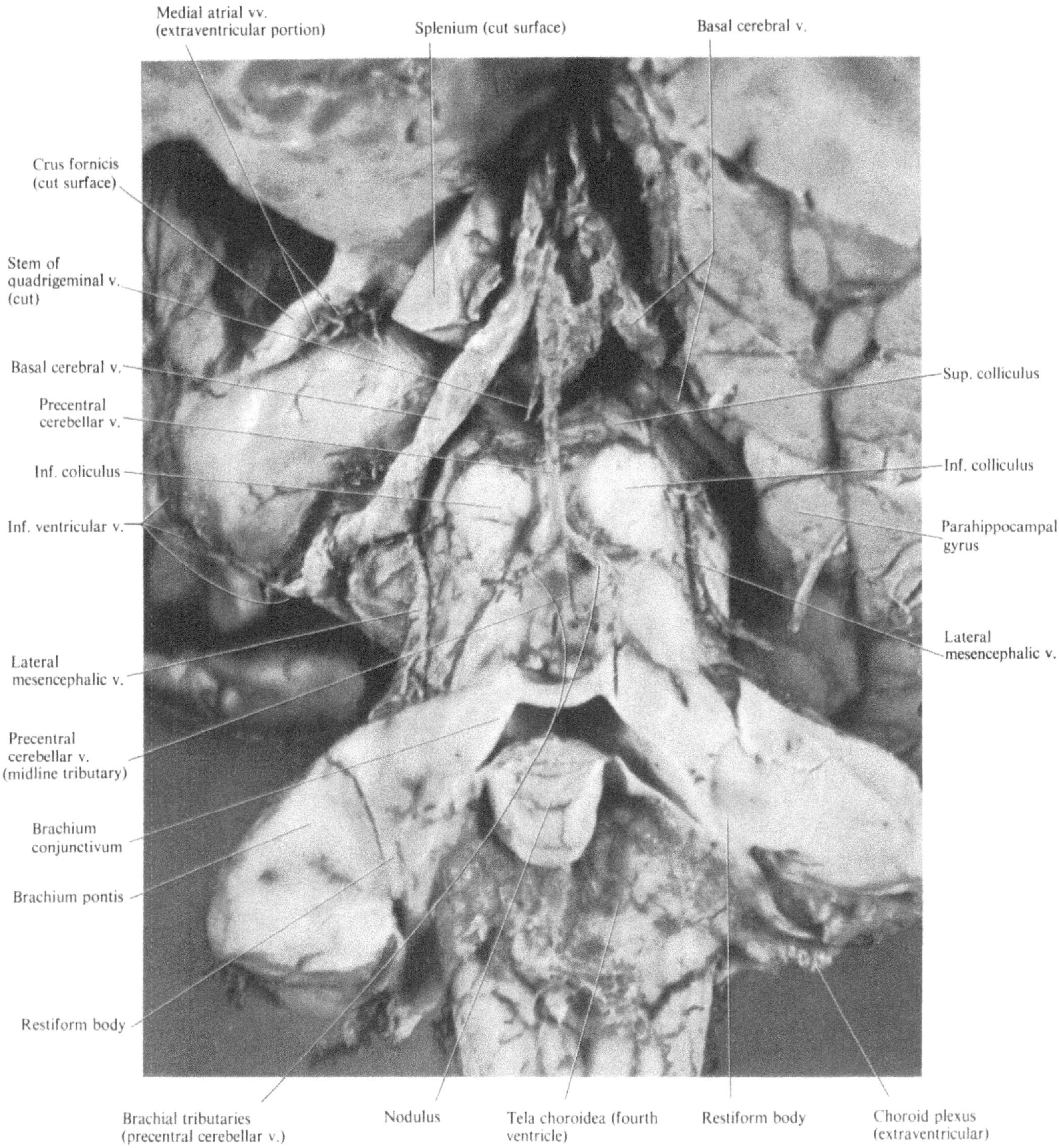

Fig. 121 B. Injected specimen showing the course of the posterior part of the basal cerebral vein, view from behind
Same specimen as in Fig. 121 A. In addition, the cerebellum and right occipital pole have been removed, exposing the posterior aspect of the mesencephalon, the medulla oblongata and the cavity of the fourth ventricle
(Courtesy of HUANG and WOLF. Charles C. Thomas, 1965)

Fig. 122A. Radiograph of an injected specimen, submentovertical view

The specimen has been divided in the mid-sagittal plane. The anterior and posterior communicating veins and the posterior ends of the right internal cerebral and basal cerebral veins are therefore severed.

On the right (R), the inferior striate veins, particularly those of the anterocentral group (arrow), are prominent. The olfactory vein, which joins the anterior cerebral vein, opens into the deep middle cerebral vein. The peduncular vein (two arrowheads), partly obscured by the superimposed direct lateral subependymal vein, joins the second segment of the basal cerebral vein slightly more posteriorly than usual. Apart from the temporal tip subependymal vein, two other subependymal veins are seen in the temporal horn—one is located medially to the tail of the caudate nucleus (terminal tributary) and the other lies on the lateral border of the temporal horn (transverse caudate or anterior temporal tributary). A prominent superior striate vein opens into the terminal tributary (on the anterior wall of the atrium). The posterior longitudinal hippocampal vein (three arrowheads), which is continuous anteriorly with the anterior longitudinal hippocampal vein, drains posteromedially to open into a combined stem of the medial temporal cortical and medial atrial subependymal veins.

On the left (L), the anterior cerebral vein, medial to the junction with the olfactory vein, is hypoplastic. The temporal tip subependymal vein, unlike that on the right side, drains not into the inferior ventricular vein but into the second segment of the basal cerebral vein. One medial atrial vein (M_1) forms a venous trunk with the occipitotemporal, medial temporal and posterior longitudinal hippocampal veins, and drains posteromedially into the posterior end of the basal cerebral vein. Another smaller medial atrial vein (M_2) joins the posterior portion of the internal cerebral vein. The hippocampal formation is drained anteriorly by the anterior hippocampal vein and posteriorly by the posterior longitudinal hippocampal vein. The midportion of the hippocampal formation is, however, drained by the anterior longitudinal hippocampal vein, which opens into the inferior ventricular vein at the inferior end of the choroid fissure

Fig. 122A see p. 150 ▷

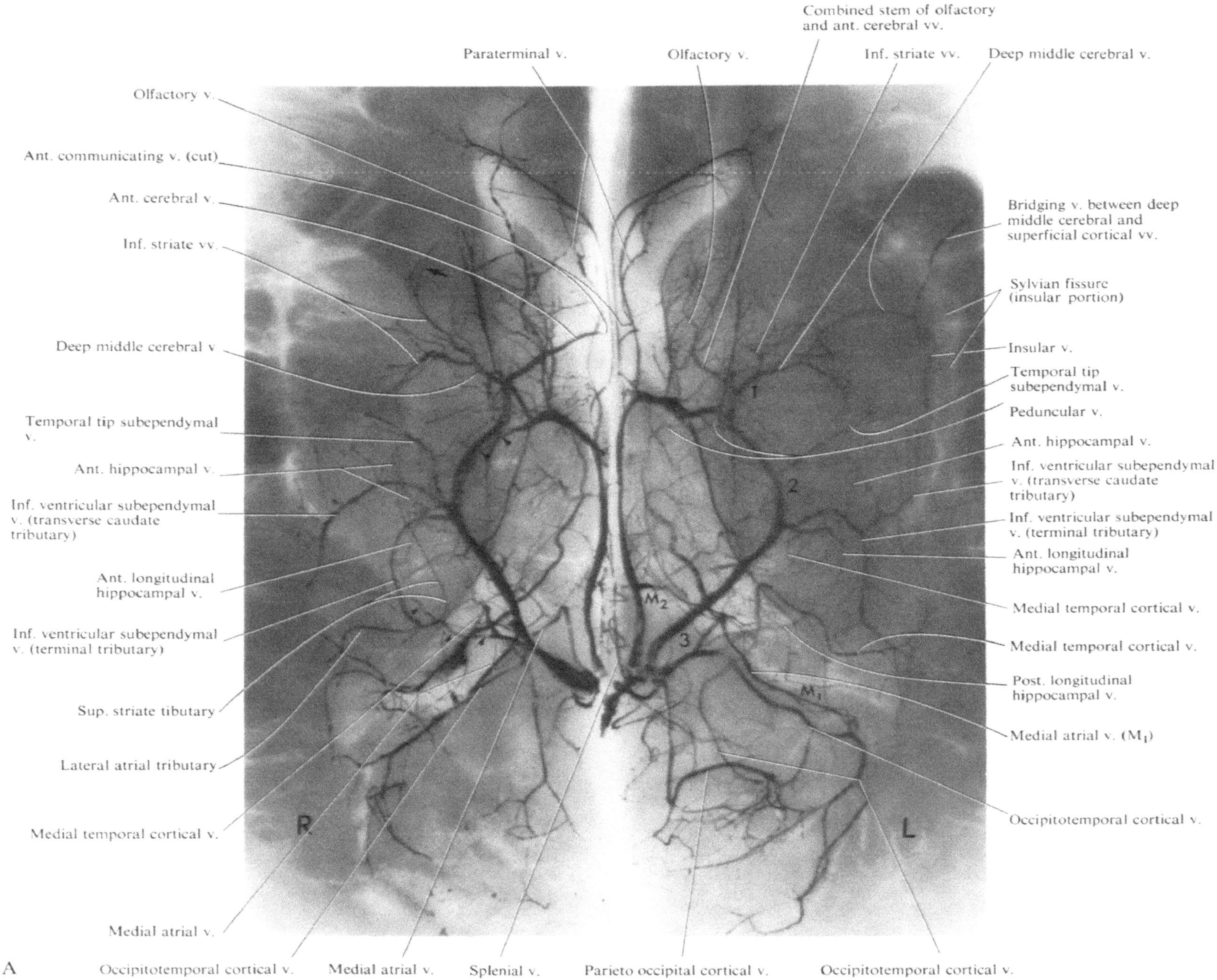
Combined stem of olfactory and ant. cerebral vv.
Paraterminal v.
Olfactory v.
Inf. striate vv.
Deep middle cerebral v.
Olfactory v.
Ant. communicating v. (cut)
Ant. cerebral v.
Inf. striate vv.
Deep middle cerebral v
Temporal tip subependymal v.
Ant. hippocampal v.
Inf. ventricular subependymal v. (transverse caudate tributary)
Ant. longitudinal hippocampal v.
Inf. ventricular subependymal v. (terminal tributary)
Sup. striate tributary
Lateral atrial tributary
Medial temporal cortical v.
Medial atrial v.
Bridging v. between deep middle cerebral and superficial cortical vv.
Sylvian fissure (insular portion)
Insular v.
Temporal tip subependymal v.
Peduncular v.
Ant. hippocampal v.
Inf. ventricular subependymal v. (transverse caudate tributary)
Inf. ventricular subependymal v. (terminal tributary)
Ant. longitudinal hippocampal v.
Medial temporal cortical v.
Medial temporal cortical v.
Post. longitudinal hippocampal v.
Medial atrial v. (M1)
Occipitotemporal cortical v.
1
2
3
M2
M1
R
L
Occipitotemporal cortical v.
Medial atrial v.
Splenial v.
Parieto occipital cortical v.
Occipitotemporal cortical v.

Fig. 122A

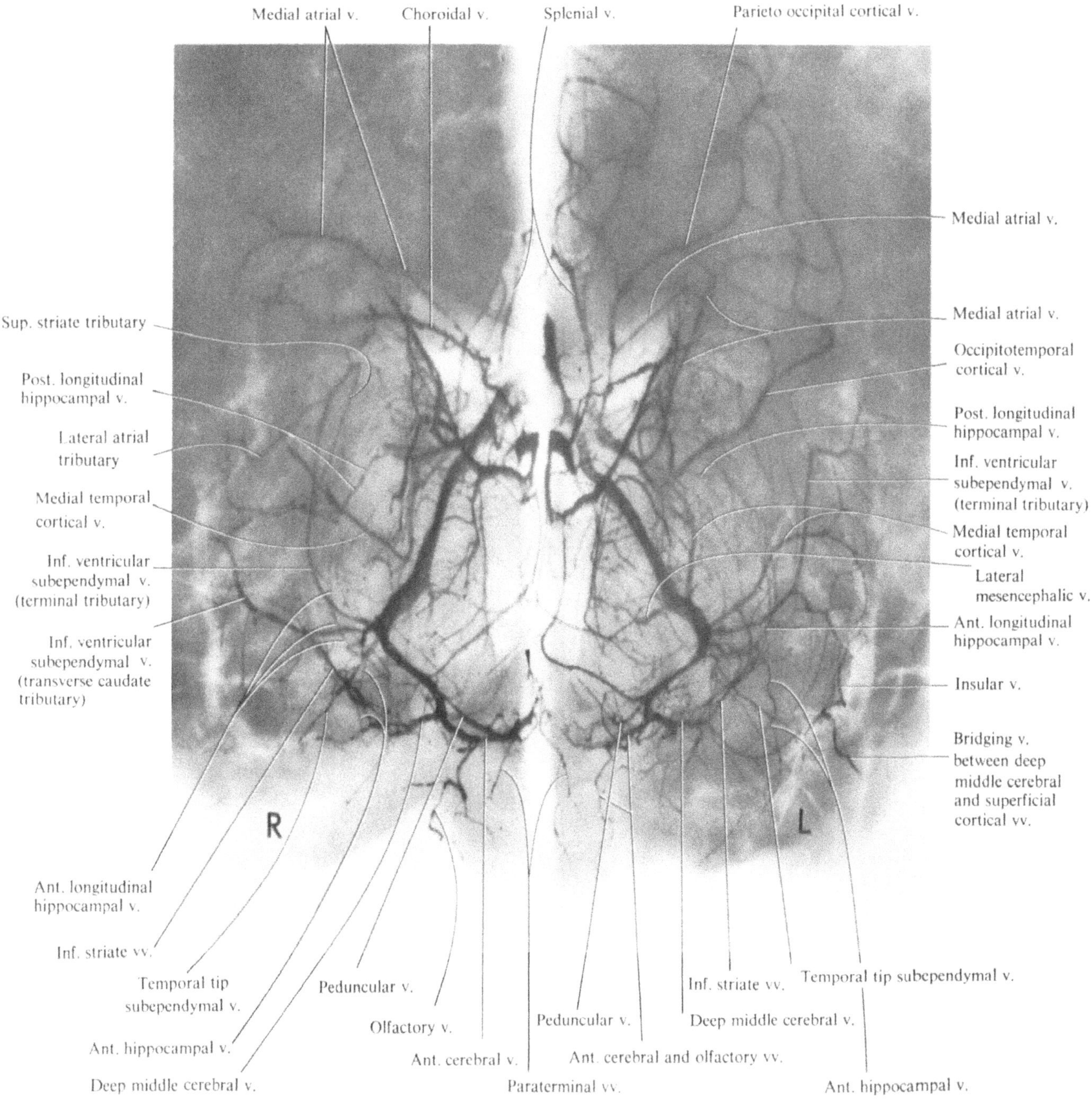

Fig. 122B. Radiograph of an injected specimen. Same specimen as in Fig. 122A semiaxial view. The pericallosal tributary (terminal segment) of the anterior cerebral vein is labelled (arrowhead)

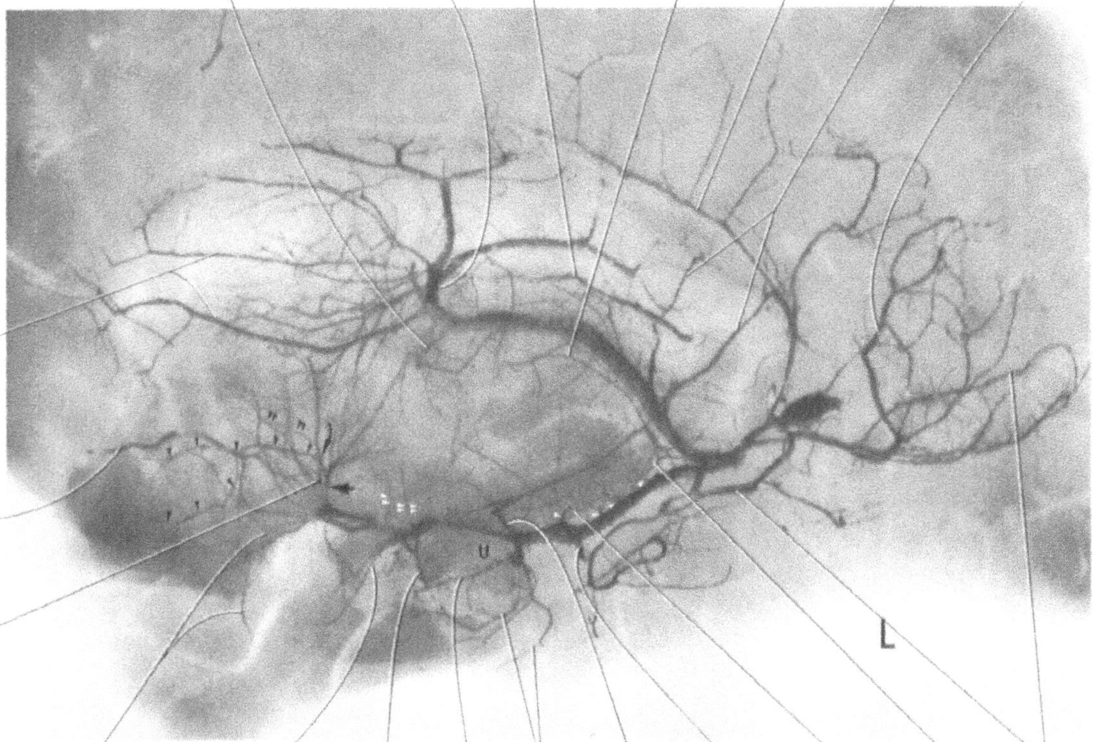

Fig. 122C. Radiograph of an injected specimen, left cerebral hemisphere. Same specimen as in Fig. 122A, lateral view

The anterior cerebral vein (large arrow), anterior communicating vein (curved arrow), terminal segment (double black arrowheads) of the anterior pericallosal vein, paraterminal vein (rows of single arrowheads) and the recurved uncus (U) are labelled. Numerous fine posterior thalamic veins (white arrowheads) and prominent premammillary veins (double white arrowheads) can also be identified

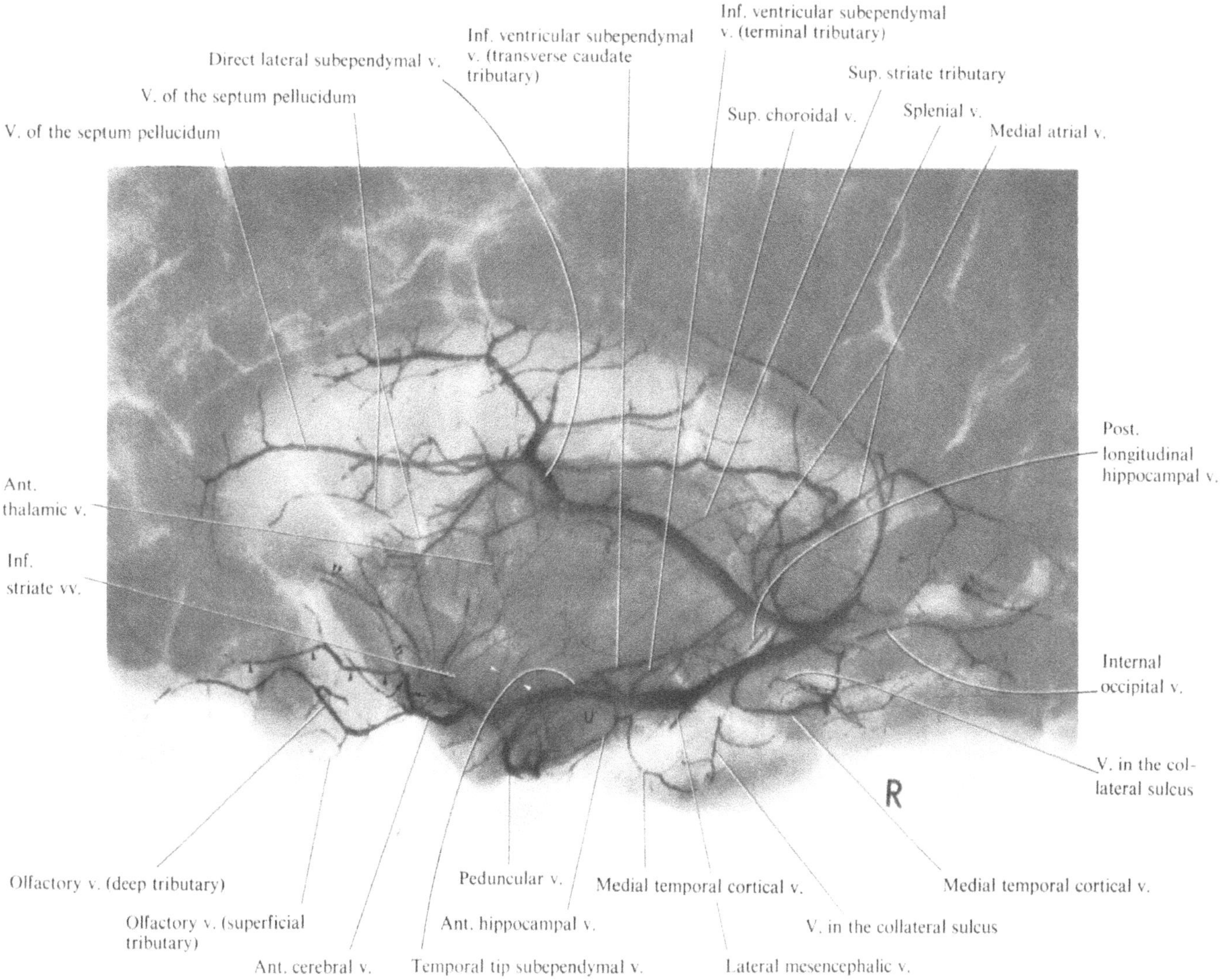

Fig. 122D. Radiograph of an injected specimen, right cerebral hemisphere. Same specimen as in Fig. 122A, lateral view
The anterior cerebral vein (arrow), anterior communicating vein (curved arrow), terminal segment (double arrowheads) of the anterior pericallosal vein, paraterminal vein (rows of single black arrowheads) and the recurved uncus (U) are labelled. The premammillary veins (white arrowheads) can also be identified

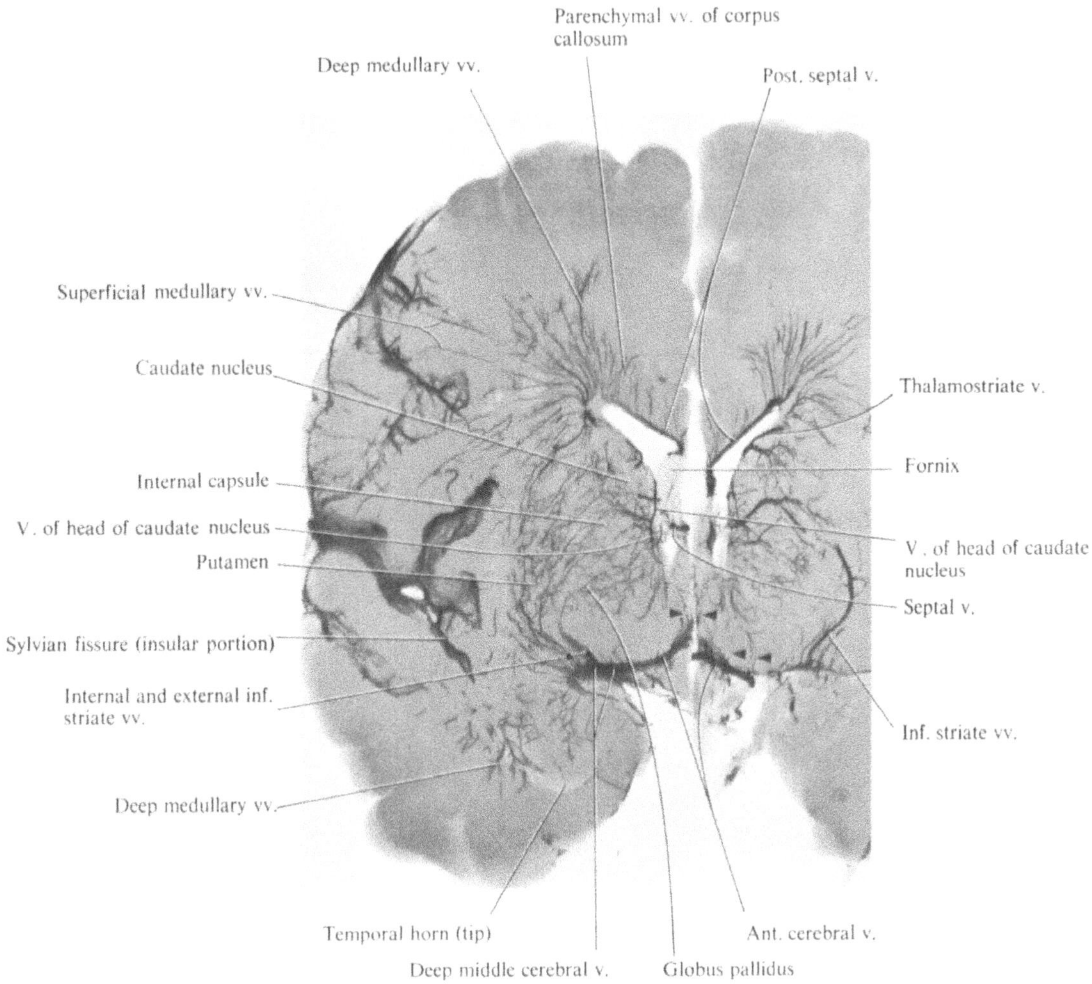

Fig. 123. Radiograph of a coronal slice of an injected specimen, at the level of the anterior perforated substance, showing the course of the internal and external inferior striate veins.

A small gap between the two cerebral hemispheres is due to a prior section through the midsagittal plane. Fine inferior thalamic and hypothalamic tributaries are labelled (arrowheads)

▷

Fig. 124A. Prominent insular tributaries of the basal cerebral vein. Cerebral angiogram, venous phase, lateral view

The posterior insular vein and a superficial cortical vein are connected by a small bridging vein (large arrows). The anterior cerebral vein, the terminal segment of the anterior pericallosal vein and the paraterminal vein can be identified (rows of small arrows). Also labelled are the fronto-orbital tributary of the basal cerebral vein, outlining the inferior and posterior aspects of the postorbital lobule (row of single arrowheads), a tortuous anterior hippocampal vein (row of double arrowheads), outlining the recurved uncus (U), and the first (1), second (2) and third segments (3) of the basal cerebral vein

Fig. 124B. Typical basal cerebral vein. Cerebral angiogram, venous phase, semiaxial view

The inferior and superior striate veins (opposing arrowheads) are seen unusually clearly. The insular, fronto-orbital, anterior cerebral (triple arrowheads) and peduncular tributaries (single arrowhead) drain into the basal cerebral vein. The first (1), second (2) and third segments (3) of the basal cerebral veins are labelled

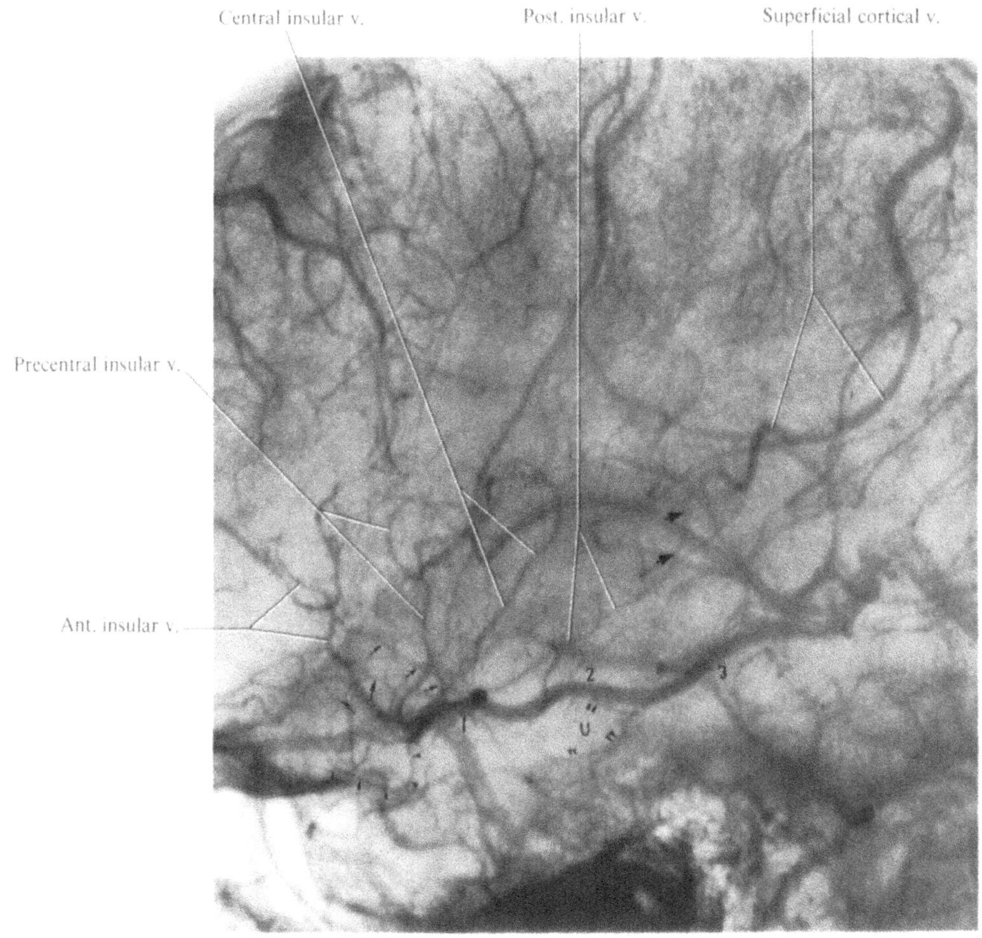

Fig. 124A

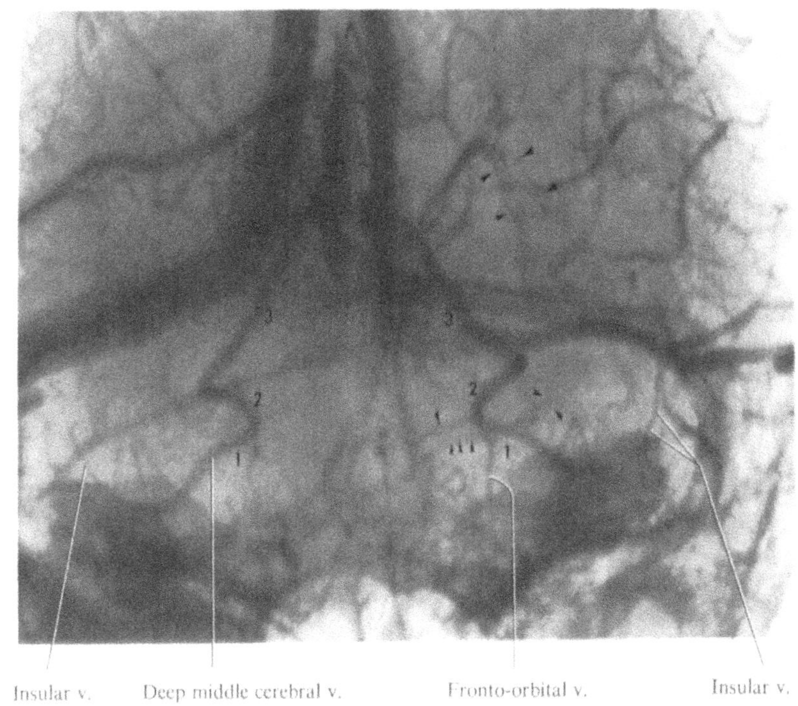

Fig. 124B

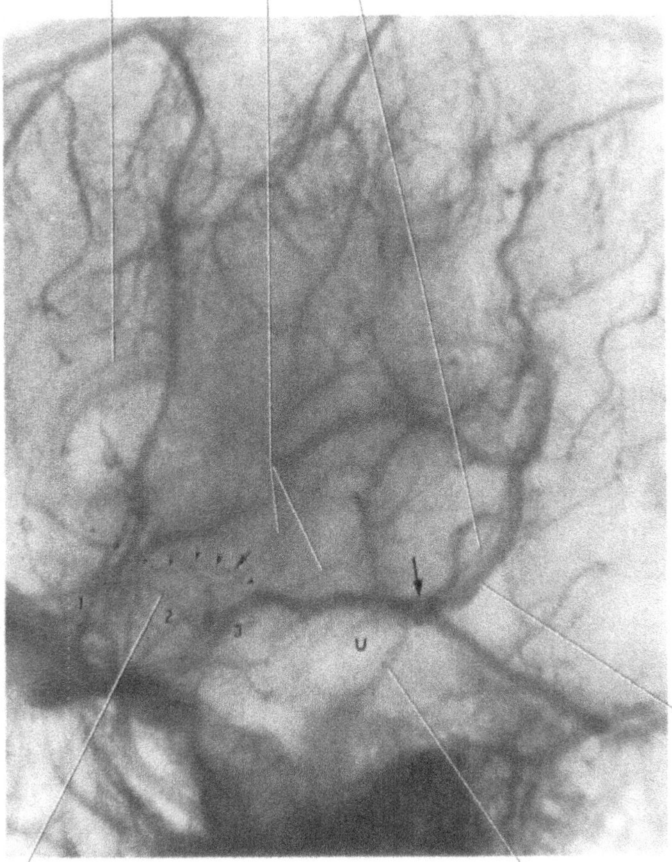

Fig. 125A

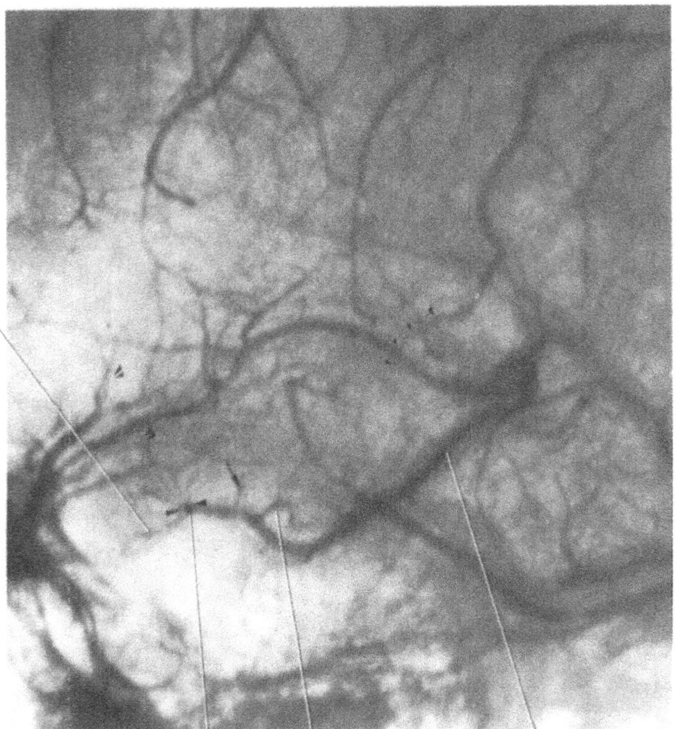

Fig. 125B

Fig. 126. Prominent olfactory vein. Carotid angiogram, venous phase, anteroposterior view
The first or ascending fissural (1), second or descending fissural (2) and third or retrofissural segments (3) of the olfactory vein can be identified. The medial position of the posterior part of the second segment (2) suggests a medial course of the olfactory vein in relation to the olfactory trigone. The anterior cerebral vein, joining the olfactory vein, is labelled

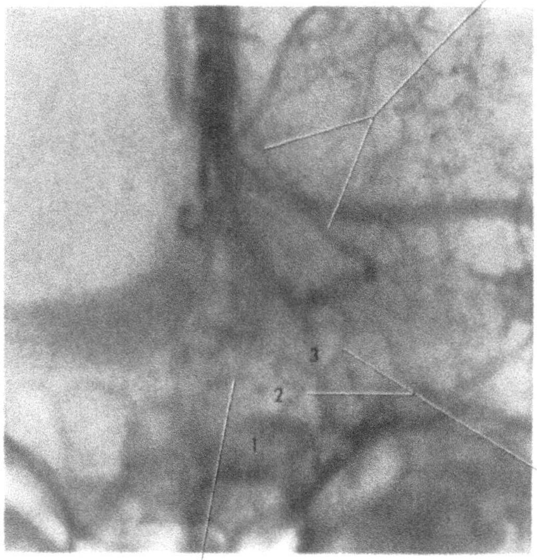

◁

Fig. 125 A. Prominent olfactory, anterior cerebral and terminal tributaries of the basal cerebral vein. Carotid angiogram, venous phase, lateral view
A characteristic sinuous course of the first or ascending fissural (1), second or descending fissural (2) and third or retrofissural segments (3) of the olfactory vein is noted. A typical obtuse angle is formed between the anterior cerebral and the paraterminal veins (row of arrowheads), at the level of the lower border of the subcallosal sulcus (small arrow). The pericallosal vein, above the corpus callosum (supracallosal segment), drains upwards to join the cortical veins on the medial aspect of the hemisphere. The inferior ventricular and anterior hippocampal veins join the basal cerebral vein at the inferior end (large arrow) of the choroid fissure. The recurved uncus (U) is also labelled

Fig. 125 B. Prominent inferior striate and peduncular tributaries of the basal cerebral vein. Cerebral angiogram, venous phase, lateral view
Numerous inferior striate veins converge towards the anterior perforated substance (two opposing arrowheads). The anterocentral group of these veins can also be seen (double arrowheads). A prominent peduncular vein, originating from the interpeduncular fossa, runs laterally around the anterior aspect of the cerebral peduncle (seen as a dense dot) to join the basal cerebral vein. Slightly anteriorly to this peduncular vein, a prominent premammillary vein (arrow) joins the basal cerebral vein. A vein (row of single arrowheads) located in the posterior end of the posterior limiting sulcus drains outwards to join a superficial cortical vein

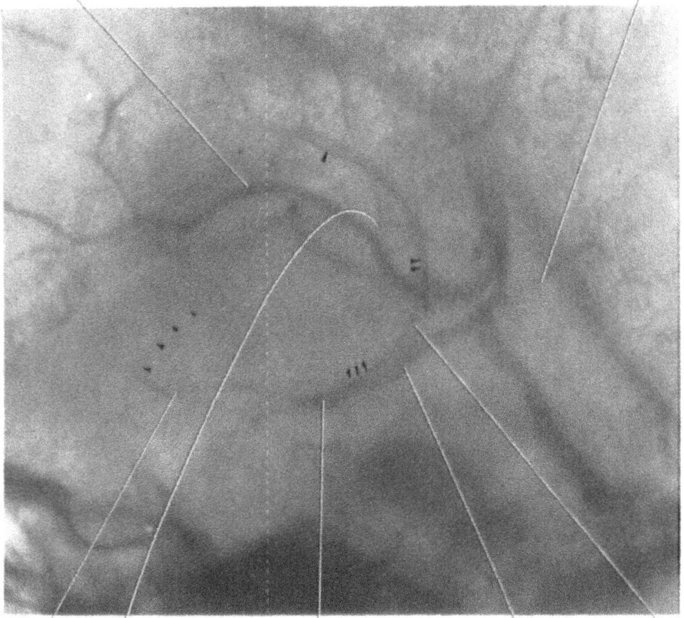

Fig. 127A. Prominent inferior ventricular vein. Carotid angiogram, venous phase, lateral view

The inferior ventricular vein begins on the lateral wall of the body of the lateral ventricle, below the caudate nucleus (single arrowhead). It then runs backwards, downwards and forwards in an arcuate fashion, convex posteriorly, travelling on the anterior wall of the atrium (double arrowheads) and on the roof of the temporal horn (triple arrowheads). This vein then turns medially (seen as a dense dot), emerging from the inferior end of the choroid fissure to join the basal cerebral vein. Note the unusual crossing of the tributaries of the direct lateral subependymal vein, under the inferior ventricular subependymal vein, in the posterior portion of the body of the lateral ventricle

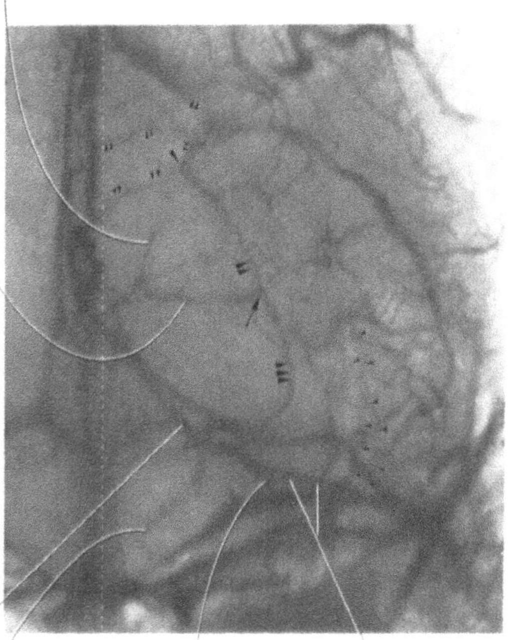

Fig. 127B. Prominent inferior ventricular vein. Same case as in Fig. 127A, anteroposterior view

The prominent inferior ventricular vein originates on the lateral wall of the body of the lateral ventricle and runs along its inferolateral angle (single arrowhead). The walls of the lateral ventricle, outlined by subependymal veins, are indicated by multiple double arrowheads. The further course of the inferior ventricular vein on the anterior wall of the atrium (double arrowheads) and on the roof of the temporal horn (triple arrowheads) is also shown. Note the crossing (arrow) of the inferior ventricular vein over the tributaries of the direct lateral subependymal vein. The central and precentral insular veins (rows of small arrowheads) are well shown

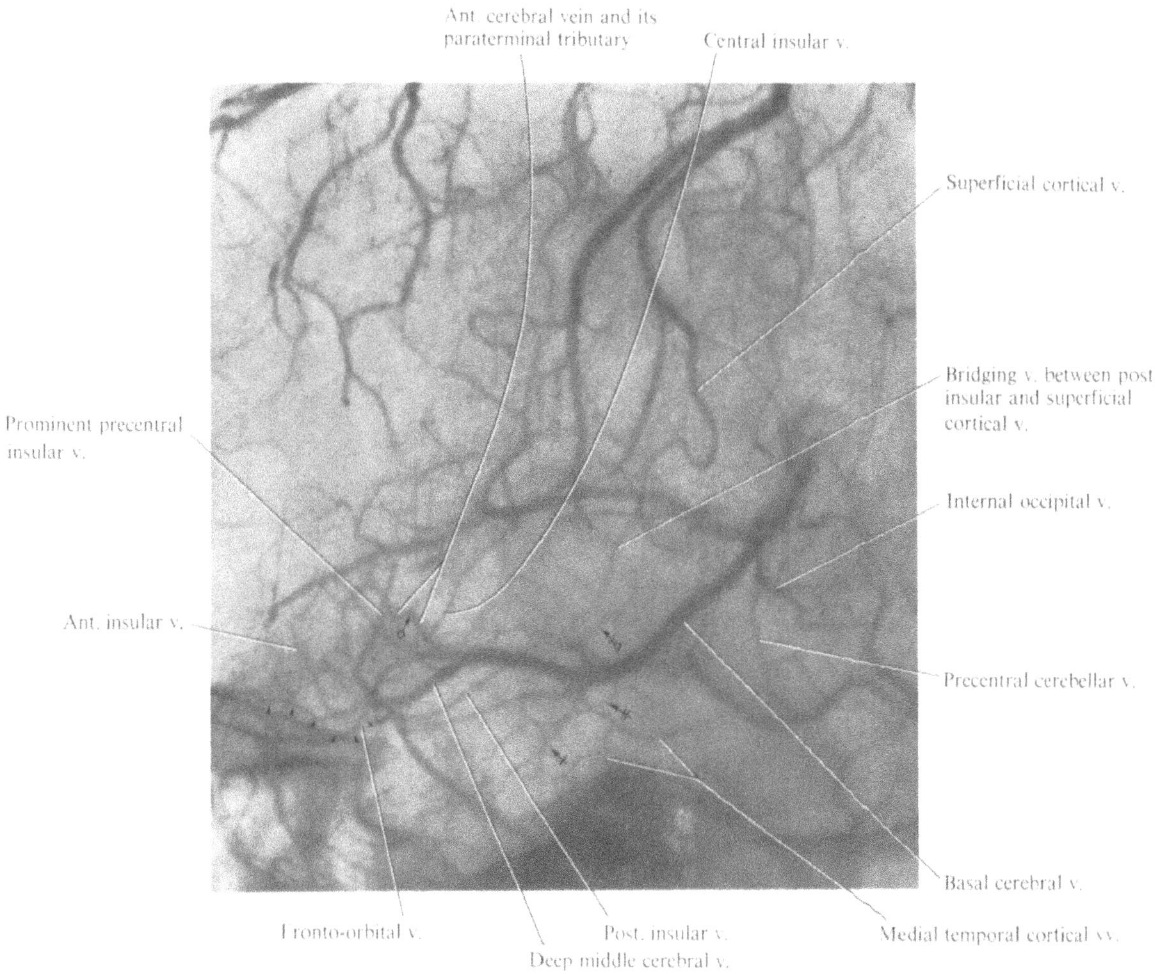

Fig. 128. Prominent medial temporal tributaries of the basal cerebral vein. Cerebral angiogram, venous phase, lateral view
Medial temporal tributaries of the basal cerebral vein run medially on the inferior surface and then superiorly on the medial surface of the hippocampal gyrus, to join the basal cerebral vein, with the anterior hippocampal (↟), anterior longitudinal hippocampal (⇞) and inferior ventricular subependymal veins (↟). The anterior cerebral vein and the site of the anterior communicating vein (↑) can be identified. A small fronto-orbital vein (row of single arrowheads) is labelled

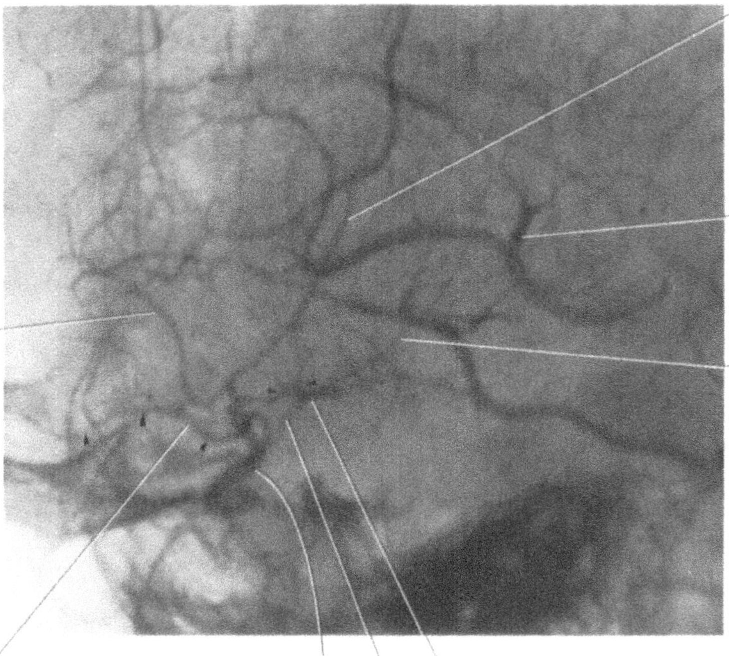

Fig. 129 A

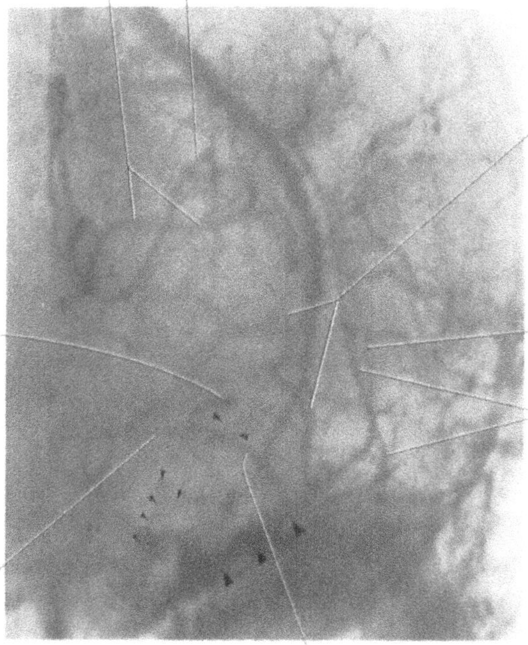

Fig. 129 B

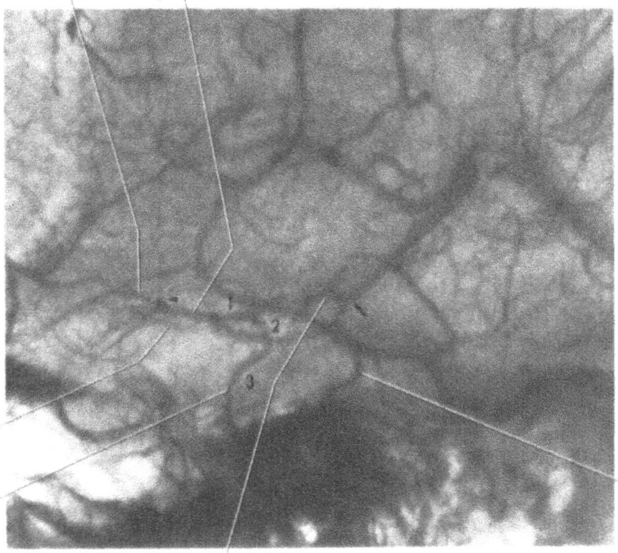

Fig. 130 A. Prominent anterior pontomesencephalic and anastomotic lateral mesencephalic veins. Cerebral angiogram, venous phase, lateral view
The anterior pontomesencephalic vein outlines the roof (1) and posterior wall (2) of the interpeduncular cistern and the posterior wall (3) of the pontine cistern. The anastomotic lateral mesencephalic vein shows the location of the lateral mesencephalic sulcus. The temporal tip subependymal vein is unusually prominent and joins (arrow) the basal cerebral vein, slightly behind the inferior end of the choroid fissure. The apex of the star-shaped inferior striate veins (single arrowhead) shows the location of the anterior perforated substance

◁

Fig. 129 A. Uncal (or medial vallecular) vein with prominent insular tributaries replacing the anterior portion of the basal cerebral vein. Carotid angiogram, venous phase, lateral view
The prominent posterior insular, central insular, and anterior insular veins unite to form a single trunk in the Sylvian vallecula. This trunk is also joined by a prominent olfactory vein (three arrowheads) and opens into the cavernous sinus via the uncal vein. The first segment of the basal cerebral vein, receiving inferior striate tributaries (two opposing arrowheads), drains into the uncal vein through a bridging vein
(Courtesy of Huang and Wolf, 1974. C.V. Mosby Co)

Fig. 129 B. Uncal (or medial vallecular) vein with prominent insular tributaries replacing the anterior portion of the basal cerebral vein. Same case as in Fig. 129 A, anteroposterior view
The anterior insular, central insular and posterior insular veins outline the anterior limiting, central and posterior limiting sulci of the insula. The olfactory (row of small arrowheads), inferior striate (two opposing arrowheads) and uncal veins (row of large arrowheads) are labelled

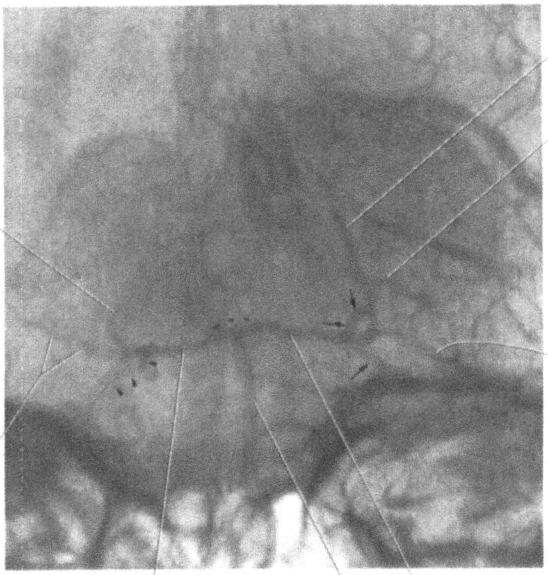

Fig. 130 B. Prominent anterior pontomesencephalic and anastomotic lateral mesencephalic veins. Same case as in Fig. 130 A, anteroposterior view
Several inferior thalamic veins (fine arrowheads), emerging from the interpeduncular fossa to join the posterior communicating vein, between the two prominent peduncular veins, can be identified. The supratentorial, mesencephalic and infratentorial segments (row of arrows) of the anastomotic lateral mesencephalic vein are seen on the left. The temporal tip subependymal vein, running posteromedially, joins the basal cerebral vein slightly more posteriorly than usual.
In addition, there is an anomalous vein (row of large arrowheads) which runs posteriorly, inferiorly and laterally on the lateral aspect of the cerebral peduncle, to join the brachial tributary of the petrosal vein.

▷

Fig. 131 A. Prominent anastomotic lateral mesencephalic vein draining primarily the first and second segments of the basal cerebral vein into the posterior fossa. Cerebral angiogram, venous phase, lateral view
The anastomotic lateral mesencephalic vein receiving the central and posterior insular, olfactory (row of 5 arrowheads), fronto-orbital, anterior cerebral (2 double arrowheads), peduncular (curved arrow), temporal tip subependymal and anterior hippocampal veins (row of 4 arrowheads) drains infratentorially. Two posterior mesencephalic and two accessory posterior mesencephalic veins are also seen but they are poorly connected with the anastomotic lateral mesencephalic vein

Fig. 131 B. Prominent anastomotic lateral mesencephalic vein connecting the third segment of the basal cerebral vein with the superior petrosal sinus. Carotid angiogram, venous phase, lateral view
The supratentorial (1), mesencephalic (2) and infratentorial segments (3) of the anastomotic lateral mesencephalic vein are labelled. Although the anterior part of the basal cerebral vein is poorly visualized, the uncal and anterior pontomesencephalic veins are still faintly identifiable

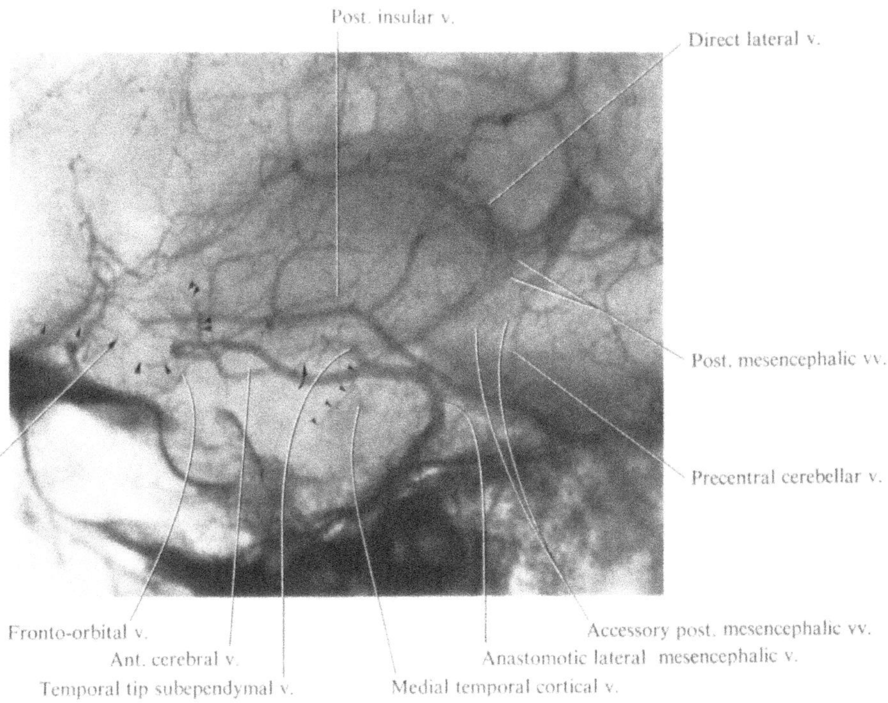

Fig. 131 A

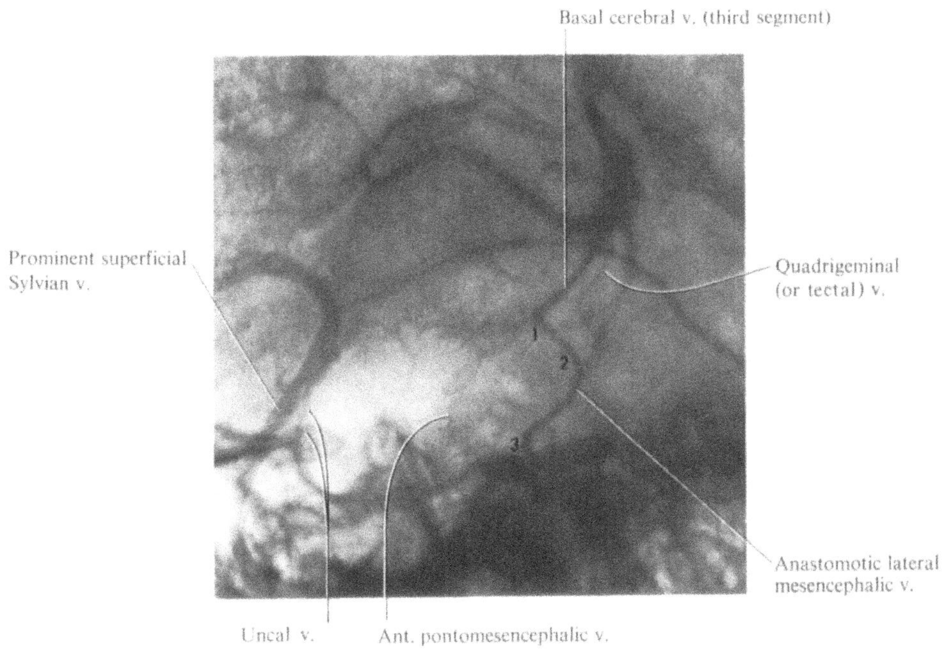

Fig. 131 B

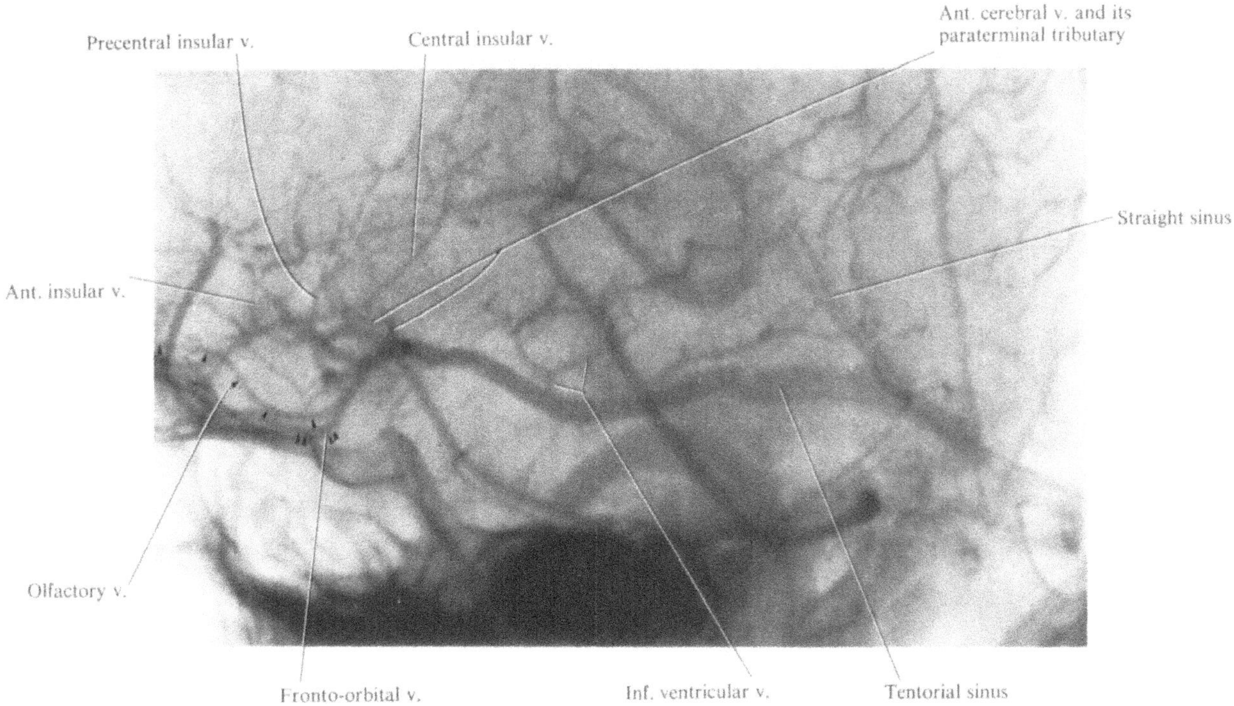

Fig. 132A

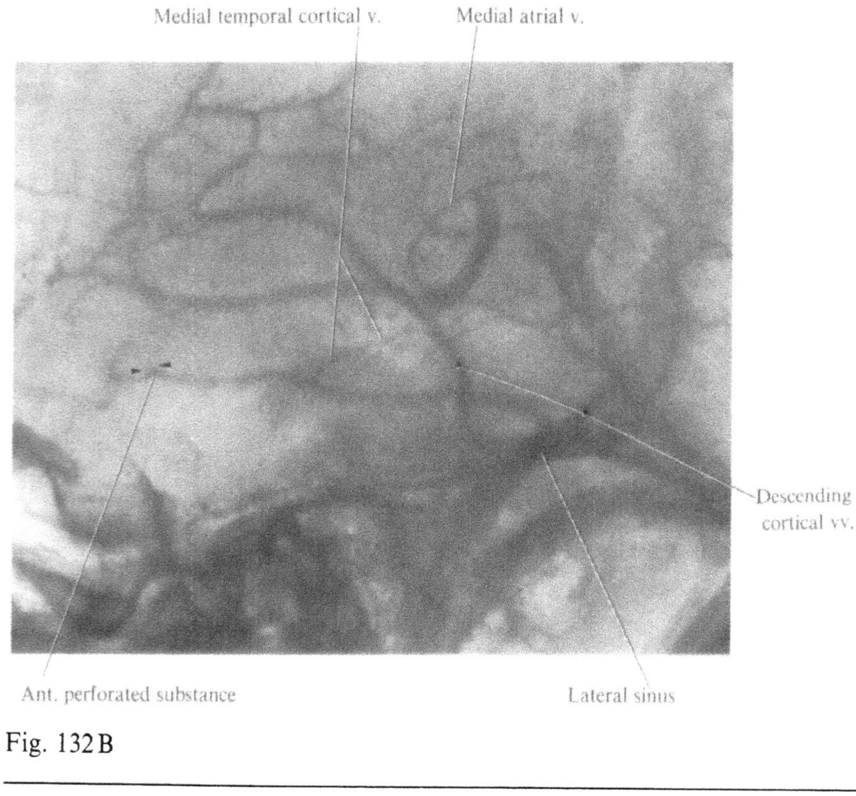

Fig. 132B

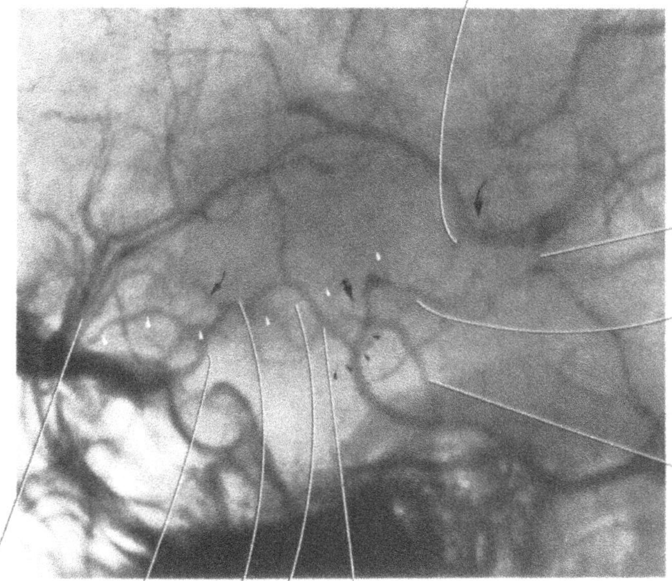

Fig. 133 A. Multiple drainage (fragmented form) of the basal cerebral vein. Carotid angiogram, venous phase, lateral view
The faintly visualized posterior insular vein drains antero-inferiorly (row of white arrowheads) to join the superficial Sylvian vein, along the greater wing of the sphenoid. Veins on the undersurface of the anterior perforated substance drain antero-inferiorly to join the uncal vein. The second segment of the basal cerebral vein, receiving inferior ventricular subependymal (⍏), temporal tip subependymal and anterior hippocampal veins (row of black arrowheads) drains downwards into the posterior fossa, via the anastomotic lateral mesencephalic vein. The posterior mesencephalic vein, derived from the third segment of the basal cerebral vein, on the other hand, drains backwards and upwards to join the posterior end of the internal cerebral vein. Note the laminar flow within the great cerebral vein, indicating the point of junction (large curved arrow) with the two internal cerebral veins. The internal occipital vein, however, drains into the great cerebral vein. The anterior cerebral vein is also labelled (small curved arrow)

◁

Fig. 132 A. Basal cerebral vein draining posteromedially into the straight sinus via a tentorial sinus. Carotid angiogram, venous phase, lateral view
The prominent basal cerebral vein, receiving the olfactory (row of single arrowheads), fronto-orbital (2 double arrowheads), insular, anterior cerebral and inferior ventricular veins, drains into the midportion of the straight sinus, following a short course within the tentorium

Fig. 132 B. Basal cerebral vein draining posterolaterally into the lateral sinus. Carotid angiogram, venous phase, lateral view
The anomalous basal cerebral vein begins at the anterior perforated substance, where it receives the inferior striate veins (arrowheads). In its posterior course towards the lateral sinus, the vein receives a medial temporal tributary which imitates the course of the more superiorly located inferior ventricular vein

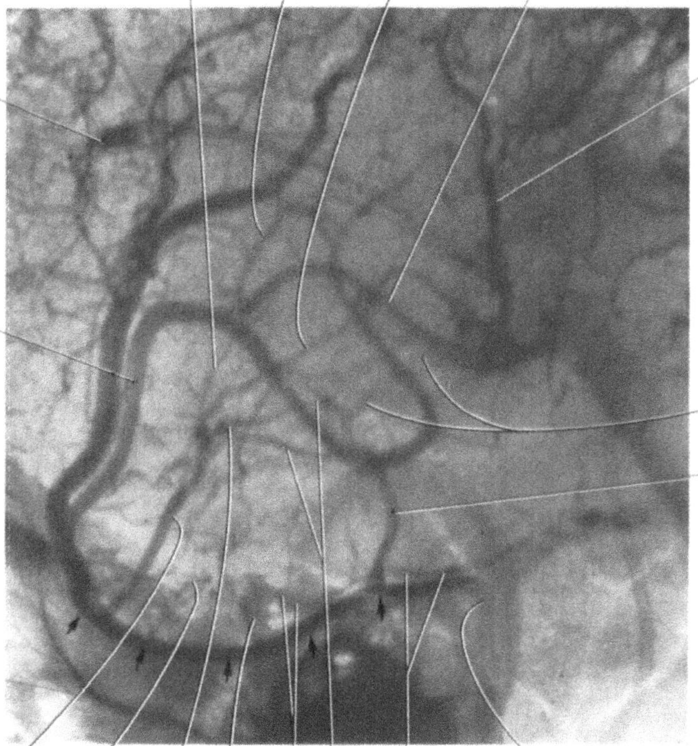

Fig. 133 B. Various segments of the basal cerebral vein and the superficial Sylvian vein draining independently into a tentorial sinus. Carotid angiogram, venous phase, lateral view

The unusually prominent superficial Sylvian, the uncal, and the anastomotic lateral mesencephalic veins drain posterolaterally into a tentorial sinus (arrows)

▷

Fig. 134 A. Drainage of the first segment of the basal cerebral vein into the second and third segments of the basal cerebral vein of the opposite side, via the posterior communicating vein. Carotid angiogram, venous phase, anteroposterior view see also Fig. 136 E

The insular and inferior striate veins, draining into the deep middle cerebral vein, are labelled (rows of arrowheads)

Fig. 134 B. Supratentorial (or Galenic) drainage of the petrosal vein and its tributaries. Vertebral angiogram, venous phase, semiaxial view

The supratentorial (1), mesencephalic (2) and infratentorial segments (3) of the anastomotic lateral mesencephalic vein are labelled on each side. On the right (reader's left), the petrosal vein and its tributaries—the postclival vein, the vein of the great horizontal fissure, the inferior hemispheric vein and the transverse pontine vein—converge to drain supratentorially, into the posterior mesencephalic vein, via the third, second and then first segments of the anastomotic lateral mesencephalic vein.

On the left (reader's right), the anastomotic lateral mesencephalic vein connects the posterior mesencephalic vein with the superior petrosal sinus

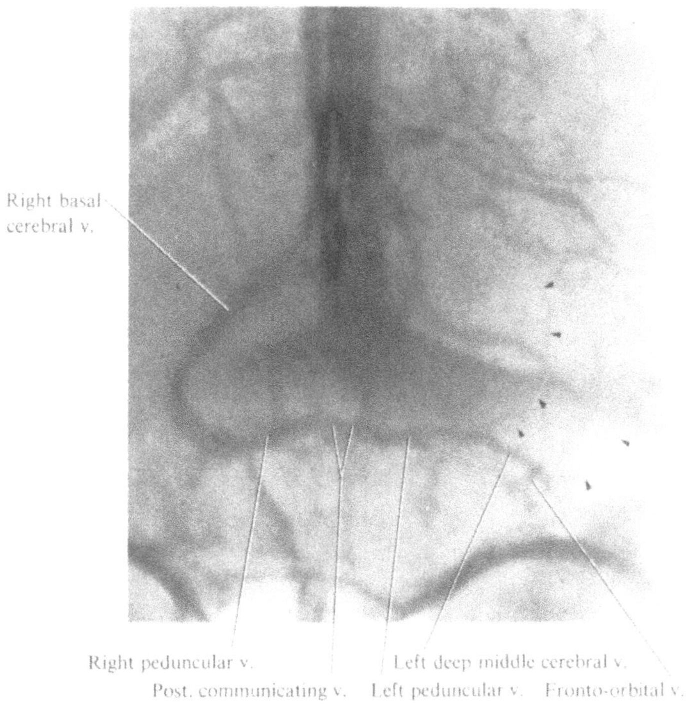

Fig. 134A

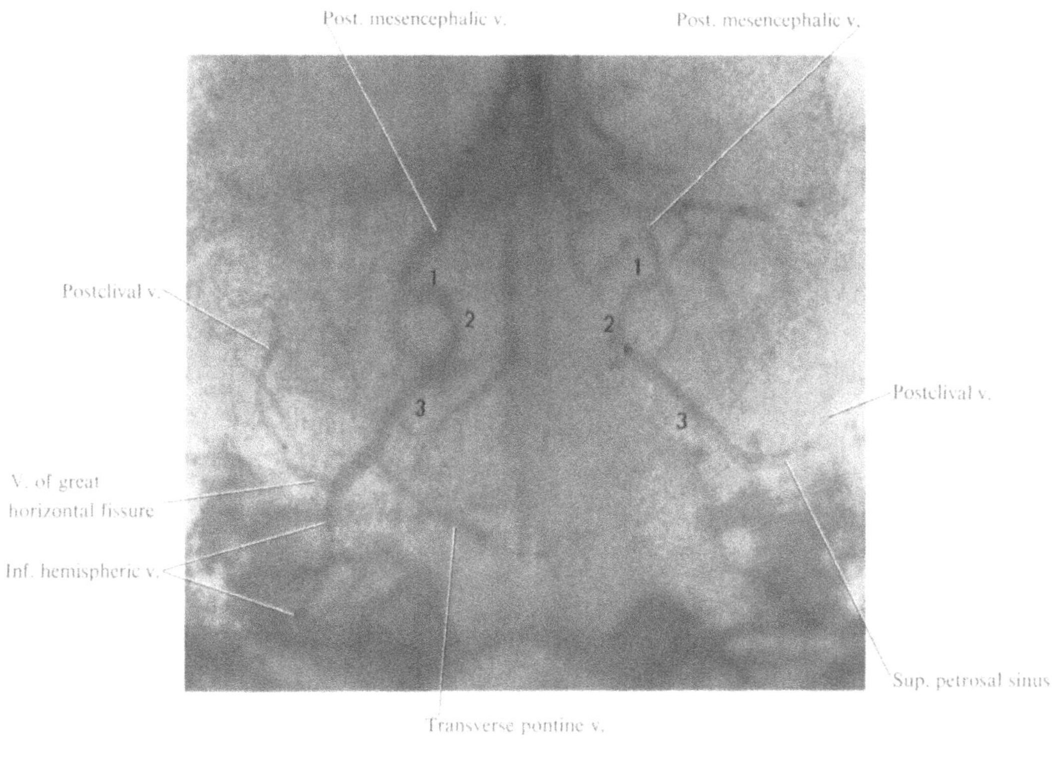

Fig. 134B

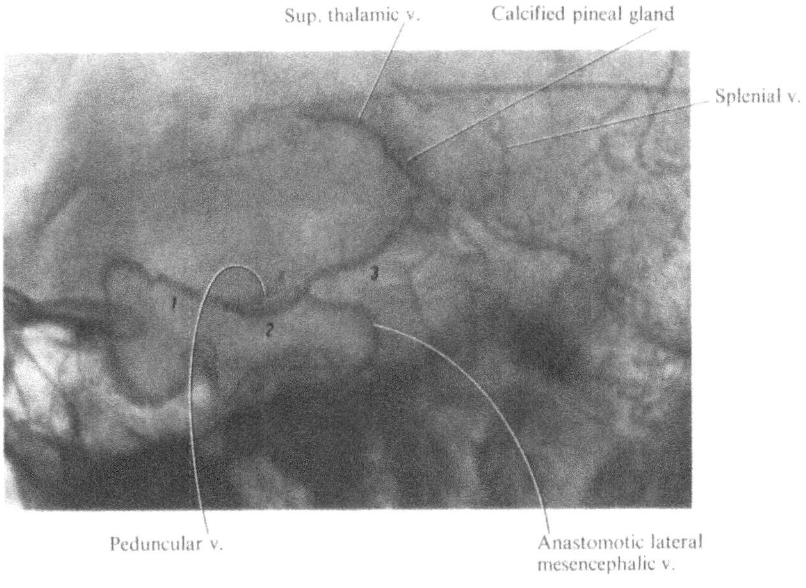

Fig. 134C. Infratentorial drainage of the superior thalamic vein via the third segment of the basal cerebral vein and the anastomotic lateral mesencephalic vein. Cerebral angiogram, venous phase, lateral view

The first (1) and second segments (2) of the basal cerebral vein join the anastomotic lateral mesencephalic vein. The third segment (3) of the basal cerebral vein, receiving the superior and inferior thalamic veins (the latter vein being unlabelled), runs forwards, instead of backwards, and opens into the anastomotic lateral mesencephalic vein. Note the location of the superior thalamic vein below the level of the calcified pineal gland.

Fig. 135. Diagram of the possible anatomic variations in the course of the basal cerebral vein

A. Typical normal course of the basal cerebral vein and its tributaries (complete form). Drawing of the precentral insular vein omitted

B. Drainage into the posterior part of the internal cerebral vein. Note the course of the internal cerebral vein medial to the pulvinar (arrow)

C. Low arcuate course below the uncus

D. High horizontal course

E. Meandering course

F. Zig-zag course

(Courtesy of HUANG and WOLF, 1974. C.V. Mosby Co, modified)

▷

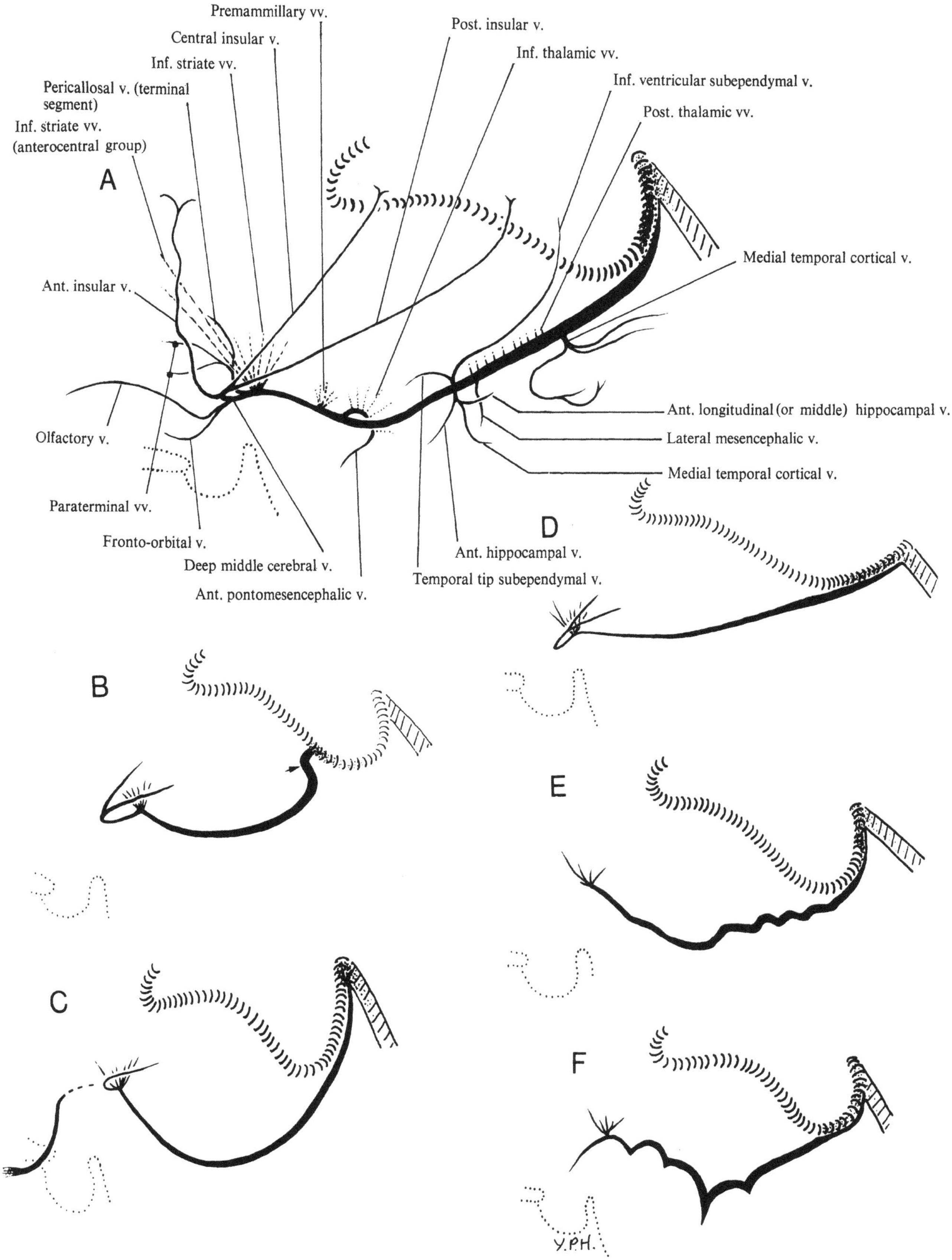

Premammillary vv.
Post. insular v.
Central insular v.
Inf. thalamic vv.
Inf. striate vv.
Inf. ventricular subependymal v.
Pericallosal v. (terminal segment)
Post. thalamic vv.
Inf. striate vv. (anterocentral group)
A
Medial temporal cortical v.
Ant. insular v.
Ant. longitudinal (or middle) hippocampal v.
Lateral mesencephalic v.
Olfactory v.
Medial temporal cortical v.
Paraterminal vv.
D
Fronto-orbital v.
Ant. hippocampal v.
Deep middle cerebral v.
Temporal tip subependymal v.
Ant. pontomesencephalic v.
B
E
C
F
Y.P.H.

Fig. 135

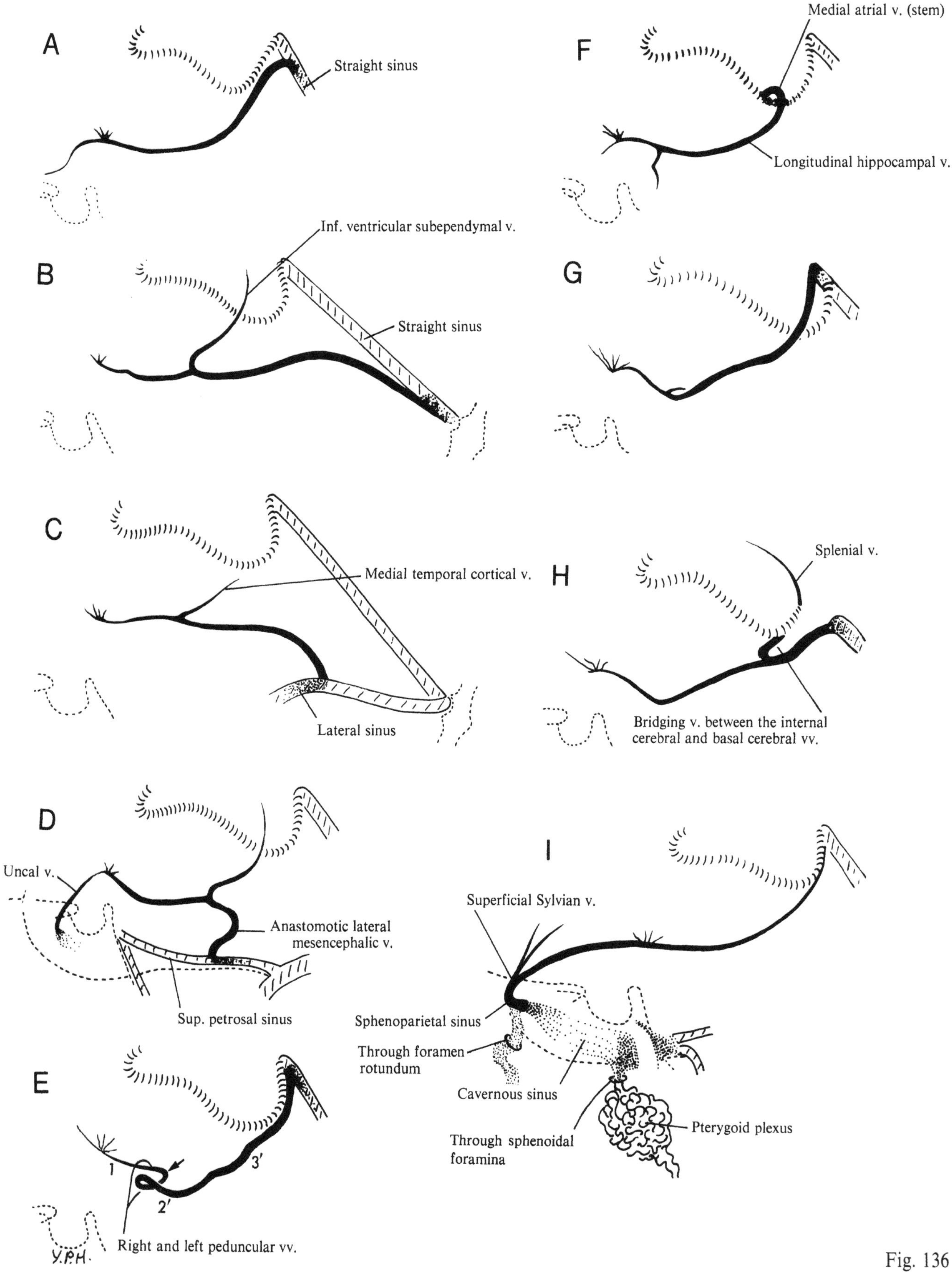
A
Straight sinus
F
Medial atrial v. (stem)
Longitudinal hippocampal v.
B
Inf. ventricular subependymal v.
Straight sinus
G
C
Medial temporal cortical v.
Lateral sinus
H
Splenial v.
Bridging v. between the internal cerebral and basal cerebral vv.
D
Uncal v.
Anastomotic lateral mesencephalic v.
Sup. petrosal sinus
E
1
2′
3′
Right and left peduncular vv.
Y.P.H.
I
Superficial Sylvian v.
Sphenoparietal sinus
Through foramen rotundum
Cavernous sinus
Through sphenoidal foramina
Pterygoid plexus

Fig. 136

Fig. 136. Diagram of the possible anatomic variations in drainage of the basal cerebral vein

A. Drainage into the anterior portion of the straight sinus

B. Drainage into the posterior portion of the straight sinus

C. Drainage into the lateral sinus

D. Drainage into the superior petrosal sinus via the anastomotic lateral mesencephalic vein

E. Drainage into the opposite basal cerebral vein via the posterior communicating vein (arrow)

F. Drainage into the internal cerebral vein via the longitudinal hippocampal and medial atrial veins

G. Drainage into the straight sinus anterior to the distal end of the great cerebral vein

H. Unusual drainage of the internal cerebral vein into the straight sinus via the basal cerebral vein

I. Drainage into the sphenoparietal sinus

(Courtesy of HUANG and WOLF, 1974. C.V. Mosby Co, modified)

Fig. 137. Diagram of the possible segmentation and multiple drainage pathways of the basal cerebral vein

A. Failure of anastomosis between the first and second segments resulting in the formation of the uncal vein

B. Failure of anastomoses between the first and second segments and between the second and third segments, resulting in the formation of the uncal, anastomotic lateral mesencephalic and posterior mesencephalic veins

C. Failure of anastomoses between the first and second segments, between the second and third segments and between the anterior and posterior parts of the second segment, resulting in the formation of the uncal, anterior pontomesencephalic, anastomotic lateral mesencephalic and posterior mesencephalic veins

D. Another form of multiple drainage similar to that seen in Fig. 137C – drainage into the uncal, lateral anterior pontomesencephalic, anastomotic lateral mesencephalic, quadrigeminal, posterior longitudinal hippocampal and medial atrial veins

E. Accessory basal cerebral vein or separate posterior mesencephalic vein

F. Drainage of the first segment into the posterior part of the straight sinus via a tentorial sinus (shaded). Note an unusual drainage of the superior thalamic vein into the posterior mesencephalic vein. This latter vein opens into the Galenic system

G. Posterolateral drainage of the first segment into the transverse sinus and posteromedial drainage of the second and third segments into the great cerebral vein

H. Drainage of the first segment and the anterior part of the second segment into the superior petrosal sinus via the anterior pontomesencephalic vein. Posterolateral drainage of the posterior part of the second segment into the lateral sinus via a tentorial sinus (shaded) is also shown

I. Drainage of the superficial Sylvian, uncal and anastomotic lateral mesencephalic veins into the lateral sinus, via a prominent inferior temporal cortical vein and tentorial sinus (shaded)

J. Supratentorial (or Galenic) drainage of the petrosal vein and its tributaries, via the anastomotic lateral mesencephalic and posterior mesenphalic veins

(Courtesy of HUANG and WOLF, 1974. C.V. Mosby Co, modified)

Fig. 137 see p. 172 ▷

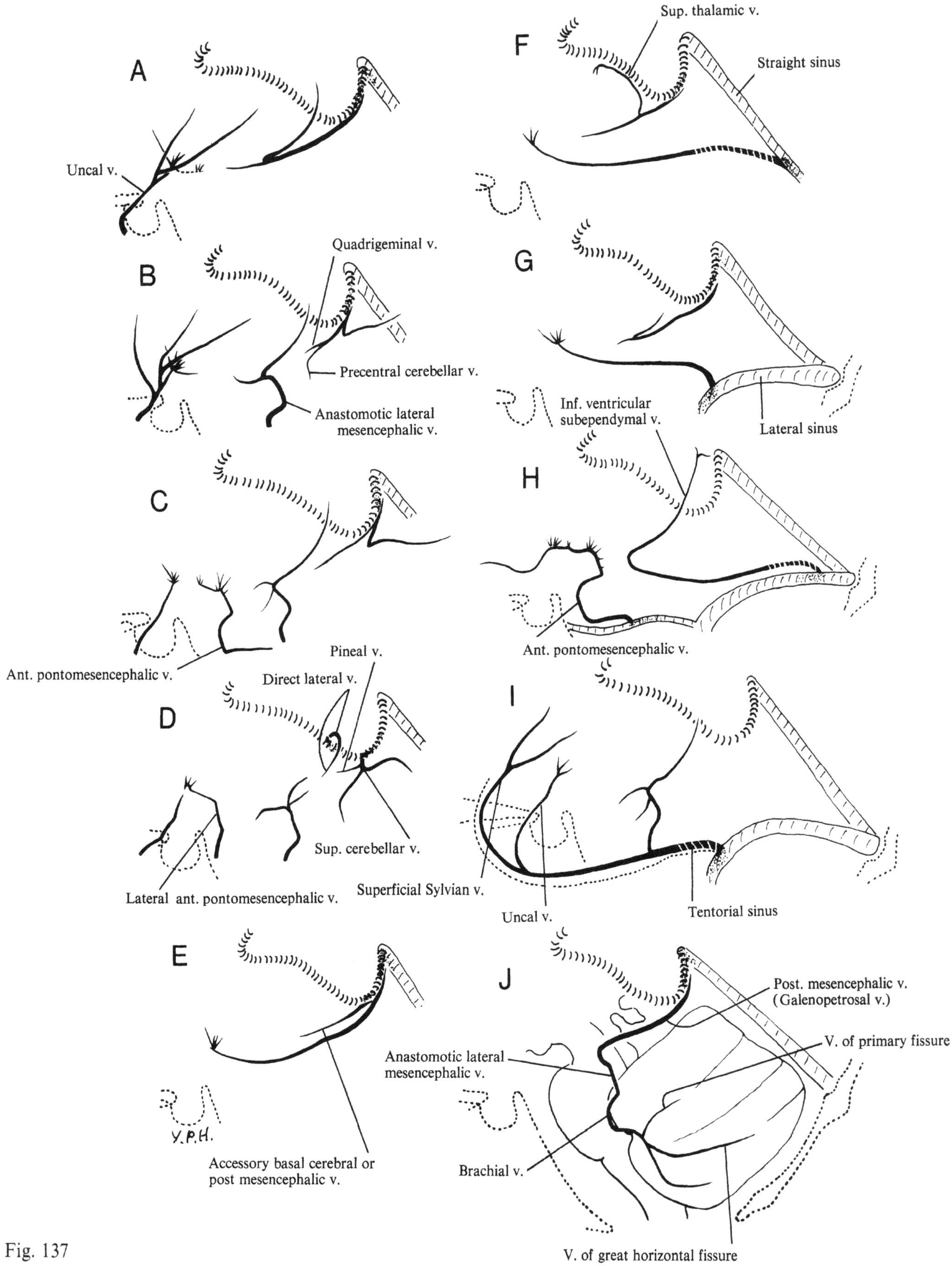

A
Uncal v.
B
Quadrigeminal v.
Precentral cerebellar v.
Anastomotic lateral mesencephalic v.
C
Ant. pontomesencephalic v.
D
Pineal v.
Direct lateral v.
Sup. cerebellar v.
Lateral ant. pontomesencephalic v.
Superficial Sylvian v.
E
Y.P.H.
Accessory basal cerebral or post mesencephalic v.
F
Sup. thalamic v.
Straight sinus
G
Inf. ventricular subependymal v.
Lateral sinus
H
Ant. pontomesencephalic v.
I
Uncal v.
Tentorial sinus
J
Post. mesencephalic v. (Galenopetrosal v.)
V. of primary fissure
Anastomotic lateral mesencephalic v.
Brachial v.
V. of great horizontal fissure

Fig. 137

PART 2

MESENCEPHALIC REGION, DIENCEPHALIC REGION, AND BASAL GANGLIA

Introduction

At first glance it might appear arbitrary to include the mesencephalon, diencephalon and basal ganglia in the same chapter. However, evaluation of a deep tumor involving the basal ganglia, the third ventricle, or pineal region requires orientation by means of morphologic changes in the third ventricle, the lenticulostriate arteries, thalamoperforate arteries, posteromedial and posterolateral choroidal arteries and the internal cerebral veins. In a similar way, the presence of a mass lesion in the cerebral hemisphere requires the exclusion of a deep extension of the tumor, which might contraindicate surgery.

The principal basal ganglia (caudate nuclei, lentiform nuclei and thalamus) present a topographic similarity in their relationship to the third ventricle. Likewise, the suprasellar cisterns form a veritable cisternal envelope around the chiasmatic and infundibular recesses of the anterior end of the third ventricle. Similar reasoning includes the study of the aqueduct of Sylvius with the posterior end of the third ventricle.

Although the cisterns of the mesencephalic region (in particular the cistern of the vein of Galen) constitute a cisternal extension of the posterior end of the third ventricle, they shall be included in the discussion of the posterior fossa. The cisterns of the posterior fossa combine with those of the tentorial incisure to form a morphologic unit which is so coherent that it would be hard to separate them.

While it might seem logical to include the study of the lateral ventricles in this chapter (since their relationships to the deep nuclei are so close), they combine with the cerebral hemispheres to form a similar coherent unit. It is for this reason that they are not included in this chapter.

The significance, inherent difficulties, and prerequisite finesse of clinical or angiographic evaluation of lesions in the region under consideration, make us hesitant to present the anatomic relationships which can be defined by neuroradiologic examinations.

Contrast ventriculography permits detailed evaluation of the major constituents of the third ventricle *in vivo*. However, angiographically there is no possibility of identifying the vascularization of all the diencephalic and mesencephalic structures. We have included vessels with a minimum caliber of 100 microns, since it should be possible (at least with magnification techniques) to identify these vessels angiographically. The vascularization of the optic chiasm, the hypothalamus and the quadrigeminal plate has been deliberately omitted as their arterial supply is by vessels that are too small to be identified.

Angiographic emphasis has been placed upon the perforating arteries which can be visualized by carotid or vertebral angiography. These vessels include the lenticulostriate arteries and the recurrent artery of Heubner from the carotid system, and the thalamoperforate arteries and posteromedial and posterolateral choroidal arteries from the vertebrobasilar system. Finally, the evaluation of the internal cerebral vein and its tributaries naturally relates to this region.

Chapter 1
Third Ventricle and Suprasellar Cisterns

I. Anatomic Study of the Third Ventricle and Suprasellar Cisterns

1. Third Ventricle

Tela choroidea of the third ventricle
Cistern of the velum interpositum

The third ventricle is a single midline cavity, located below the fornix and the tela choroidea of the third ventricle and between the two halves of the thalamus. It communicates with the lateral ventricles through the foramina of Monro, and with the fourth ventricle through the aqueduct of Sylvius. Its length is 20 mm and transverse diameter is 1.5 mm. The third ventricle may be described as funnel-shaped, having two lateral surfaces, an anterior and a posterior wall, a base which is superiorly placed and an apex which is inferiorly placed (Figs. 138–142).

The lateral surfaces of the third ventricle are divided by the hypothalamic sulci into two parts. The upper part corresponds to the thalamus while the inferior part relates to the region of the hypothalamus, the infundibulum and the tuber cinereum. The hypothalamic sulcus extends from the foramen of Monro to the aqueduct of Sylvius. The two foramina of Monro (or interventricular foramina) are symmetrical channels situated between the anterior columns of the fornix and the anterior pole of the thalamus. They measure 5 mm in length and 3 mm transversely.

The base of the third ventricle is elongated in the anteroposterior direction. Anteriorly it is bounded by the opening between the anterior columns of the fornix and posteriorly by the pineal body and its lateral attachments, the habenulae. In between, the base of the third ventricle is formed by ependymal lining which is covered by tela choroidea.

The anterior wall is directed anteriorly and inferiorly. Its direction is almost vertical. Superiorly to inferiorly it is formed by the anterior columns of the fornix, the anterior commissure, the lamina terminalis, the optic recess and the optic chiasm.

The posterior wall also slopes anteriorly and inferiorly. Superiorly to inferiorly it is formed by the attachment of the pineal body, the posterior commissure and the opening of the aqueduct of Sylvius. Beneath the orifice of the aqueduct one finds the upper end of the cerebral peduncles, the mammillary bodies and the tuber cinereum. Above the aqueduct two posterior recesses of the third ventricle are present, the suprapineal and pineal recesses.

The apex of the third ventricle is formed by the infundibular recess which continues inferiorly as the pituitary stalk.

In ***the cavity of the third ventricle*** is the massa intermedia (grey commissure), which is of variable size and shape. This is where the two halves of the thalamus, on either side of the ventricle, touch in the midline. No nerve fibres cross between the two halves of the thalamus, via this commissure.

The tela choroidea of the third ventricle is formed by the coalescence of two leaves of the pia mater. The superior one arises from the splenium of the corpus callosum, the inferior one arises from the quadrigeminal bodies. These two leaves insinuate themselves into the choroidal fissure, to lie below the fornix and on the roof of the third ventricle. The tela choroidea is triangular in shape with its base located posteriorly. Laterally, it rests against the medial extraventricular surfaces of the two halves of the thalamus. In its midportion it forms the roof of the third ventricle. It thickens on both sides of the midline to form the choroid plexus of the third ventricle which is continuous with that of the lateral ventricles, through the foramina of Monro.

The cistern of the velum interpositum is the space situated between the two leaves of the tela choroidea. It communicates posteriorly and superiorly with the cistern of the corpus callosum, and posteriorly and inferiorly with the cistern of the vein of Galen or the quadrigeminal cistern. The two internal cerebral veins run in this cistern.

2. Suprasellar Cisterns

Interpeduncular cistern
Chiasmatic cistern
Cistern of the lamina terminalis

At the base of the brain, anterior to the cerebral peduncles and around the optic chiasm, several cisterns communicate to form a large lake of cerebrospinal fluid. These cisterns are, from posteriorly to anteriorly, the interpeduncular cistern, the chiasmatic cistern and the cistern of the lamina terminalis (Figs. 143–146).
The interpeduncular cistern is situated in the fossa between the two cerebral peduncles. The chiasmatic cistern extends backwards from the subfrontal region, and is arbitrarily divided posteriorly, from the interpeduncular cistern, by a line from the anterior margin of the mammillary bodies to the dorsum sellae. This cistern is traversed by the optic chiasm and the optic nerves, which divide it into prechiasmatic and postchiasmatic compartments. Laterally, the chiasmatic cistern has a wide communication with the cistern of the Sylvian fissure. The cistern of the lamina terminalis is located in the midline in front of the lamina terminalis.

The interpeduncular cistern is bounded posterosuperiorly by the posterior perforated substance and the anterior aspect of the cerebral peduncles. The roof of this cistern is made up of the mammillary bodies and the tuber cinereum. The interpeduncular cistern communicates inferiorly with the pontine cistern, between the posterior clinoid processes and the anterior surface of the pons. Laterally, the interpeduncular cistern is continuous with the crural cisterns, which are located anteriorly to the lateral aspects of the cerebral peduncles. The interpeduncular cistern may be arbitrarily limited anteriorly by a plane which passes through the anterior border of the mammillary bodies and the dorsum sellae. This cistern contains the tip of the basilar artery, the origins of the posterior cerebral and superior cerebellar arteries, the posterior communicating arteries and the thalamoperforate arteries. Anteriorly to the interpeduncular cistern is a clival plexus of veins and posteriorly to it is the interpeduncular portion of the anterior pontomesencephalic vein complex. On either side of the midline, the interpeduncular cistern is traversed by the third and sixth cranial nerves.

The chiasmatic cistern. This space extends from the interpeduncular cistern to the subfrontal region. Its lateral boundaries are formed by the two hippocampal gyri. This cistern is crossed by both the pituitary stalk and the optic nerves. The optic chiasm divides the cistern into two compartments; the prechiasmatic which is elongated anteroposteriorly and the postchiasmatic which extends from the chiasm to the diaphragma sellae.
Anteriorly, in frontal section, the optic nerves form the lateral borders of the prechiasmatic portion. Along the outer aspect of each optic nerve one finds the pericarotid cistern and the region of the anterior perforated substance. Laterally, the chiasmatic cistern is continuous with the cistern of the Sylvian fissure. In addition to the nervous elements which cross the chiasmatic cistern, the cistern is closely related to the internal carotid arteries and their branches forming the anterior aspect of the circle of Willis, and also to the roof of the cavernous sinus.

The cistern of the lamina terminalis. Lying anteriorly to the third ventricle, the cistern of the lamina terminalis is continuous inferiorly with the chiasmatic cistern. It is limited posteriorly by the anterior commissure and the lamina terminalis and contains the first portions of the anterior cerebral arteries and also the anterior communicating artery.

II. Radiologic Study of the Third Ventricle and Suprasellar Cisterns

The radiologic evaluation of the third ventricle has been the subject of numerous studies [Bull (1956), Robertson (1957), Lindgren (1951), Ruggiero (1953)]. During encephalography, evaluation of the third ventricle commences with the patient seated in the upright position. Filling occurs via the aqueduct of Sylvius and air outlines the base and upper part of the posterior wall of the third ventricle, and also the pineal and suprapineal recesses (Fig. 147).
The anterior portion of the third ventricle is seldom visualized until the patient is placed in the brow-up position. When this is done, air fills the optic and infundibular recesses, the foramina of Monro and the frontal horns of the lateral ventricles (Fig. 147).
If the third ventricle is to be studied by gas ventriculography, the reverse steps are followed, i.e., the anterior end of the third ventricle is studied first, with evaluation of its posterior portion being performed subsequently (Ziedses des Plantes, 1950).
Certain authors have proposed selective insufflation of the third ventricle by means of a catheter guided through a ventriculostomy with the aid of a fine chain (Corrales, 1973). Finally, the third ventricle may be opacified with oily or water-soluble contrast media. It is this method which is most frequently used for localization of the anterior and posterior commissures prior to sterotactic surgery.

DAVIDOFF and DYKE (1951), and ORLEY (1949) found the anteroposterior length of the third ventricle measured 26 mm. The average distance between the anterior and posterior commissures was 25 mm in the study of TALAIRACH and SZIKLA (1967). The height of the third ventricle, as measured in the lateral projection, varies between 12 mm and 16 mm.

In RUGGIERO's study the width of the normal third ventricle varied between 5 mm and 15 mm. DAVIDOFF and DYKE (1951), never found the normal width to exceed 9 mm.

RUGGIERO and CASTELLANO (1953) proposed a precise method for localizing the posterior end of the third ventricle (Fig. 151). A line is constructed tangentially to the lower part of the posterior wall of the third ventricle and perpendicular to the plane of the clivus. This line transects the junction of the posterior end of the third ventricle and aqueduct of Sylvius at the level of the uncus.

GREITZ and LOFSTEDT (1954) described an indentation of the posterior wall of the third ventricle caused by ectatic elongation of the basilar artery.

The lateral projection provides the best detail of the third ventricle because of its sagittal orientation. In this projection one can identify the foramina of Monro, the impressions of the anterior and posterior commissures, the outline of the massa intermedia, the posterior wall and its junction with the aqueduct, and also the optic, infundibular, pineal and supra-pineal recesses (Figs. 147, 148, 150). The last recess is extremely variable in its development, form and dimensions.

The works of DAVIDOFF and DYKE (1951), DILENGE (1955), and LILIEQUIST (1959) have greatly assisted the radiologic study of the suprasellar cisterns, but the hypocycloidal tomographic studies of METZGER (1967) and his collaborators have provided the best images of this region and the most information about possible variations.

The suprasellar cisterns may be arbitrarily divided by a plane which passes between the anterior border of the mammillary bodies and the dorsum sellae. In front of this plane is the chiasmatic cistern, containing the pituitary stalk, and behind is the interpeduncular cistern.

At its name implies, *the interpeduncular cistern* fills the region between the cerebral peduncles, and outlines the mammillary bodies arteriorly. It may also show anteriorly a thin membrane, first described by KEY and RETZIUS (1875) and later identified radiologically by LILIEQUIST (1959). Laterally the interpeduncular cisterns are continuous with the crural cisterns which lie along the anterolateral surfaces of the cerebral peduncles. Frontal and lateral tomograms of this region frequently outline the shadows of the basilar trunk, the origins of the posterior cerebral and superior cerebellar arteries, and occasionally, the shadows of the oculomotor nerves.

The chiasmatic cistern extends to the posterior surface of the frontal lobes. From this region it continues forwards as the cistern of the lamina terminalis. In the lateral projection, the chiasmatic cistern is traversed by the optic chiasm and, more posteriorly, by the pituitary stalk.

The portion of the chiasmatic cistern in front of the optic chiasm and between the two optic nerves has a quadrangular shape. Further posteriorly the shape is that of a triangle, with a concave base, corresponding to the diaphragma sellae.

Above the chiasmatic cistern are the anterior recesses of the third ventricle. Posteriorly to the pituitary stalk, the chiasmatic cistern is continuous with the anterior part of the interpeduncular cistern.

In frontal tomograms, METZGER (1967) has shown that it is possible to study in great detail the anatomic structures in this region. Anteriorly, the cuts show first the optic nerves and then the chiasm. Further posteriorly is the pituitary stalk with the infundibular recess of the third ventricle above it. Finally, the optic tracts can be identified as they pass backwards on either side of the third ventricle.

In lateral tomograms air outlines the optic nerves and the carotid siphons.

Recently, GREPE (1974) proposed the use of a water-soluble contrast material (Metrizamide), for the study of the fine details of the chiasmatic region.

Anatomic familiarity with this region and the availability of hypocycloidal tomography realizes the expectations of LINDGREN (1957), who wanted to be able "to search this region with X-rays like an anatomist with his scalpel in the course of a dissection".

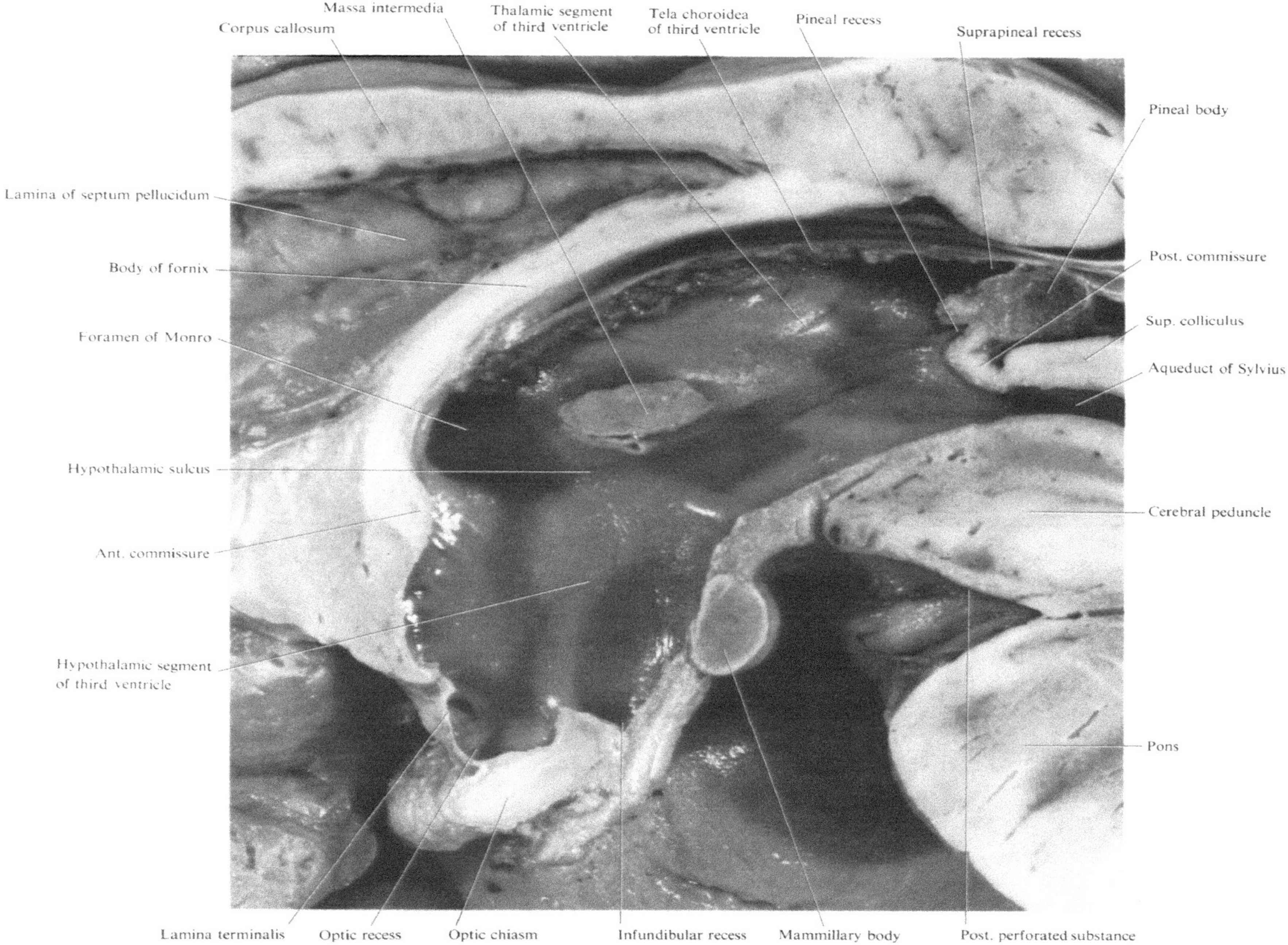

Fig. 138. Sagittal section through the third ventricle

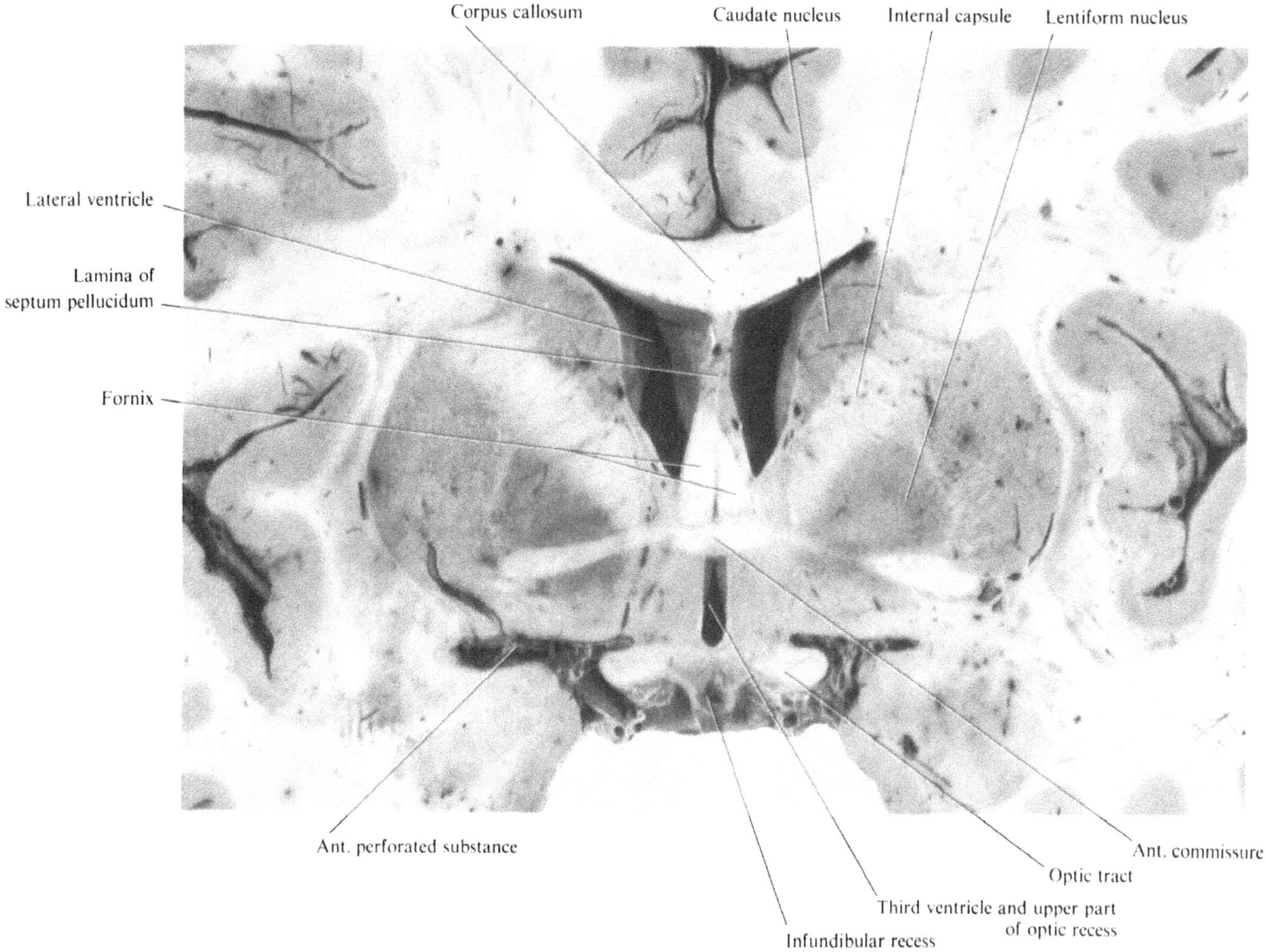

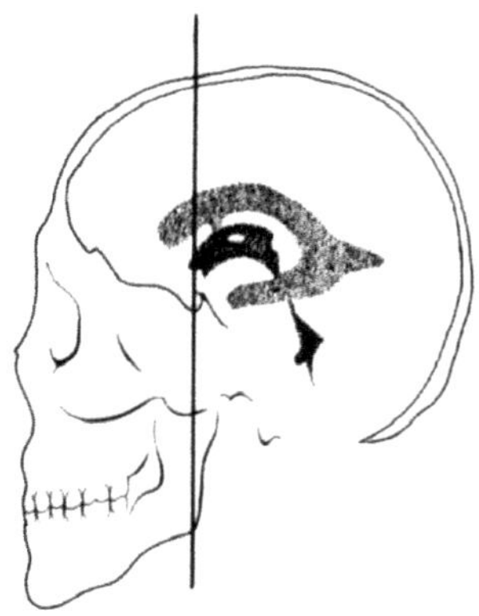

Fig. 139. Frontal section through the anterior part of the third ventricle

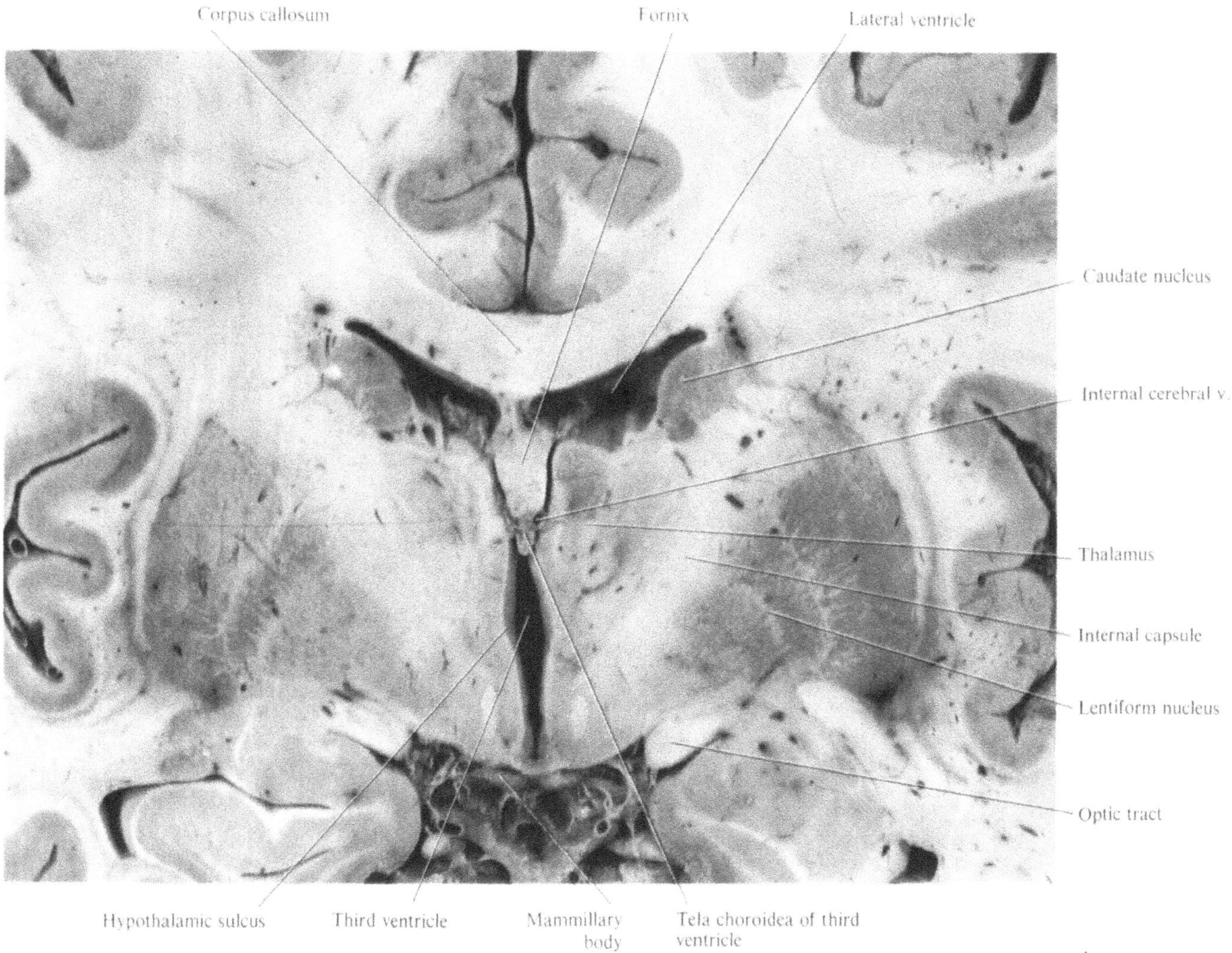

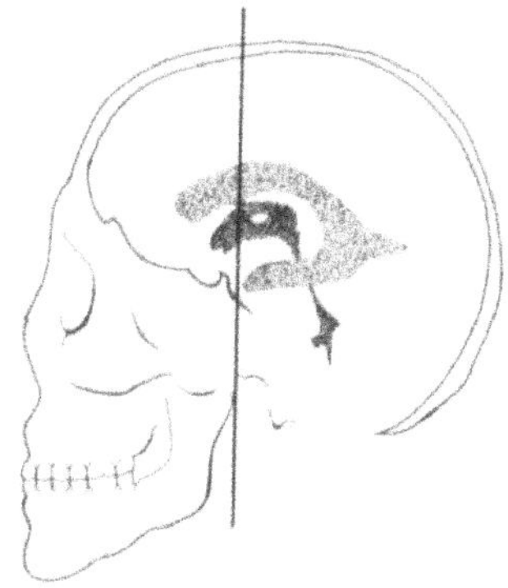

Fig. 140. Frontal section through the middle part of the third ventricle

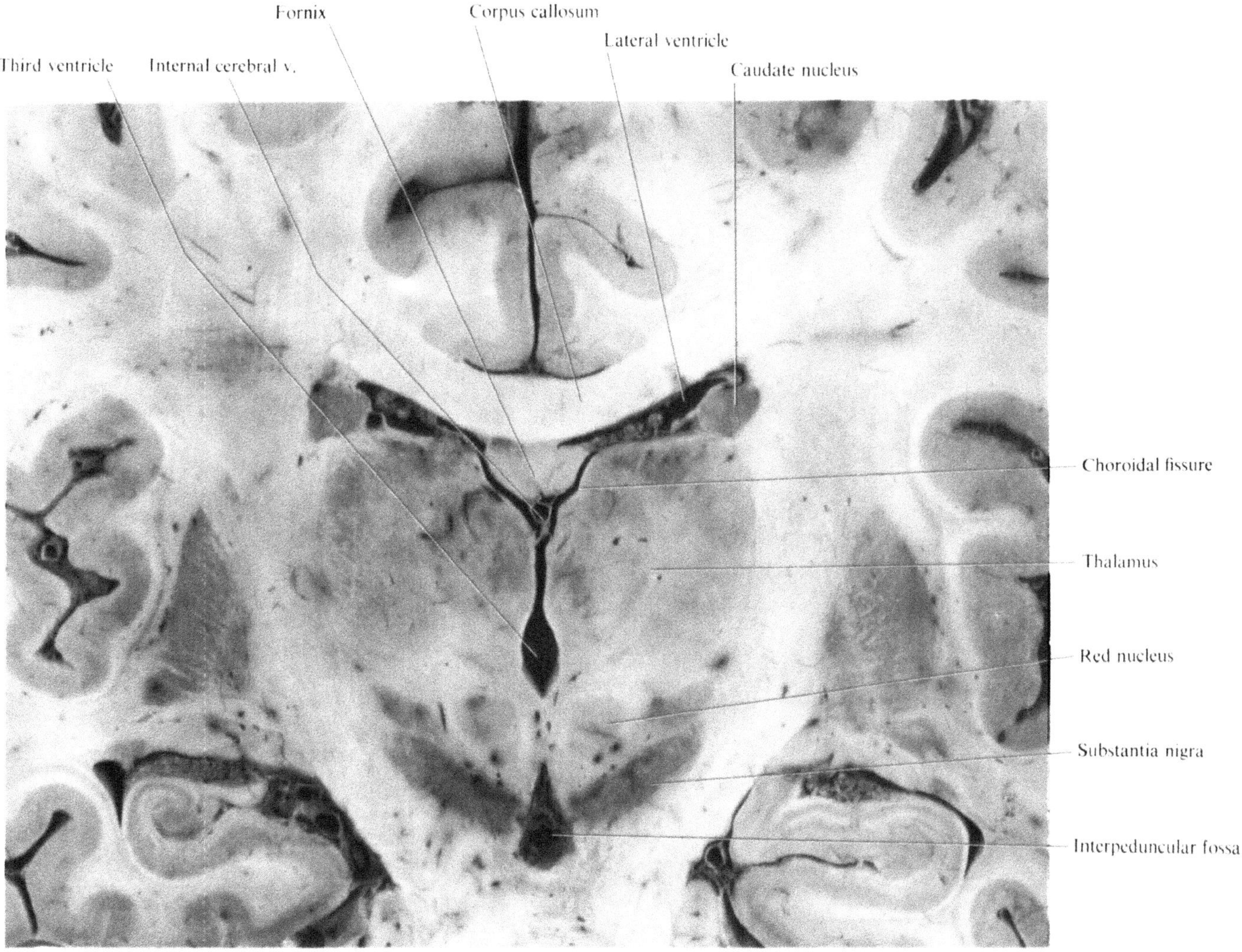

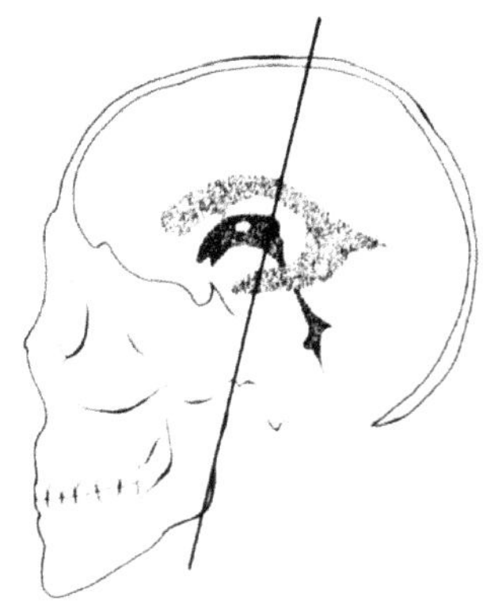

Fig. 141. Frontal section through the posterior part of the third ventricle

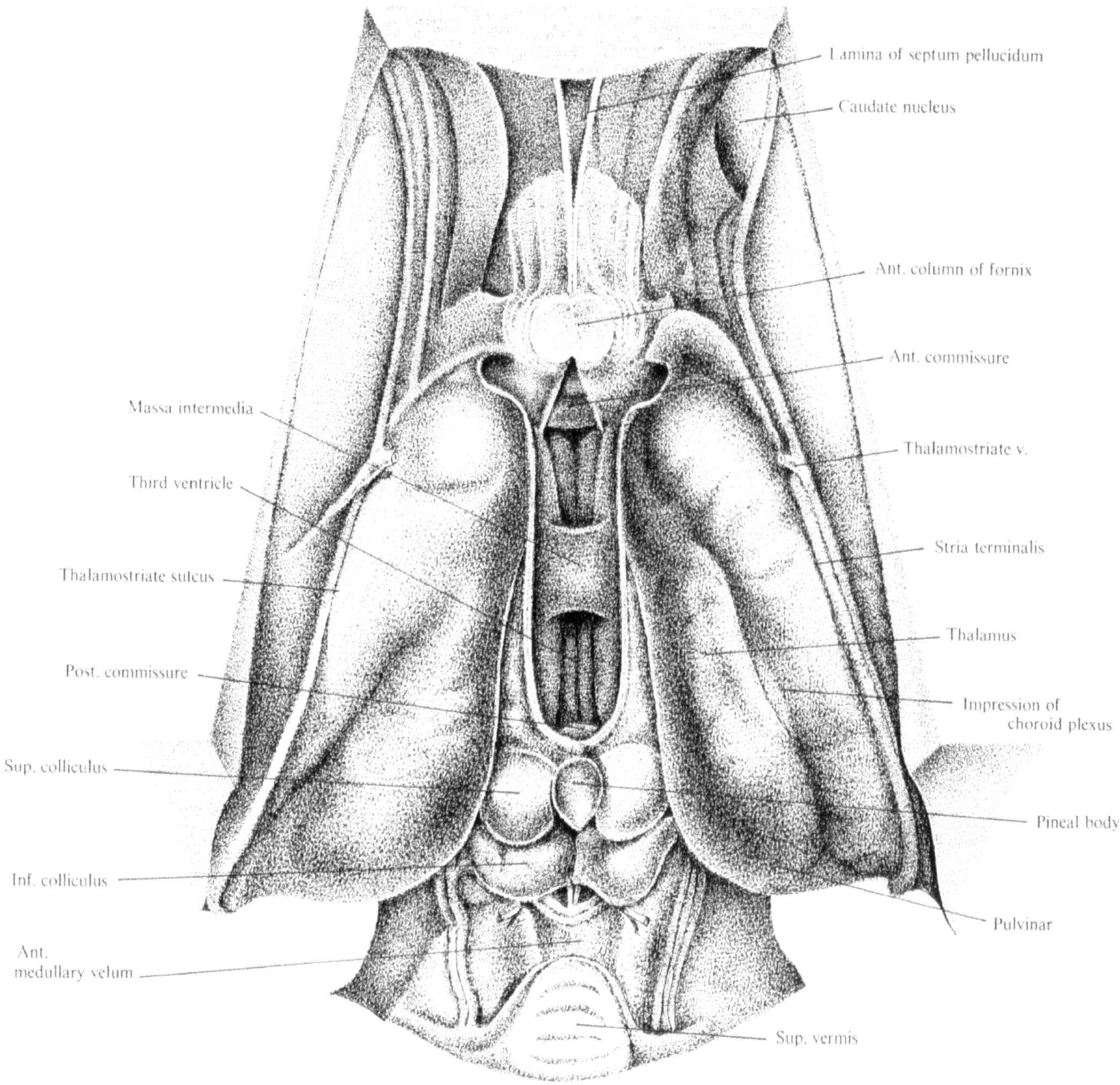

Fig. 142. Third ventricle viewed from above (according to TESTUT, 1948)

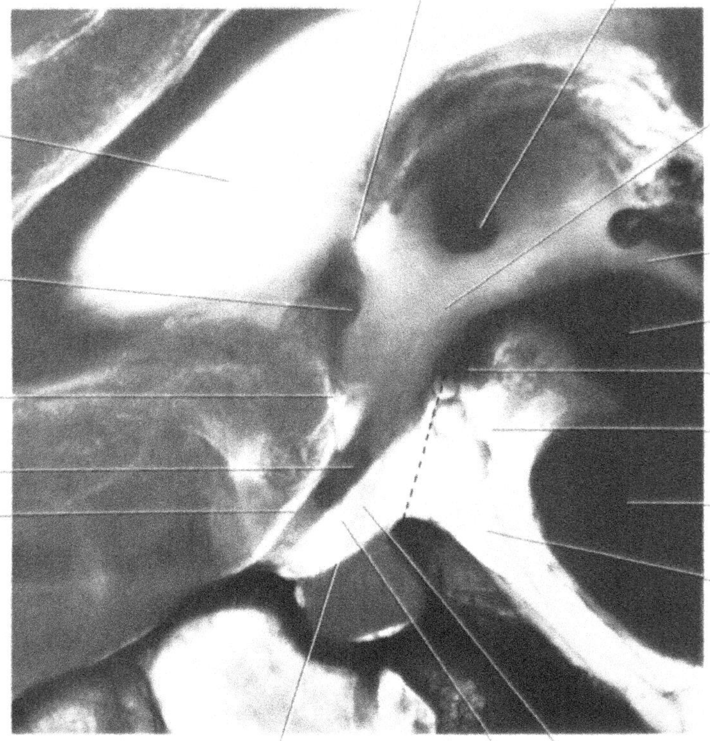

Fig. 143. Sagittal section through the suprasellar cisterns. The dotted line marks the boundary between chiasmatic and interpeduncular cisterns

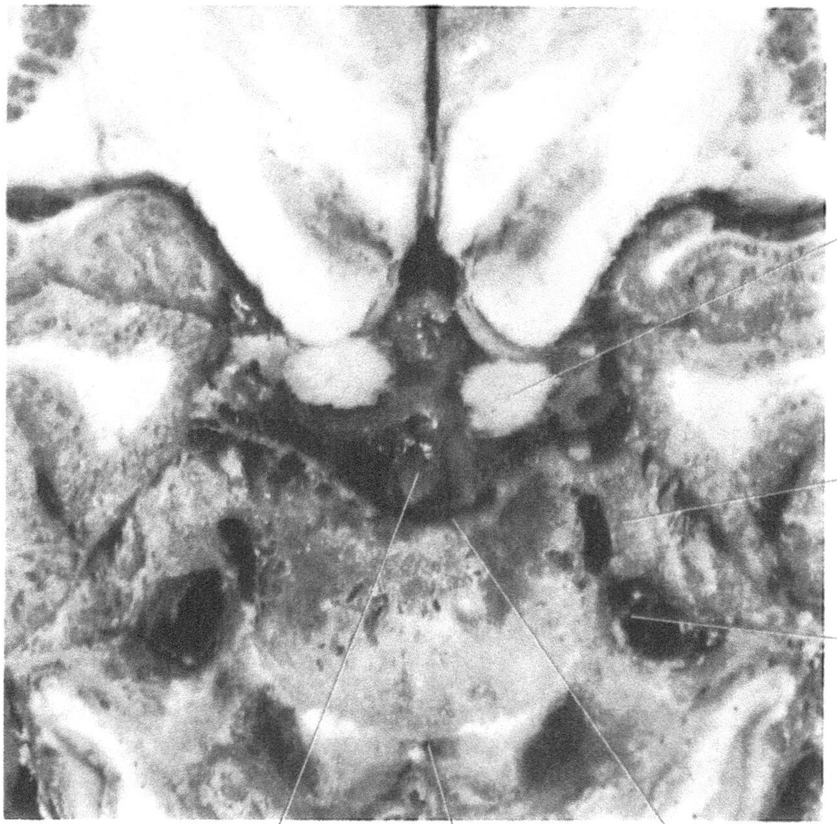

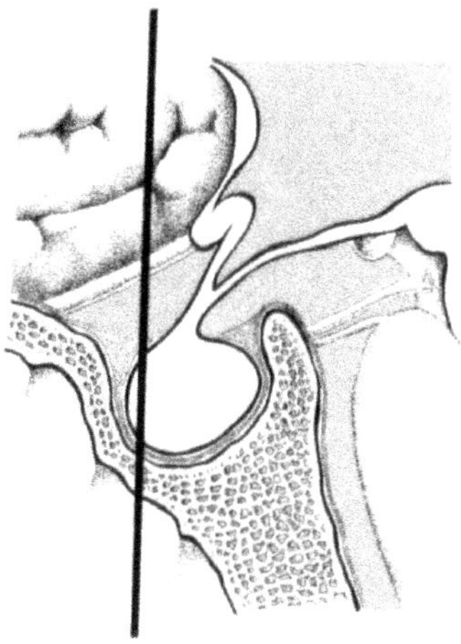

Fig. 144. Frontal section through the anterior part of the suprasellar cistern

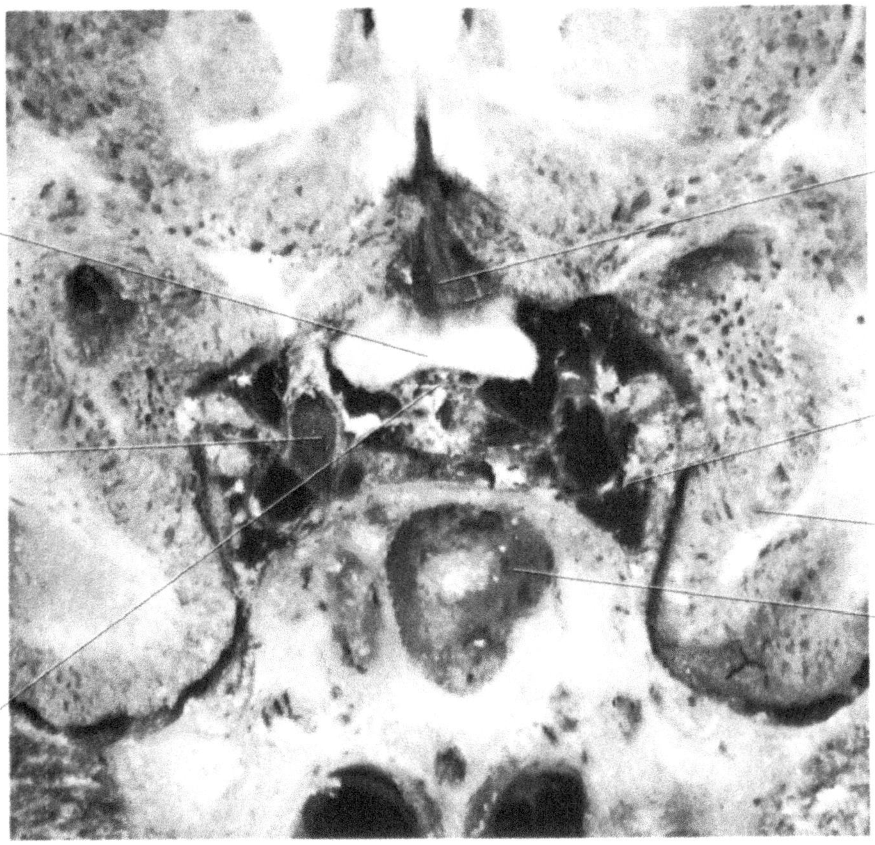

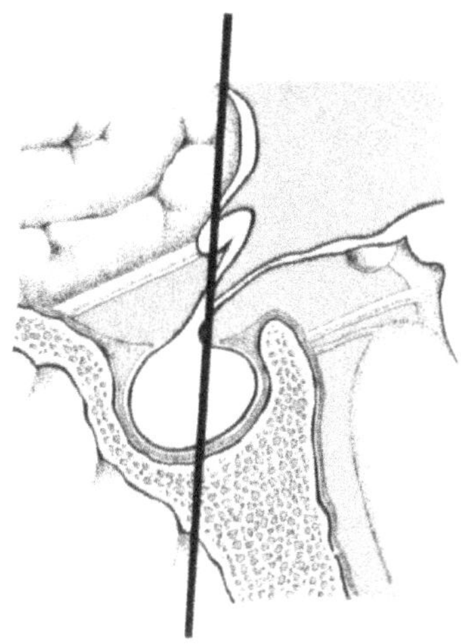

Fig. 145. Frontal section through the optic chiasm

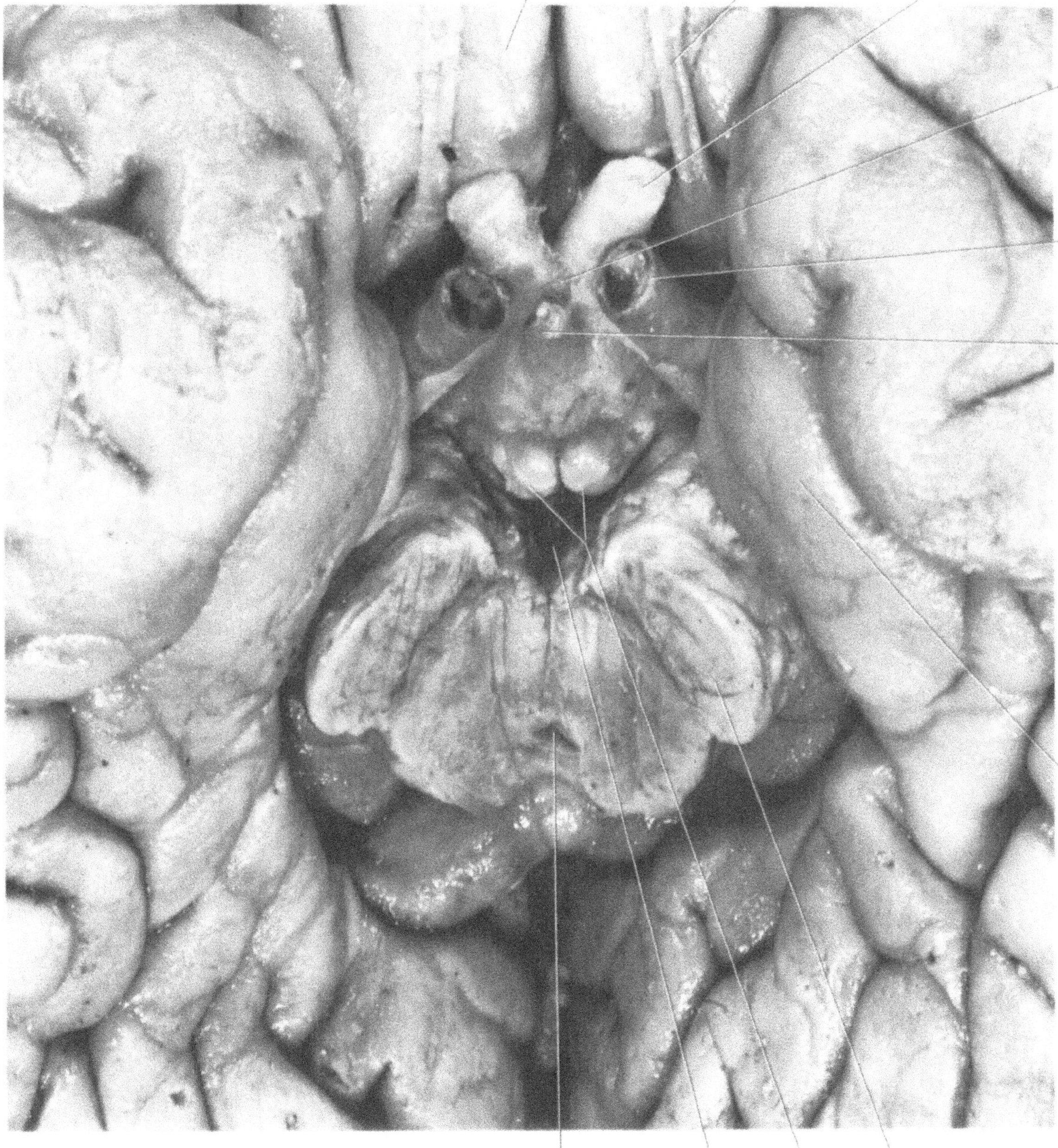

Fig. 146. Inferior surface of the brain, showing structures in the region of suprasellar cisterns

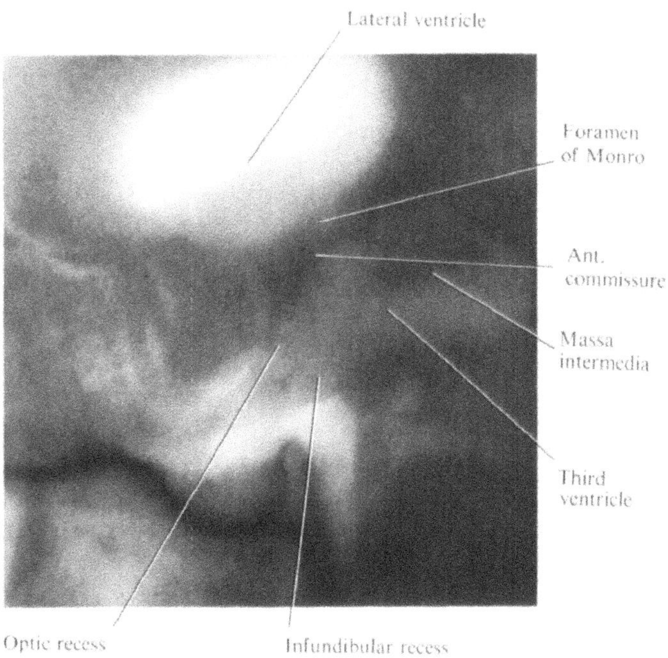

Fig. 147 A. Anterior recesses of the third ventricle

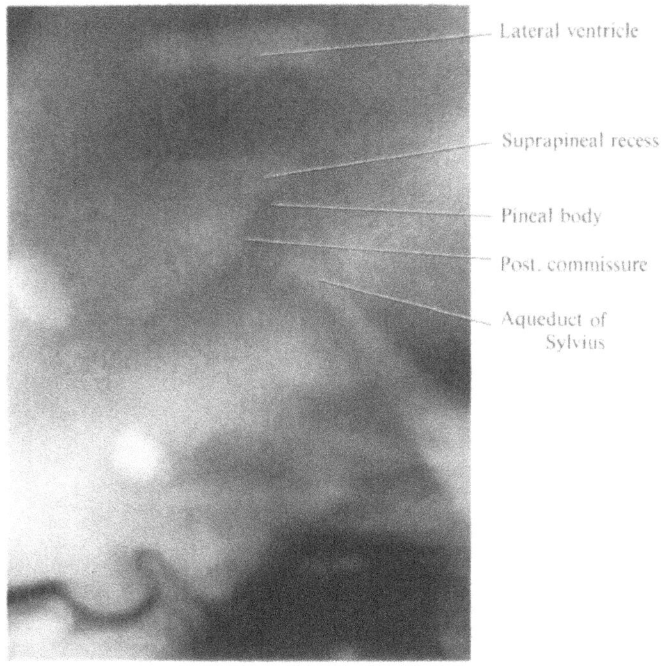

Fig. 147 B. Posterior part of the third ventricle

Fig. 147 A–B. Pneumoencephalograms, midline sagittal tomograms, showing

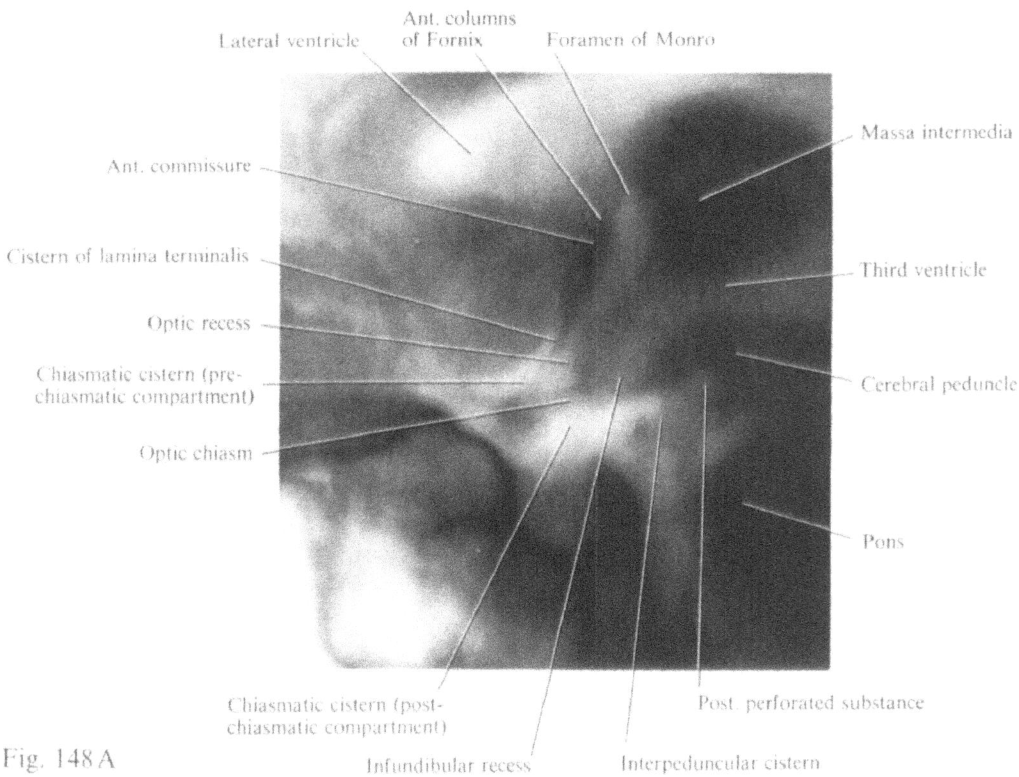

Fig. 148 A

Fig. 148 A–D. Pneumoencephalograms, midline sagittal tomograms ▷

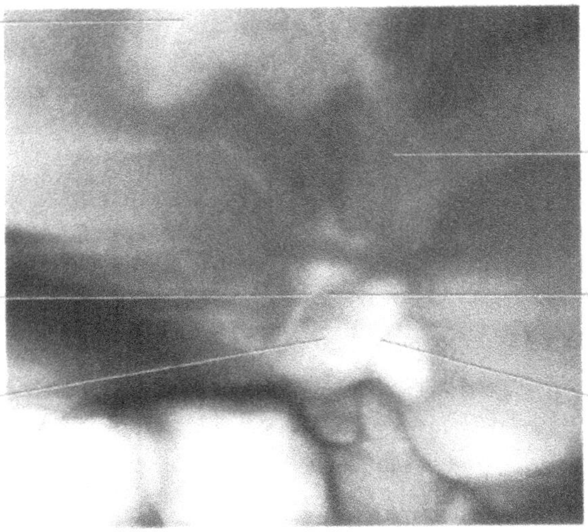

Fig. 148 B

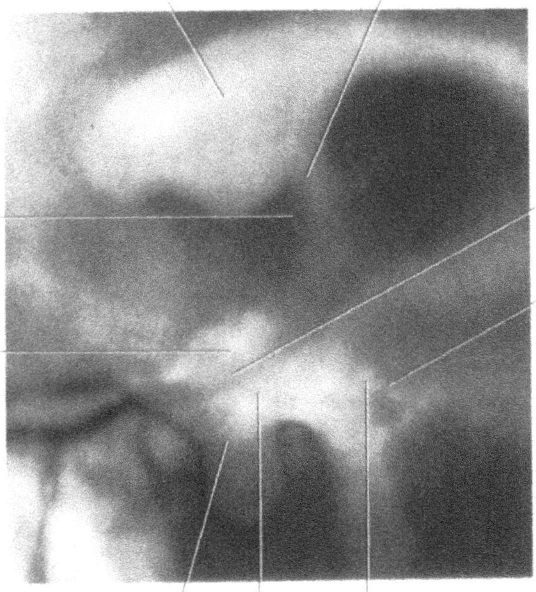

Fig. 148 C

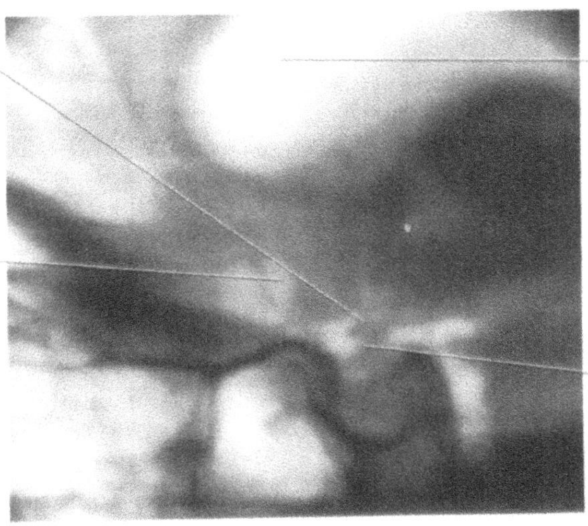

Fig. 148 D

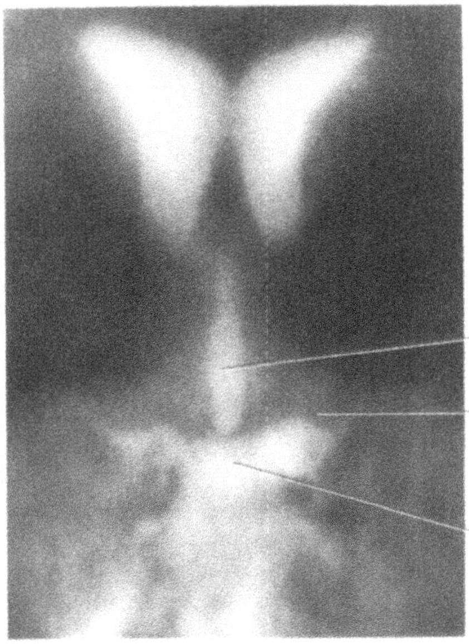

Fig. 149 A

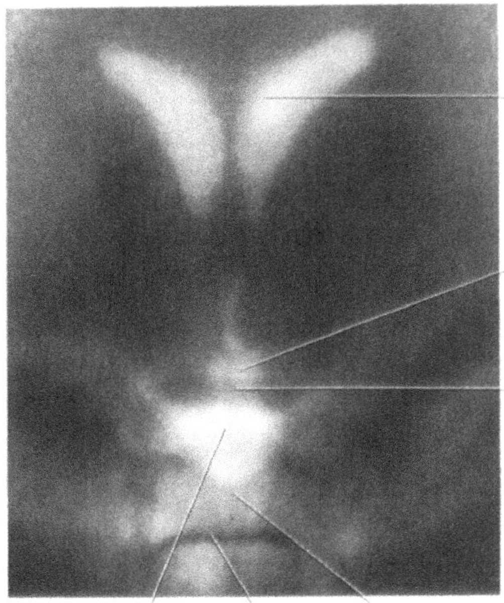

Fig. 149 B

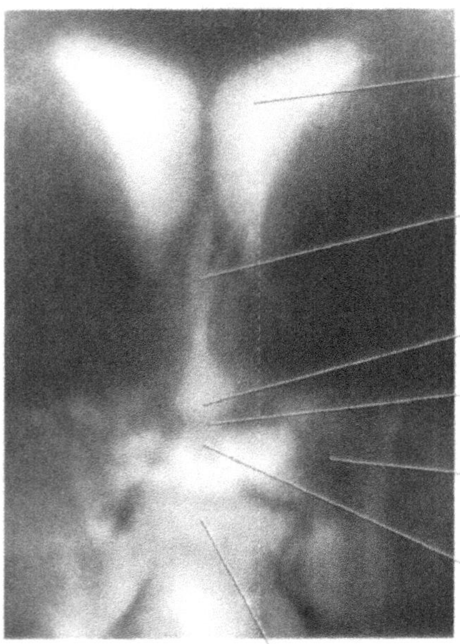

Fig. 149 C

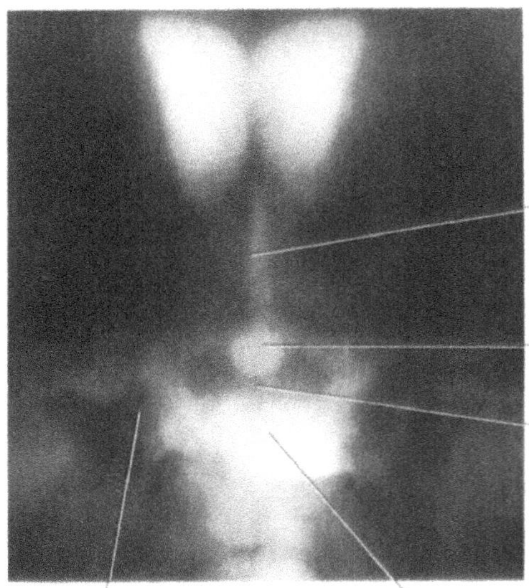

Fig. 149 D

Fig. 149 A–E. Pneumoencephalograms, frontal tomograms ▷

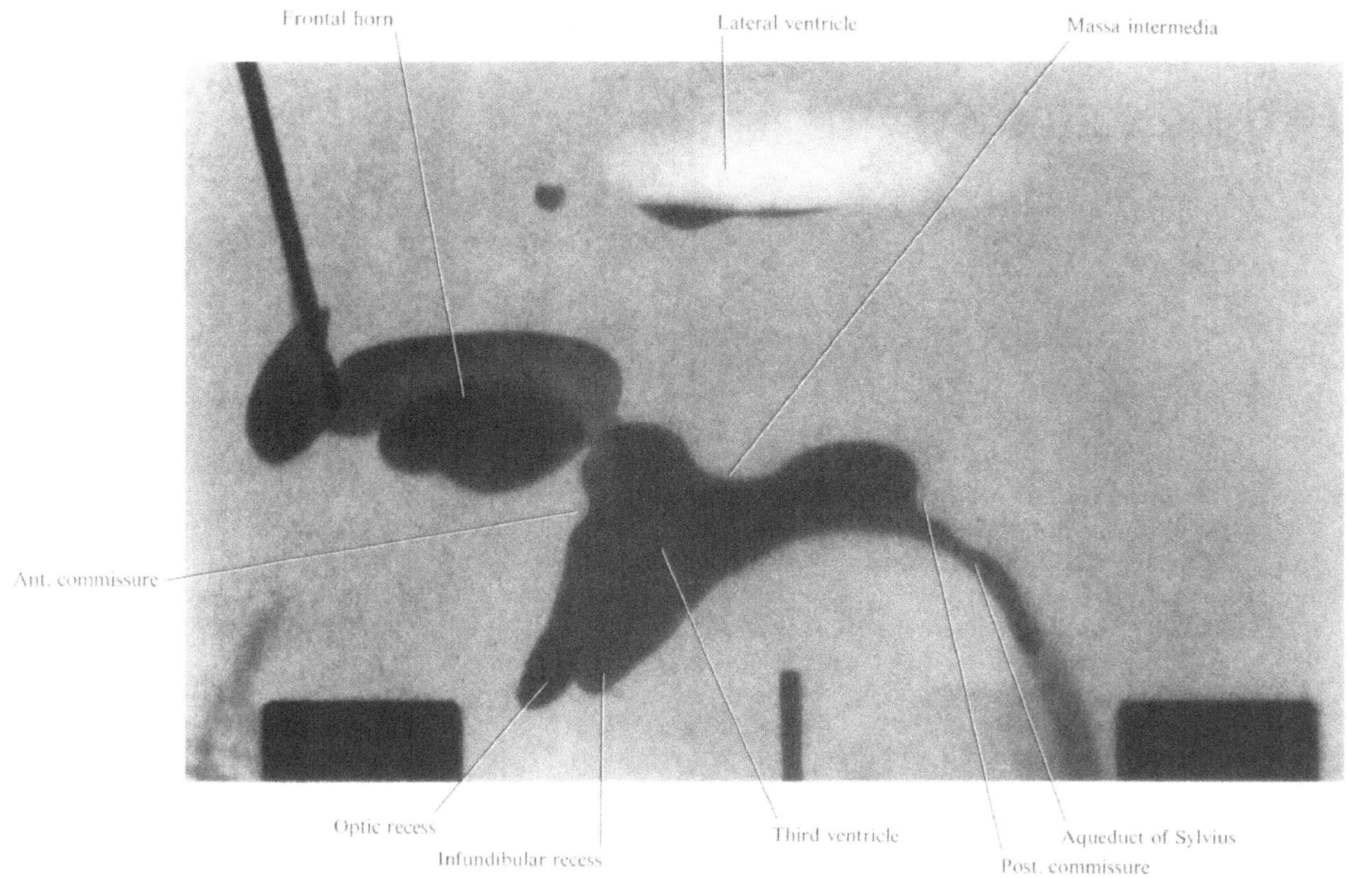

Fig. 150. Pantopaque ventriculogram, lateral projection

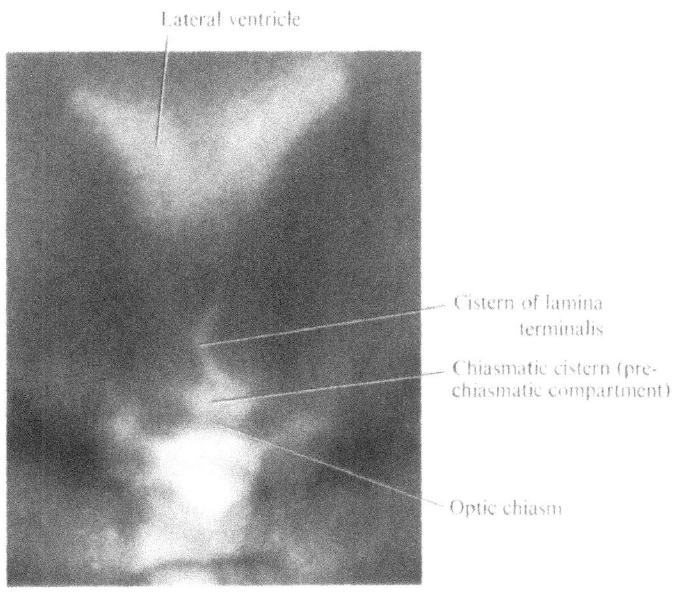

Fig. 149 E

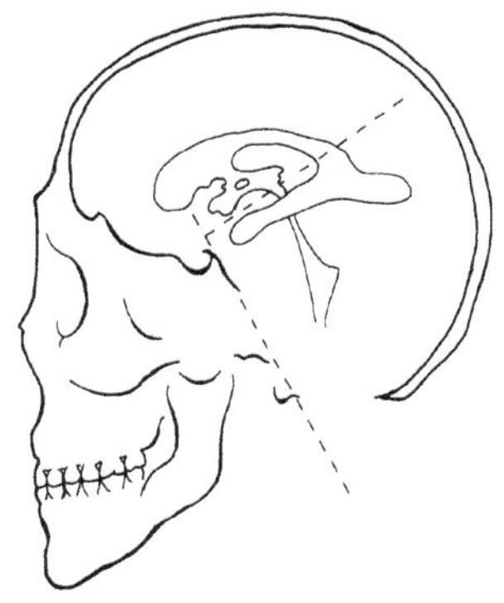

Fig. 151. Schematic representation of the method of Ruggiero and Castellano (1953) for localization of the posterior end of the third ventricle.
A line tangential to the lower part of the posterior wall of the third ventricle, and perpendicular to the clivus, passes through the posterior end of the third ventricle

Chapter 2

Aqueduct of Sylvius

I. Anatomic Study of the Aqueduct of Sylvius

The aqueduct of Sylvius represents the communication between the third and fourth ventricles. It is 15 to 18 mm long and 1 to 2 mm in diameter. Its shape is like the neck of a swan. Posteriorly, its relations are, from superiorly to inferiorly, the posterior commissure, the superior and inferior colliculi and the anterior medullary velum. Its floor is the midbrain, and contains the nuclei of the third and fourth cranial nerves (Fig. 153).

II. Radiologic Study of the Aqueduct of Sylvius

During pneumoencephalography air fills the aqueduct of Sylvius while the patient is in the sitting position. It can also be visualized by opaque ventriculography. The radiologic appearence of the aqueduct has been studied in detail by LINDGREN and DI CHIRO (1953) (Figs. 152, 154). It has the characteristic shape of the neck of a swan, exhibiting a curve which is concave anteriorly and inferiorly. The diameter of the aqueduct is not constant throughout its course, and slight enlargement is frequently seen at the level of the inferior colliculi.

LYSHOLM, EBENIUS, and SAHLSTEDT (1935) proposed an original method for localization of the aqueduct (Fig. 155). On radiographs the aqueduct measures 15 to 20 mm in length and approximately 2 mm in diameter. In conjunction with the cistern of the vein of Galen, the aqueduct outlines the margins of the quadrigeminal plate.

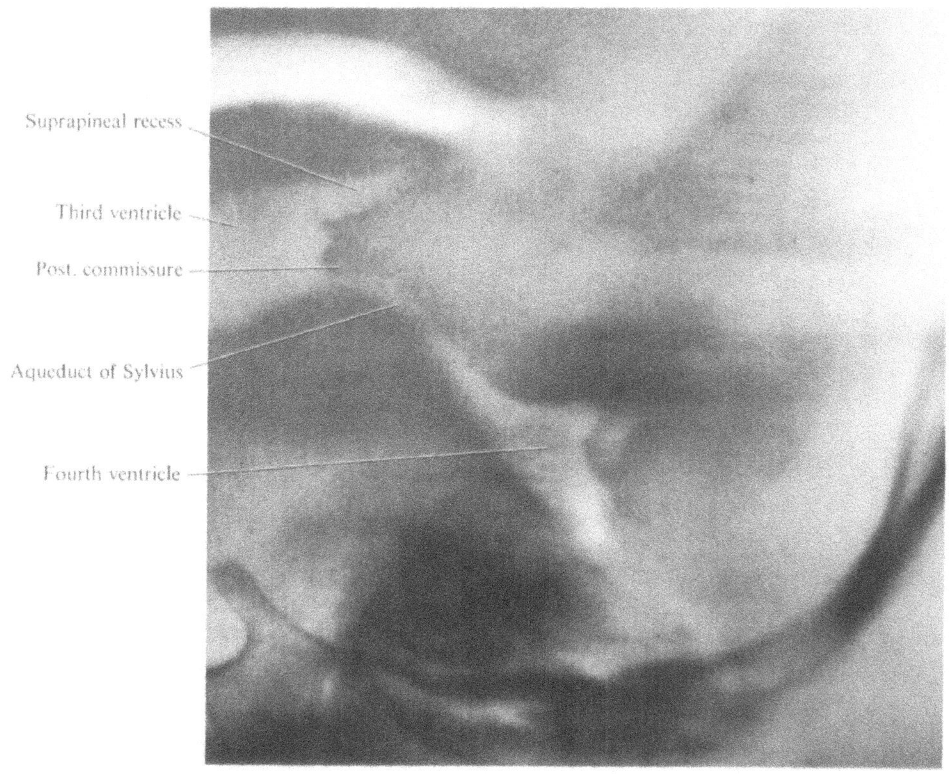

Fig. 152. Pneumoencephalogram, sagittal tomogram

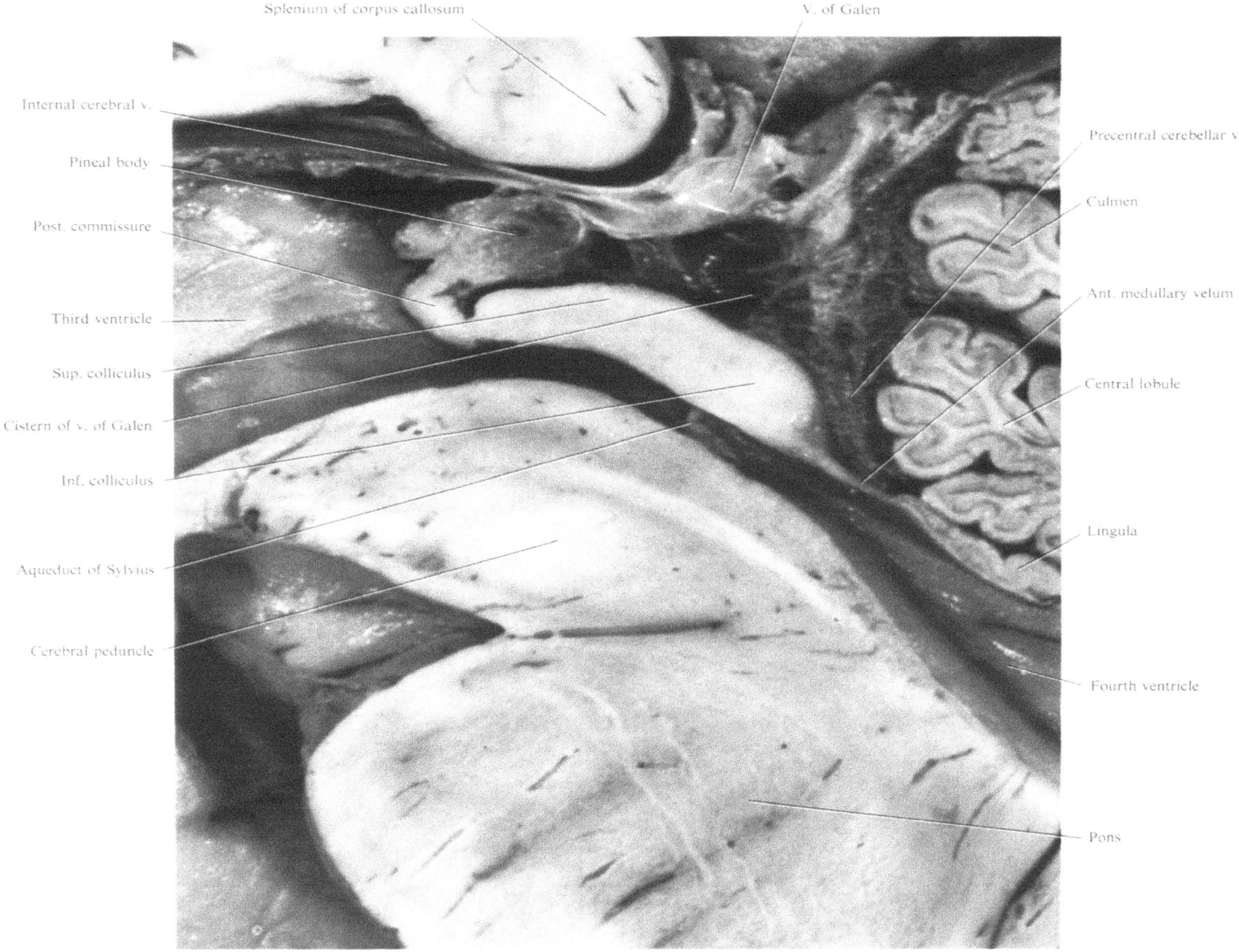

Fig. 153. Sagittal section through the mesencephalon

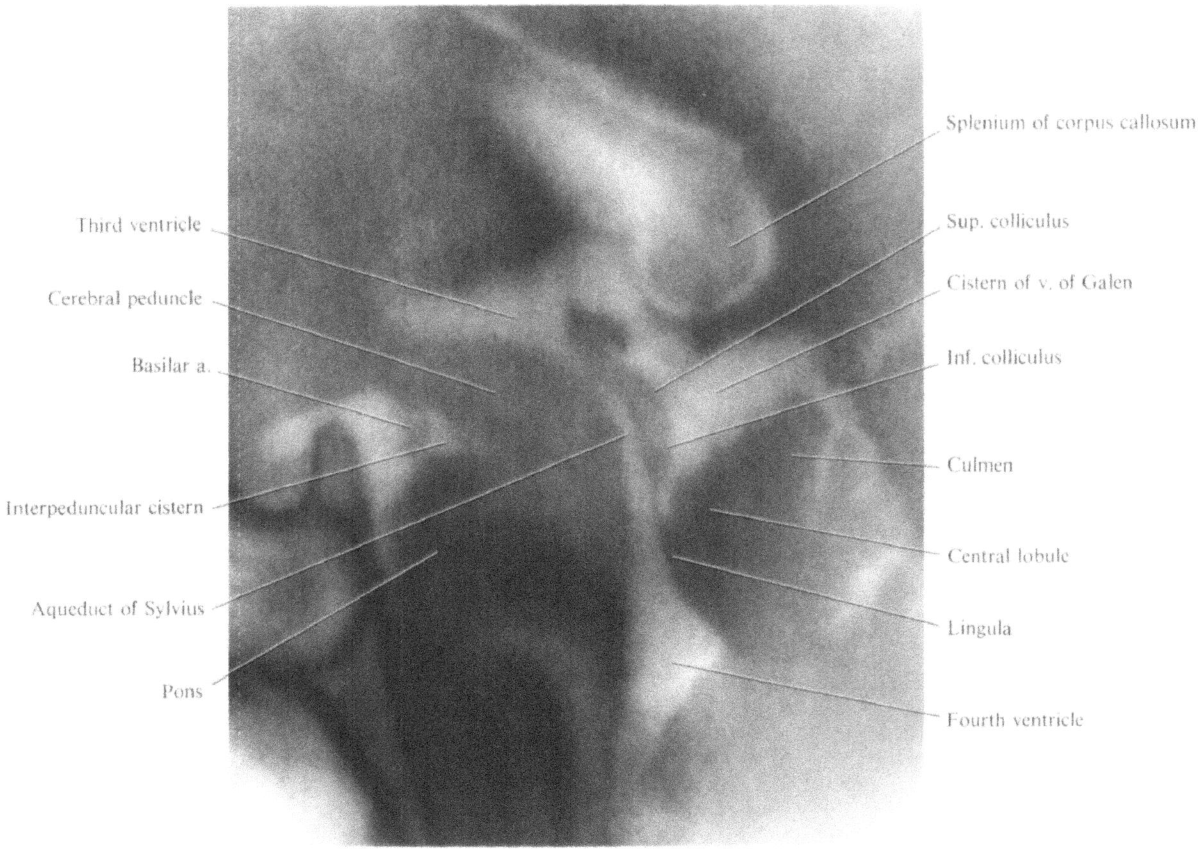

Fig. 154. Pneumoencephalogram, sagittal tomogram

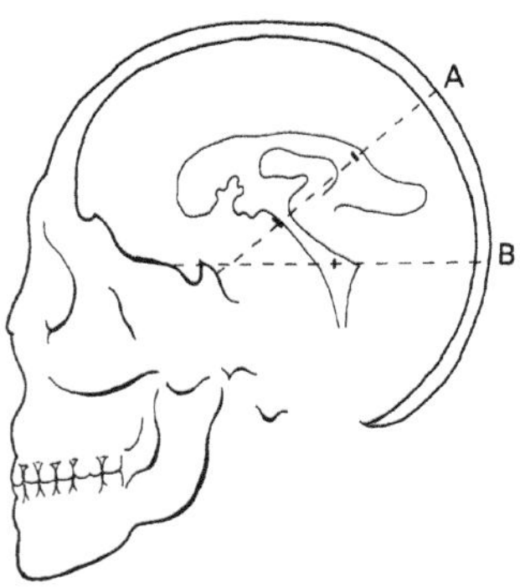

Fig. 155. Schematic representations of the methods of LYSHOLM *et al.* (1935) (A) and TWINNING (1939) (B) for localization of the aqueduct of Sylvius and the fourth ventricle

A. LYSHOLM *et al.* (1935). A line perpendicular to the clivus at the posterior clinoid process, localizes the aqueduct at the junction of its proximal and middle thirds

B. TWINNING. The midpoint of a line from the tuberculum to the torcular, approximately locates the floor of the fourth ventricle

Chapter 3

Arteries of the Basal Ganglia and the Posterior Choroidal Arteries

I. Anatomic Study of the Perforating Arteries of the Basal Ganglia and of the Posterior Choroidal Arteries

The vascularization of the lentiform nucleus, the caudate nucleus, the thalamus and the internal capsule is provided by perforating arteries which arise from the anterior, middle and posterior cerebral arteries and the anterior choroidal arteries. The carotid branches supply the nuclei of telencephalic origin (caudate and lentiform) while the vertebrobasilar branches supply the diencephalic nuclei (thalamus).

Numerous anatomic works have been dedicated to the study of these vessels. In 1874, DURET, influenced by Charcot, made a precise description of the lenticulostriate arteries, which arise from the middle cerebral artery. In the same year, HEUBNER described the system of perforating arteries arising from the anterior cerebral artery. The majority of the early works dedicated to the anterior, middle, or posterior cerebral arteries, or the choroidal arteries, dealt with the origin and distribution of these perforating arteries: BEEVOR (1907), SHELLSHEAR (1920), ABBIE (1924), FOIX and HILLEMAND (1925), AITKEN (1929).

More recently the vascularization of the basal ganglia has been studied by LAZORTHES, POULHES and GAUBERT (1956), OSTROWSKI (1960), LAZORTHES (1961), HERMAN (1963), KAPLAN (1969), LAZORTHES, SALAMON and COMBALBERT (1971), PERCHERON (1971), PLETS, DE REUCK, VAN DER ECKEN and VAN DEN BERGH (1971), and most recently by GEREBTZOFF, ZIEGEH and DUCHESNE (1973).

Finally, numerous angiographic treatises include anatomic sections dealing with the special angiographic anatomic correlations which can be identified.

Since the perforating arteries are readily subdivided by their carotid or vertebrobasilar origins, we shall use that approach in the description of their anatomy.

1. Perforating Branches of the Carotid System

(Anterior cerebral artery, middle cerebral artery, anterior choroidal artery.)

a) Perforating Branches of the Anterior Cerebral Artery (Figs. 156–160)

These arteries have been the subject of a recent study by LAZORTHES and SALAMON (1971). We shall limit our discussion to those arteries of such a diameter that can be angiographically identified, at least by magnification techniques.

A fine series of parallel arteries arise from the origin and horizontal segment of the anterior cerebral artery. They supply the medial part of the globus pallidus and the hypothalamus and are called the medial striate arteries (to differentiate them from the lenticulostriate arteries from the middle cerebral artery).

One branch, from the proximal anterior cerebral artery, has a caliber slightly larger than the medial striate arteries, and differs in its course by running laterally, parallel to the anterior cerebral artery, to enter the brain at the anterior perforated substance. This artery was originally described in 1874 by HEUBNER and consequently bears his name. Together with the lenticulostriate arteries, it supplies the middle and lateral portions of the lentiform nucleus, the head of the caudate nucleus and the anterior limb of the internal capsule.

b) Perforating Branches of the Middle Cerebral Artery (Figs. 156–160)

These lenticulostriate arteries have been well described by DURET (1874). They arise from the middle cerebral artery as it passes beneath the anterior perforated substance. These vessels can be divided into medial and lateral groups by their origin and size.

The medial lenticulostriate arteries are the smaller branches. They supply a portion of the lentiform region, namely the medial portion of the putamen and the area beneath the globus pallidus.

The lateral lenticulostriate arteries are larger in caliber and also longer. Since they originate more laterally on the horizontal segment of the middle cerebral artery, they must pass slightly medially to penetrate the anterior perforated substance. This causes the inferior portion of their characteristic S-shape: a slight curve concave laterally. The superior portion presents a wider radius of curvature, concave medially.
The lateral lenticulostriate arteries usually number between 6 and 8, and the largest (the artery of Charcot) has a diameter of between 250 and 400 μ. They run across the lateral surface of the lentiform nucleus, parallel to the external capsule. In the lateral projection their distribution is fan-like.
There are no apparent anastomoses between the lateral lenticulostriate arteries and the insular arteries. The vascular territory of the lateral lenticulostriate arteries is extensive, and includes the region beneath the globus pallidus, the anterior limb of the internal capsule, the head of the caudate nucleus, the lateral part of the lentiform nucleus and the external capsule.

c) Branches of the Anterior Choroidal Artery
(Figs. 159, 160)

The distal ramifications of these arteries participate in the vascularization of several of the nuclear formations, especially the putamen, the internal capsule, the caudate nucleus, the amygdaloid body and the lateral geniculate body (see Part 1, Chapt. 3).

2. Perforating Branches of the Vertebrobasilar System
(Figs. 157–160)

These arteries, as described by FOIX and HILLEMAND (1925), can be morphologically divided into three groups; the paramedian arteries, the short circumferential arteries and the long circumferential arteries.
At the level of the thalamic nuclei the paramedian arteries are the thalamoperforate arteries (pre- and retro-mammillary) which arise from the posterior communicating artery and the termination of the basilar trunk. The short circumferential arteries are represented by the thalamoperforate arteries (thalamogeniculate arteries) arising from the posterior cerebral artery. Finally, the long circumferential arteries are the posteromedial and posterolateral choroidal arteries.
LAZORTHES and SALAMON (1971) modified this classification of the thalamic arteries, not only for the sake of simplicity, but to more closely approximate the neurosurgical and angiographic findings. They distinguish a group of inferior thalamic arteries, corresponding to the thalamoperforate pedicle of FOIX and HILLEMAND (1925), a group of posterior thalamic arteries, corresponding to the thalamogeniculate pedicle, and a group to the superior thalamus, represented by the posteromedial and posterolateral choroidal arteries.

a) Arteries to the Inferior Surface of the Thalamus
(Fig. 158) (syn. Thalamoperforate, inferior thalamic)

These arteries originate from the posterior communicating artery and the proximal posterior cerebral artery. Of these, the group which arises from the posterior cerebral artery is the most constant. These fine branches measure between 200 and 400 μ in diameter. They have an extra-cerebral course of about 5 mm and then pass upwards, on either side of the third ventricle, to a height of approximately 15 mm.
In our laboratory, GEORGE *et al.* (1975) demonstrated the possibility of distinguishing between the premammillary and retromammillary branches. This distinction provides additional information about the walls of the third ventricle, which has obvious diagnostic significance.
Finally, it is possible to include with the thalamoperforate arteries a group of branches, with a horizontal course, which vascularize the cerebral peduncles. These are the mesencephalic arteries of the inferior thalamic group (LAZORTHES and SALAMON, 1971).
The arteries to the inferior surface of the thalamus supply its anterior nuclei.

b) Arteries to the Posterior Surface of the Thalamus
(Fig. 157) (syn. Thalamogeniculate, posterior thalamic, pulvinarian pedicle)

These arteries arise from the posterior cerebral artery as it lies close to the pulvinar region of the thalamus. There are generally 8 to 10 branches, approximately 300 μ in diameter, which have an ascendant course with a curve concave anteriorly.
The arteries to the posterior surface of the thalamus supply the pulvinar region and the posterolateral ventral nucleus.

c) Arteries to the Superior Surface of the Thalamus
(Fig. 158) (syn. Posteromedial and posterolateral choroidal arteries)

The two posterior choroidal arteries arise from the circumpeduncular portion of the posterior cerebral artery.
Generally the ***posterolateral choroidal artery*** arises slightly anteriorly to the posteromedial choroidal artery and follows the posterior contour of the pulvinar. After providing branches to the optic tract and lateral geniculate

body, it enters the choroidal fissure. The artery then changes course and follows the choroid plexus of the lateral ventricle, supplying this structure and anastomosing with its counterpart, the anterior choroidal artery.
In the studies of GALLOWAY and GREITZ (1960) there were almost always two branches of the posterolateral choroidal artery, one anterior and the other posterior. The posterior of these two branches was usually the largest.

The posteromedial choroidal artery arises from the posterior cerebral artery a few millimeters behind the posterolateral choroidal artery. Its ascendant course follows the contours of the medial and lateral geniculate bodies, which causes its characteristic appearance, like that of the numeral 3, when seen on lateral angiograms.
The posteromedial choroidal artery enters the choroidal fissure and supplies the choroid plexus of the third ventricle. It also provides between one and three thalamic arterioles, which vascularize the anterior nucleus of the thalamus.

II. Radiologic Study of the Perforating Arteries of the Basal Ganglia and of the Posterior Choroidal Arteries

Angiography of the lenticulostriate, thalamoperforate and posterior choroidal arteries has been the subject of numerous treatises. The first precise description of the lenticulostriate arteries and the study of their displacement in deep cerebral hemorrhage was the subject of the work of ANDERSEN (1958). WESTBERG (1966) aroused interest in these arteries by his casts, and dedicated a treatise to the angiographic study of the recurrent artery of HEUBNER (1872).
We have also studied the angiography of the lenticulostriate arteries and their displacement by cerebral tumors and hemorrhages.
The angiography of the perforating branches of the vertebrobasilar system was the subject of DILENGE'S work (1965) on the conditions required for opacification of the thalamoperforate arteries. HARA and FUJINO (1966) also studied these vessels. BRICOUT and GUIOT (1964) demonstrated the courses of the thalamic arteries and raised interest in their study as related to stereotactic neurosurgery.
LAZORTHES and SALAMON (1971) studied the thalamic arteries and their displacement by tumors of the basal ganglia. LOFGREN (1958) studied the posterior choroidal arteries, which were also the subject of the very precise work of GALLOWAY and GREITZ (1960). GEORGE, SALAMON and KRICHEFF (1975) aroused interest in the use of magnification techniques in the study of tumors of the third ventricular region.

Angiographic evaluation of the arteries to the basal ganglia is generally performed with magnification and includes both carotid angiography (for evaluation of the caudate and lenticular branches) and vertebral angiography (for evaluation of the thalamic branches).
On frontal carotid angiograms, the lenticulostriate arteries are visible as 5 or 6 fine branches arising from the superior surface of the middle cerebral artery (Figs. 161, 162). They pass upwards, with a slight curve concave laterally, followed by a more pronounced curve concave medially. The more lateral of these arteries locate the lateral extent of the lentiform nucleus, the external capsule, and the head of the caudate nucleus.
It is difficult, even with magnification, to identify the medial lenticulostriate arteries, or the medial striate arteries which arise from the anterior cerebral artery. On the other hand, opacification of the recurrent artery of Heubner is easy to identify, due to its large diameter. It is distinguished from the anterior choroidal artery by its origin from the anterior cerebral artery, and its lateral course origin prior to its entry into the anterior perforated substance with the lenticulostriate arteries.
By employing threefold magnification, it is occasionally possible to separate the images of the lenticulostriate arteries from those of the middle cerebral artery and its branches in the lateral projection.
Displacement of the lenticulostriate arteries always possesses diagnostic significance, whether it is medial or lateral displacement. It is thus important to localize their position in the frontal plane using the method of ANDERSEN (1958) or that of SALAMON *et al.* (1966) (Fig. 165).
While the evaluation of the perforating branches of the carotid system is most informative in the frontal projection, the study of the perforating branches of the vertebrobasilar system is best accomplished in the lateral projection. This view allows the separation of the arteries to the inferior, posterior and superior surfaces of the thalamus.
Magnification angiography of the thalamoperforate arteries was the subject of a precise study by GEORGE *et al.* (1975), who demonstrated the potential for differentiating those branches arising from the posterior communicating artery from those of posterior cerebral artery origin. Both of these groups of arteries, after a short extracerebral course, penetrate the brain at the posterior perforated substance.
Occasionally, magnification angiograms allow the identification of the branches to the mesencephalon (Figs. 163, 164). While the arteries to the posterior surface of the thalamus usually opacify poorly, the posteromedial and posterolateral choroidal arteries almost invariably opacify well and exhibit characteristic courses (Figs. 163, 164).

The posterolateral choroidal artery arises first, projects higher, and exhibits the characteristic curve, concave anteriorly due to the back of the pulvinar. Its termination indicates the floor of the body of the lateral ventricle. The posteromedial choroidal artery presents the characteristic appearance, of the figure 3, due to its relationship to the geniculate bodies. It terminates at the level of the choroid plexus of the third ventricle and consequently identifies the level of the roof of that structure. The methods of LOFGREN (1958) (Fig. 165) and, more recently, PACHTMAN, HILAL and WOOD (1974) permit the study of displacements of this vessel.

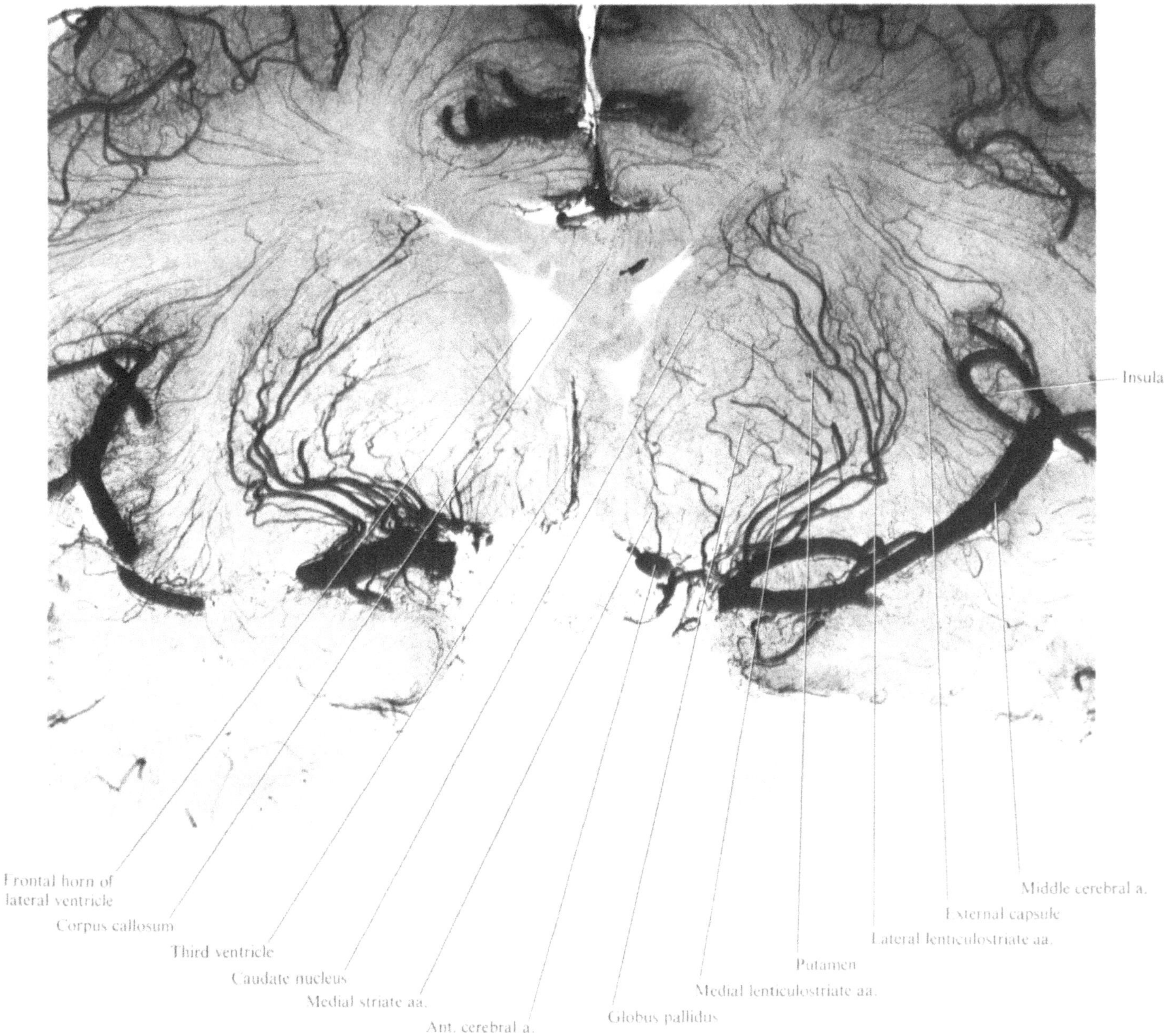

Fig. 156. Perforating arteries of the carotid system, frontal section through the basal ganglia

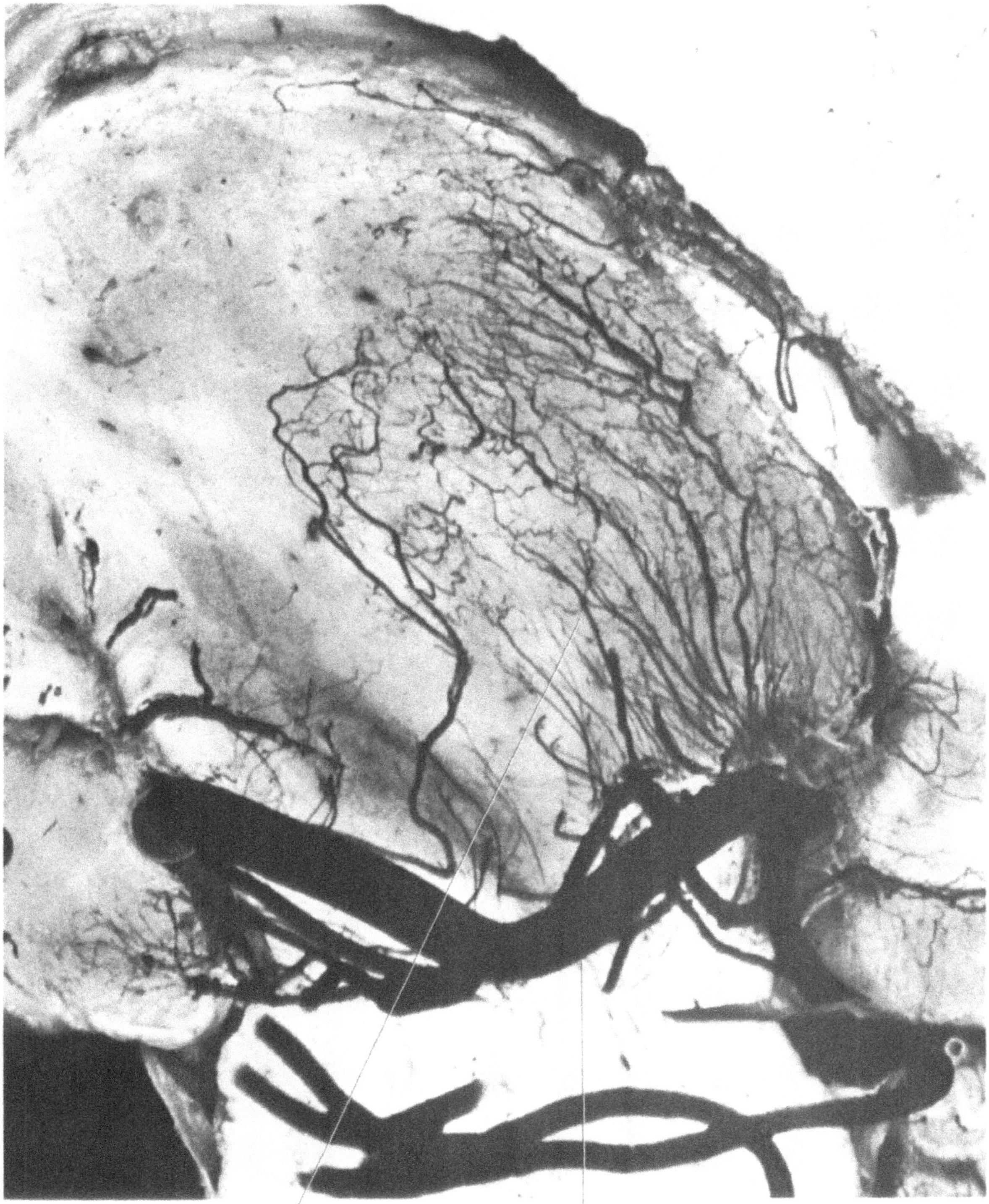

Fig. 157. Perforating arteries of the vertebrobasilar system, parasagittal section of the thalamus, through the circumpeduncular portion of the posterior cerebral artery, showing thalamogeniculate arteries

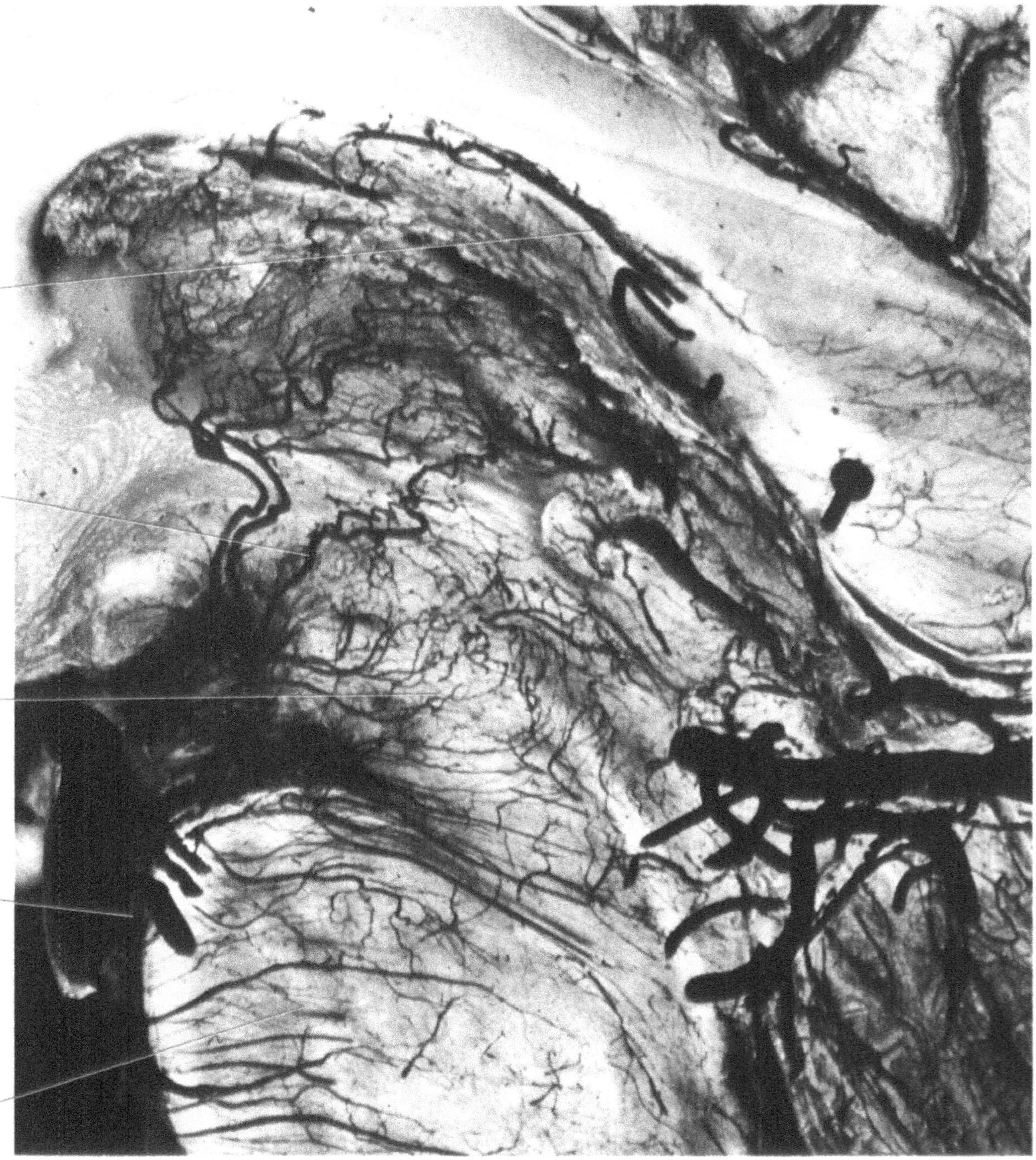

Fig. 158. Perforating arteries of the vertebrobasilar system, midline sagittal section showing the distribution of the thalamoperforate arteries. It can also be seen on this section that the most posterior branches supply the mesencephalon. Note also a segment of the posterolateral choroidal artery and the medial perforating arteries of the pons

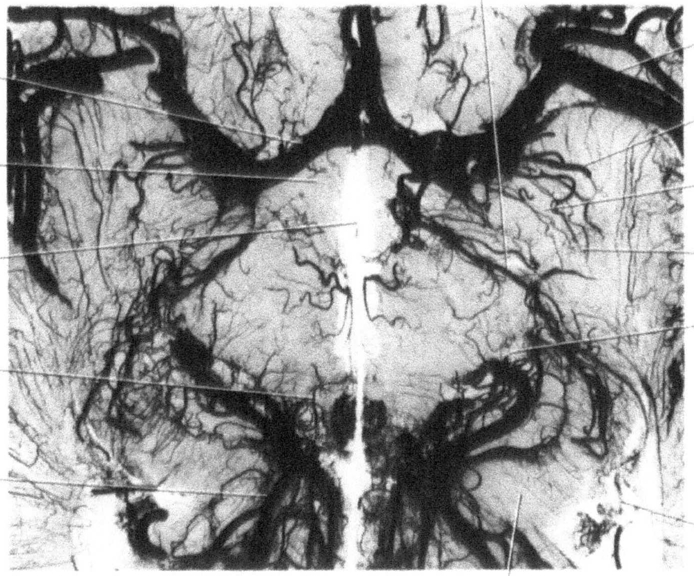

Fig. 159. Horizontal section of an injected brain

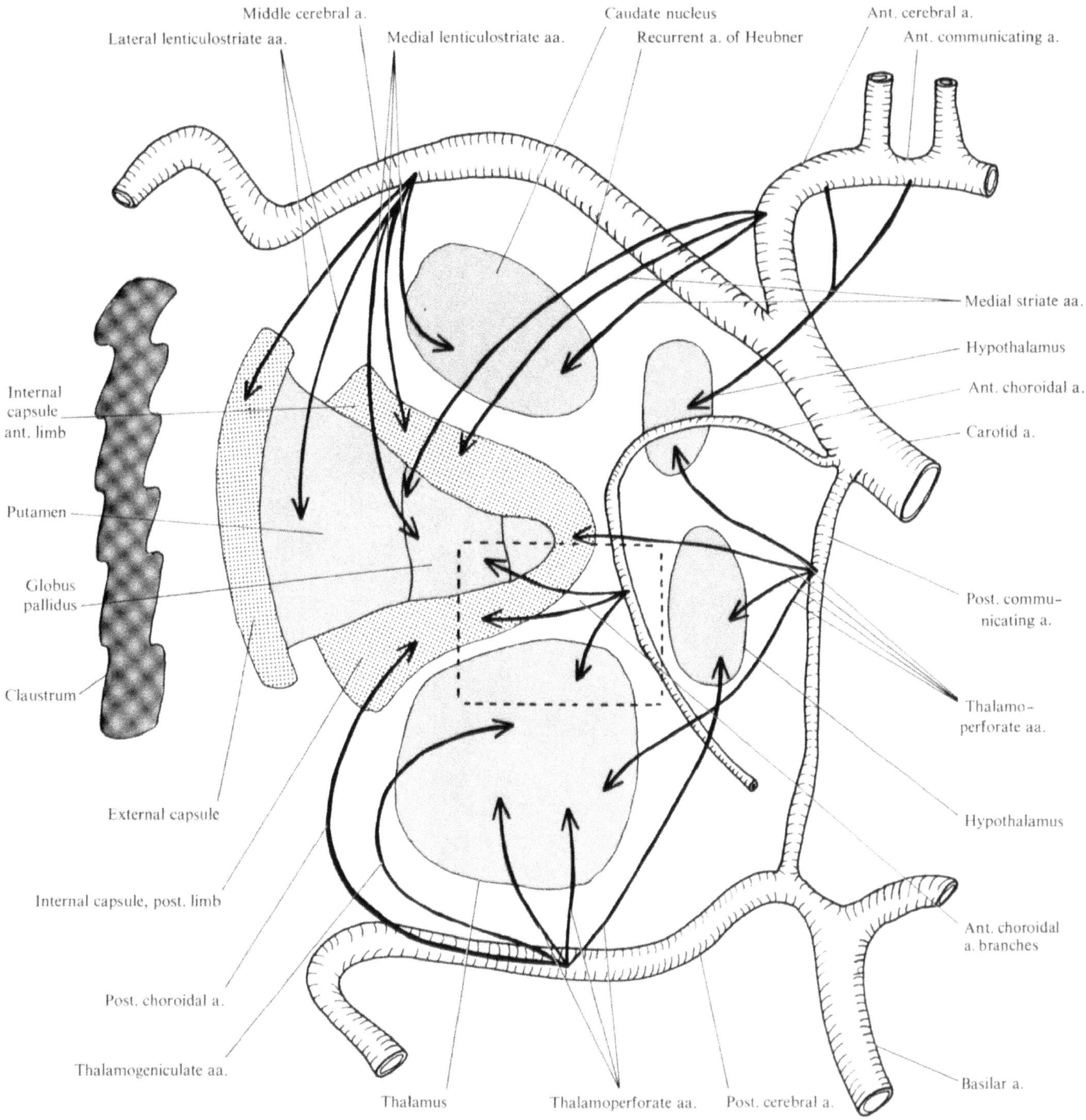

Fig. 160. Schematic representation of the origin and distribution of the arteries to the basal ganglia (after FOIX and HILLEMAND, 1925)

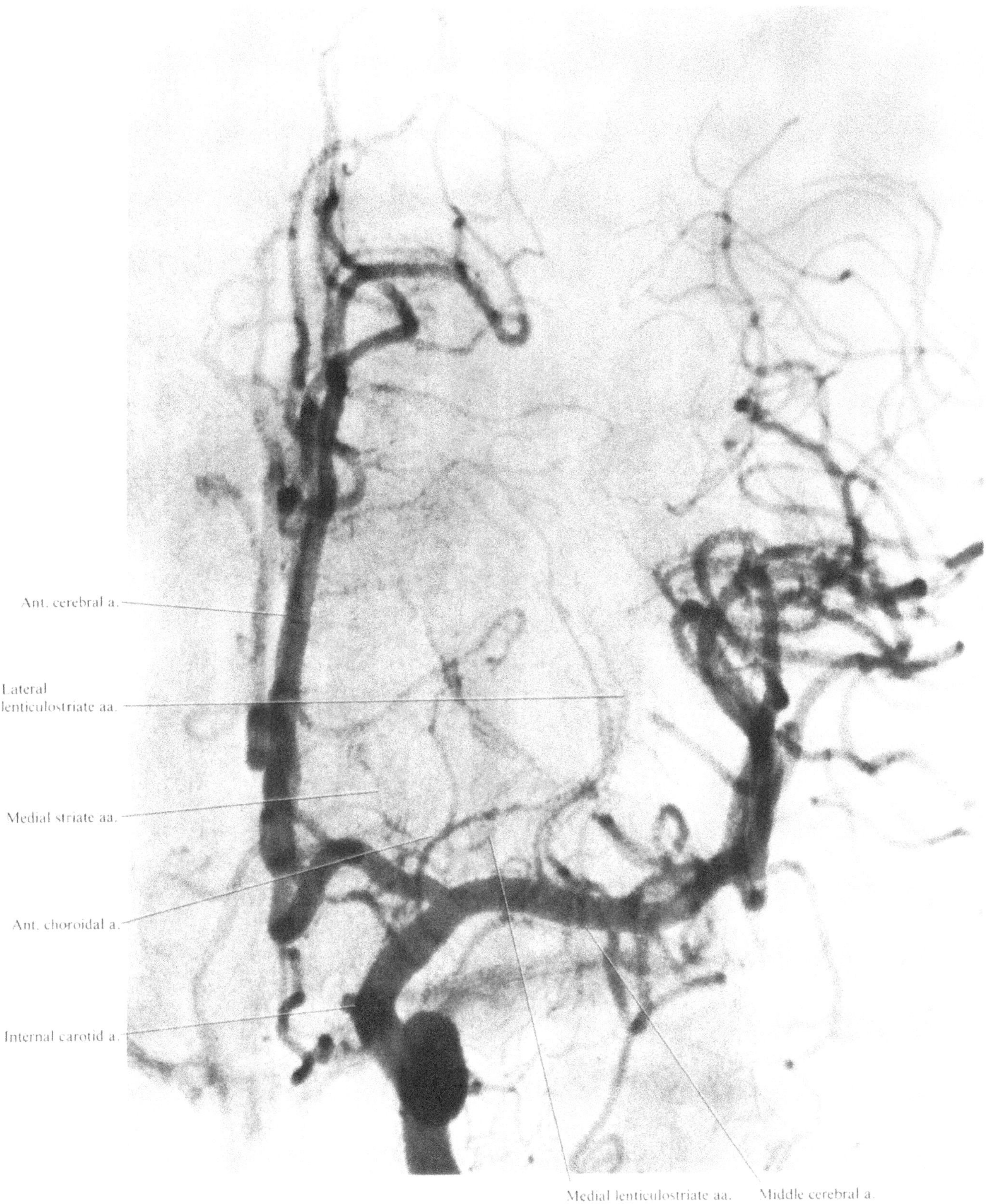

Fig. 161. Carotid angiogram, frontal projection (× 2.5 magnification)

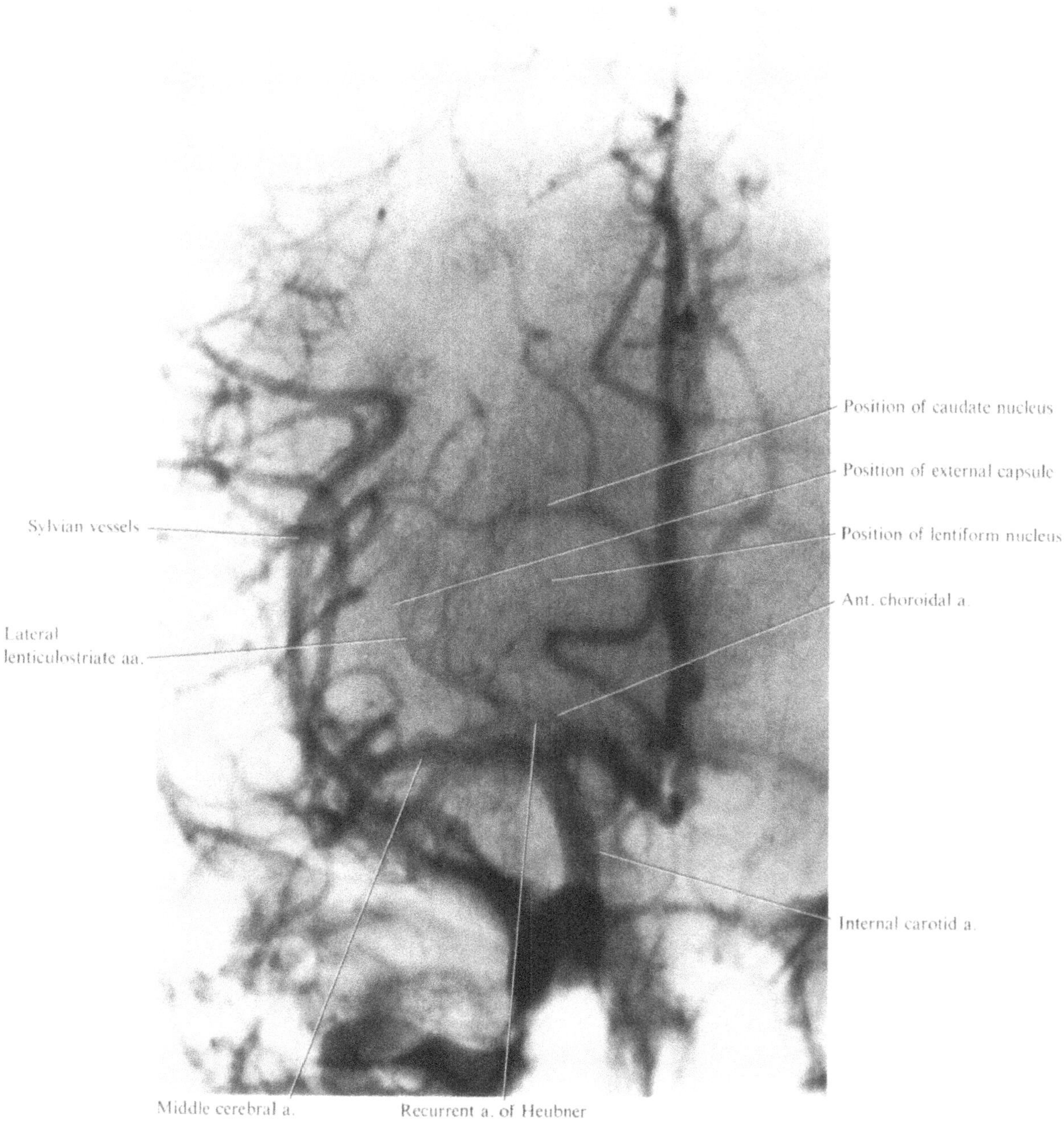

Fig. 162A

Fig. 162A–C. Carotid angiograms, frontal projection ▷

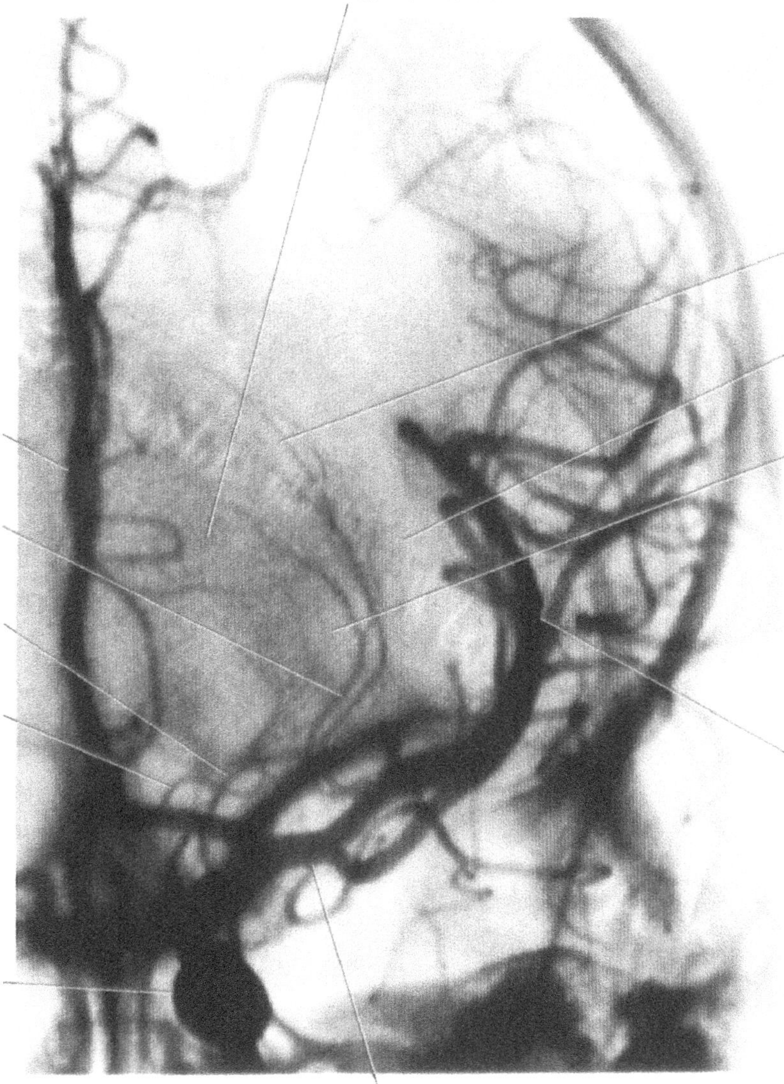
Position of caudate nucleus
Ant. choroidal a.
Position of external capsule
Ant. cerebral a.
Position of lentiform nucleus
Lateral
lenticulostriate aa.
Ant. choroidal a.
Recurrent a. of Heubner
Sylvian vessels
Internal carotid a.
Middle cerebral a.

Fig. 162 B

▷

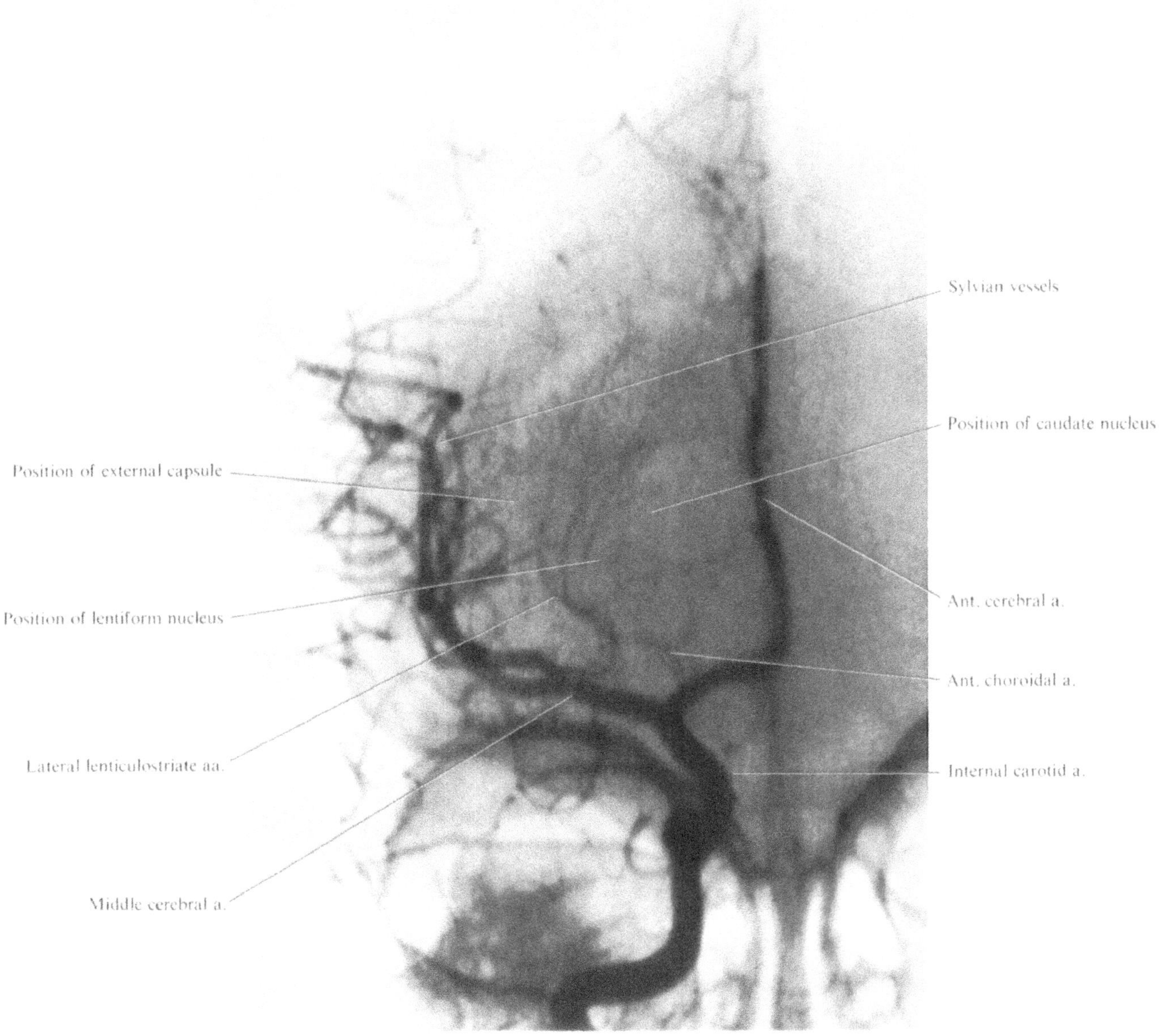
Sylvian vessels
Position of caudate nucleus
Position of external capsule
Ant. cerebral a.
Position of lentiform nucleus
Ant. choroidal a.
Lateral lenticulostriate aa.
Internal carotid a.
Middle cerebral a.

Fig. 162C

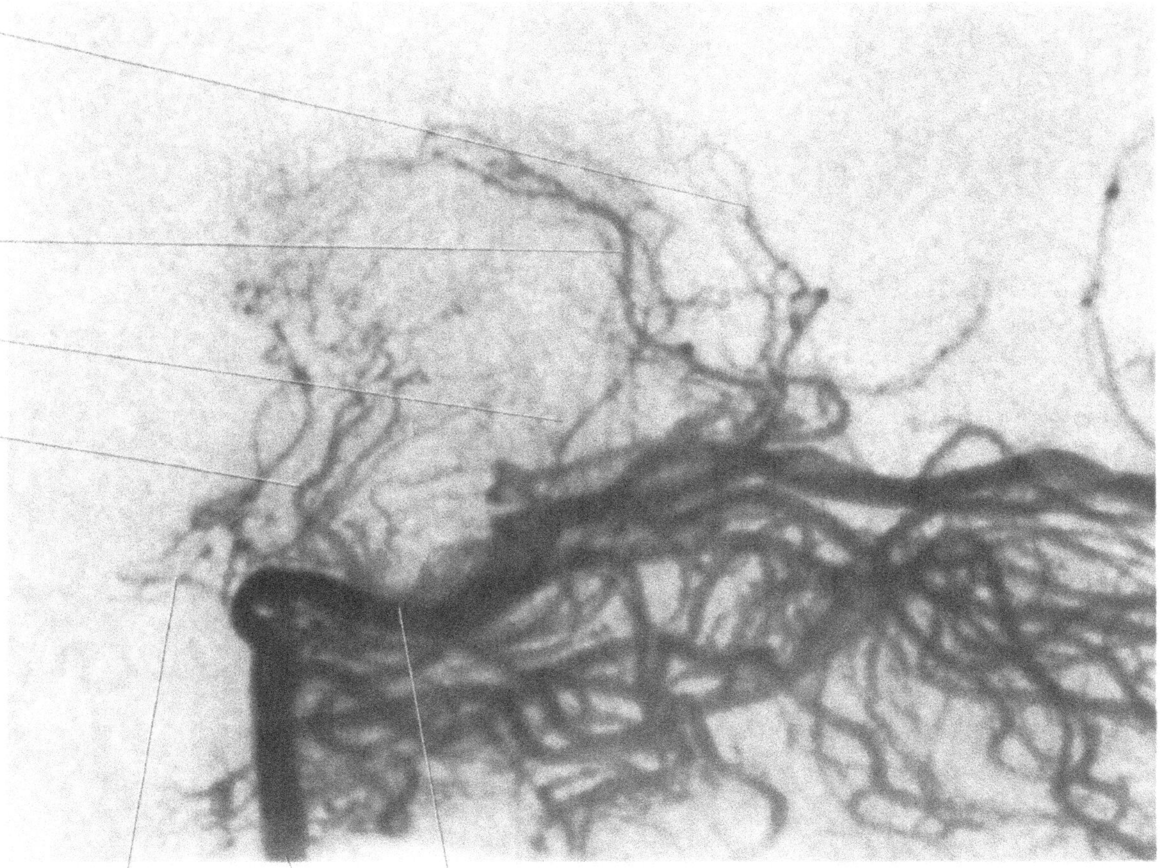

Fig. 163. Lateral vertebral angiogram (× 2.5 magnification)

Fig. 164A

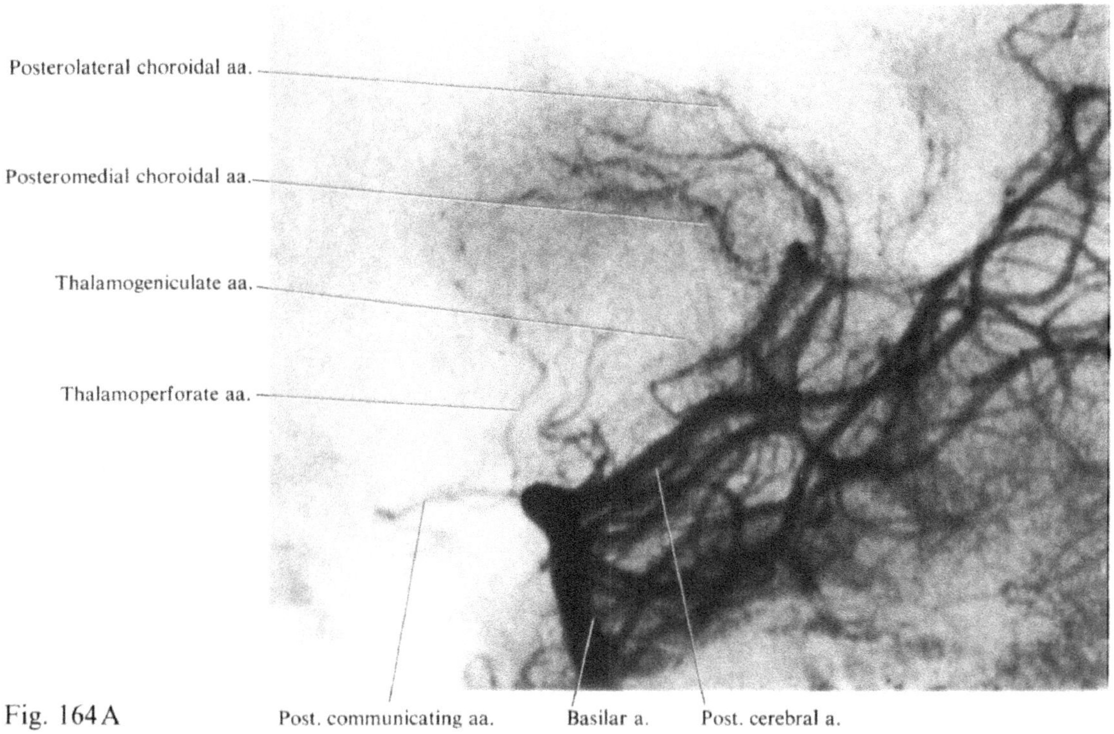

Fig. 164B

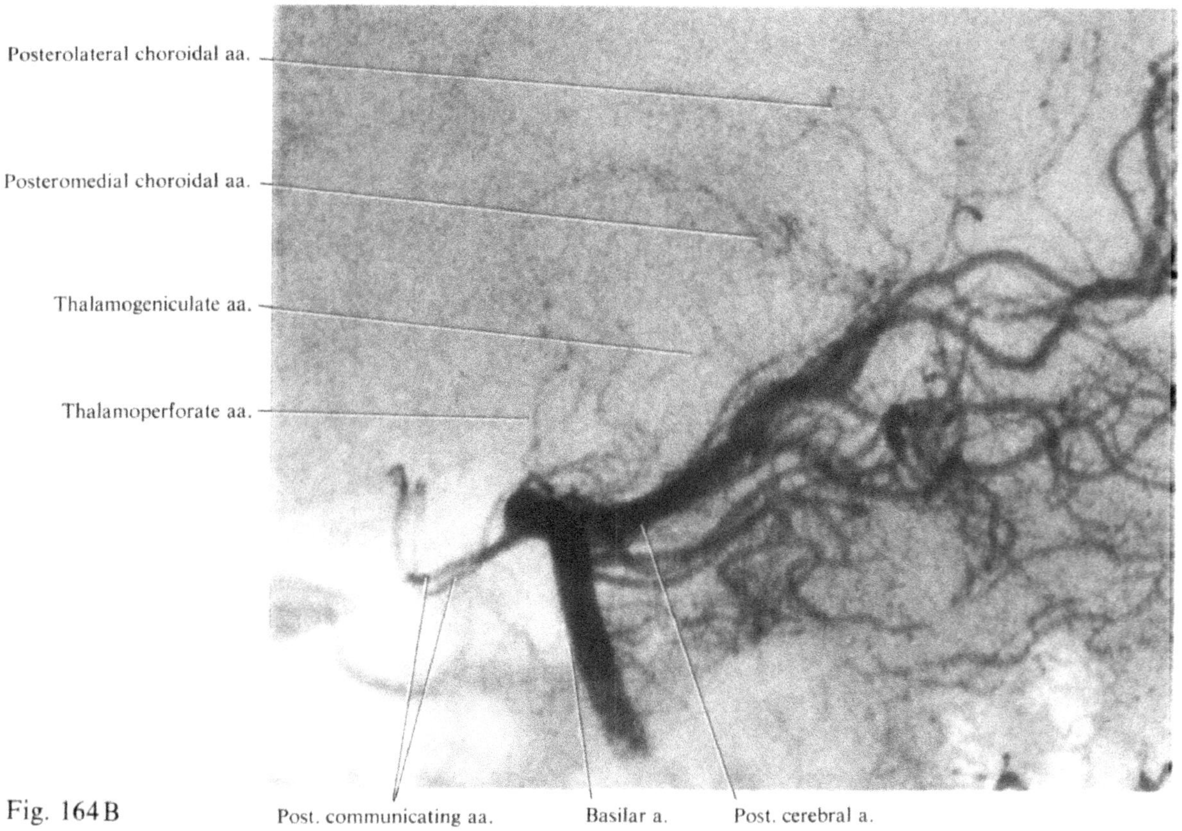

Fig. 164A–B. Lateral vertebral angiograms (×2.5 magnification)

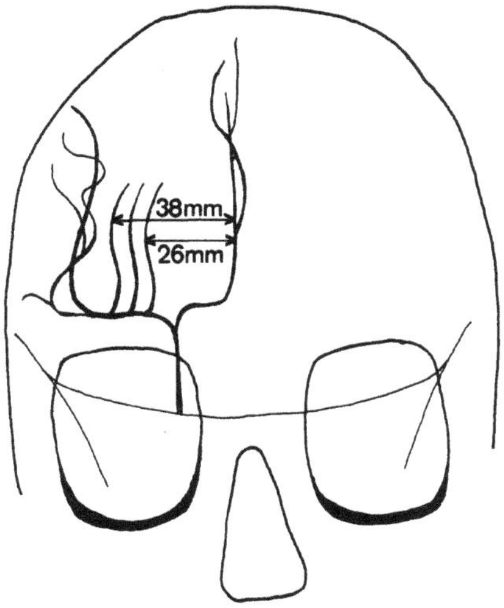

A. The most medial lenticulostriate arteries are 26 mm from the midline while the most lateral are 38 mm from it (ANDERSEN, 1958)

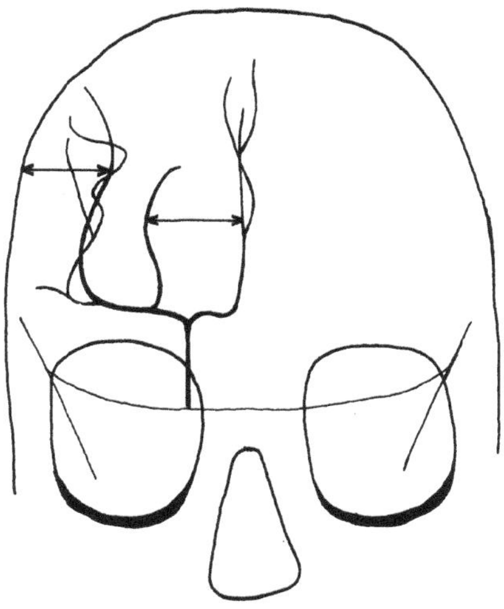

B. The distance from the most lateral lenticulostriate arteries to the midline approximates to the distance from the deep insular branches of the middle cerebral artery to the inner table (SALAMON *et al.*, 1966)

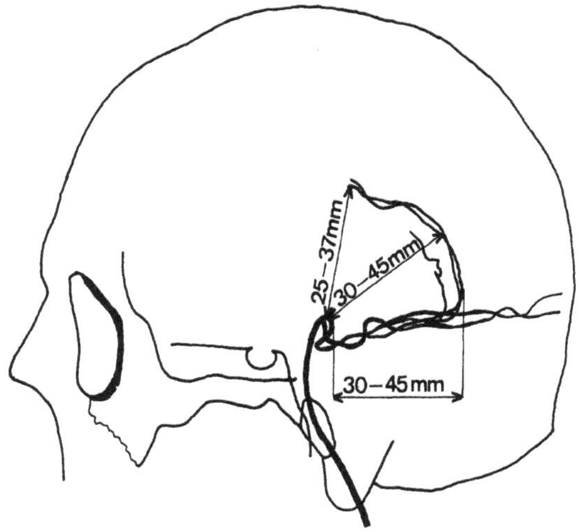

C. The distances shown are from the posterior choroidal arteries to the basilar trunk (LOFGREN, 1958)

Fig. 165. Method of ANDERSEN (1958) (A) and SALAMON *et al.* (1966) (B) for locating the lenticulostriate arteries and the method of LOFGREN (1958) (C) for locating the posterior choroidal arteries

Chapter 4
Deep Cerebral Veins

The deep cerebral venous system may be said to consists of the two internal cerebral veins and their tributaries—the subependymal, deep medullary, superior striate and choroidal veins. The basal cerebral vein, sometimes included in the deep venous system, is described elsewhere (Part 1, Chap. 4, p. 128).

A. Internal Cerebral and Great Cerebral Veins
(Figs. 166–168)

The internal cerebral vein, sometimes called the small cerebral vein of Galen (LAZORTHES, 1961) begins by the confluence of the septal, thalamostriate, anterior thalamic and superior choroidal veins at the posterosuperior margin of the interventricular foramen (or foramen of Monro). The combined stem, the internal cerebral vein, then runs backwards in the cistern of the velum interpositum, below the fornix and above the roof of the third ventricle. In a typical form it runs posteriorly, taking an S-shaped course, first posterosuperiorly and then posteroinferiorly, before turning upwards and backwards to join the great cerebral vein. Anteriorly, the two internal cerebral veins are located on either side of the midline. Their medial borders should be located no more than 2 mm from the midsagittal plane in normal cases. Posteriorly, the two internal cerebral veins are slightly separated. When the thalamostriate and septal veins join the internal cerebral veins posteriorly to the interventricular foramen, the internal cerebral vein appears short; whereas when the thalamostriate vein loops forwards and downwards; anteriorly to the interventricular foramen, the internal cerebral vein appears longer (Fig. 167). A communication between the two internal cerebral veins or a loop in their posterior course, before joining the great cerebral vein has been observed. The course of the internal cerebral vein is otherwise relatively constant. Other tributaries which may join the internal cerebral vein are the superior thalamic, medial posterior thalamic, posterior septal, medial atrial, direct lateral, internal occipital, splenial, and, in some instances, the quadrigeminal, precentral cerebellar and superior vermian veins.

The great cerebral vein is formed by the union of the two internal cerebral veins. It runs backwards and upwards around the posterior aspect of the splenium of the corpus callosum and joins the anterior end of the straight sinus, usually at an acute angle. When the straight sinus is short and low in position, the great cerebral vein may take a more horizontal course.
The basal cerebral vein, which runs around the midbrain, may join either the great cerebral vein or the posterior portion of the internal cerebral vein. Other tributaries which may join the great cerebral vein are the splenial, internal occipital, medial posterior thalamic, superior thalamic, quadrigeminal, precentral cerebellar and superior vermian veins. Variations in the course of the internal cerebral vein and the great cerebral vein are shown in Fig. 167.

B. Subependymal Veins of the Lateral Ventricle

Major tributaries of the internal cerebral vein, the subependymal veins, have been studied by BEKOV (1965), BEN AMOR and WACKENHEIM (1973), BROWNING (1884), FERNER (1958), HASSLER (1966), JOHANSON (1954), KAPLAN and FORD (1966), ROSA and VIALE (1971), STEIN and ROSENBAUM (1974), STEPHENS and STILWELL (1969), WOLF and HUANG (1964), and ZIMMER and ANNES (1966). Although some of the subependymal veins are located in the temporal horn and drain into the basal cerebral vein, they will be discussed in this chapter.
During embryologic development, the posterior part of the lateral ventricle is bent inferiorly and, then anteriorly to form the temporal horn. Posterior protrusion of the lateral ventricle results in the formation of the occipital horn and the occipital lobe. The roof of the frontal horn and the roof of the body of the lateral ventricle are continuous with the floor of the temporal horn and are located outside the C-shaped choroid fissure. On the other hand, the floor of the frontal horn and the floor of the body of the lateral ventricle are connected with

the roof of the temporal horn and lies inside the curve of the choroid fissure (Figs. 169–175).

The original telencephalic vesicles are thin-walled structures and consist of the ependymal, mantle and marginal layers. During embryologic development, the cerebral cortex is formed by migration of neuroblasts from the subependymal mantle layer. With development of the thalamus and basal ganglia and intrusion of the fornix and corpus callosum, it is likely that the original site of migration of neuroblasts becomes compressed and confined to narrow band-like areas, around the anterior and superior angles of the frontal horn, the lateral angle of the body and the lateral part of the roof of the temporal horn. It is therefore natural to presume that the medullary veins, which drain the white matter, converge towards and concentrate in the areas described above. In the atrium and occipital horn, the original site of neuroblast migration is not compressed and the cells remain located subependymally, diffusely scattered over the superior and lateral aspects of the ventricular wall.

Development of the choroid fissure eventually divides the subependymal veins of the lateral ventricle into two groups – the medial and lateral groups – since these veins leave the ventricle by penetrating its wall either on the outside (medial group) or inside (lateral group) of the semicircular choroid fissure (WOLF and HUANG, 1964). The medial group originates from the lateral angle of the lateral ventricle, receiving deep medullary veins, and runs along the roof and medial wall of the lateral ventricle. These veins drain the deep white matter of the cerebral hemisphere and leave the lateral ventricle by passing deep to the fornix and tenia choroidea. The lateral group of subependymal veins also originates from the lateral angle of the lateral ventricle. This group drains not only the medial portion of the deep white matter but also the deep basal nuclei, by running along the lateral wall and the floor of the lateral ventricle. The lateral group leaves the lateral ventricle by passing deep to the stria terminalis, lamina affixa and tenia choroidea (Figs. 168–179). From the embryologic point of view, it is interesting to find that the subependymal veins do not leave the lateral ventricle through the choroid fissure. The medial group leaves by passing deep to the fornix, whereas the lateral group emerges by running deep to the stria terminalis, lamina affixa and tenia choroidea (Figs. 170–176).

The *non-crossing rule* (STEIN and ROSENBAUM, 1974) – subependymal veins that cross each other cannot lie in the same plane – is very useful in distinguishing medial from lateral groups of subependymal veins. The only exception is seen with the longitudinal caudate veins, described later.

I. Medial Group of the Subependymal Veins
(Figs. 170–173, 175, 176, 177A and B, 178A and B, 179–186)

The medial group of the subependymal veins includes the septal, the posterior septal (or direct medial), the medial atrial and the transverse hippocampal subependymal veins.

1. Septal Vein
(Figs. 168, 172A, 173, 176, 177A, 178A, 179–181, 187)

The septal vein, or the vein of the septum pellucidum, arises as multiple tributaries from the anterior angle of the frontal horn. They first run posteromedially on the anterior wall of the frontal horn, behind the genu of the corpus callosum (callosal segment). When they reach the anteromedial corner (septal point) (ZIMMER and ANNES, 1966) of the frontal horn they turn backwards to run along the septum pellucidum (septal segment). The stem of the septal vein, formed by the progressive union of these tributaries, continues backwards along the lower border of the septum pellucidum. It then runs around the lateral border of the anterior column of the fornix (columnar segment) and joins the internal cerebral vein at the posterosuperior margin of the interventricular foramen (foramen of Monro), together with the anterior thalamic, thalamostriate, and superior choroidal veins. Instead of coursing around the anterior column of the fornix, the septal vein may pass through it in some cases (STEIN and ROSENBAUM, 1974).

Veins travelling medially along the roof of the frontal horn and inferiorly along the septum pellucidum, may join either the stem of the septal vein or the posterior septal vein, which will be described below. The course of the septal vein varies; it may be straight, convex or concave superiorly, or a combination of these. In the case of a bifid or duplicated septal vein, the terms, superior and inferior septal veins, may be more applicable (Figs. 168, 176, 188C).

2. Posterior Septal Vein
(Figs. 170, 177A, 178A, 181, 183, 184)

The posterior septal vein usually begins in the lateral angle of the frontal horn or body of the lateral ventricle. It runs posteromedially or, rarely, anteromedially along the roof and then inferiorly or posteroinferiorly along the medial wall of the lateral ventricle. After passing between the two fornices, it usually joins the internal cerebral vein from above, some distance behind the interventricular foramen. When the posterior septal vein joins the internal cerebral vein adjacent to the interventricular foramen, it may run laterally to the fornix. The posterior septal vein, also called the *direct medial vein* (WOLF and HUANG, 1964), has also been designated the *roof vein* (STEPHENS and STILWELL, 1969).

There are many veins on the roof of the lateral ventricle. Anteriorly, roof veins drain into the septal vein. More posteriorly, in the region of the body of the lateral ventricle, roof veins open into the posterior septal or the anomalous septal vein. Further posteriorly still, in the atrium, roof veins unite with tributaries of the medial atrial vein, which will be described below. A vein running along the medial wall of the body of the lateral ventricle may, on rare occasions, drain into the direct lateral vein through a roof vein. Similarly, a vein coursing along the lateral wall very occasionally opens into the medial atrial vein through a roof vein. According to STEPHENS and STILWELL (1969), roof veins drain the more inferior and lateral portions of the deep white matter and do not drain the basal ganglia.

The *anomalous septal vein* combines features of both the septal and posterior septal veins (Figs. 177B, 178B, 179, 182A and B, 186, 188A, 189, 192B, 192E, 193, 195B) (BEKOV, 1965; JOHANSON, 1954; WOLF and HUANG, 1964). It begins in the anterior angle of the frontal horn and travels posteromedially, and somewhat superiorly, on the posterior aspect of the genu of the corpus callosum. Upon reaching the medial wall of the frontal horn, the vein turns backwards to run along the upper part of the rapidly tapering septum pellucidum. It then turns downwards onto the posterior portion of the septum pellucidum, passing between the two fornices, to join the internal cerebral vein well behind the interventricular foramen. The point of union with the internal cerebral vein is, however, variable. In some cases the junction lies behind but near the interventricular foramen (Figs. 182A and C, 183A, 186, 189, 192B, 192E); in others the junction lies a long way posteriorly. The anomalous septal vein may even join the stem of the medial atrial vein, near the posterior beak of the splenium of the corpus callosum (POIRIER *et al.*, 1921) to form the *septo-atrial vein* (Figs. 177B, 178B, 188A, 193). Unlike other subependymal veins, the septal and medial atrial veins drain almost exclusively the white and not the grey matter of the cerebral hemisphere. The circulation time of these veins (WHITE and GREITZ, 1970) is therefore prolonged (Fig. 195).

3. Medial Atrial Vein

(Figs. 168, 169, 172A, 173, 175, 176, 177A and B, 178A and B, 179, 180, 182–186, 188A and C, 190, 192A, B and F, 193, 194)

This group of veins has been designated the *vein of the posterior horn* (BROWNING, 1884; JOHANSON, 1954), the *internal vein of the atrium and posterior horn* (BEKOV, 1965) and the *posterior paraventricular vein* (BEKOV, 1965).

The medial atrial vein usually receives tributaries from the medial aspect of the atrium (atrial or medial atrial tributaries) and also tributaries from the medial wall or roof of the occipital horn (veins of the posterior horn or occipital tributaries). Also, not infrequently, tributaries originating from the medial wall of the body of the lateral ventricle (posterior septal tributaries) join the stem of the medial atrial vein. The posterior septal tributary, which may be absent when the posterior septal vein is prominent, usually begins in the lateral angle of the body of the lateral ventricle. It passes posteromedially along the roof and then posteroinferiorly along the medial wall of the lateral ventricle. It then penetrates the brain substance, passing medially, deep to the fornix, to become extraventricular in the cistern of the velum interpositum and joins the stem of the medial atrial vein described below. The atrial tributary arises more posteriorly on the roof of the atrium. It runs medially on the roof and then downwards on the medial wall of the atrium. The occipital tributary originates from the walls of the occipital horn, runs medially and upwards on the roof, and then antero-inferiorly on the medial wall of the atrium.

The posterior septal, atrial and occipital tributaries then converge towards the upper part of the rapidly disappearing hippocampus, anterior to the calcar avis and the bulb of the occipital horn (ventricular segment). After running over the hippocampus and penetrating the attached portion of the posterior column of the fornix (Figs. 168, 172A, 175, 176, 177A and B, 178A and B, 179), the atrial and occipital tributaries of the medial atrial vein leave the ventricle. They now lie in the subarachnoid space between the posterior pillar of the fornix and the anterior surface of the inferior fasciculus of the corpus callosum, which is the lateral extension of the posterior beak of the splenium (Figs. 175, 176). In this subarachnoid space they join the stem of the medial atrial vein. This venous stem (extraventricular segment) runs medially, superiorly and anteriorly, successively receiving its more anteriorly and medially located tributaries. The venous stem is also joined by the posterior septal tributary and then opens into the posterior portion of the internal cerebral vein.

On the lateral venogram this venous stem has a typical terminal curve, convex anteriorly, corresponding to the contour of the antero-inferior surface of the splenium of the corpus callosum and the lateral extension of its inferior fasciculus. In the anteroposterior projection the stem takes a gently curved course, convex superiorly. The course of the occipital tributary of the medial atrial vein is characteristic and, therefore, requires comment. It runs in the roof of the occipital horn, upwards and forwards. At the level of the occipito-atrial junction, the vein makes an abrupt but characteristic antero-inferior turn, to run on the medial wall of the atrium. Because of its characteristic course on the lateral venogram, the occipital tributary may be more appropriately be called the *vein of the posterior horn* (Figs. 168, 175, 177A and B, 178A and B, 179, 182C, 183, 184, 186A, 188C, 190A and B, 192A, B and F, 193, 194). In the anteroposterior projection, ventricular segments of all of these tributaries of the medial atrial vein show typical multiple curves, convex superiorly and medially. The vertical limbs of the atrium and the adjacent portion of the lateral ventricle of these curved veins outline various parts of the medial wall, whereas their horizontal limbs outline the roof. Since the medial wall of the occipito-atrial portion of the ventricle runs anteromedially as it is traced forwards, the vertical limb of an anteriorly located medial atrial tributary lies more medially in the anteroposterior projection than that of a posteriorly located tributary (Figs. 178A and B, 180, 185, 186). Also the horizontal limb of a posterior septal tributary of the medial atrial vein shows a more horizontal course and a more acute angulation as it turns downwards towards the midline.

Although the number of tributaries of the medial atrial vein is variable and ranges from 0 to 6, usually there are 2 or 3. These tributaries, however, may join independently the internal cerebral, the great cerebral or the basal cerebral veins (Figs. 176, 184, 188C).

The *posterior longitudinal hippocampal vein*, described in the chapter on the basal cerebral vein (p. 131), lies adjacent to the dentate gyrus and runs posteromedially and superiorly to join the stem of the medial atrial vein (Fig. 175). Other veins that may join the medial atrial vein include the internal occipital, the medial temporal, the splenial and the anomalous septal veins. Not infrequently, the direct lateral vein joins the stem of the medial atrial vein in the cistern of the velum interpositum, to form the *common atrial vein*. This acts as a common stem for both the medial and the lateral groups of subependymal veins and drains into the internal cerebral vein (Figs. 182A, 190, 192A and C, 194A). It is also not uncommon to see the *septo-atrial vein*, which is formed by the union of the anomalous septal and medial atrial veins (Figs. 177B, 178B, 182B, 188A, 193A). Drainage of the direct lateral vein into the medial atrial vein, or vice versa, through a roof vein, is, however, rare (Figs. 192C, 194B).

4. Transverse Hippocampal Subependymal Veins
(Figs. 171, 172A, 173, 175, 177A, 178A, 179)

These multiple short subependymal tributaries, located on the floor of the temporal horn, arise from the lateral border of the hippocampus (Huang and Wolf, 1974; Padget, 1956; Wolf and Huang, 1964). They run medially under the ependyma and above the alveus. After piercing the alveus and running medially, under the attachment of the fimbria, these *transverse hippocampal subependymal tributaries* emerge from the fimbriodentate sulcus, to join the anterior or posterior longitudinal hippocampal vein at right angles (Figs. 171, 172A, 173, 175, 177A, 178A, 179). Posteriorly, transverse hippocampal subependymal veins are not present and are replaced by tributaries of the medial atrial vein, particularly the occipital tributary. Similarly, numerous, fine, short *transverse hippocampal pial veins*, originating from the depth of the hippocampal sulcus, also join the anterior or posterior longitudinal hippocampal vein at right angles. The *anterior longitudinal hippocampal vein*, thus formed, runs anteriorly to join the stem of the inferior ventricular vein at the level of the inferior end of the choroid fissure. The *posterior longitudinal hippocampal vein*, formed in a similar fashion, drains posteromedially and superiorly to open into the stem of the medial atrial vein. In some cases it opens into the posterior portion of the basal cerebral vein. The anterior and posterior longitudinal hippocampal veins, running along the corrugated gyrus, frequently communicate with each other (Figs. 171, 175, 177A, 178A, 179). It is rare, however, for this channel to become so prominent as to replace the basal cerebral vein (Fig. 175) (Huang and Wolf, 1974; Wolf and Huang, 1964) (see Fig. 136F, Chap. 4). Transverse hippocampal veins, either pial or subependymal, are usually too fine and too small to be of any diagnostic value.

II. Lateral Group of the Subependymal Veins
(Figs. 168, 170, 171, 172B, 174, 177C and D, 178C and D, 179, 187–192)

While the medial group of subependymal veins drains the deep white matter of the hemisphere, the lateral group drains both the deep white and the deep grey matter. Along the lateral angle of the lateral ventricle, the lateral group drains the deep white matter and the superolateral part of the basal ganglia. Since the thalamus is derived

from the diencephalon, the subependymal veins of the lateral ventricle do not drain this structure.
Included in the lateral group are the thalamostriate, the direct lateral and the inferior ventricular veins.

1. Thalamostriate Vein

(Figs. 168, 174, 177C and D, 178D, 179–181, 182A, 183, 186–188, 190B, 192B–F, 193)

The thalamostriate vein drains the white matter of the frontoparietal region and the superior and anterior parts of the corpus striatum. It does not, however, drain the thalamus (FISCHER, 1966; GIUDICELLI *et al.*, 1970).
The definition of the thalamostriate vein varies. The most widely accepted description of this vein is that it begins in the region of the anterior wall of the atrium or in the inferolateral wall of the body of the lateral ventricle, in the linea terminalis. It passes anteriorly and medially, beneath the stria terminalis, receiving several transverse caudate tributaries on its way towards the interventricular foramen. At the level of the interventricular foramen, the thalamostriate vein runs around the anterior tubercle of the thalamus and receives the vein from the head of the caudate nucleus. The thalamostriate vein then passes medially and joins the internal cerebral vein at the posterosuperior margin of the interventricular foramen, together with the superior choroidal, septal and superior thalamic veins (Figs. 179, 180, 181A, 187, 195A). The confluence of these veins at the interventricular foramen has been designated by others the *anterior paraventricular vein* (Fig. 179) (BEKOV, 1965).
The angle formed by the thalamostriate vein and the internal cerebral vein is often referred to as the *venous angle* and is important angiographically. Topometric studies of the venous angle and internal cerebral vein, therefore, are many (FISCHER, 1966; KRAYENBÜHL and RICHTER, 1952; LIN *et al.*, 1955; MOKROHISKY, 1956; POTTS and TAVERAS, 1963; RING, 1959; WOLF *et al.*, 1955). However, it should be noted that when the thalamostriate vein joins the internal cerebral vein posteriorly to, or anteriorly to, the interventricular foramen, a false venous angle is created (MOKROHISKY, 1956).
As described above, there are several veins running parallel to and beneath the stria terminalis. It seems proper to call these veins *terminal veins*. They may be present in the anterior part of the body of the lateral ventricle, joining the stem of the thalamostriate vein (superior terminal vein). They may also be in the upper part of the atrium, opening into the direct lateral vein (middle terminal vein), or in the temporal horn, joining the inferior ventricular vein (inferior terminal vein). Since a *superior terminal vein* is usually short and frequently not the largest tributary of the thalamostriate vein, it seems appropriate to describe the latter vein as running from the junction between the superior terminal vein and the most prominent anteriorly located caudate vein (i.e., the anterior caudate vein) to the interventricular foramen, where it is joined by the septal vein to become the internal cerebral vein.
The veins that drain into the transverse caudate veins are the *longitudinal caudate veins* of SCHLESINGER (Figs. 166, 168, 174, 179, 180, 186, 192B, 193A, 196, 197) (BEKOV, 1965a; KAPLAN and FORD, 1966; SCHLESINGER, 1939; STEIN and ROSENBAUM, 1974; STEPHENS and STILWELL, 1969; WOLF and HUANG, 1963, 1964). They lie subependymally along the lateral angle of the frontal horn and body of the lateral ventricle. In the body they usually are short, draining either forwards or backwards above the caudate nucleus, and may overlap each other, i.e., one may see, on cross-section, several longitudinally orientated veins in the lateral angle of the body of the lateral ventricle. Therefore, the *non-crossing rule* (WOLF and HUANG, 1964) – subependymal veins that cross each other cannot lie in the same plane – does not hold here (Fig. 190B). They receive superior striate veins from part of the head and body of the caudate nucleus, the upper part of the putamen, the internal capsule, and the claustrum as well as numerous fine deep medullary veins from the lower part of the frontoparietal region (STEPHENS and STILWELL, 1969).
These longitudinal caudate veins join the *transverse caudate veins* at various levels (Figs. 166, 168, 172B, 174, 177C and D, 178C and D, 179–183, 188C). The latter veins, in turn, run downwards, crossing the body of the caudate nucleus in parallel arcs and unite with the terminal tributary of the thalamostriate vein.
A caudate vein adjacent to the lateral angle of the lateral ventricle, above the head of the caudate nucleus, is, however, frequently large and long. This is often referred to as the *anterior caudate vein* (WOLF *et al.*, 1955; WOLF and HUANG, 1964) and is, in reality, a combination of a prominent longitudinal and transverse caudate vein, originating from the frontal horn (Figs. 166, 174, 177C and D, 178C and D, 179–183, 185–187, 188A and C, 190B, 192–196). Quite frequently the anterior caudate vein is so prominent that it becomes the chief tributary of the thalamostriate vein. Although the anterior caudate vein usually joins the anterior portion of the thalamostriate vein, it may open directly into the internal cerebral vein (Fig. 188A), the direct lateral vein (Figs. 184, 189, 195B), or even the low-running septal vein, passing below the internal cerebral vein (WOLF and HUANG, 1964).
In contrast to the anterior caudate vein described above, *veins of the head of the caudate nucleus* originate from the ventricular aspect of the head of the caudate nucleus.

They converge posteriorly to form one or two trunks which, in turn, join the stem of the thalamostriate vein (Figs. 166, 172B, 177C and D, 178C and D, 179, 180, 187A, 192E, 195A). Since they run posteriorly over the head of the caudate nucleus, these veins may also be included with the group of transverse caudate veins. For this reason, they have also been included with the anterior caudate veins (WOLF and HUANG, 1964), or referred to as the *antero-inferior caudate vein* (STEIN and ROSENBAUM, 1974). Since they mainly drain the head of the caudate nucleus, the term *veins of the head of the caudate nucleus* is most appropriate. However, when they are prominent and reach the anterior angle of the frontal horn, they may receive blood from the deep white matter of the frontal lobe. The longitudinal caudate segment of the anterior caudate vein usually meets a septal vein in this angle.

2. Direct Lateral Vein

(Figs. 170, 172B, 174, 176, 177C, 178C, 179, 180, 182A, 184, 188B, 189A, 190, 192A, C and D, 194A, 195)

The direct lateral vein, described by BROWNING in 1884, begins as several tributaries originating from the lateral angle of the body and from the anterior or lateral wall of the atrium of the lateral ventricle. They converge inferiorly and medially, crossing the caudate nucleus and passing under the stria terminalis, lamina affixa and tenia choroidea to become extraventricular, in the cistern of the velum interpositum. As they run medially, they unite at various points, to form a single trunk that crosses further medially over the thalamus (*suprathalamic direct lateral vein*) (Figs. 170, 176, 177C, 179, 184, 189, 195). Not infrequently a single trunk is formed behind the thalamus (*retrothalamic direct lateral vein*) which runs medially to join the posterior portion of the internal cerebral vein or, in rare cases, the posterior portion of the basal cerebral vein (Figs. 190A and B). Recognition of both supra- and retrothalamic veins is important angiographically, since these veins outline respectively the superior and posterior surfaces of the thalamus, or the floor of the body of the lateral ventricle and anterior wall of the atrium.

Not infrequently a vein running adjacent to the stria terminalis joins the direct lateral vein (Figs. 172B, 177C, 180, 190A, 192A and B). This middle terminal vein may communicate with the superior terminal tributary of the thalamostriate vein or the inferior terminal tributary of the inferior ventricular vein (Fig. 192A).

The direct lateral vein may also drain into the stem of the medial atrial vein in the cistern of the velum interpositum to form the *common atrial vein* (Figs. 180, 190, 192A and C, 194). The latter vein has also been designated the *posterior paraventricular vein* (Fig. 179) (BEKOV, 1965a; KAPLAN and FORD, 1966). In rare cases the direct lateral vein may open into the medial atrial vein, or vice versa, through a roof vein (Figs. 192C, 194B).

3. Inferior Ventricular Vein

(Figs. 166, 171, 172B, 174, 177C and D, 178C and D, 179, 180, 184–186, 191, 192A, E and F, 193) (PADGET, 1956; WOLF and HUANG, 1964)

The inferior ventricular vein arises from the lateral wall of the body of the lateral ventricle, usually above the caudate nucleus. First it runs posteriorly, then inferolaterally and then antero-inferiorly in a continuous smooth curve, travelling on the anterolateral wall of the atrium and in the roof of the temporal horn, lateral to the tail of the caudate nucleus. At the level of the inferior end of the choroid fissure, the vein makes an abrupt but smooth medial turn and crosses the undersurface of the tail of the caudate nucleus. It receives a subependymal tributary from the roof of the anterior part of the temporal horn *(the anterior temporal vein)*, occasionally a small vein lying adjacent to the stria terminalis *(inferior terminal vein)* and almost invariably a small vein from the choroid plexus of the temporal horn *(inferior choroidal vein)*. After passing above the stria terminalis, lamina affixa and tenia choroidea, the vein becomes extraventricular (Figs. 171, 174, 178C and D, 179, 191). Further medially, in the subarachnoid space, the uncal cortical vein, the anterior (or uncal) hippocampal vein (HUANG and WOLF, 1974) and the anterior longitudinal hippocampal vein join this extraventricular segment (Figs. 180, 187A) (see Part 1., Chap. 4, p.150). The stem of the inferior ventricular vein, which leaves the temporal horn, indicates the location of the inferior end of the choroid fissure *(the inferior choroidal point)* and is therefore important angiographically (see Part 1., Chap. 4, p. 130).

Much less frequently, the inferior ventricular (subependymal) vein may run medially and parallel to the tail of the caudate nucleus – the *inferior terminal vein* (Figs. 174, 179, 192A). This can be compared with the terminal tributary of the direct lateral or thalamostriate vein. Although any of the adjacent terminal tributaries may occasionally unite (Fig. 192A), a continuous terminal vein extending from the interventricular foramen down to the inferior end of the choroid fissure is extremely rare.

It should be noted that the inferior ventricular (subependymal) vein drains mainly the white matter of the hemisphere (WHITE and GREITZ, 1970). However, the inferior terminal vein may drain the posterosuperior part of the basal ganglia (Fig. 180).

Since transverse hippocampal veins are too small to be identified angiographically, all tributaries which originate from the lateral wall or roof of the temporal horn and which join the inferior ventricular vein or the inferior terminal vein, may be designated simply *temporal veins* (Figs. 177C and D, 178C and D, 179, 180, 182A, 187A, 192B, E and F). Depending on their location in the temporal horn, they can be further subdivided into the *anterior and posterior temporal veins*. Among the tributaries of the former vein, the *temporal tip vein* is important angiographically because it delineates the tip of the temporal horn. When a tributary begins in the lateral wall of the atrium, it may be designated a lateral atrial tributary regardless of whether it terminates in the inferior ventricular vein, the direct lateral vein or the posterior part of the basal cerebral vein.

C. Choroidal Veins of the Lateral Ventricle

(Figs. 168, 170, 171, 179, 180, 186, 187B, 188A, 192B, 193A)

The choroid plexus of the lateral ventricle is drained by the *superior* and, to a much lesser extent, the *inferior choroidal veins* (BEN AMOR *et al.*, 1971; PADGET, 1956; TAKAHASHI and OKUDERA, 1972). The former vein runs anteromedially, along the lateral border of the choroid plexus, taking a spiral course and opens into the anterior end of the internal cerebral vein, the stem of the thalamostriate vein, or the septal vein (Fig. 180). The inferior choroidal vein is smaller in caliber and joins the inferior ventricular vein at the inferior end of the choroid fissure. Since the choroid plexus of the lateral ventricle is formed by invagination through the choroid fissure, of the pia and the accompanying arteries and veins it is not surprising to see a choroidal vein leave the choroid fissure through a point other than its superior end (superior choroidal point or interventricular foramen) or its inferior end (inferior choroidal point). In fact, in Fig. 168B it is seen that the right superior choroidal vein joins the internal cerebral vein some distance behind the interventricular foramen by passing through the *true* choroid fissure. This is unlike the subependymal veins, which never leave the lateral ventricle this way.

TAKAHASHI and OKUDERA (1972), have also described a *connecting vein* linking the glomus of the atrium with the medial atrial vein, in the cistern of the velum interpositum. Not infrequently, the vein of the choroid plexus of the posterior temporal horn and atrium drains upwards and forwards, to join the posterior part of the internal cerebral vein directly or indirectly, through the stem of the direct lateral vein. The term *middle choroidal vein* may be more appropriate in these cases. It is interesting to find, however, on the left side in Fig. 168B, that a vein originating from the glomus runs superiorly and medially to join one of the subependymal tributaries of the medial atrial vein, not within the subarachnoid space, the cistern of the velum interpositum, but within the cavity of the lateral ventricle. A similar connecting vein between the glomus and one of the tributaries of the direct lateral vein, in the atrium, has also been observed by the author. From the embryologic viewpoint it is rather difficult to explain the presence of the *intraventricular* connecting vein, seen on the left side of Fig. 168B, in contradistinction to the usual *subarachnoid* connecting veins, already described. As with the superior choroidal vein, the inferior choroidal vein may join the longitudinal hippocampal or basal cerebral vein, some distance behind the inferior end of the choroid fissure. Although choroidal veins are usually poorly seen, choroidal blushes are observed frequently during vertebral angiography (Figs. 186, 187B, 188A, 192, 193A), particularly in the Towne projection. They are of great value in angiographic diagnosis when visualized on both sides.

D. Veins of the White Matter of the Cerebral Hemisphere—Medullary Veins

(Figs. 166, 168, 170, 171, 173, 179, 180, 182C, 184, 186, 193, 194B, 196, 197)

The medullary veins have been studied by DURET (1874), HOOSHMAND *et al.* (1974), HUANG and WOLF (1964), KAPLAN (1959), PFEIFER (1930), and SCHLESINGER (1939). The medullary veins may be divided into those draining superficially to join the superficial cortical veins (superficial medullary veins) and those draining deeply to open into the subependymal veins (deep medullary veins).

The *superficial medullary veins* begin 1 to 2 cm below the cortical grey matter and have a surprisingly straight course towards and through the cortex, to join the superficial cortical veins. The *deep medullary veins*, on the other hand, pass deeply and converge towards the lateral angle of the frontal horn and body of the lateral ventricle, the lateral wall of the atrium and the lateral part of the roof of the temporal horn. More specifically, the deep medullary veins, from the depths of the anterior part of the frontal lobe, run backwards to join the vein of the septum pellucidum and the anterior caudate vein, along the anterolateral angle of the frontal horn. Deep medullary veins from the remainder of the frontal lobe and from the anterior parietal lobe, converge inferiorly and medially towards the lateral angle of the body of the lateral ventricle and open into the thalamostriate, posterior septal, direct lateral and medial atrial subependymal veins. The veins from the posterior parietal and occipital lobes stream inferiorly, anteriorly and medially, towards the occipital horn, as well as towards the superior and lateral wall of the atrium, where they join the medial atrial, the lateral atrial and the direct lateral subependymal veins. The veins from the lateral posterior temporal lobe run anteriorly, superiorly and medially, to join the inferior ventricular, direct lateral and lateral atrial veins, along the lateral wall of the atrium and the superolateral wall of the posterior part of the temporal horn. The deep medullary veins from the anterior part of the temporal lobe, however, run backwards to open into the temporal veins, including the temporal tip subependymal veins along the anterior and lateral aspects of the temporal horn. According to SCHLESINGER, there are anastomotic veins that connect the deep and superficial medullary veins. Not infrequently, continuous venous channels, extending from the cortex down to the ependyma, may be observed (transcerebral veins) (KAPLAN, 1959).

Under normal conditions, on a cerebral angiogram, the superficial medullary veins are difficult to distinguish from the superficial cortical veins, located deep in the sulci. On the other hand, deep medullary veins are more easily identified. Not infrequently, short segments of the deep medullary veins may be identified near the tip of the frontal horn and along the lateral angle of the body and atrium of the lateral ventricle. With magnification cerebral angiography, longer segments of many deep medullary veins may be observed in more than 50% of cases (STEIN and ROSENBAUM, 1974).

Veins of the corpus callosum are prominent posteriorly (Figs. 176, 180, 187A, 188B, 192A, 195, 197). The *posterior pericallosal vein* or *splenial vein* begins on the dorsal surface of the posterior one-third of the corpus callosum (BELLEWICZ and BEN AMOR, 1971; BEN AMOR and WACKENHEIM, 1973; ROSA and VIALE, 1971). It runs posteriorly in the pericallosal cistern or on the medial aspect of the cingulate gyrus (supracallosal segment), receiving, at right angles, numerous, fine, short parenchymal tributaries from the corpus callosum and cortical tributaries of the adjacent gyri. The splenial vein then runs around the posterior border of the splenium (splenial segment) and joins the anterior end of the straight sinus, the great cerebral vein, the basal cerebral vein, the internal cerebral vein, the medial atrial vein or the internal occipital vein. The remaining parts of the corpus callosum are drained in a similar fashion. Penetrating veins from the body of the corpus callosum join, at right angles, longitudinally orientated short veins within the pericallosal cistern. The latter veins, in turn, unite directly with the inferior sagittal sinus or indirectly with the superior sagittal sinus via medial frontoparietal cortical veins. More anteriorly, the *anterior pericallosal vein*, draining the anterior part of the corpus callosum and adjacent gyri, runs forwards above the corpus callosum (supracallosal segment), around the genu (genual segment), and then inferoposteriorly on the medial aspect of the subcallosal gyrus, in the cistern of the lamina terminalis (terminal segment). Before turning medially at the lower end of the subcallosal gyrus, to become the anterior cerebral vein, the anterior pericallosal vein frequently receives the *paraterminal tributary* and also the *anterior communicating vein*, a short distance antero-inferiorly to the anterior commissure (see Part 1, Chap. 4, p. 129). The anterior cerebral vein joins the basal cerebral vein on the undersurface of the anterior perforated substance (Fig. 176).

E. Veins of the Gray Matter of the Cerebral Hemisphere

(Figs. 166, 169, 170, 196, 197, 198)

Because of their small size, short course and superficial location, veins of the superficial cortical grey matter are indistinguishable angiographically from the superficial cortical pial veins. Only veins draining the deep basal nuclei will therefore be discussed.

The caudate and lentiform nuclei are drained superiorly by the *superior striate veins* (HUANG and WOLF, 1964) and inferiorly by *the inferior striate veins* (HUANG and WOLF, 1974; WOLF and HUANG, 1963). These veins have been further subdivided into internal and external groups (SCHLESINGER, 1939). Though they are often indistinct, the *external superior striate veins* may be seen to run upwards in a diverging fashion (anterior tributaries run anterosuperiorly and posterior tributaries posterosuperiorly), in or adjacent to the external capsule. They drain the caudate nucleus, putamen, claustrum, internal capsule and neighboring structures. They join the veins of the head of the caudate nucleus, transverse caudate veins, posterior septal and direct lateral subependymal veins, along the anterior and lateral angles of the frontal horn and the lateral angle of the body of the lateral ventricle. Veins running more medially, in or adjacent to the external and internal medullary laminae *(internal superior striate veins)*, similarly stream upwards in a diverging fashion, to join the terminal tributaries of the thalamostriate and direct lateral veins and the veins of the head of the caudate nucleus. In some cases the superior striate veins may be found to drain into the inferior ventricular vein (Fig. 180).

The inferior striate veins, on the other hand, converge downwards, lying in the external capsule *(external inferi-*

or striate veins) and in the external and internal medullary laminae *(internal inferior striate veins)*. They drain the putamen, globus pallidus and neighboring structures, opening into the stem of the deep middle cerebral tributary of the basal cerebral vein, on the undersurface of the anterior perforated substance (see Part 1, Chap. 4, p. 128). Distinction between the external and internal striate veins may at times be exceedingly difficult, particularly in the inferior striate group, because they all converge towards the anterior perforated substance (SCHLESINGER, 1939).

Angiographically, the inferior striate veins mark the location of the anterior perforated substance, in both the anteroposterior and lateral views. A gentle curve, convex laterally, formed by the superior and inferior striate veins, in the anteroposterior view, shows the shape and location of the lateral part of the corpus striatum.

Thalamic Veins (Figs. 180, 198)

Veins draining the thalamus have been studied by BEN AMOR and WACKENHEIM (1973), FERNER (1958), GIUDICELLI and SALAMON (1970), and HASSLER (1966). GIUDICELLI and SALAMON divided the thalamic veins into four groups: anterior, superior, inferior and posterior. The largest is the *superior thalamic vein*, which originates from the midportion of the thalamus by the union of several small tributaries. This vein runs medially and, after emerging from the thalamus, turns posteriorly, running below and parallel to the internal cerebral vein, to join the posterior part of this vein or the great cerebral vein of Galen. The superior thalamic vein may, however, join the midportion of the internal cerebral vein or, in rare cases, the posterior portion of the basal cerebral vein or the stem of the medial atrial vein (Figs. 137F, 180).

The *anterior thalamic vein* runs forwards, upwards, and then backwards to join the internal cerebral or septal vein. It drains the anterior thalamus (Figs. 180, 198). The *inferior thalamic veins*, on the other hand, drain the inferior part of the thalamus and emerge from the posterior perforated substance to join the interpeduncular (or peduncular) vein. The *posterior thalamic veins* are usually too small to be seen normally (Fig. 180). They drain the posterolateral and inferior portions of the thalamus into the posterior mesencephalic or basal cerebral veins.

The *epithalamic veins* (SCHLESINGER, 1939), also called the *medial posterior thalamic veins* (HUANG and WOLF, 1974a), the *latero-epiphyseal veins* (DUVERNOY, 1975) or the *superior pineal veins* (TAMAKI *et al.*, 1973), drain the epithalamic and adjacent areas of the posteromedial part of the thalamus, i.e., the pineal gland, posterior commissure, habenular commissure and the neighboring portion of the thalamus (Fig. 176). These veins emerge from the area lateral to the habenular trigone. They frequently form a small venous stem on each side and drain into the internal cerebral vein, basal cerebral vein or great cerebral vein. The small venous stem on each side may unite before opening into those veins described above.

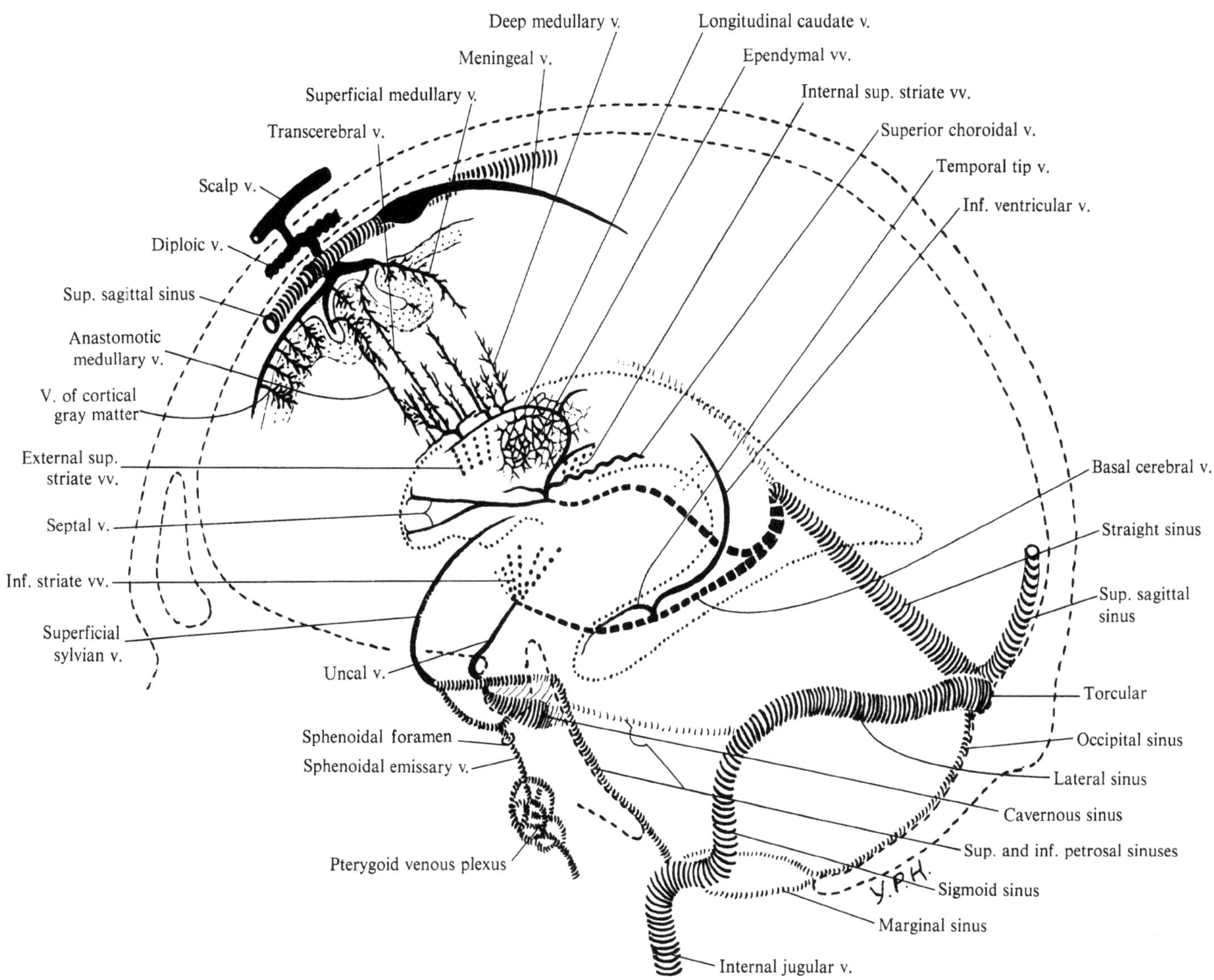

Fig. 166. Schematic diagram showing the general features of the cranial venous system
Veins originating in the superficial portion of the grey and white matter drain into the superficial cortical veins and then into the superficial dural sinuses. On the other hand, veins from the deep grey and white matter and from the choroid plexuses of the lateral ventricles, run deeply to join the deep dural sinuses (inferior sagittal sinus and straight sinus). The drainage from the dural sinuses is, for the most part, via the internal jugular vein, although some drain through the foramina of the middle cranial fossa and join the external jugular venous system via the pterygoid venous plexus. Communications between the dural sinuses and the diploic and scalp veins are also shown

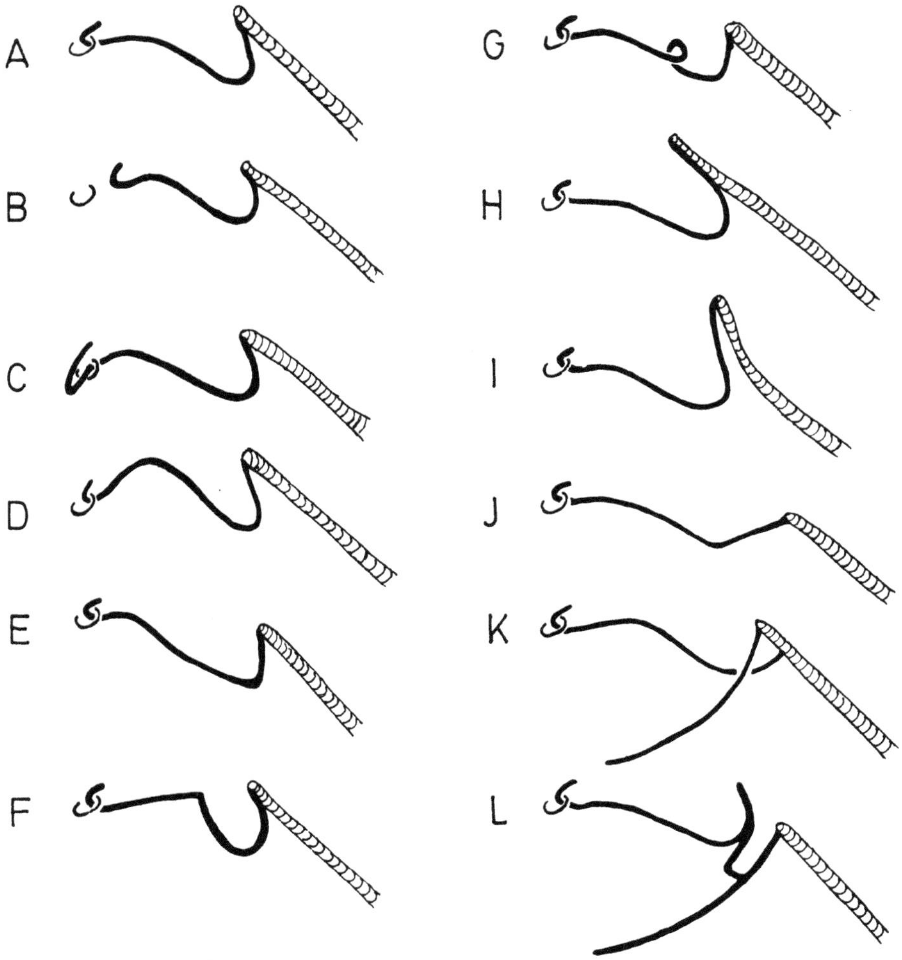

Fig. 167. Diagram of the possible anatomic variations in the course of the internal cerebral and great cerebral veins

A. Typical normal course. The thalamostriate vein joins the internal cerebral vein at the posterosuperior margin of the interventricular foramen

B. Thalamostriate vein joining the internal cerebral vein behind the interventricular foramen

C. Thalamostriate vein joining the internal cerebral vein anteriorly to the interventricular foramen

D. High arched internal cerebral vein

E. Angular course at the junction between the internal cerebral and great cerebral veins

F. Angular course at the midportion of the internal cerebral vein

G. Loop formation

H. Distal end of the great cerebral vein located far anteriorly

I. Distal end of the great cerebral vein located far superiorly

J. Posterior tilting or unfolding of the great cerebral vein

K. Internal cerebral vein joining the straight sinus posteriorly to the basal cerebral vein

L. Great cerebral vein joining the straight sinus indirectly through the basal cerebral vein

Fig. 168. Injected specimen showing the subependymal veins of the lateral ventricles, view from above ▷

Figs. 168 A and 168 B see pp. 221–222

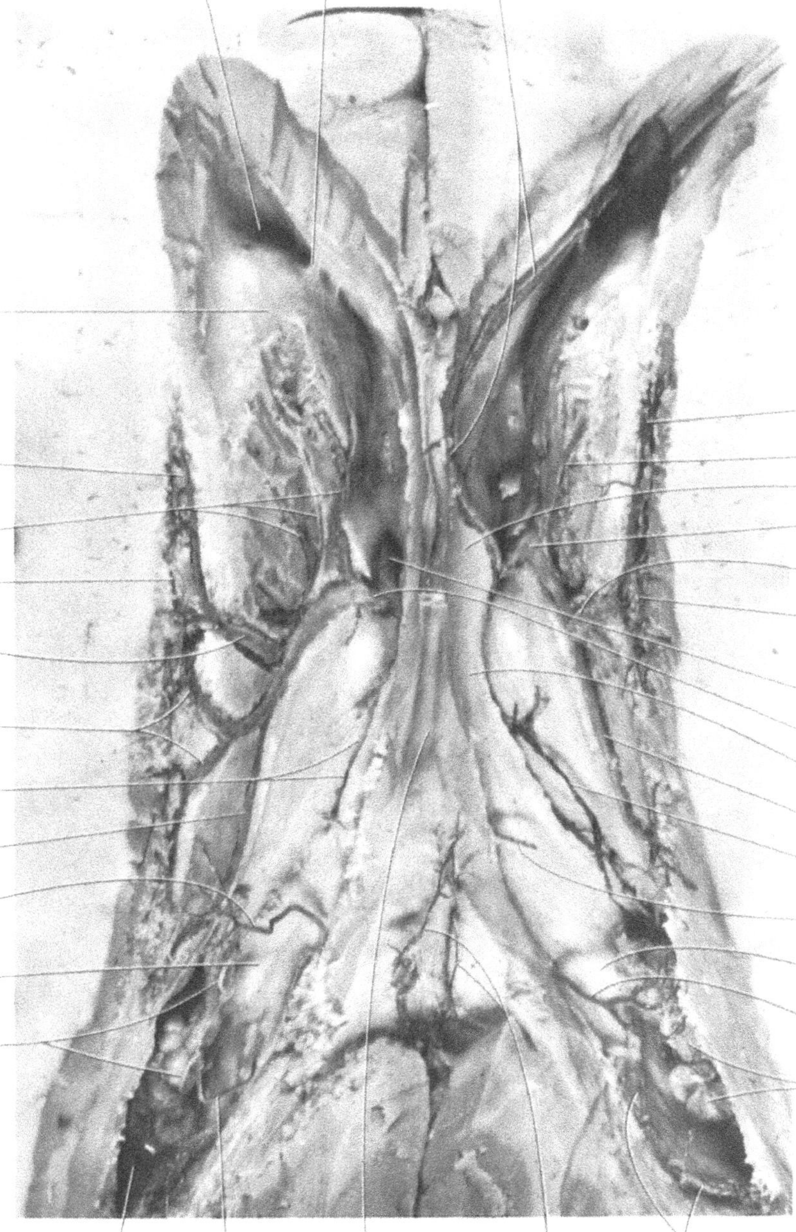

Fig. 168A. The roofs of the lateral ventricles and the ependymal covering of individual subependymal veins were removed, exposing these veins in the frontal horns, bodies and atria of the lateral ventricles. The central portion of the corpus callosum was left intact. The choroid plexuses in the regions of the bodies of the lateral ventricles have also been removed, to show the superior choroidal vein running under the tenia fornicis (right) and a medial atrial vein draining the choroid plexus (left). The thalamostriate veins on each side receive the veins of the head of the caudate nucleus, the transverse caudate veins and the superior terminal veins. Note many fine, longitudinally orientated veins, running along the lateral angles of the lateral ventricles and receiving deep medullary tributaries at right angles. These are most prominent in the region of the bodies of the lateral ventricles. Note also the asymmetry of the thalamostriate veins – the right one loops further forwards around the anterior tubercle of the thalamus. The splenial veins run backwards over and around the splenium of the corpus callosum

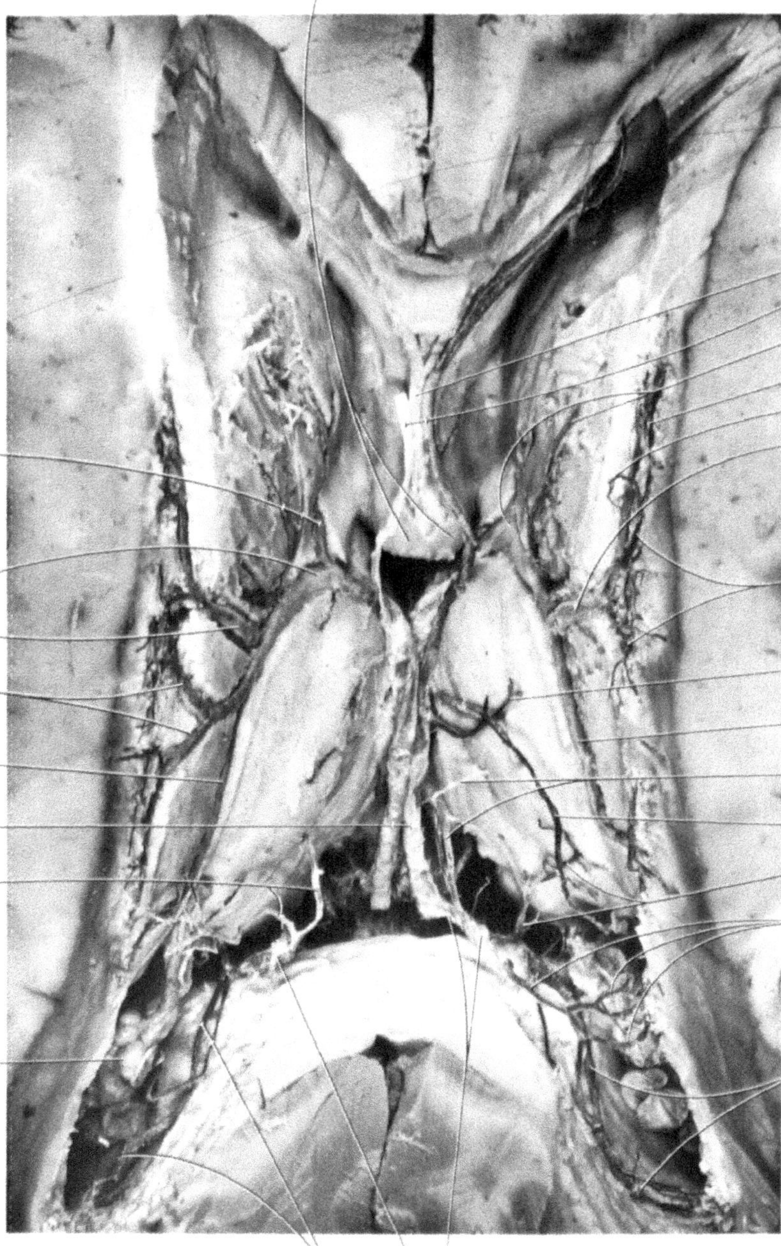

Fig. 168 B. Same specimen. In addition to the structures removed in Fig. 168 A, the central portion of the corpus callosum and the fornix have also been cut away, to expose the internal cerebral veins and their tributaries, located in the cistern of the velum interpositum. Although the superior choroidal vein frequently joins the stem of the thalamostriate vein or the anterior end of the internal cerebral vein, in this specimen the right superior choroidal vein, after passing medially through the choroid fissure, some distance behind the interventricular foramen, joins the midportion of the internal cerebral vein. The choroid plexus within the atrium on the left, drains partly into one of the medial atrial tributaries, via a connecting vein lying not in the cistern of the velum interpositum, but in the ventricular cavity. Note on the right, a tributary of the septal vein running not on the septum pellucidum but on the ventricular side of the rostrum of the corpus callosum; it is therefore more laterally located. The left septal vein is only partly filled with the injection material

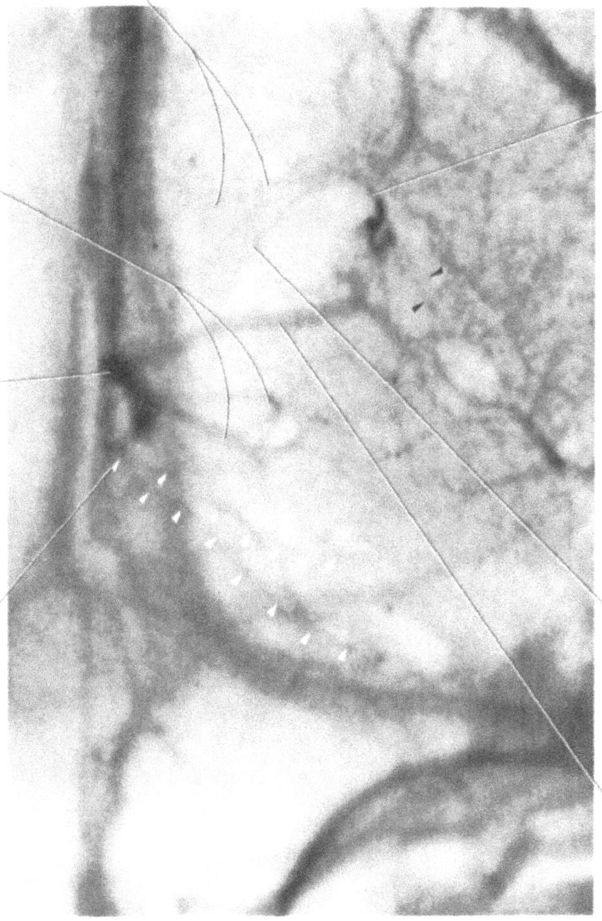

Fig. 169. Subependymal veins outlining the walls of the body of the left lateral ventricle. Carotid angiogram, venous phase, anteroposterior view
The posterior septal vein outlines the roof and the medial wall, while the lateral (intraventricular) portion of the direct lateral vein marks the lateral wall and the lateral part of the floor of the body of the lateral ventricle. The medial (extraventricular) portion of the direct lateral vein runs over the superior surface of the thalamus in the cistern of the velum interpositum. Posteriorly, the medial atrial vein indicates the location of the medial wall of the atrium. More anteriorly, veins of the head of the caudate nucleus and their tributaries show the lateral wall of the frontal horn, whereas the septal vein (rows of white arrowheads) marks the medial and anterior walls. The external superior striate veins (black arrowheads) can also be identified

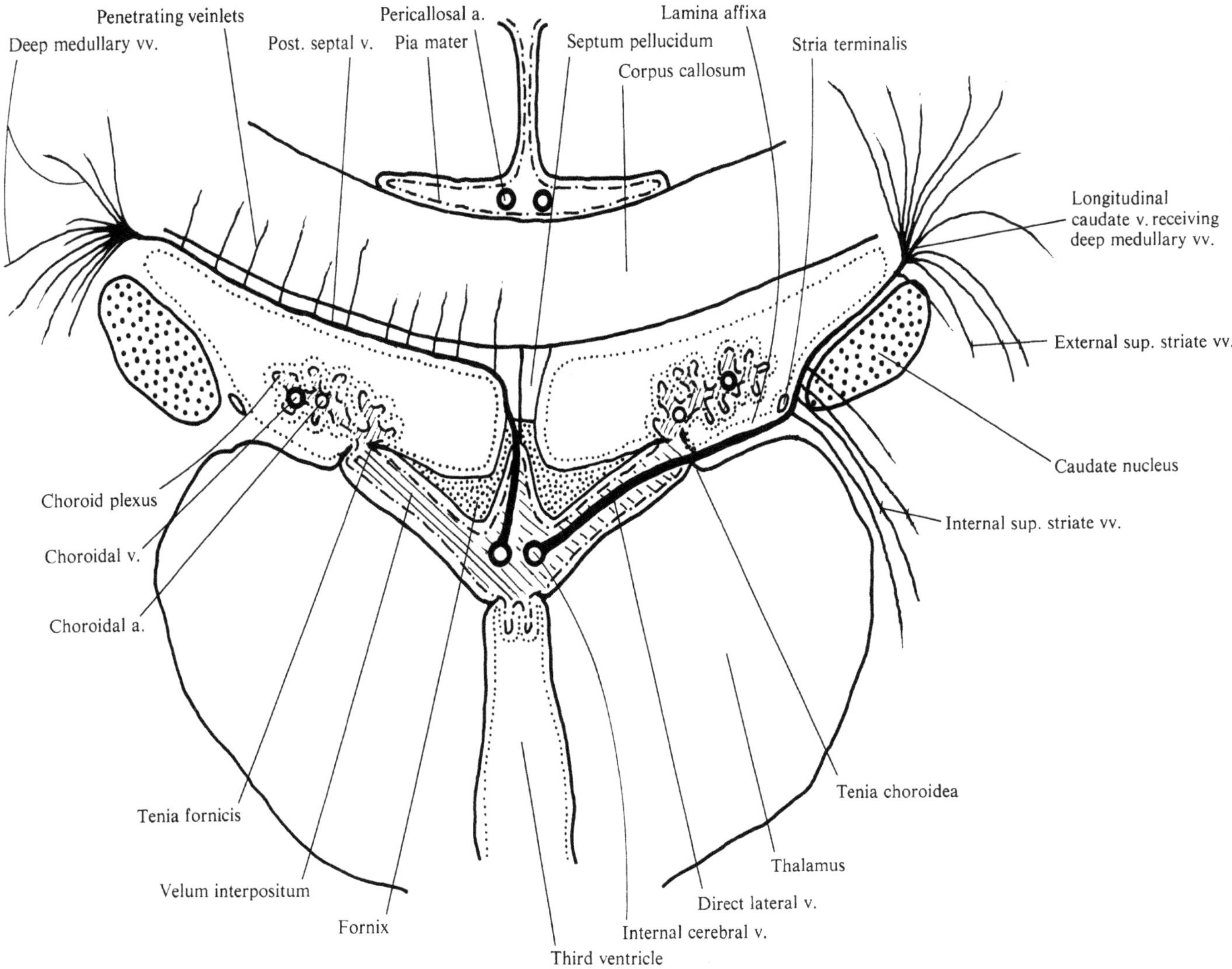

Fig. 170. Diagram showing the medial and lateral groups of subependymal veins in coronal section through the bodies of the lateral ventricles. The posterior septal vein receives numerous fine deep medullary veins, that converge towards the lateral angle of the lateral ventricle. The posterior septal vein then runs medially along the roof of the lateral ventricle, receiving tiny perforating veinlets from the corpus callosum. Upon reaching the medial wall, the vein turns to pass downwards on the rapidly tapering septum pellucidum, before passing between the two bodies of the fornix to join the internal cerebral vein in the cistern of the velum interpositum. Similarly, longitudinal caudate tributaries of the direct lateral vein receive deep medullary veins and external superior striate veins, at the lateral angle of the lateral ventricle. The direct lateral vein then runs inferiorly and medially, receiving internal superior striate veins. The vein passes under the stria terminalis, lamina affixa and tenia choroidea, before entering the cistern of the velum interpositum, where it joins the internal cerebral vein. Note that the deep medullary veins, converging towards the lateral angle of the lateral ventricle, may drain either into the medial or lateral subependymal venous system

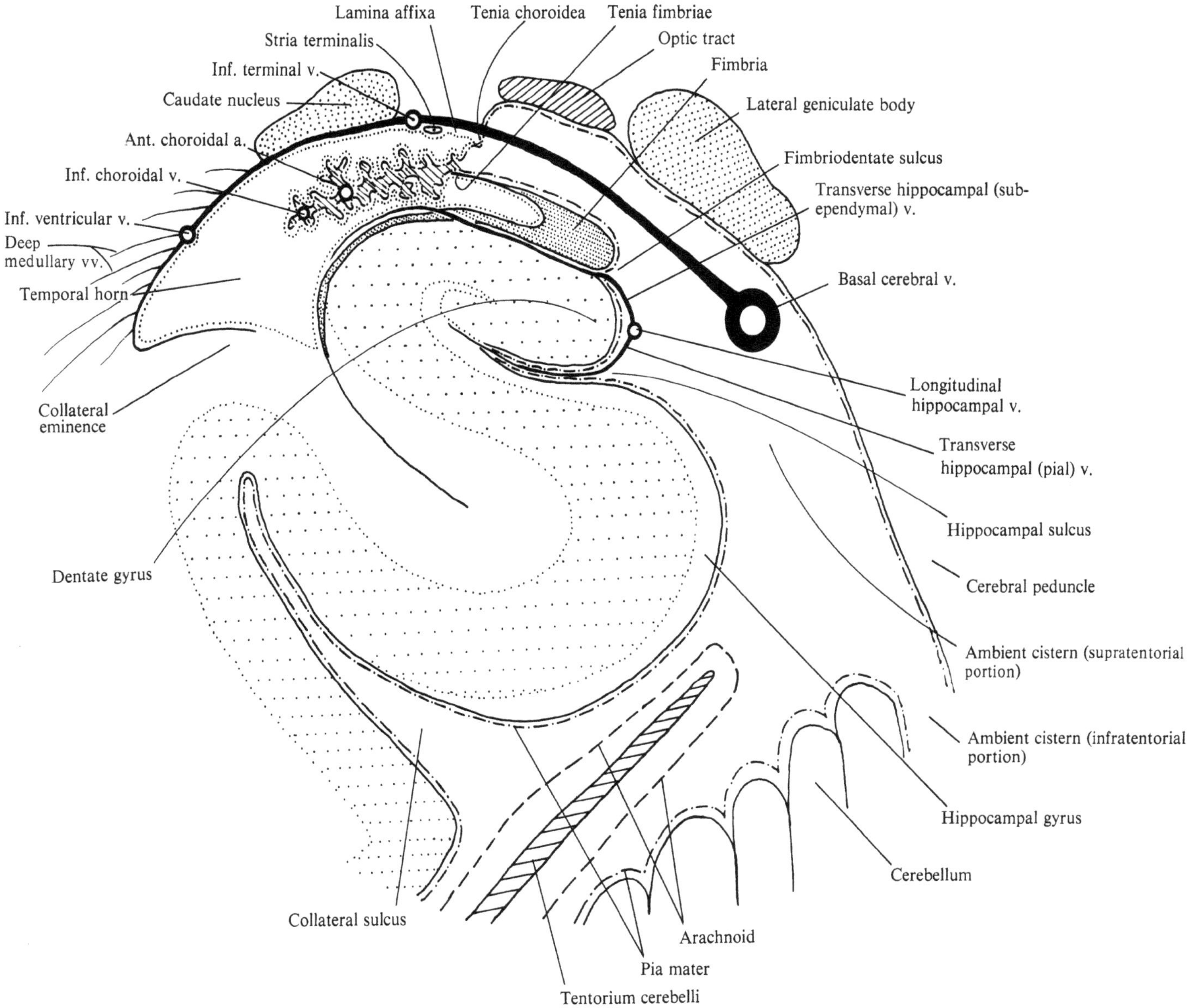

Fig. 171. Diagram showing the medial and lateral groups of subependymal veins in coronal section through the midtemporal horn. Small transverse hippocampal subependymal and pial veins join the longitudinal hippocampal vein at right angles. Note that a tributary originating from the collateral eminence runs around the lateral angle of the temporal horn, first laterally and then superomedially, receiving small deep medullary veins to join the inferior ventricular vein. The latter vein courses anteriorly and then medially to leave the inferior end of the choroid fissure, after passing deeply above the stria terminalis, lamina affixa and tenia choroidea. Although these vessels are located in different planes, they are shown as a continuous venous channel. The inferior terminal vein, which lies medially to the tail of the caudate nucleus, may be present in addition to the inferior ventricular vein and may entirely replace it; it is, therefore, shown in the diagram. The mode of exit of the transverse hippocampal subependymal veins is similar to that of the posterior septal vein, while the inferior ventricular vein resembles the thalamostriate vein

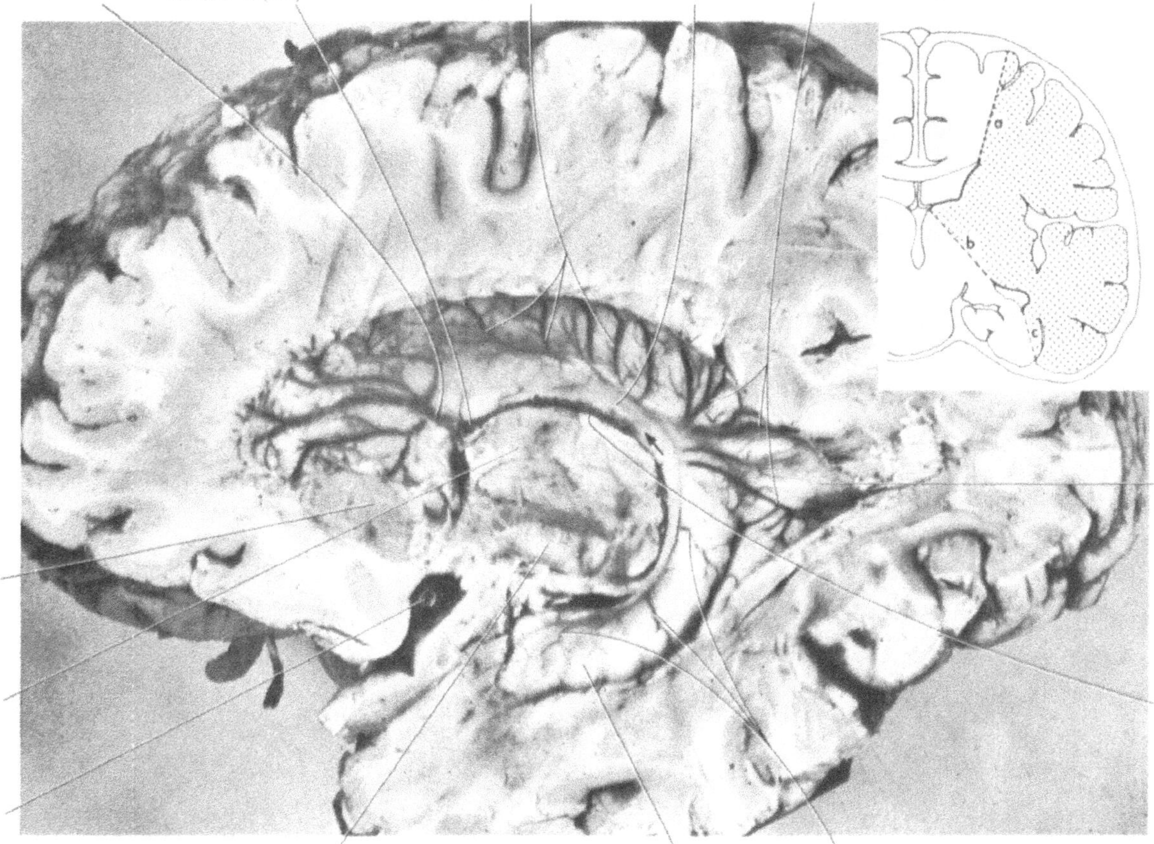

Fig. 172A

Fig. 172. Photographs of an injected specimen, showing the medial and lateral groups of subependymal veins of the lateral ventricle. The insert shows how the left cerebral hemisphere was cut, to separate the medial from the lateral groups of subependymal veins—incision (*a*) from the superior surface to the lateral angle of the ventricle, incision (*b*) between the tenia thalami and temporal horn, and incision (*c*) from the temporal horn to the inferior surface. Fig. 172A is a view of the medial portion (unshaded) of the cut brain as seen from the lateral aspect. Fig. 172B shows the medial aspect of the remaining lateral portion (shaded) of the same hemisphere

Fig. 172A. Medial group of subependymal veins. Several prominent tributaries of the septal vein, running on the superior, anterior and inferomedial walls of the frontal horn, converge to form a single trunk, before turning around the lateral aspect of the column of the fornix, to join the anterior end of the internal cerebral vein. More posteriorly, veins running on the roof and medial wall of the body of the lateral ventricle (posterior septal tributaries), and other veins running on the medial wall of the atrium and occipital horn (atrial and occipital tributaries), converge towards the posterior part of the body of the lateral ventricle. The posterior septal tributaries pass between the two bodies of the fornix, while the atrial and occipital tributaries run over the hippocampus and then pass deeply, behind the crus fornicis, to become extraventricular. On dissection, these posterior septal, atrial and occipital tributaries were found to form a common venous trunk, the septo-atrial vein, which ran medially, to join the posterior portion of the internal cerebral vein. Several tiny transverse hippocampal subependymal veins are seen to run medially over the hippocampus. They also run below the fimbria of the fornix (to become extraventricular and join the longitudinal hippocampal vein)

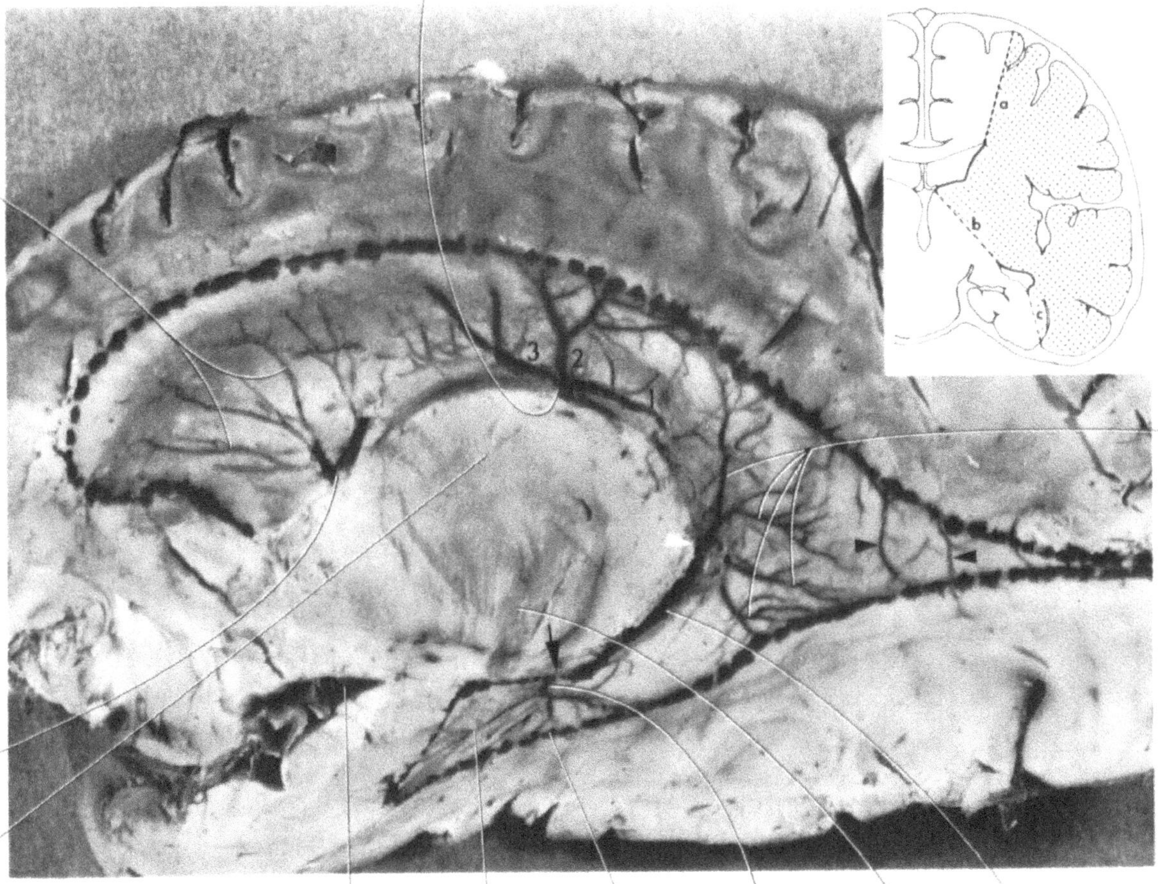

Fig. 172B. Lateral group of subependymal veins. The most prominent vein in this specimen is the direct lateral vein which has three main tributaries: (1) one running in the stria terminalis – the middle terminal tributary; and the other two (2,3) running downwards and backwards on the lateral wall of the body of the lateral ventricle, crossing the body of the caudate nucleus – the transverse caudate tributaries. They all unite to form a single trunk that runs further medially on the superior surface of the thalamus (suprathalamic direct lateral vein). The inferior ventricular vein is also prominent and receives the lateral atrial tributaries, which converge towards the anterior wall of the atrium (white arrowhead). This vein then runs downwards and forwards along the roof of the temporal horn, in this case laterally to the tail of the caudate nucleus. Anteriorly, at the level of the inferior end of the choroid fissure (black arrow), it is joined by the anterior temporal vein and drains medially into the basal cerebral vein. Cut veins, draining into the occipital tributary of the medial atrial vein, are seen on the lateral aspect of the occipital horn (opposing black arrowheads). Note the prominent veins of the head of the caudate nucleus

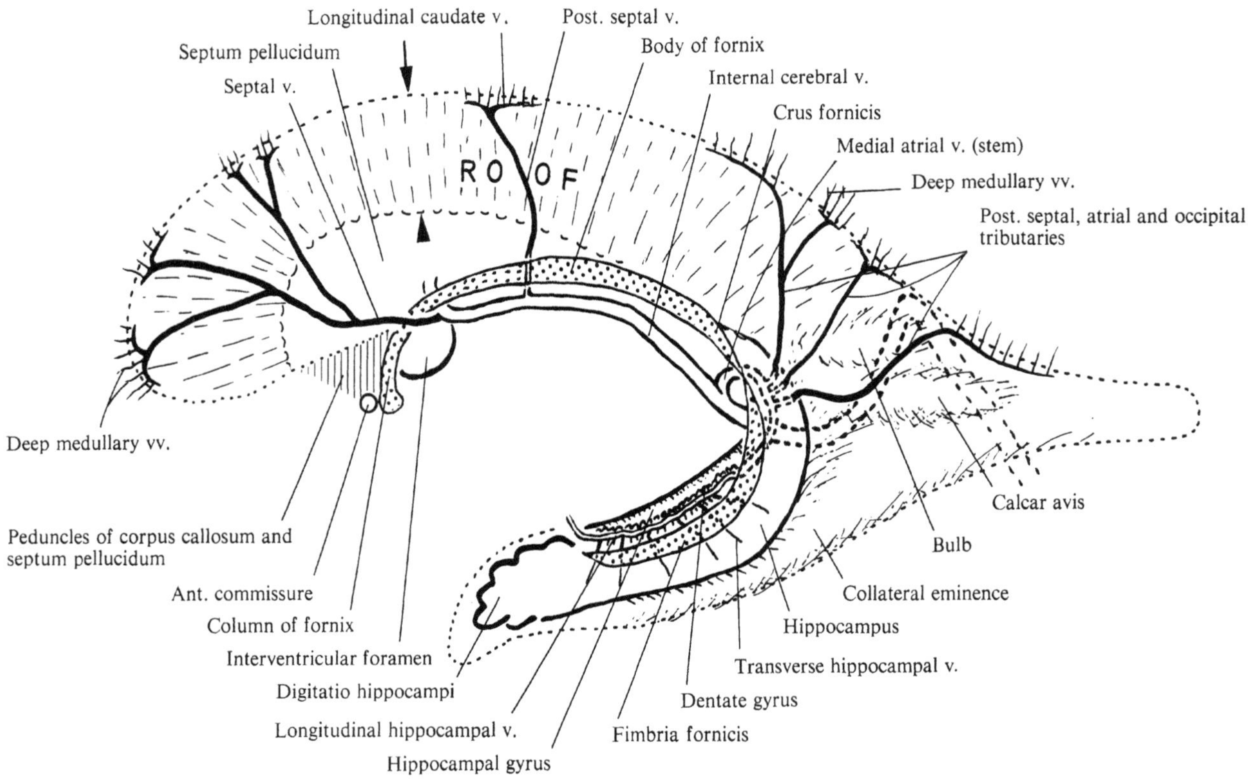

Fig. 173. Anatomic diagram showing the *medial group* of subependymal veins, viewed from the lateral aspect
The intraventricular segments of the subependymal veins are shown with solid lines and the extraventricular segments with empty lines. The superolateral corner (lateral angle) and superomedial corner (medial angle) of the lateral ventricle are indicated (arrow and arrowhead respectively). The intervening roof is coarsely shaded. The anterior part of the septal vein is related to the posterior aspect of the genu of the corpus callosum (callosal segment), whereas the posterior part of the vein is related to the septum pellucidum (septal segment) and the column of the fornix (columnar segment). Similarly, the upper part of the posterior septal vein lies on the undersurface of the body of the corpus callosum (callosal segment), whereas its lower part is related to the septum pellucidum (septal segment) and the body of the fornix (corporal segment). The stem of the medial atrial vein receives the posterior longitudinal hippocampal vein, which runs posterosuperiorly and medially along the dentate gyrus. Transverse hippocampal subependymal and pial veins join the longitudinal hippocampal vein at right angles. (Reprinted by permission of WOLF and HUANG, 1964)

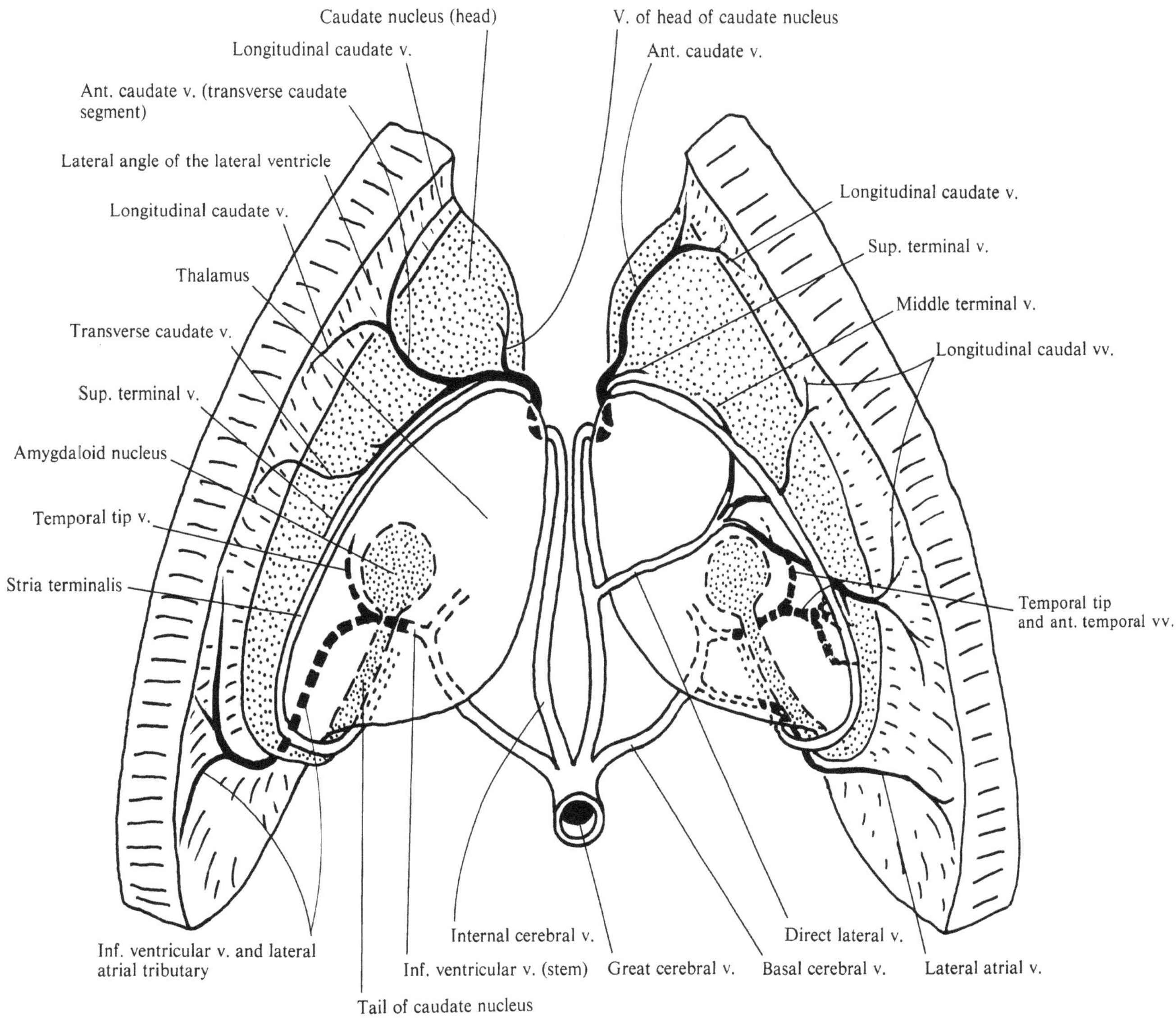

Fig. 174. Anatomic diagram showing the *lateral group* of subependymal veins, viewed from above and behind

The intraventricular segments of the subependymal veins are shown with solid lines and the extraventricular segments with empty lines. On the left (reader's left), the thalamostriate vein receives the longitudinal and anterior caudate veins, the superior terminal vein and the vein of the head of the caudate nucleus. More posteriorly, the inferior ventricular vein receives tributaries from the lateral and anterolateral walls of the atrium. This vein then runs laterally to the tail of the caudate nucleus and leaves through the inferior end of the choroid fissure. On the right (reader's right), the direct lateral vein, receiving tributaries from the lateral wall of the body of the lateral ventricle, runs medially above the thalamus to join the midportion of the internal cerebral vein. More posteriorly, the lateral atrial vein runs anteromedially on the lateral wall of the atrium and then anteroinferiorly on the roof of the temporal horn, medial to the tail of the caudate nucleus (a variation of the inferior terminal vein). This vein then turns medially to join the basal cerebral vein behind the inferior end of the choroid fissure. (Reprinted by permission of WOLF and HUANG, 1964)

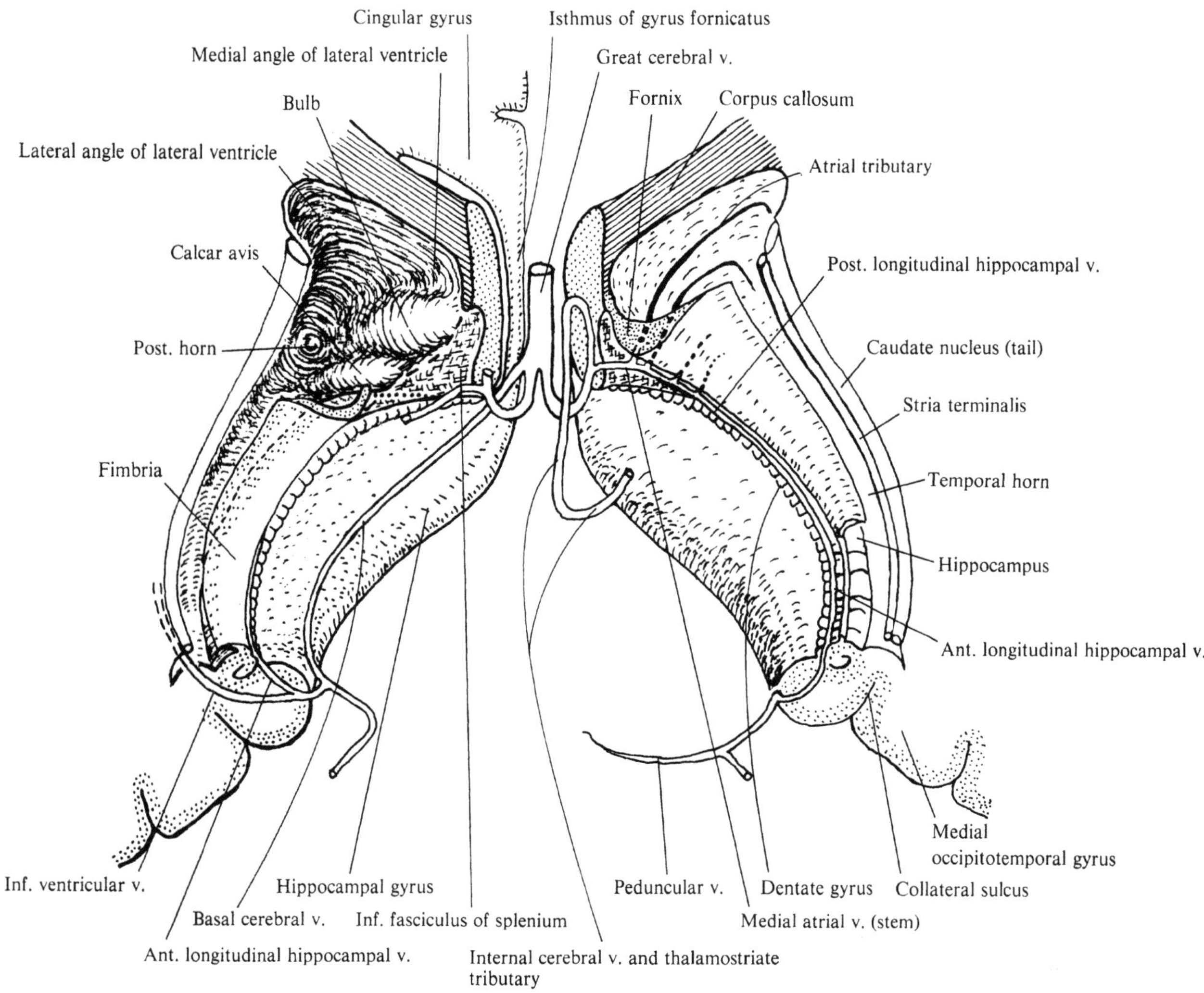

Fig. 175. The medial atrial veins and the veins of the hippocampal formation, showing their relationships to the surrounding anatomic structures, view from the front

Part of the splenium of the corpus callosum has been removed to show the great cerebral vein and its tributaries. The longitudinal hippocampal vein, running along the dentate gyrus, joins posteriorly the stem of the medial atrial vein, and anteriorly the inferior ventricular vein. The longitudinal hippocampal vein receives the transverse hippocampal subependymal and pial veins. Note the subarachnoid space between the crus fornicis and the inferior fasciculus of the splenium of the corpus callosum, the fornicosplenial space. Medial atrial subependymal tributaries, running on the roof and medial wall of the atrium and occipital horn, leave the ventricle by passing medially behind the crus fornicis, to enter the fornicosplenial space, where they join the stem (extraventricular segment) of the medial atrial vein. This stem runs medially to open into the posterior part of the internal cerebral vein. (Reprinted by permission of Wolf and Huang, 1964)

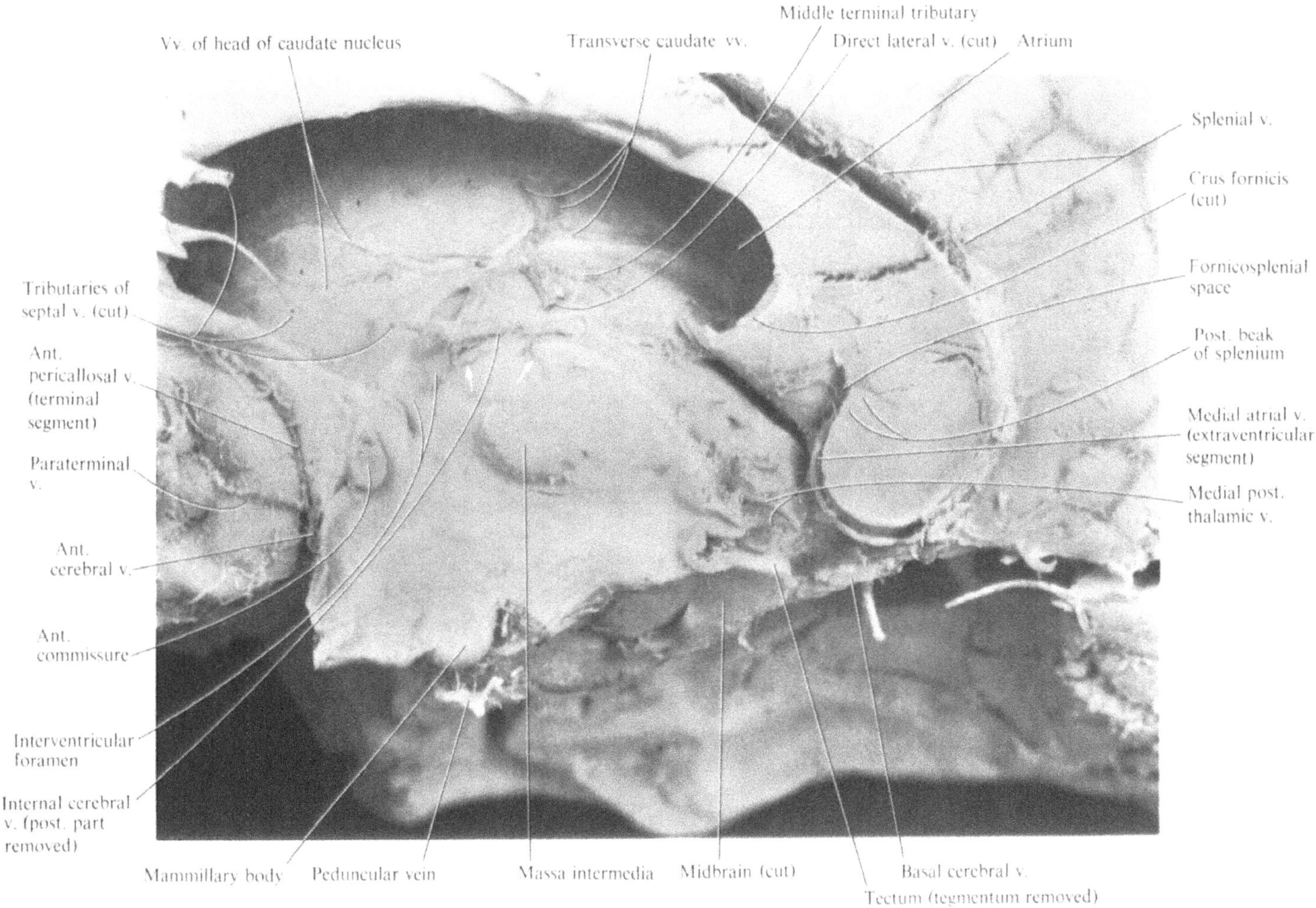

Fig. 176. Midsagittal section of an injected specimen showing the extraventricular segment (stem) of the medial atrial vein, and its relationship to the crus fornicis and the posterior beak of the splenium of the corpus callosum. The posterior two-thirds of the internal cerebral vein and the septum pellucidum have been removed. The stem of the medial atrial vein takes a typically curved course, convex anteriorly, before draining into the internal cerebral or great cerebral vein. The anterior curve corresponds to the contour of the antero-inferior surface of the splenium of the corpus callosum and its lateral extension. Small subependymal tributaries (white arrows) from the third ventricle, draining into the anterior and midportions of the internal cerebral vein, can be identified. The medial posterior thalamic vein (or epithalamic vein), emerging from the region lateral to the habenular trigone, can be identified.

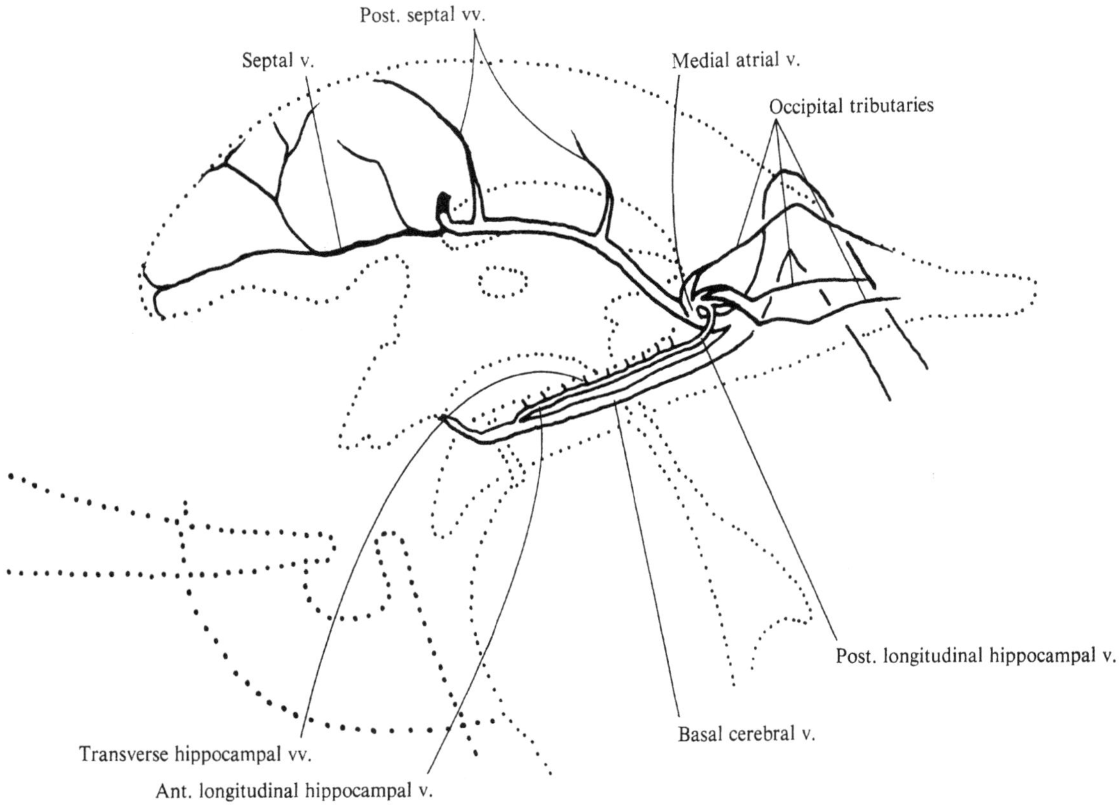

Fig. 177A

▷

Fig. 177. Diagram showing the course of the *medial group* (Fig. 177A and B) and *lateral group* (Fig. 177C and D) of subependymal veins as they might be seen on a lateral angiogram. Corresponding anteroposterior views are shown in Fig. 178. The intraventricular segments of the subependymal veins are shown with solid lines and the extraventricular segments with empty lines. (Reprinted by permission of WOLF and HUANG, 1964)

Fig. 177A. *Medial group* of subependymal veins showing the septal vein, posterior septal veins, medial atrial vein and transverse hippocampal veins

Fig. 177B. *Medial group* of subependymal veins showing the septo-atrial vein

Fig. 177C. *Lateral group* of subependymal veins showing the vein of the head of the caudate nucleus, the direct lateral vein, the lateral atrial vein and the anterior temporal vein

Fig. 177D see p. 234

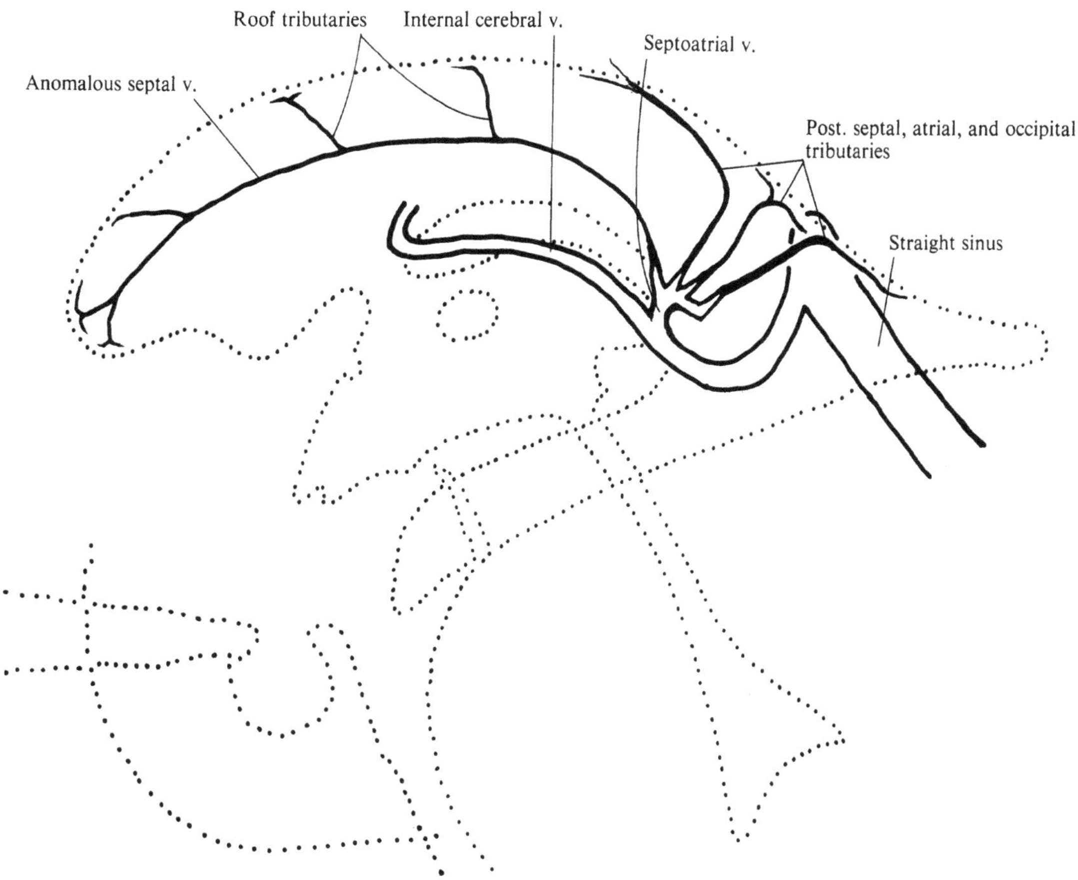

Fig. 177B

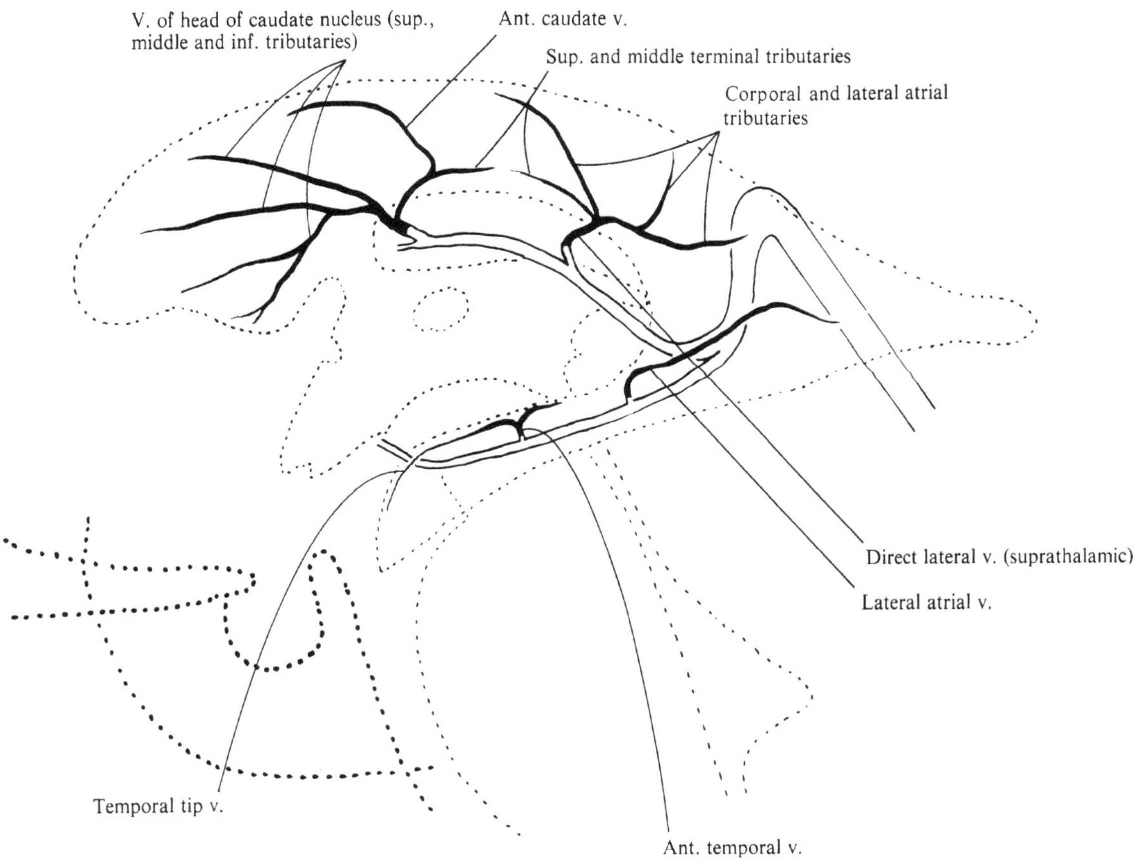

Fig. 177C

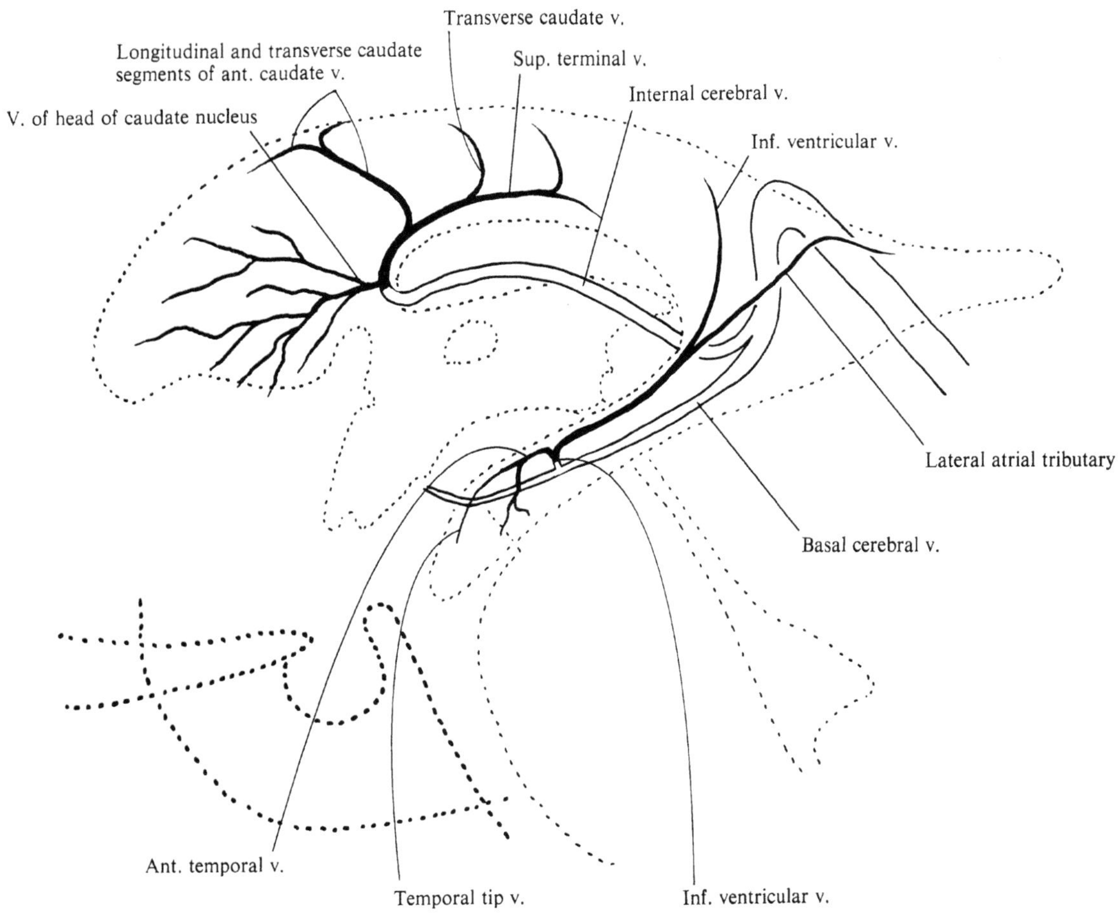

Fig. 177 D. *Lateral group* of subependymal veins showing the anterior caudate vein, the inferior ventricular vein, the temporal tip vein and the vein of the head of the caudate nucleus

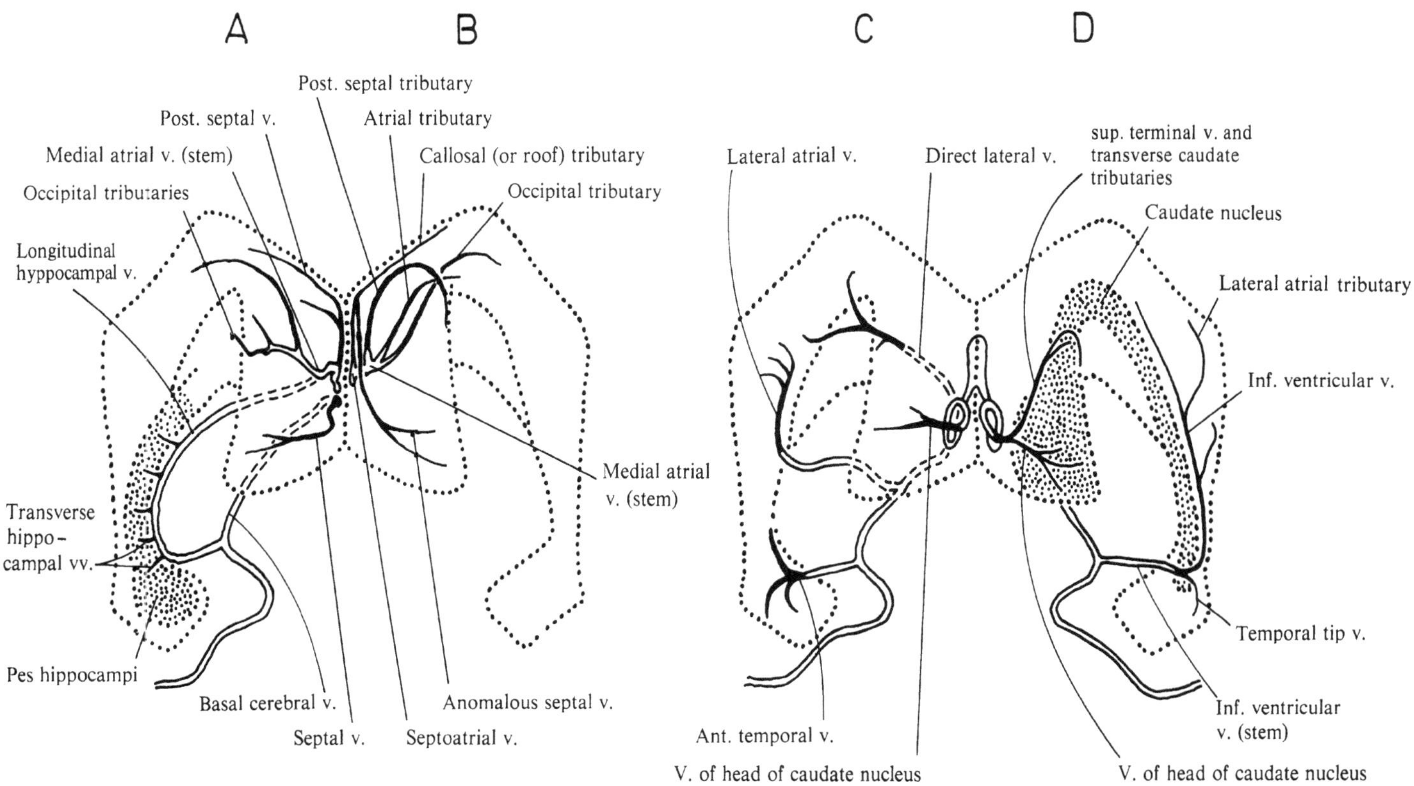

Fig. 178. Diagram showing the course of the *medial group* (A and B) and *lateral group* (C and D) of subependymal veins as they might be seen on an anteroposterior angiogram. Corresponding lateral views are shown in Fig. 177. The intraventricular segments of the subependymal veins are shown with solid lines and the extraventricular segments with empty lines

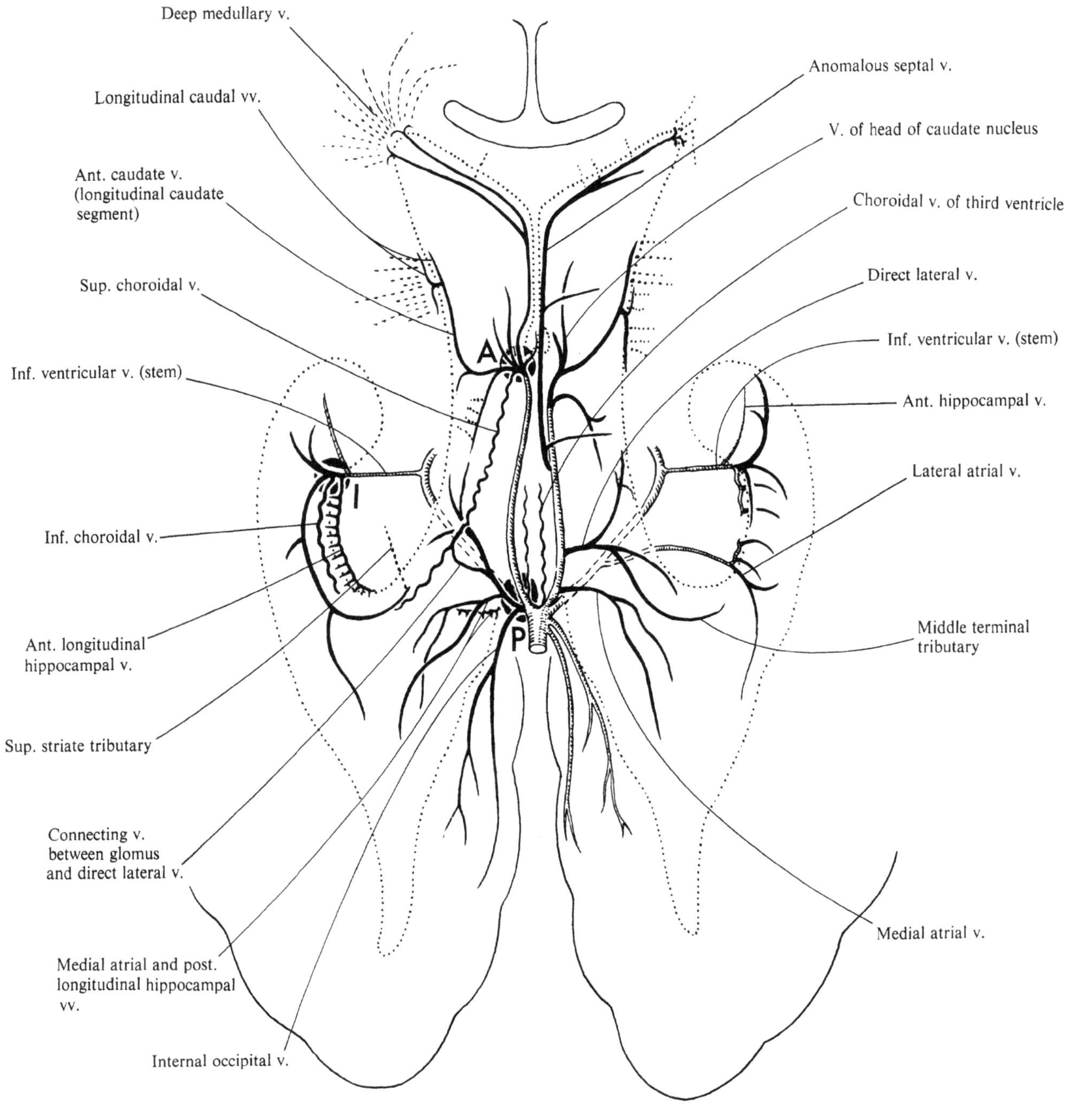

Fig. 179. Diagrammatic representation of the subependymal veins of the lateral ventricle, showing the three major sites of confluence of veins. Anteriorly (A), the septal vein, thalamostriate vein, anterior thalamic vein and superior choroidal vein converge towards the interventricular foramen and join the anterior end of the internal cerebral vein. Posteriorly (P), the direct lateral vein, medial atrial vein, posterior longitudinal hippocampal vein, a connecting vein from the glomus and sometimes the internal occipital vein, unite medially to the atrium and then join the posterior part of the internal cerebral, basal cerebral or great cerebral vein. Inferiorly (I), the inferior ventricular vein, inferior choroidal vein, anterior longitudinal hippocampal vein and anterior hippocampal vein join to form a single trunk, in the region medial to the inferior end of the choroid fissure. Not infrequently, the uncal cortical vein opens into the stem of the inferior ventricular vein

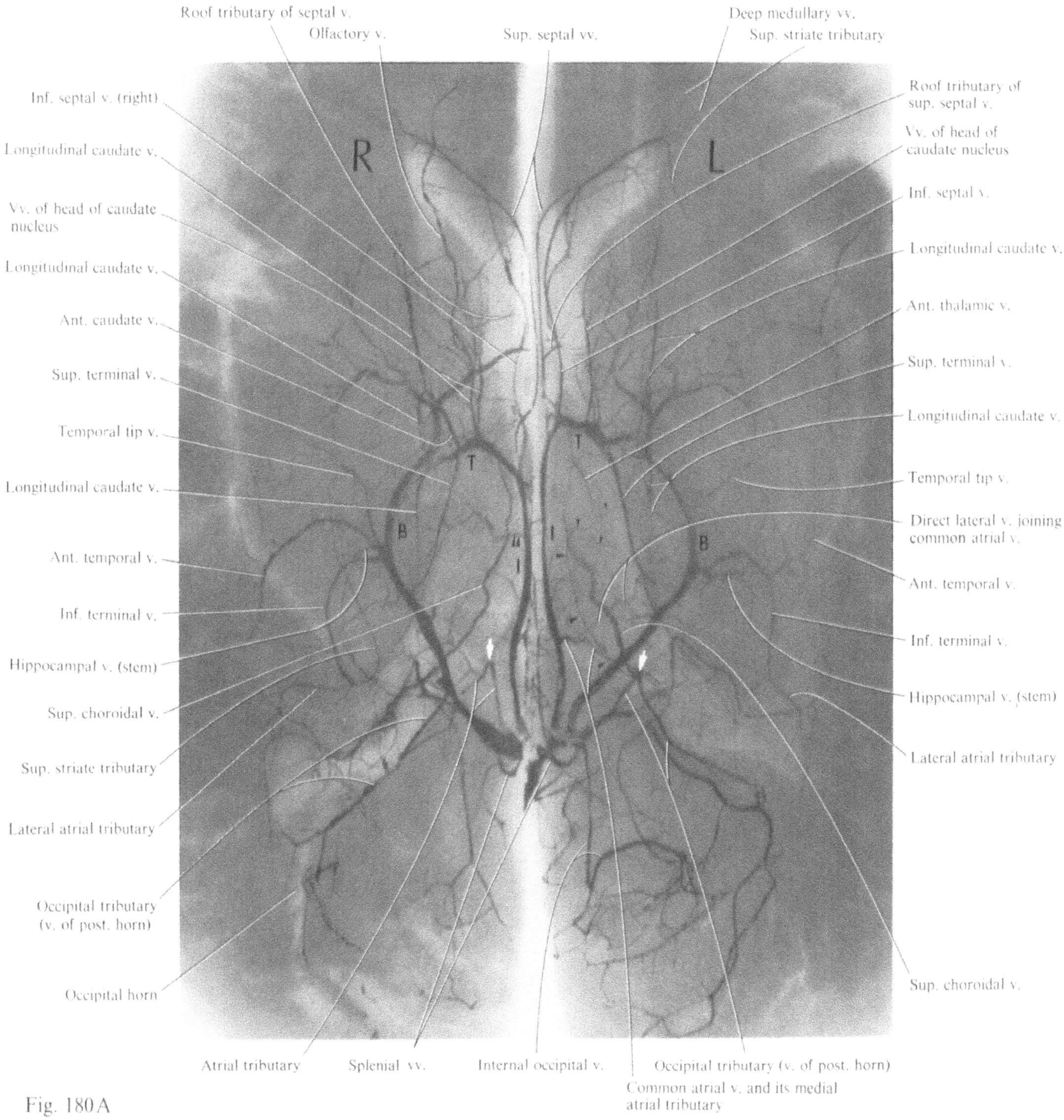

Fig. 180A

▷

Fig. 180. Radiographs of an injected specimen showing the course of the subependymal veins in the submentovertical (Fig. 180A), Towne (Fig. 180B) and lateral (Fig. 180C and D, right and left hemispheres are labelled R and L) views

There are two septal veins on each side—one running higher than the other. On the right, the superior septal vein is larger than the inferior one, whereas on the left the superior one is the smaller. The superior septal vein begins at the anterolateral and superior corner of the frontal horn and runs posteriorly along the midportion of the septum pellucidum. The inferior septal vein begins at the anterolateral and inferior corner of the frontal horn and runs posteriorly in contact with the more lateral

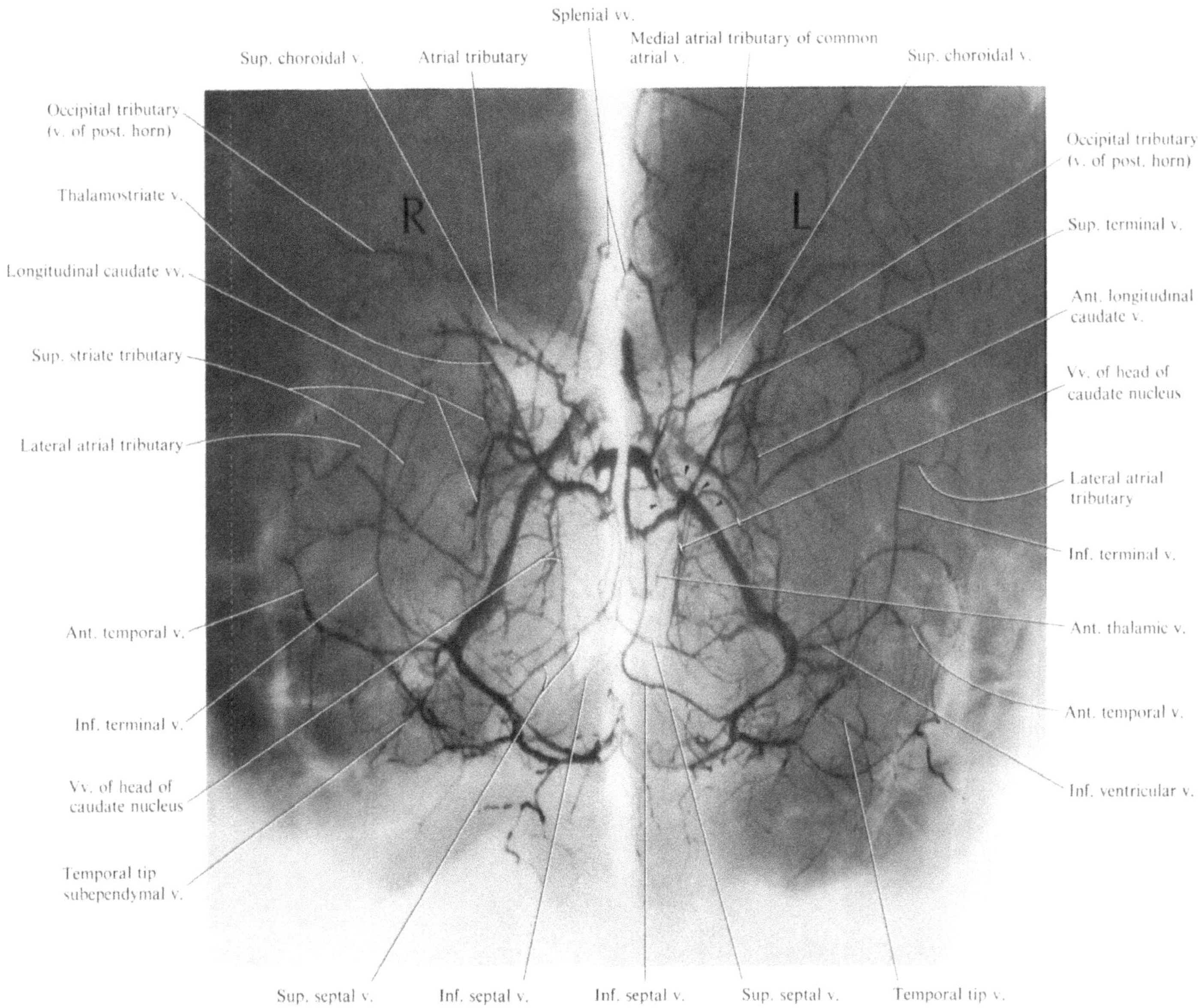

Fig. 180B

Fig. 180 (continued)

portion of the genu and rostrum of the corpus callosum. Therefore, the inferior septal veins are, as seen in this specimen, located more laterally than the superior ones (Fig. 180A and B). On the left, a roof tributary opens into the posterior part of the superior septal vein. Anteriorly, together with deep medullary veins, a prominent superior striate vein (Fig. 180A–C) drains into the inferior septal vein on the same side. There are two medial atrial veins on each side—the anterior one is the smaller and runs on the medial wall of the atrium (medial atrial tributary), whereas the posterior one is the larger and begins in the occipital horn (occipital tributary or vein of the posterior horn). On the left, the medial atrial tributary drains into the posterior part of the internal cerebral vein, whereas the vein of the posterior horn opens into the posterior end of the basal cerebral vein. On the right, both the medial atrial tributary and the vein of the posterior horn join the posterior end of the basal cerebral vein. The two thalamostriate veins are slightly asymmetric: on the left, this vein joins the internal cerebral vein at the level of the interventricular foramen, whereas on the right, it opens into the internal cerebral vein a short distance behind the foramen. The veins of the head of the caudate nucleus are prominent

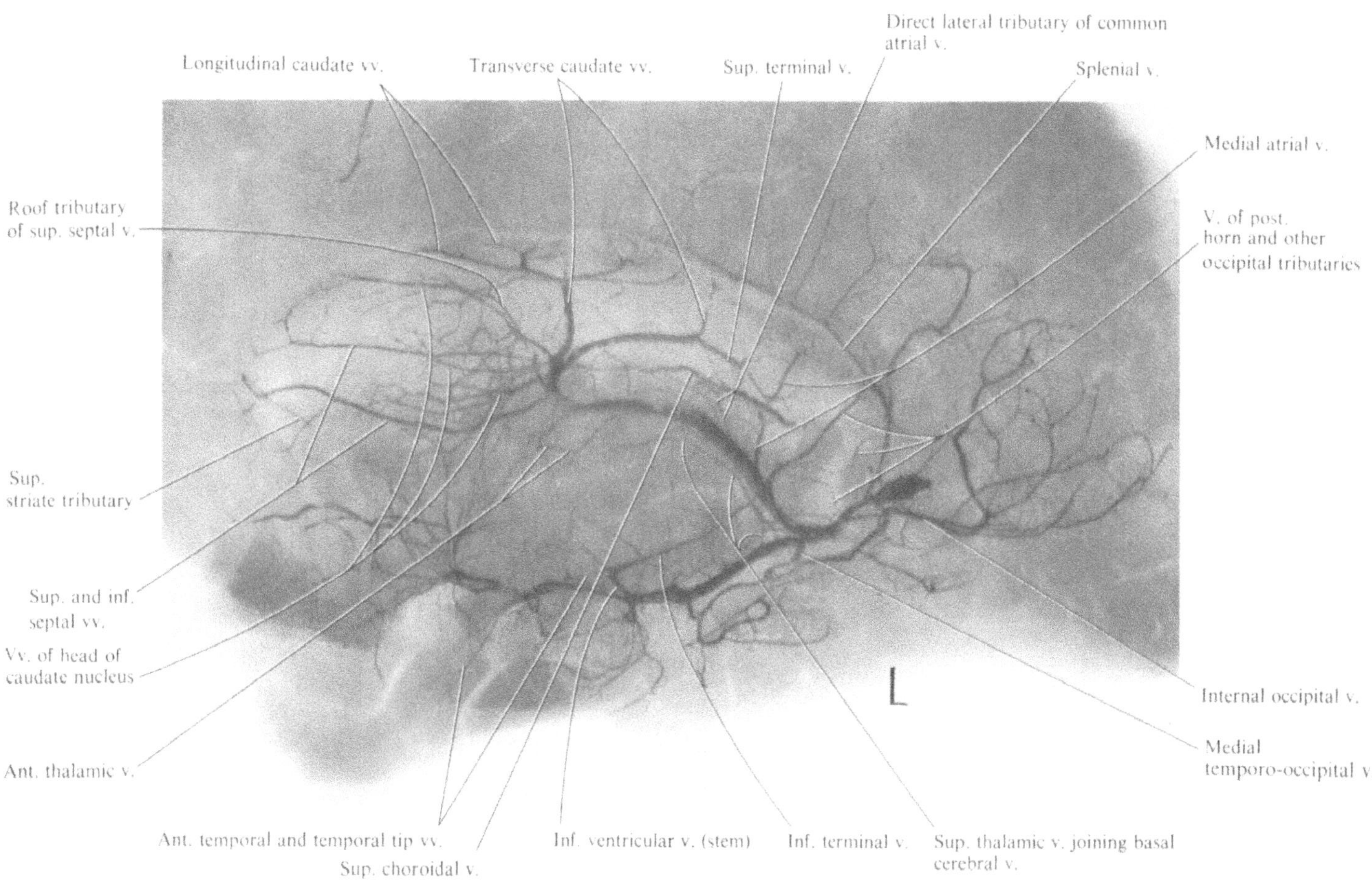

Fig. 180C

Fig. 180 (continued)

on both sides. The superior choroidal vein joins the stem of the thalamostriate vein on each side. Note the hairpin course of the vein of the posterior horn on each side (white arrows), in the submentovertical view (Fig. 180A). This is caused by the extraventricular segment of the vein, where it runs around the antero-inferior aspect of the inferior fasciculus of the splenium of the corpus callosum, behind the crus fornicis. Note the arcuate course, convex anteriorly, of the extraventricular segment of this vein, before it joins the posterior part of the internal cerebral vein (Fig. 180C and D). In the temporal horn, the inferior ventricular vein runs medially to the tail of the caudate nucleus on each side (inferior terminal vein). On the left, the inferior terminal vein receives the anterior temporal and lateral atrial tributaries. These begin, respectively, in the inferolateral corner of the temporal horn and on the lateral wall of the atrium and then pass medially, crossing the undersurface of the tail of the caudate nucleus. On the right, in the posterior part of the temporal horn and in the atrium, the inferior terminal vein receives a superior striate and a lateral atrial tributary. More anteriorly, originating from the anterolateral wall of the temporal horn, is the anterior temporal vein, which runs medially to join the basal cerebral vein independently of the inferior terminal vein.

The superior thalamic vein drains into the basal cerebral vein on the left (row of single arrowheads), whereas on the right, it drains directly into the midportion of the internal cerebral vein (double arrowhead) (Fig. 180A, B and D). The two anterior thalamic veins are also asymmetric: on the right, this vein joins the inferior septal vein (Fig. 180D), whereas on the left, it takes a recurved course to join the anterior part of the internal cerebral vein (Fig. 180C). The basal cerebral vein (B), the internal cerebral vein (I) and the thalamostriate vein (T) are labelled in Fig. 180A

Fig. 180D see p. 240 ▷

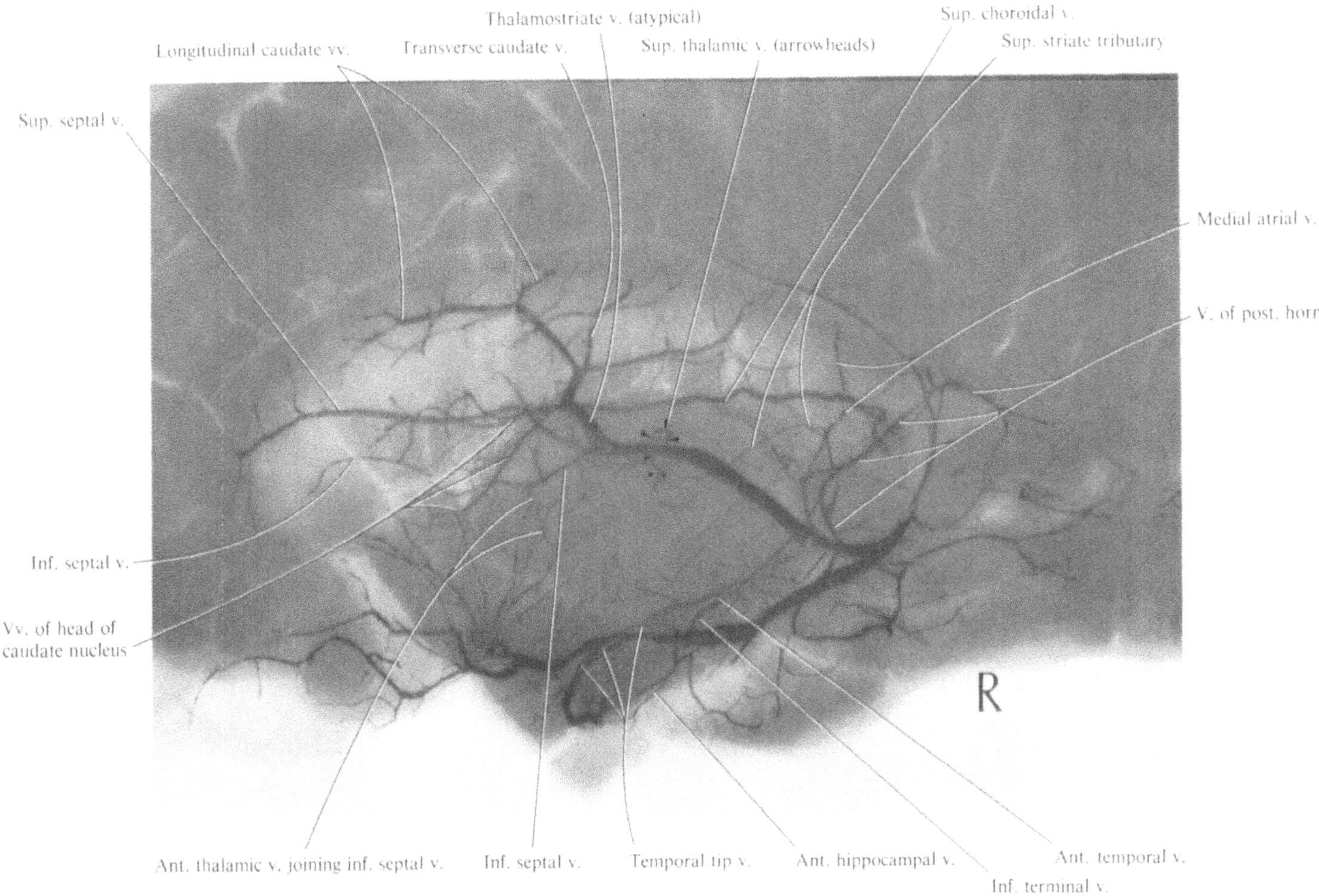

Fig. 180D

Fig. 181. Typical septal vein. Carotid angiogram, venous phase

Fig. 181A. Lateral view. The superior septal vein and its tributaries are more prominent than the inferior septal vein. The two veins unite near the interventricular foramen. The posterior septal vein (row of single white arrowheads) runs downwards to join the anterior portion of the internal cerebral vein. The thalamostriate vein (unlabelled arrow) has an unusually prominent superior terminal tributary into which several transverse caudate veins drain. More posteriorly, the posterior septal and atrial tributaries (four single black arrowheads) of the medial atrial vein converge downwards to form a venous trunk. This venous stem is later joined by a middle terminal vein (black double arrowhead) to form the common atrial vein. The anterior thalamic vein is faintly visualized (white double arrowheads)

Fig. 181B. Anteroposterior view, same case. The superior and inferior septal veins (rows of arrowheads) can be identified. The thalamostriate vein and its terminal and transverse caudate tributaries outline the lateral wall and floor of the body of the lateral ventricle, while the posterior septal vein outlines the roof and medial wall. The roof tributary of the superior septal vein is also labelled (upper-most three black arrowheads)

▷

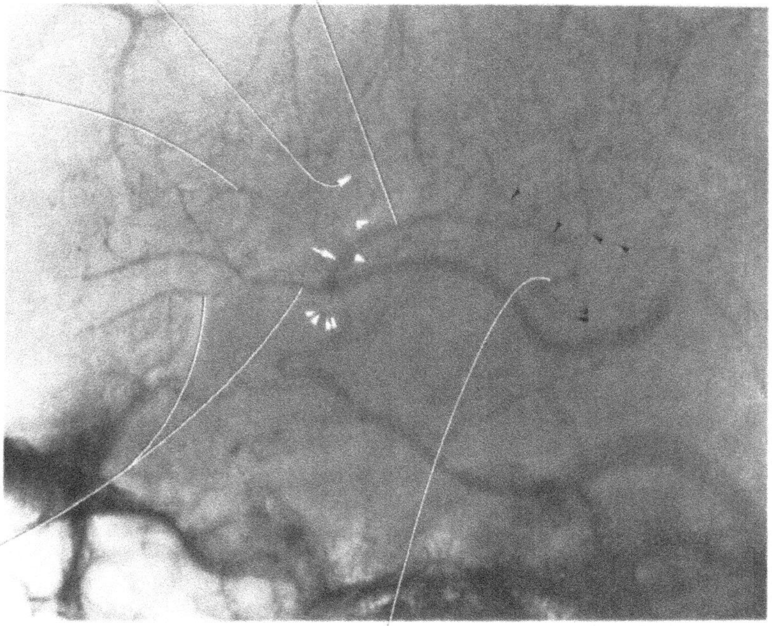

Fig. 181A

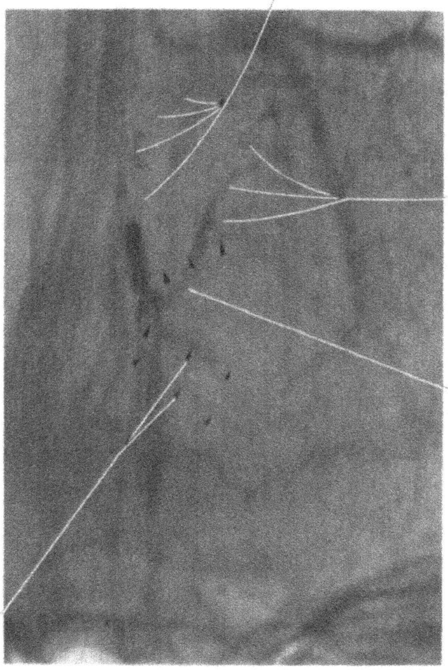

Fig. 181B

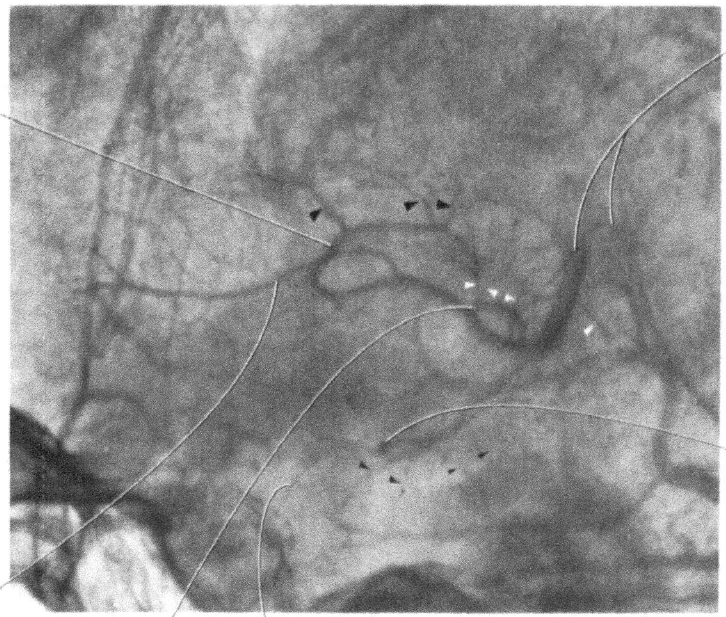

Fig. 182 A

▷

Fig. 182. Variations in the course of the septal vein. Carotid angiogram, venous phase, lateral views, 3 cases

Fig. 182 A. Anomalous septal vein. The anomalous septal vein joins the anterior portion of the internal cerebral vein some distance behind the interventricular foramen. Several transverse caudate tributaries (large black arrowheads) join the superior terminal tributary of the thalamostriate vein. More posteriorly, the vein of the posterior horn is joined by several direct lateral tributaries (white arrowheads) and form the common atrial vein. In the temporal horn, tributaries of the anterior temporal vein (small black arrowheads) including its temporal tip tributary unite to form a stem that leaves via the inferior end of the choroidal fissure

Fig. 182 B. Septo-atrial vein. The anomalous septal vein runs backwards along the upper border of the septum pellucidum, receiving roof or callosal tributaries, and joins the stem of the medial atrial vein to form the septo-atrial vein. The most posterior tributary of the medial atrial vein, which may be called either the occipital tributary or the vein of the posterior horn, can be identified

Fig. 182 C. Septal vein running below the internal cerebral vein. The septal vein runs backwards below the internal cerebral vein, in the cistern of the velum interpositum and joins the midportion of this vein. The prominent superior terminal vein begins in the lateral wall of the atrium (white arrowheads) and receives several transverse caudate tributaries (black arrowheads). Note the typical vein of the posterior horn. Numerous fine deep medullary veins (M), joining the longitudinal caudate veins along the lateral angle of the lateral ventricle, can be identified. Note also several longitudinal caudate veins above the head of the caudate nucleus

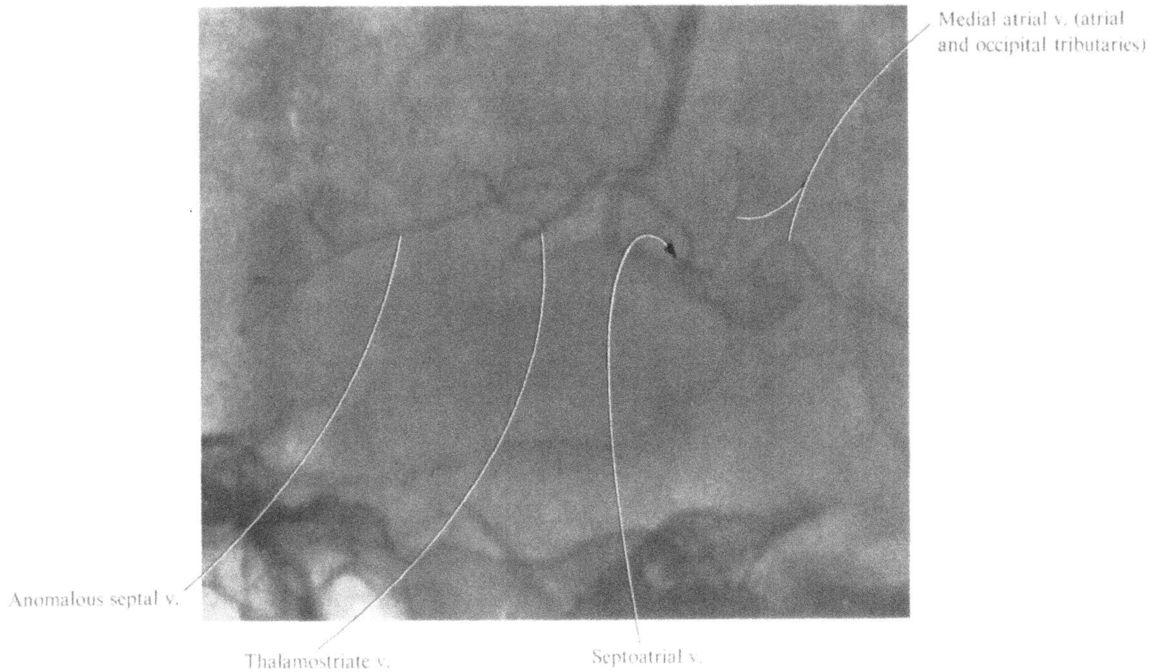

Fig. 182B

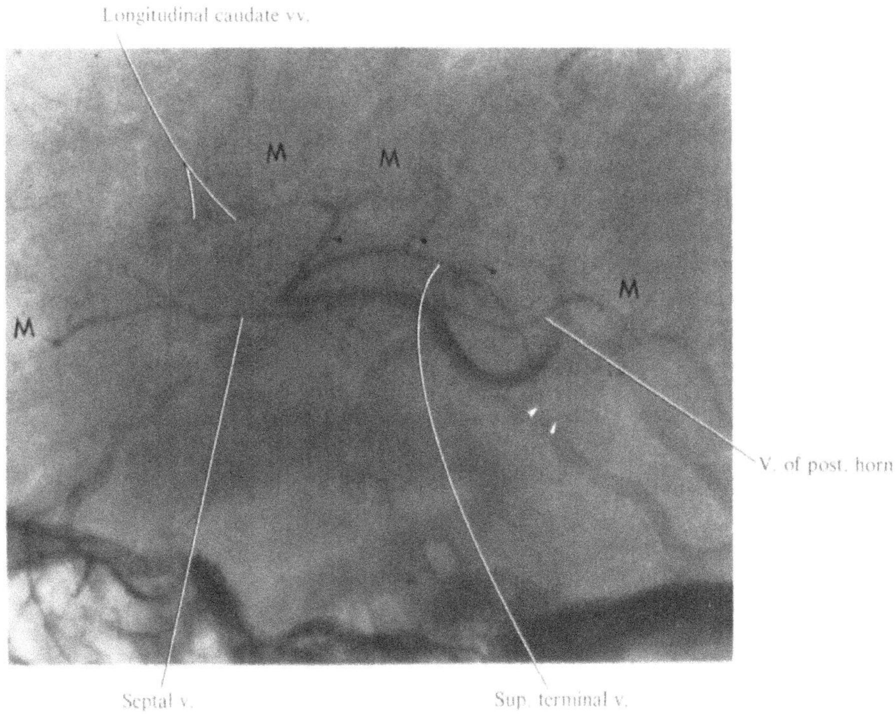

Fig. 182C

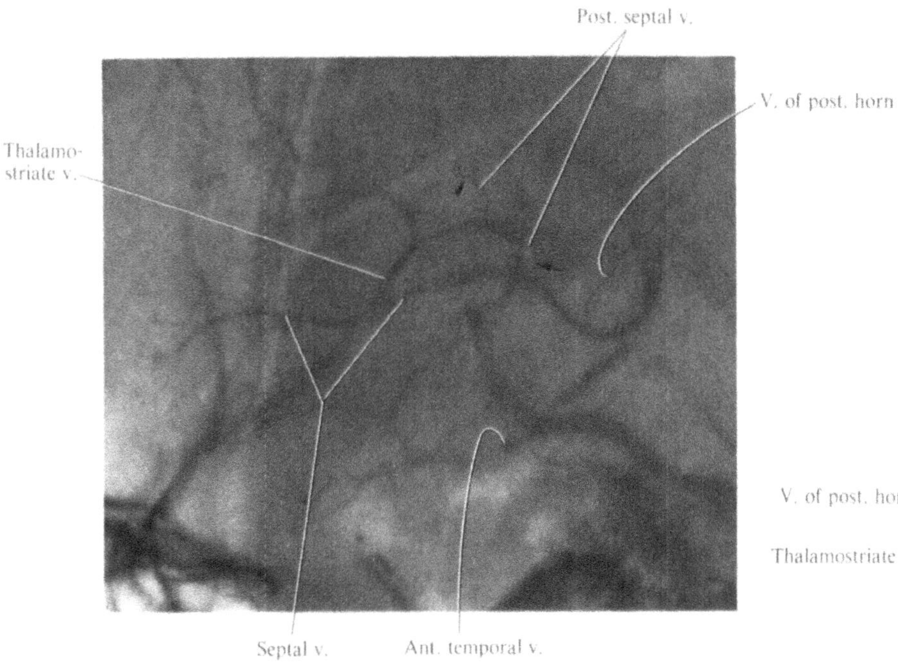

Fig. 183A

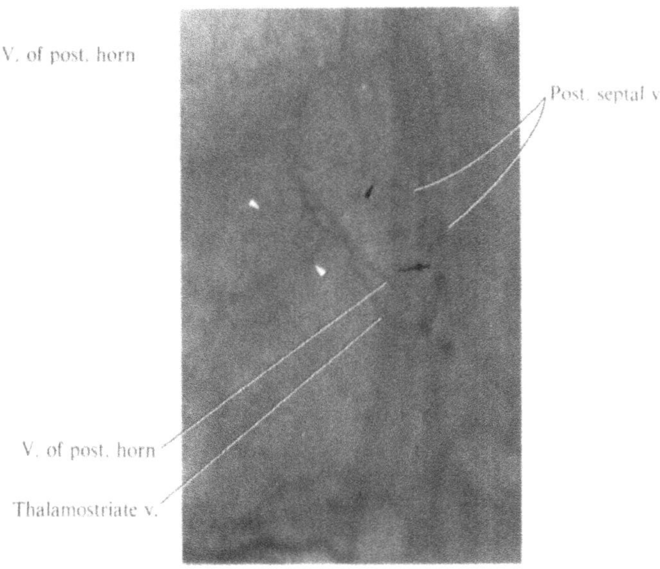

Fig. 183B

Fig. 183. Posterior septal vein. Carotid angiogram, venous phase

Fig. 183A. Lateral view. The posterior septal vein takes an undulating course, running posteromedially on the undersurface of the corpus callosum (arrowhead), on the septum pellucidum, parallel to and above the column of the fornix and then between the two bodies of the fornix (arrow), before draining into the internal cerebral vein. The septal vein runs below the internal cerebral vein

Fig. 183B. Anteroposterior view, same case. Various segments of the undulating posterior septal vein show the undersurface of the corpus callosum (black arrowhead), the septum pellucidum and the medial border of the diverging posterior pillar of the fornix (arrow). External and internal superior striate veins (white arrowheads) can also be identified

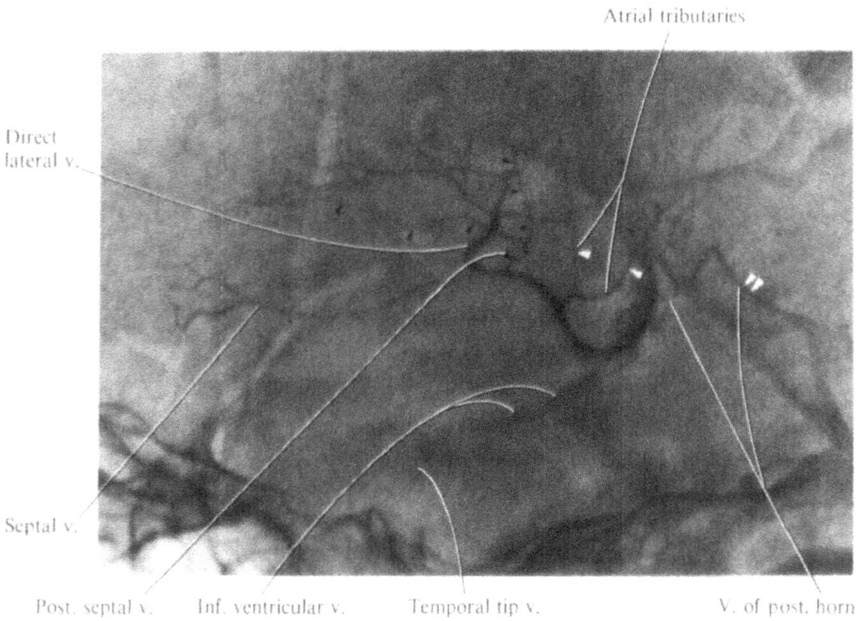

Fig. 184. Prominent posterior septal vein. Carotid angiogram, venous phase, lateral view
Tributaries of the posterior septal vein originate from the roof of the frontal horn and body of the lateral ventricle. they run posteriorly and medially on the roof and then on the septum pelludicum (black arrowheads). They unite to form a stem that passes between the two bodies of the fornix and joins the internal cerebral vein. The longitudinal caudate tributaries of the medial atrial vein (of two white single arrowheads) and the vein of the posterior horn (white double arrowhead) outline the roof of the atrium and of the occipital horn. The latter vein joins the great cerebral vein independently. The temporal tip vein marks the tip of the temporal horn

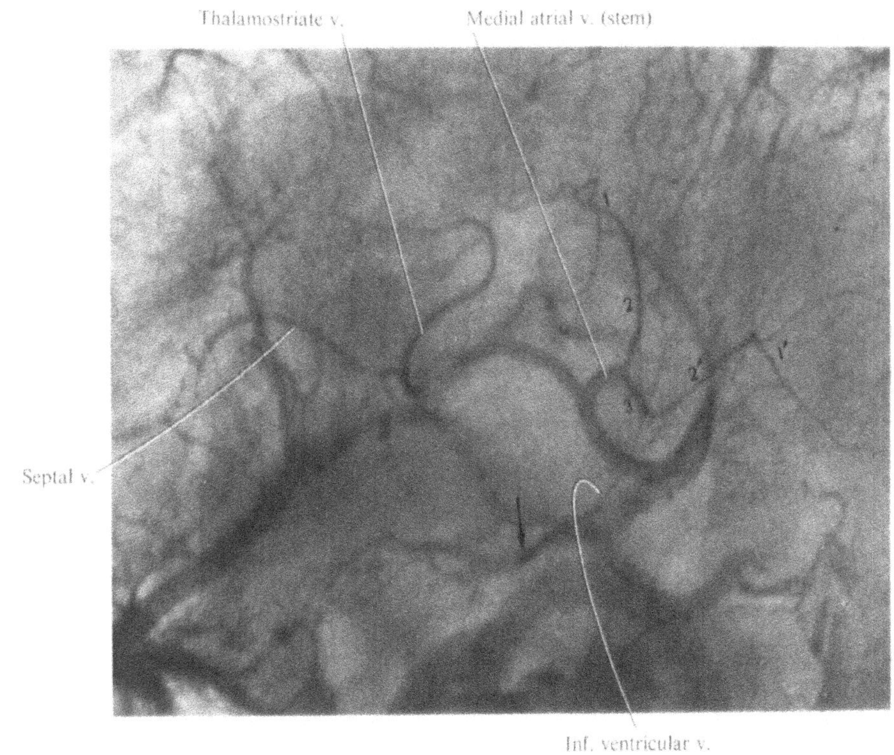

Fig. 185A

Fig. 185. Medial atrial vein. Carotid angiogram, venous phase

Fig. 185A. Lateral view. The roof (1,1′), medial atrial (2,2′) and extraventricular segments (3) of both atrial and occipital tributaries of the medial atrial vein can be identified. Note the typical angular course of the occipital tributary (vein of the posterior horn) and the typically curved course of the stem of the medial atrial vein. The septal vein takes an unusual sinuous course on the wall of the cavum septi pellucidi (see Fig. 185B) and joins the internal cerebral vein behind the interventricular foramen. The thalamostriate vein is typical and begins as the anterior caudate vein. The inferior ventricular vein joins the basal cerebral vein at the inferior choroidal point (arrow)

Fig. 185B. Anteroposterior view, same case. The roof (1,1′), medial atrial (2,2′), and extraventricular segments (3) of both atrial and occipital tributaries of the medial atrial vein, seen in Fig. 185A, can be identified. The unusual zigzag course of the septal vein is due to the large cavum septi pellucidi. The junction between the basal cerebral vein and inferior ventricular vein marks the level of the inferior end of the choroids fissure (arrow)

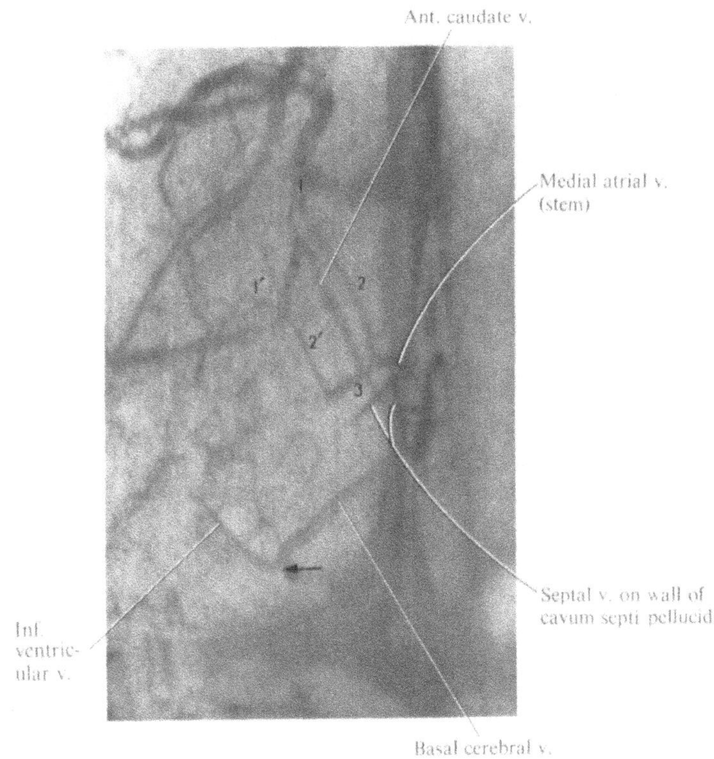

Fig. 185B

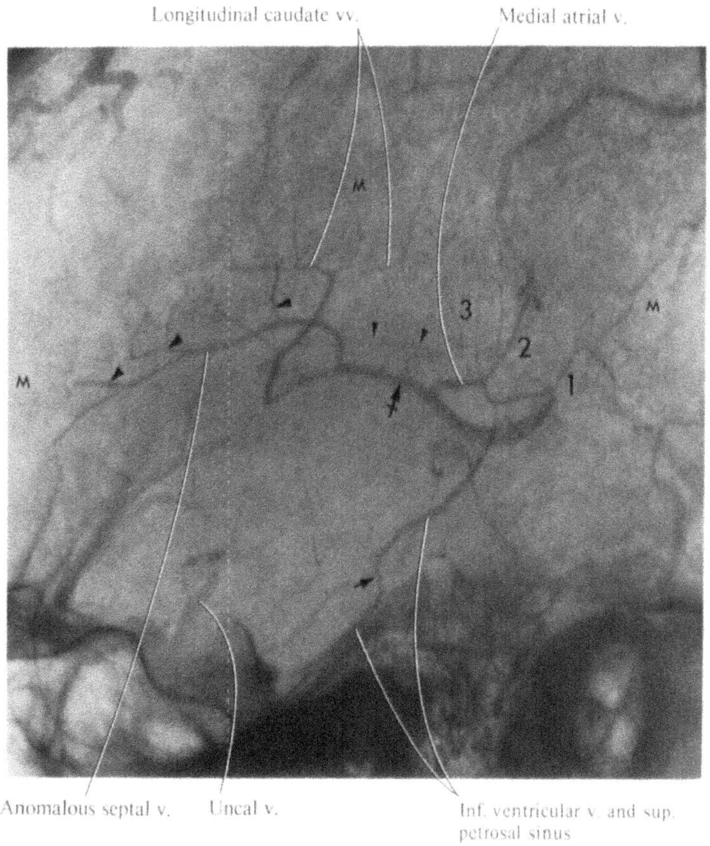

Fig. 186A

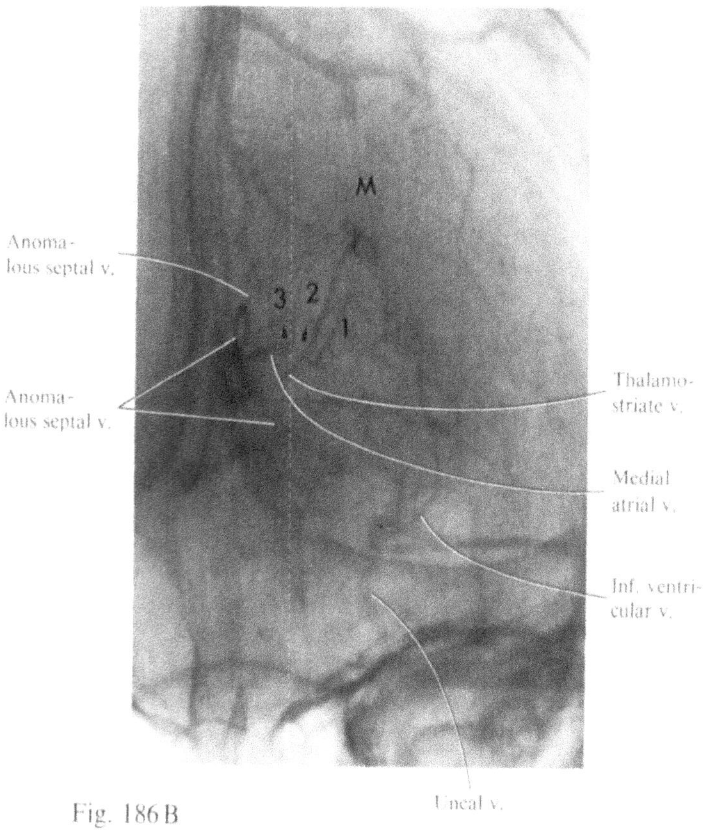

Fig. 186B

Fig. 186. Medial atrial vein. Carotid angiogram, venous phase

Fig. 186A. Lateral view. The occipital (1), atrial (2) and the posterior septal tributaries (3) of the medial atrial vein can be identified. The inferior ventricular vein is anomalous and drains into the lateral mesencephalic vein (arrow) which joins the superior petrosal sinus. Numerous deep medullary veins (M) join the longitudinal caudate veins. The anomalous septal vein begins in the usual location but runs unusually high on the medial wall of the frontal horn. Its roof tributaries are labelled (large arrowheads). A prominent connecting vein, bridging between the superior choroidal vein (small arrowheads) and the midportion of the internal cerebral vein (⇞), can be identified

Fig. 186B. Anteroposterior view, same case. The medial atrial vein and its tributaries (1, 2, 3), seen in Fig. 186A, can be identified. The anomalous septal vein, in the frontal horn, shows a long straight course as it runs unusually high to reach the upper border of the septum pellucidum. Because of its high position, the callosal segment of this vein is long. The choroidal blush (arrowheads), within the body of the lateral ventricle, is faintly seen. Deep medullary veins are labelled (M)

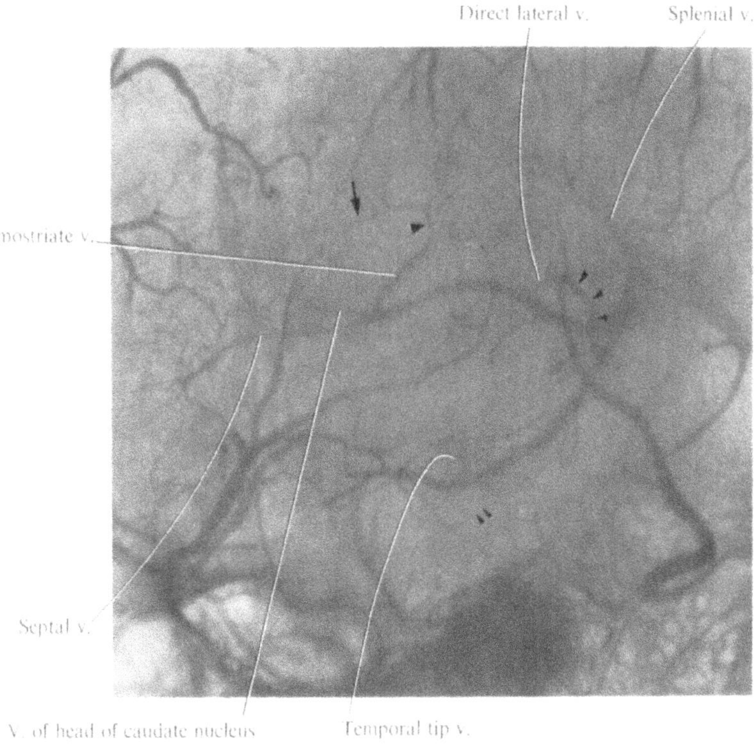

Fig. 187A

Fig. 187. Thalamostriate vein (an absent superior terminal vein). Carotid angiogram, venous phase

Fig. 187A. Lateral view. The the anterior caudate vein begins as a longitudinal caudate vein. It runs posteriorly, above the caudate nucleus (arrow), then transversely downwards (single arrowhead) over the caudate nucleus to open into the thalamostriate vein. The absence of the superior terminal vein is not unusual. A middle terminal vein (three arrowheads) joins the direct lateral vein. The anterior hippocampal vein (double arrowhead) outlines the lower border of the recurved uncus

Fig. 187B. Anteroposterior view, same case. The longitudinal caudate segment (arrow) of the anterior caudate vein marks the lateral angle of the frontal horn, whereas the septal vein marks the medial and anterior walls of the frontal horn. The direct lateral vein receives a middle terminal vein (three arrowheads). A choroidal blush (⍏) within the body of the lateral ventricle is noted. The medial angle of the frontal horn is indicated by the junction between the callosal and septal segments of the septal vein (septal point of Zimmer)

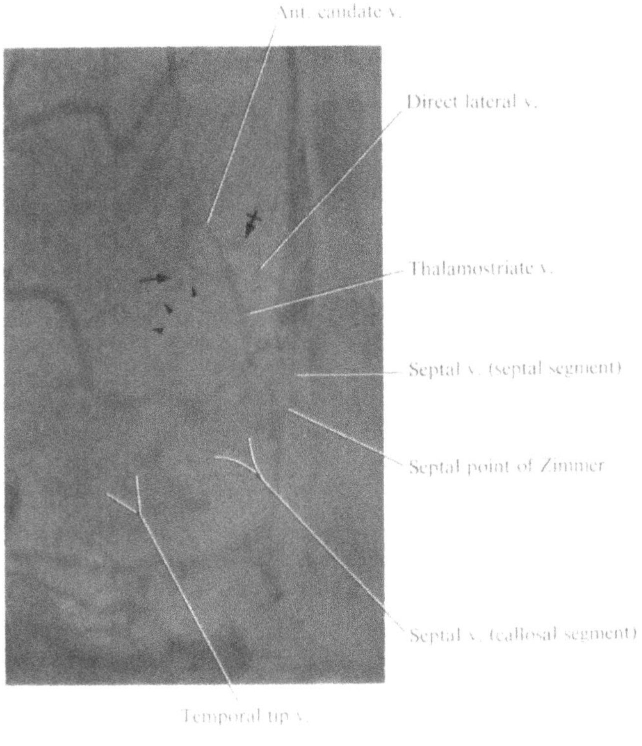

Fig. 187B

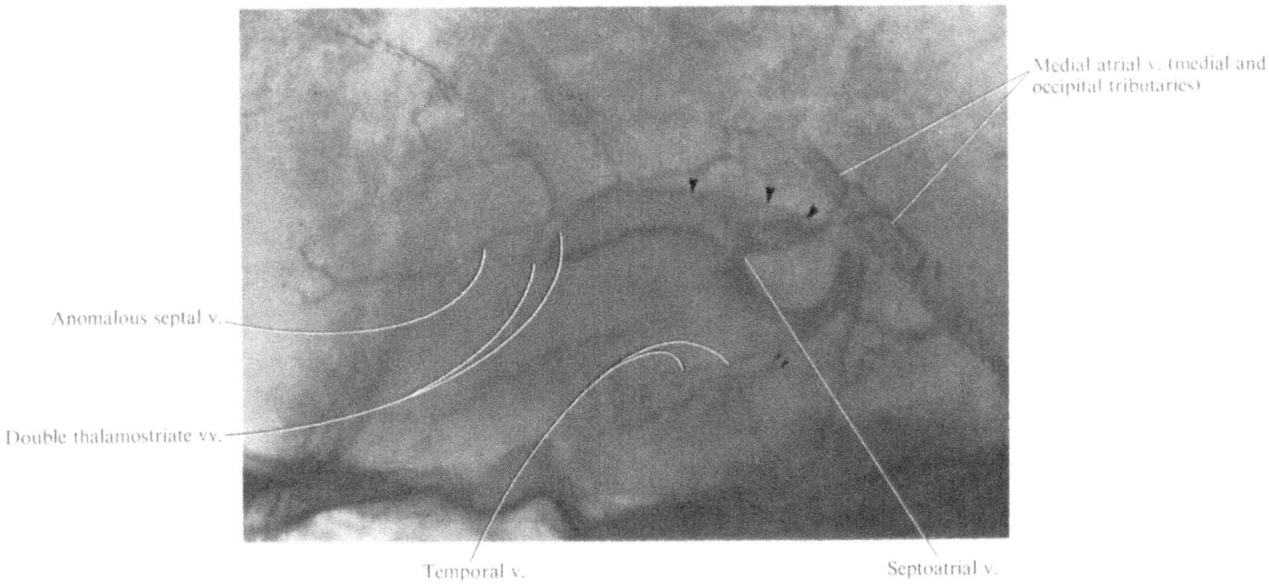

Fig. 188 A

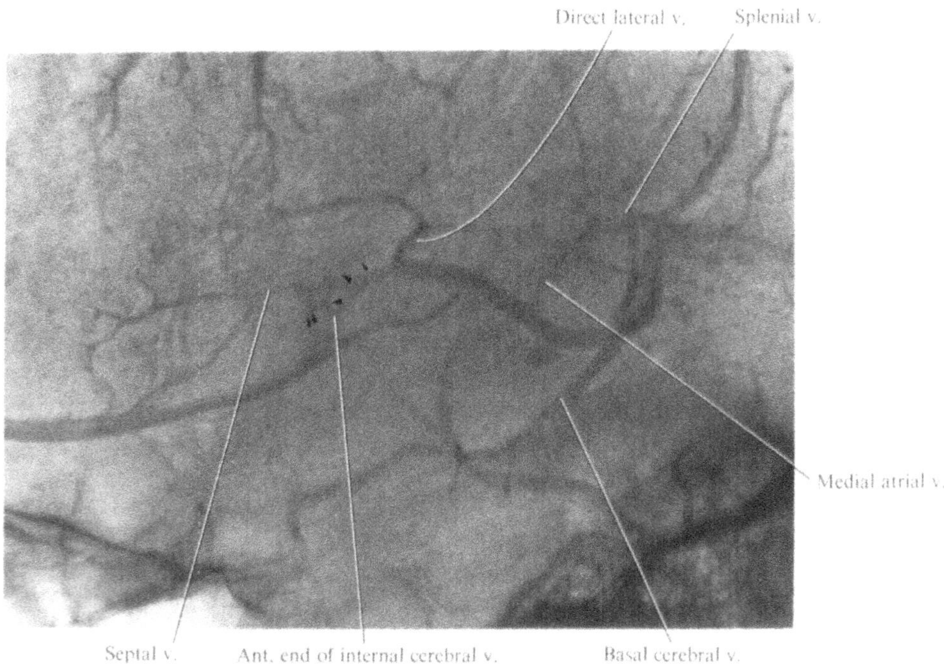

Fig. 188 B

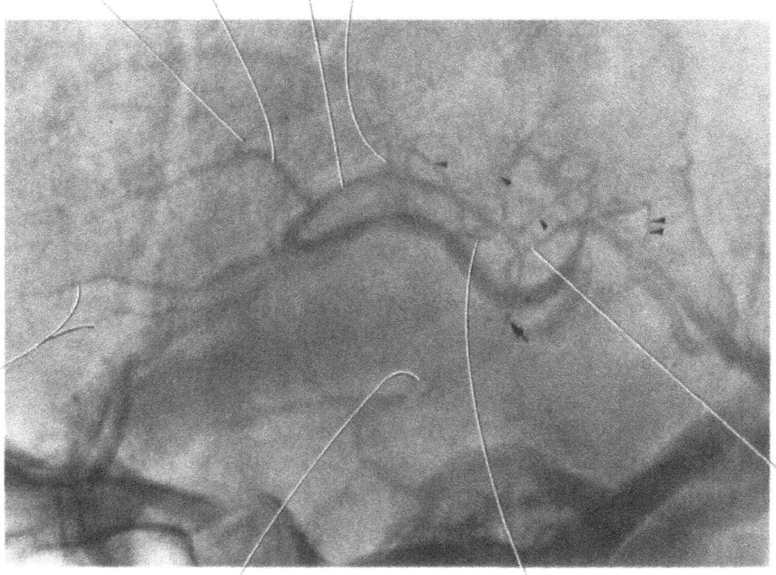

Fig. 188C

Fig. 188. Variations of the thalamostriate vein. Carotid angiogram, venous phase, lateral view, 3 cases

Fig. 188A. Double thalamostriate veins. Two thalamostriate veins make it difficult to determine the location of the interventricular foramen. The anterior one receives the anterior caudate vein; the posterior one receives the transverse caudate veins. The septo-atrial vein receives the anomalous septal vein and the stem of the medial atrial vein. The choroid plexus (large arrowheads) is clearly seen and appears to drain into the septo-atrial vein. The posterior temporal vein, originating from the lateral part of the posterior temporal horn (douple arrowhead), runs medially and anteriorly, on the roof of the temporal horn, to leave at the inferior choroidal point

Fig. 188B. The direct lateral vein simulates the displaced thalamostriate vein. It receives a large longitudinal caudate vein and replaces the usual anterior caudate vein. The anterior end of the internal cerebral vein is indicated by the poorly filled small thalamostriate vein (row of single arrowheads) and by the vein of the head of the caudate nucleus (double arrowheads)

Fig. 188C. Prominent terminal tributary of the thalamostriate vein. The middle terminal vein (arrow) continues into the superior terminal vein along the stria terminalis. One posterior septal and two atrial tributaries (three arrowheads) form the stem of the medial atrial vein. The vein of the posterior horn drains into the posterior end of the internal cerebral vein independently. Note the origin of this vein on the lateral wall of the posterior horn (double arrowheads). The superior and inferior septal veins join the internal cerebral vein respectively at and behind the interventricular foramen

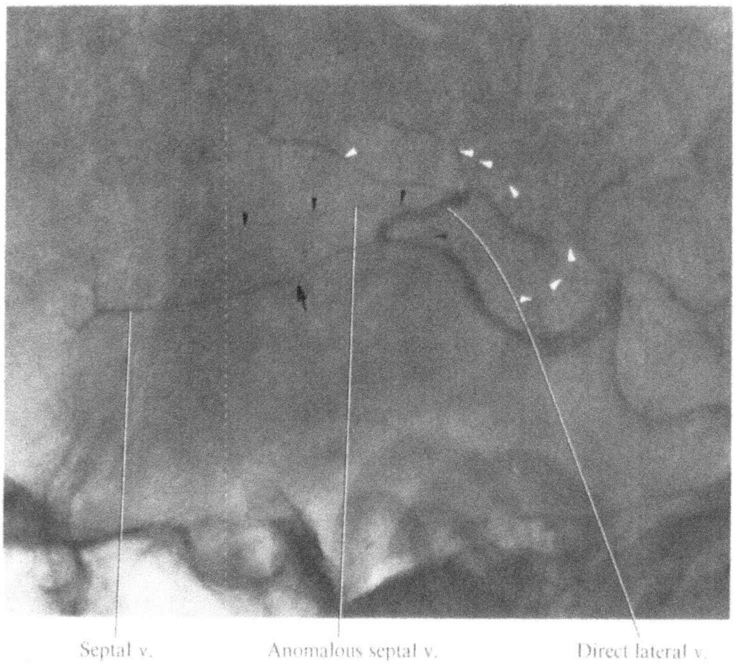

Fig. 189 A

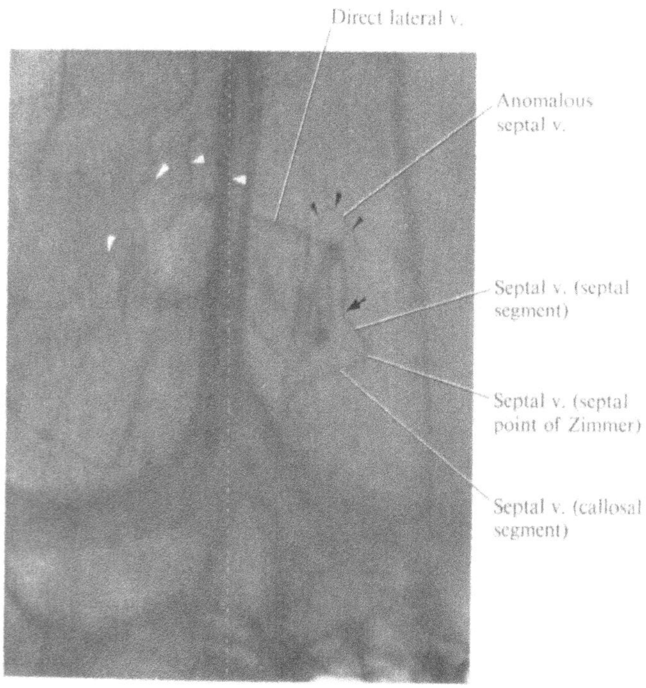

Fig. 189 B

Fig. 189. Prominent direct lateral vein. Carotid angiogram, venous phase

Fig. 189 A. Lateral view. Since the thalamostriate vein is absent, the direct lateral vein is reciprocally prominent and receives tributaries from the lateral wall of the frontal horn, body, atrium and occipital horn of the lateral ventricle (white arrowheads). Two septal veins are seen: one is anomalous (black arrowheads) and joins the midportion of the internal cerebral vein; the other opens into its anterior end at the interventricular foramen (superior choroidal point). This point can be identified by a local dip in the course from septal vein to internal cerebral vein (arrow), their being no thalamostriate vein to show it more clearly

Fig. 189 B. Slightly oblique anteroposterior view, same case. The stem of the prominent direct lateral vein marks the superior border of the thalamus. It receives tributaries from the body, atrium and temporal horn of the lateral ventricle (white arrowheads). The anomalous septal (black arrowheads) and septal veins mark the medial and anterior walls of the frontal horn. The junction (arrow) between the internal cerebral vein and its septal tributaries is indicated by a lateral bulge in the course of the septal vein around the column of the fornix (columnar segment)

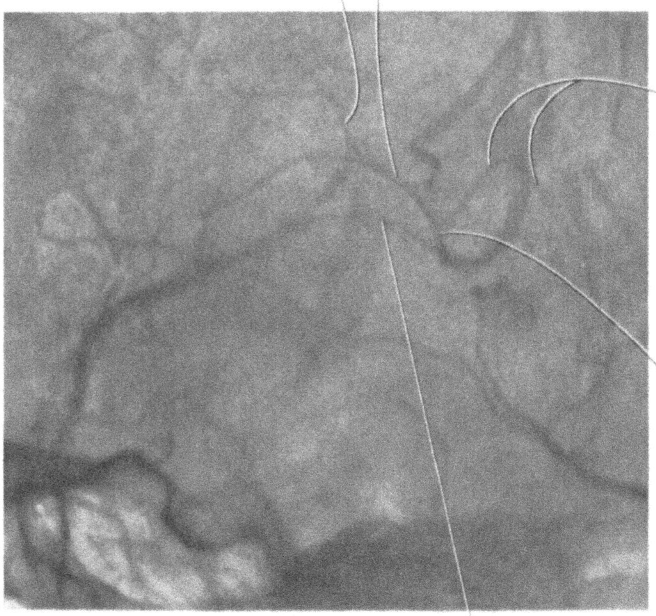

Fig. 190 A

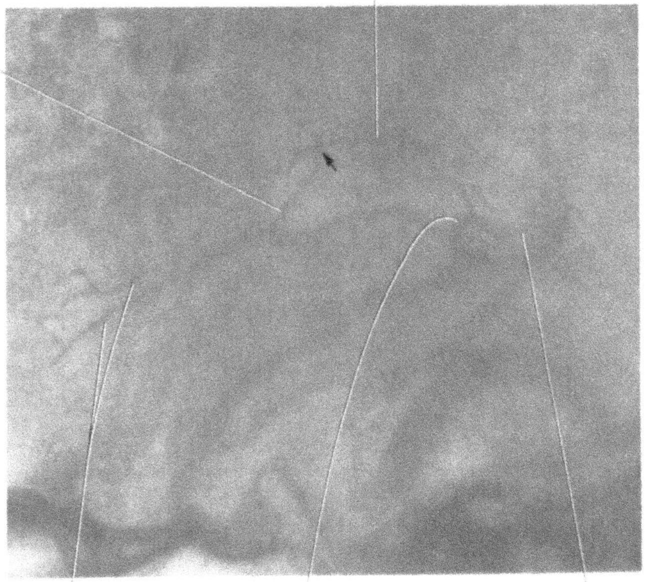

Fig. 190 B

Fig. 190. Variations of the direct lateral vein — retrothalamic direct lateral vein. Carotid angiogram, venous phase, lateral view, 2 cases

Fig. 190 A. The superior terminal vein continues backwards as the middle terminal vein and, turns medially to course behind the thalamus, and joins the posterior part of the internal cerebral vein together with the vein of the posterior horn (common atrial vein). The internal cerebral vein is unusually small

Fig. 190 B. The direct lateral vein is anomalous. It begins in the lateral angle of the anterior part of the body of the lateral ventricle and runs backwards and downwards on the lateral wall. It turns medially on the posterosuperior aspect of the thalamus and is joined by the vein of the posterior horn to form the common atrial vein. This vein then joins the posterior part of the internal cerebral vein. Note the apparent crossing (arrow) of the longitudinal caudate tributaries of the direct lateral and anterior caudate veins. (In the stereoscopic views, the longitudinal caudate tributaries of the direct lateral vein are slightly deeper within the parenchyma in both the anteroposterior and lateral views)

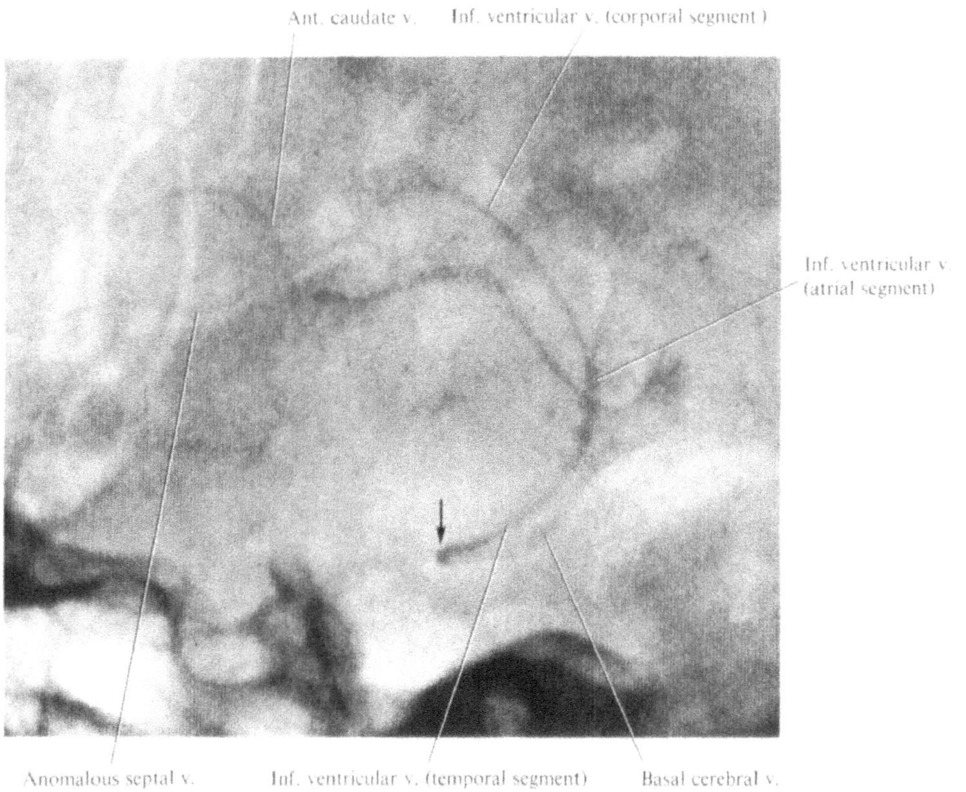

Fig. 191 A

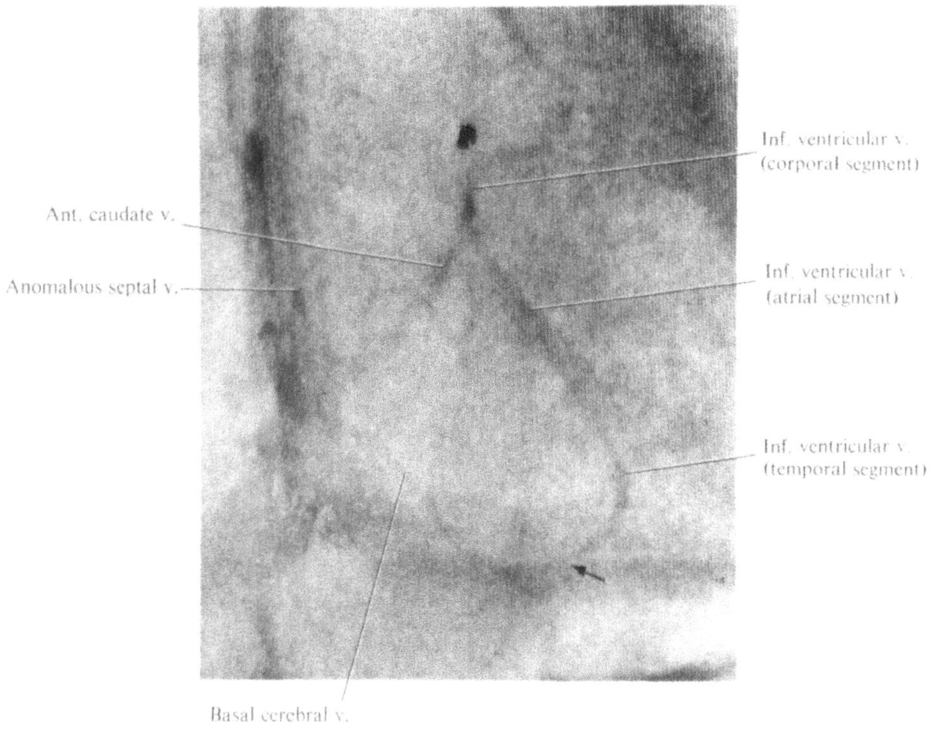

Fig. 191 B

Fig. 191. Prominent inferior ventricular vein. Carotid angiogram, venous phase, lateral (Fig. 191 A) and anteroposterior views (Fig. 191 B). The inferior ventricular vein begins in the body of the lateral ventricle and runs posteriorly above the caudate nucleus (corporal segment). It then runs inferolaterally on the lateral wall of the atrium (atrial segment) and then on the roof of the temporal horn, laterally to the caudate nucleus (temporal segment). Terminally, the vein turns medially, crossing the tail of the caudate nucleus, and leaves the temporal horn at the inferior end of the choroid fissure, the inferior choroidal point (arrow), to join the basal cerebral vein

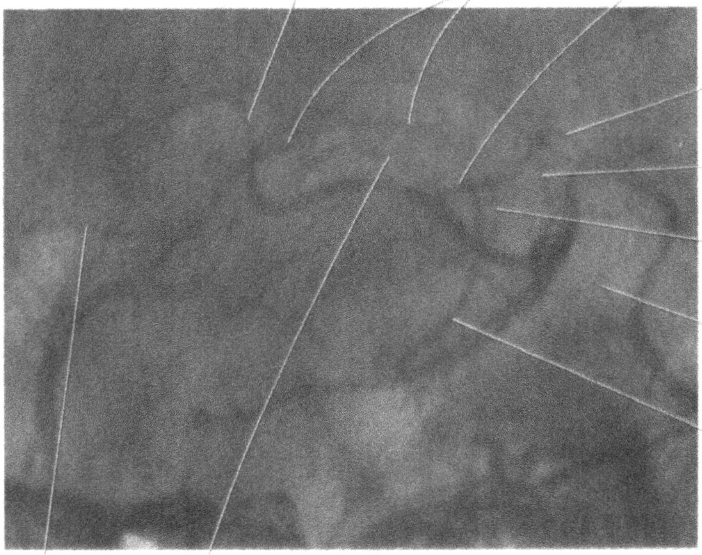

Fig. 192A

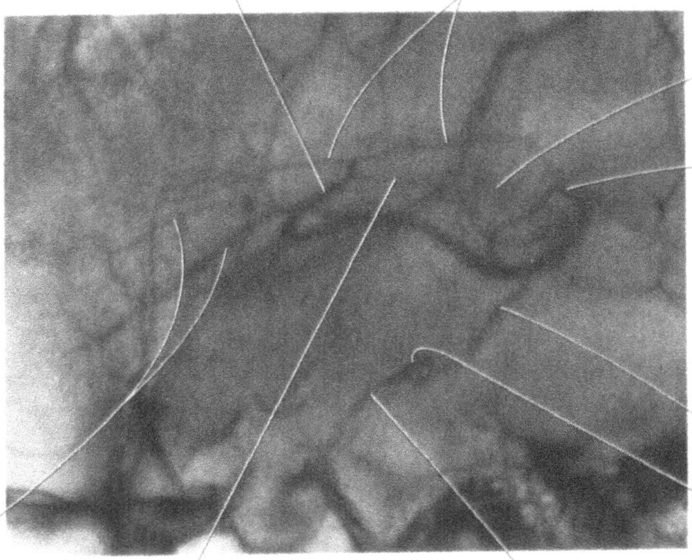

Fig. 192B

Fig. 192. Variations of the inferior ventricular vein. Cerebral angiogram, venous phase, lateral views, 6 cases

Fig. 192A. Inferior terminal vein joining the direct lateral vein. The middle and inferior terminal veins form a continuous curve and outline the course of the stria terminalis. These terminal veins connect the common atrial vein superiorly with the basal cerebral vein inferiorly. The direct lateral vein, in addition, receives the vein of the posterior horn and a small vein on the superior surface of the thalamus, to become the common atrial vein

Fig. 192B. Prominent anterior temporal vein. Major tributaries of the anterior temporal vein originate from the tip of the temporal horn (temporal tip vein). The choroid plexus in the atrium communicates with the vein of the posterior horn by fine connecting twigs

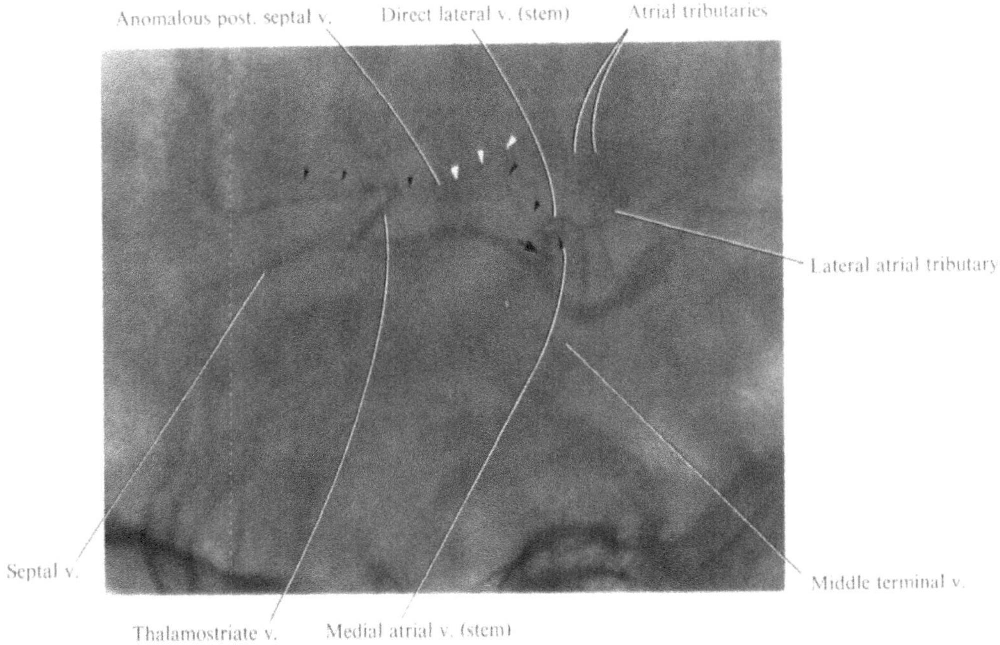

Fig. 192C. Prominent middle terminal vein. The middle terminal vein, running on the roof of the temporal horn and the anterior wall of the atrium, drains backwards and upwards (instead of downwards and forwards). It receives a lateral atrial and an anomalous posterior septal vein to form a short venous stem. This stem opens into the common atrial vein (arrow) with the medial atrial vein. The course of the posterior septal vein is unusual. It runs posteriorly on the upper part of the septum pellucidum (three black arrowheads) and then posterosuperiorly and laterally on the undersurface of the corpus callosum (white arrowheads). It then passes posteroinferiorly, on the lateral wall of the body of the lateral ventricle (two black arrowheads), before draining into the stem of the direct lateral tributary of the common atrial vein. Note the angular course of the posterior septal vein at the supero-lateral corner of the lateral ventricle

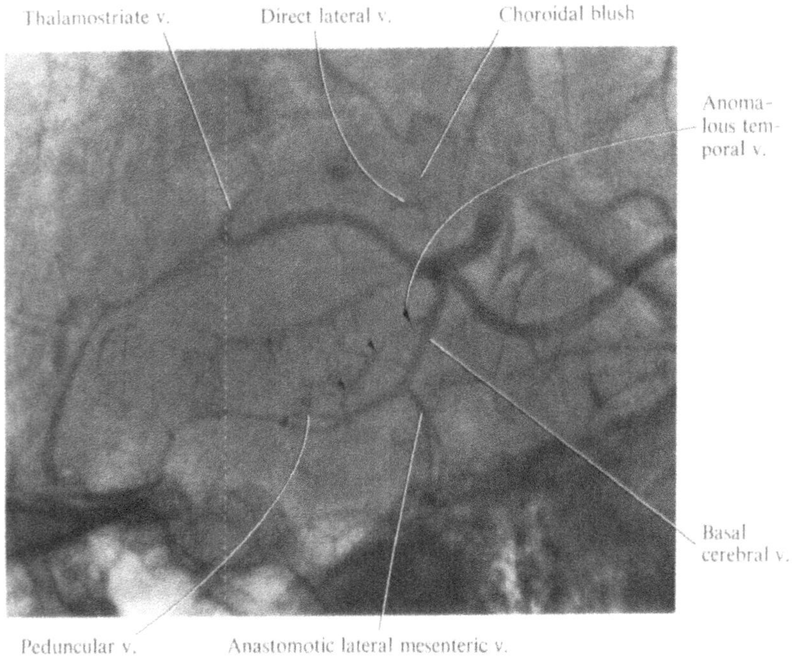

Fig. 192D. Anomalous temporal vein. A prominent temporal subependymal vein, originating from the anterior part of the temporal horn, runs posteriorly and then medially on its roof (arrowheads). In the posterior part of the temporal horn the vein emerges from the ventricle and then joins the posterior part of the basal cerebral vein. Fine connecting veins are seen joining the choroidal blush and the direct lateral vein

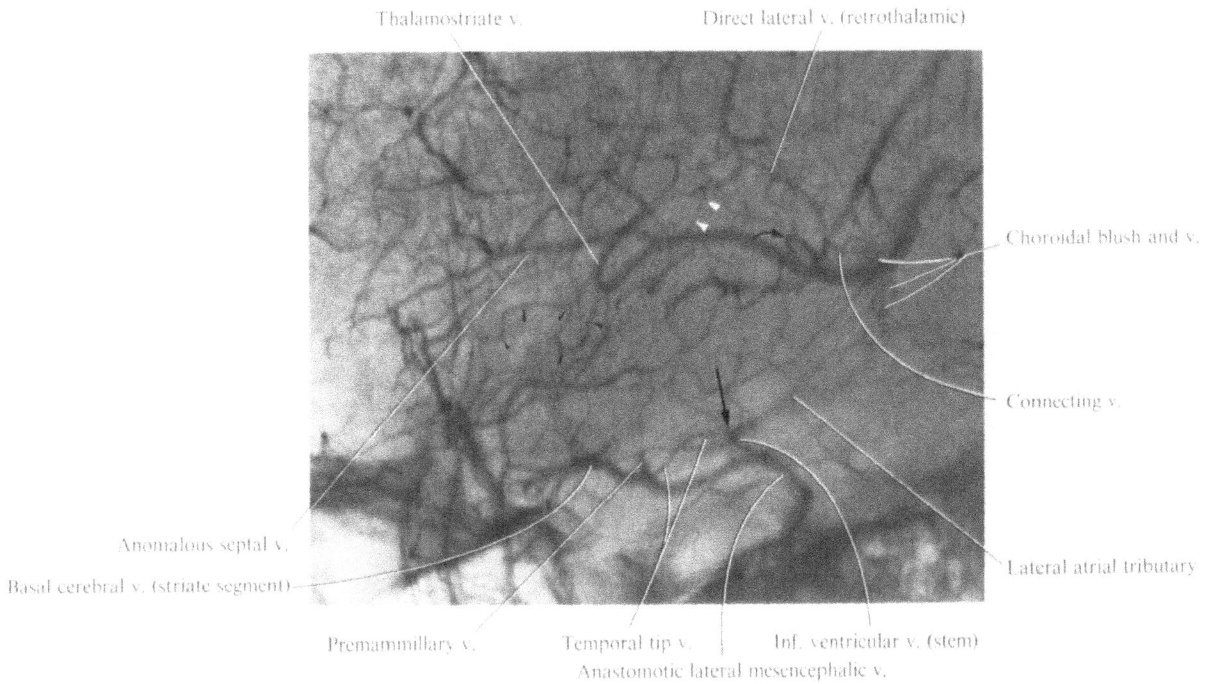

Fig. 192E. Inferior ventricular vein draining into the anastomotic lateral mesencephalic vein. The inferior ventricular vein has two tributaries: the lateral atrial tributary, originating from the lateral wall of the atrium and the temporal tip tributary, outlining the tip of the temporal horn. They unite and emerge at the inferior choroidal point (arrow) to join the anastomotic lateral mesencephalic vein. Note the unusually tortuous vein of the head of the caudate nucleus (row of arrowheads). The stem of the direct lateral vein (curved arrow) receives a tributary from the lateral wall of the body and atrium of the lateral ventricle, and also a connecting vein from the choroid plexus in the atrium. Prominent internal superior striate veins are also seen (white arrowheads)

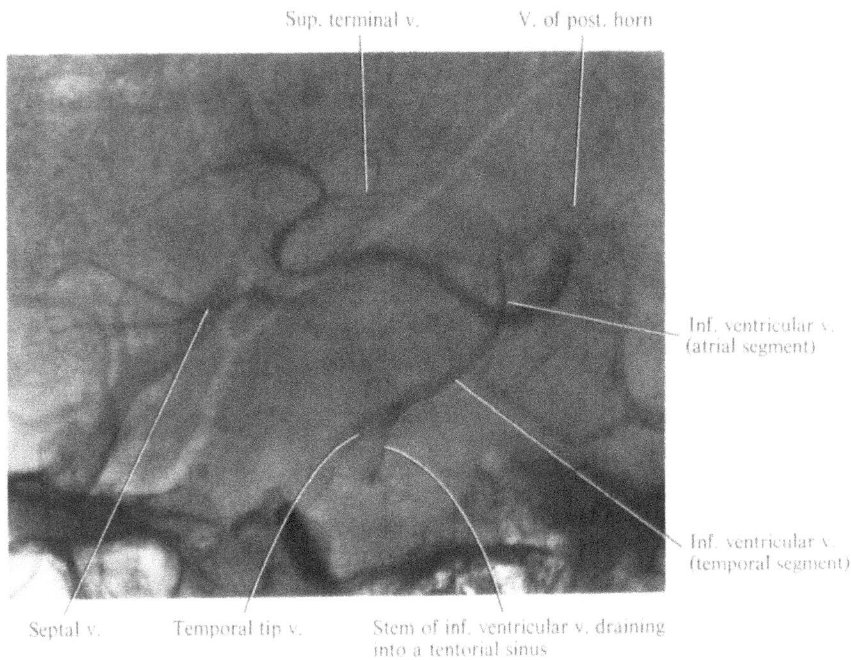

Fig. 192F. Inferior ventricular vein draining into a tentorial sinus. The inferior ventricular and temporal tip subependymal veins unite to form the stem of the inferior ventricular vein. It then runs forwards and downwards to open into a dural sinus within the tentorium. The tentorial sinus itself is not well opacified

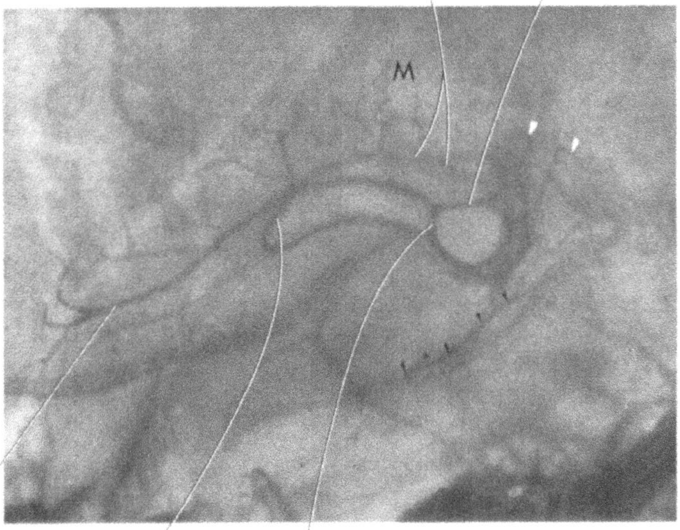

Fig. 193A

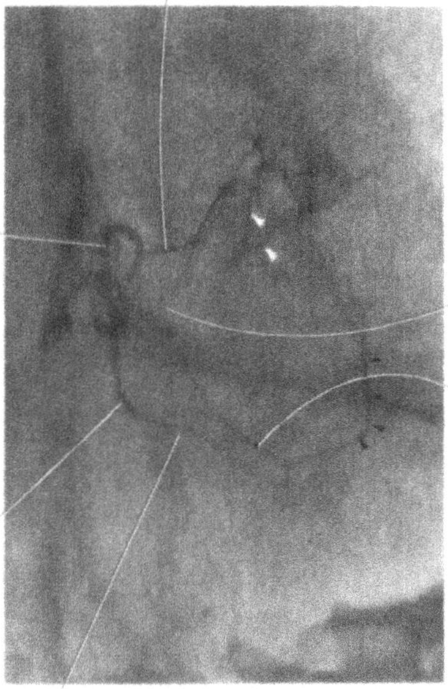

Fig. 193B

Fig. 193. Septo-atrial vein. Carotid angiogram, venous phase, lateral (Fig. A) and anteroposterior (Fig. B) views. The anomalous septal and the medial atrial veins (white arrowheads) unite to form the septo-atrial vein, which joins the posterior portion of the internal cerebral vein. Numerous medullary veins (M) join the subependymal veins along the anterior and lateral angles of the lateral ventricle. The lateral atrial tributary of the inferior ventricular vein, originating from the inferolateral border of the atrium, is seen leaving the lateral ventricle at the inferior choroidal point (row of black arrowheads). Note the angular course of the septo-atrial vein in the anteroposterior projection (see Fig. 186B)

Fig. 194. Common atrial vein. Carotid angiogram, venous phase, lateral views, 2 cases

Fig. 194A. The anomalous septal (row of black arrowheads), atrial (white arrowheads) and occipital tributaries form the stem of the medial atrial vein. This is joined by the stem of the direct lateral vein, which receives the lateral atrial and middle terminal tributaries, forming the common atrial vein (arrow)

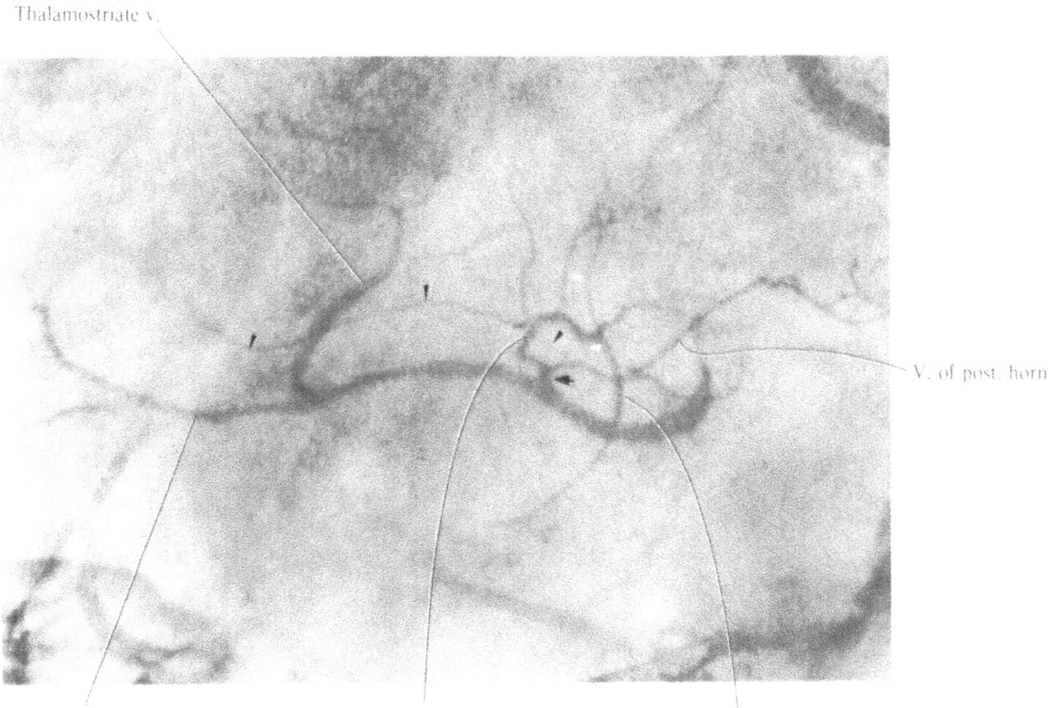

Fig. 194A

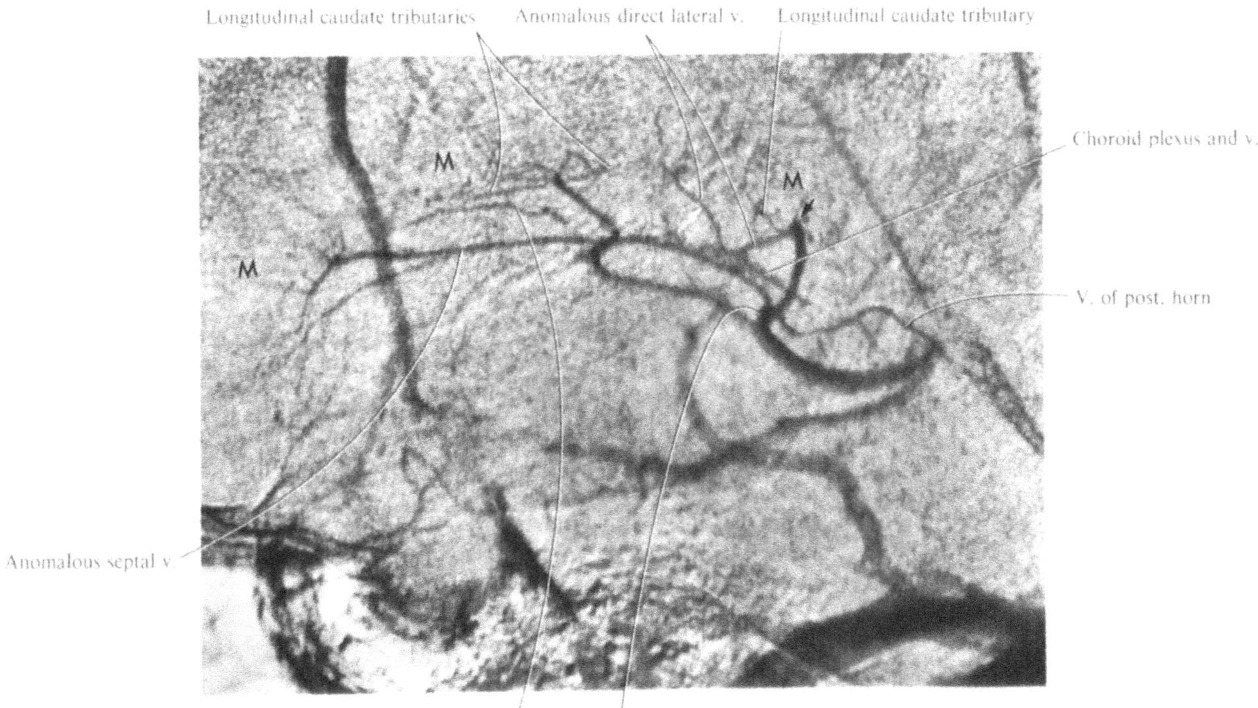

Fig. 194B

Fig. 194B. Vein of the lateral wall of the body of the lateral ventricle draining into the medial atrial vein through a roof vein. A vein on the upper part of the lateral wall of the body of the lateral ventricle (white arrow) takes a zig-zag course posteriorly. This anomalous direct lateral vein then turns medially (seen as a dense dot—black arrow) on the roof of the lateral ventricle. Upon reaching the medial wall, it runs downwards, receiving anomalous septal veins and the vein of the posterior horn, to form the common atrial vein which, in turn, opens into the internal cerebral vein. Note numerous deep medullary veins (M) joining the subependymal veins

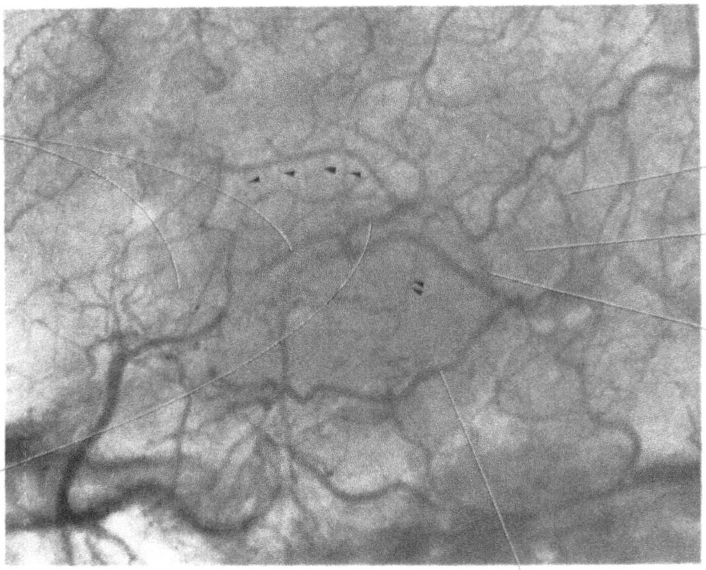

Fig. 195 A

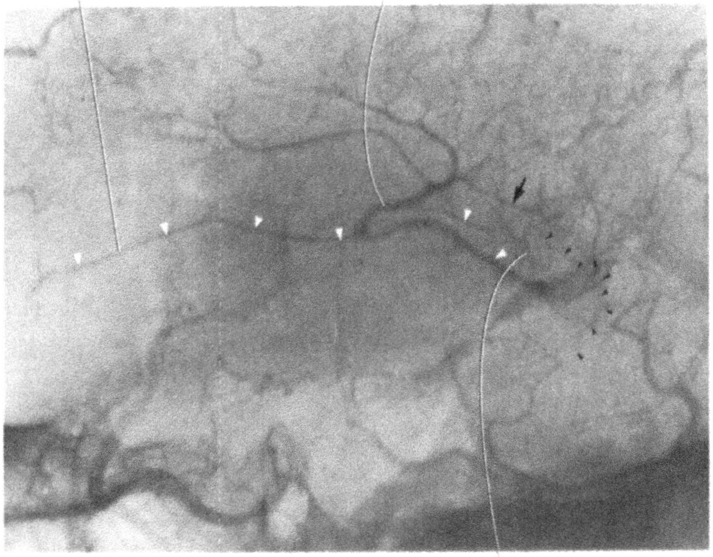

Fig. 195 B

Fig. 195. Early filling of the vein of the head of the caudate nucleus (Fig. 195 A) and late filling of the septal vein (Fig. 195 B). Carotid angiogram, venous phase, lateral views

Fig. 195 A. Early to intermediate venous phase. The basal cerebral vein, the direct lateral vein and its tributaries, including the external (arrowheads), and internal superior striate veins (double arrowheads) are well opacified. The septal vein is, however, not seen

Fig. 195 B. Late venous phase. The vein of the head of the caudate nucleus is no longer opacified. The anomalous septal vein (row of white arrowheads) is, however, well visualized and is seen running above and close to the internal cerebral vein. The lateral atrial tributary (arrow) of the direct lateral vein, receiving a choroidal vein from the atrium (black arrowheads), is clearly seen

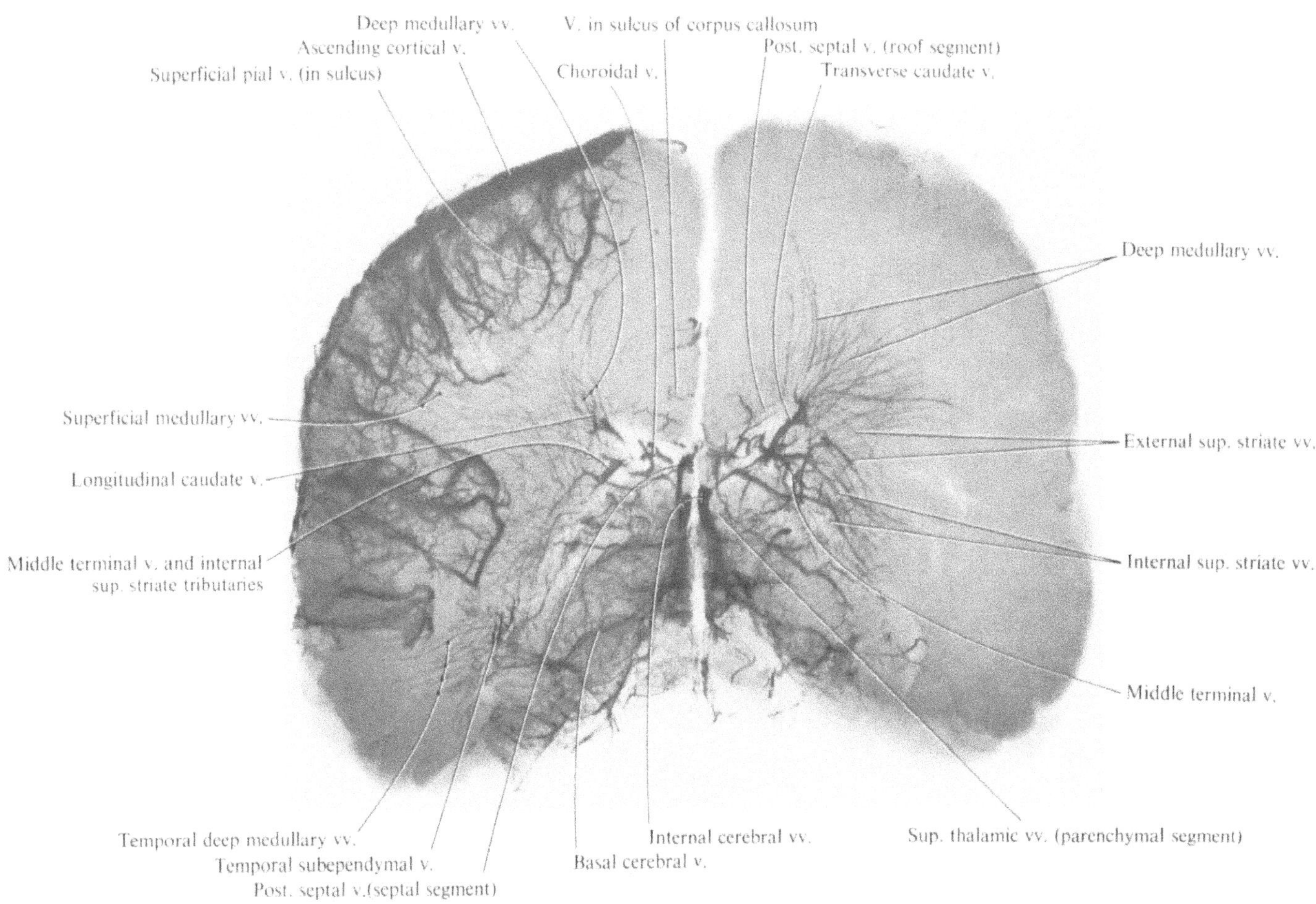

Fig. 196. Radiograph of a coronal slice of an injected specimen, showing the deep and superficial medullary veins. The slice includes the posterior part of the body and the atrium of the lateral ventricle. Numerous comparatively short superficial and relatively long deep medullary veins are seen. Deep medullary veins in the temporal lobe are, however, relatively short. Note the streaming pattern of deep medullary veins towards the lateral angle of the body, the lateral wall of the atrium and the lateral part of the roof of the temporal horn

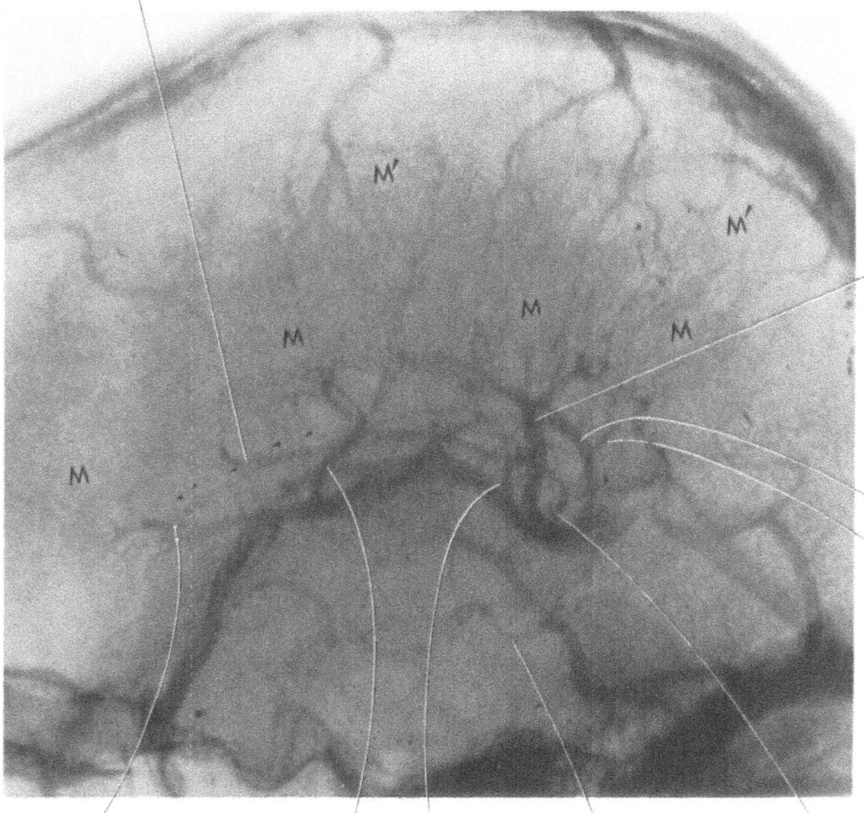

Fig. 197. Prominent medullary veins. Carotid angiogram, venous phase, lateral view

Deep medullary veins (M) are numerous, long, and prominent and stream toward the lateral angle of the lateral ventricle. They are most pronounced in the posterior frontal and parietal areas. Neither dural sinus occlusion nor space-occupying lesions were found. Superficial medullary veins (M′) are also seen. They are, however, difficult to distinguish from the superimposed pial veins within sulci. Superior striate veins (arrowheads) are also prominent in the frontal region and converge downwards and slightly backwards. Those located more posteriorly are difficult to identify

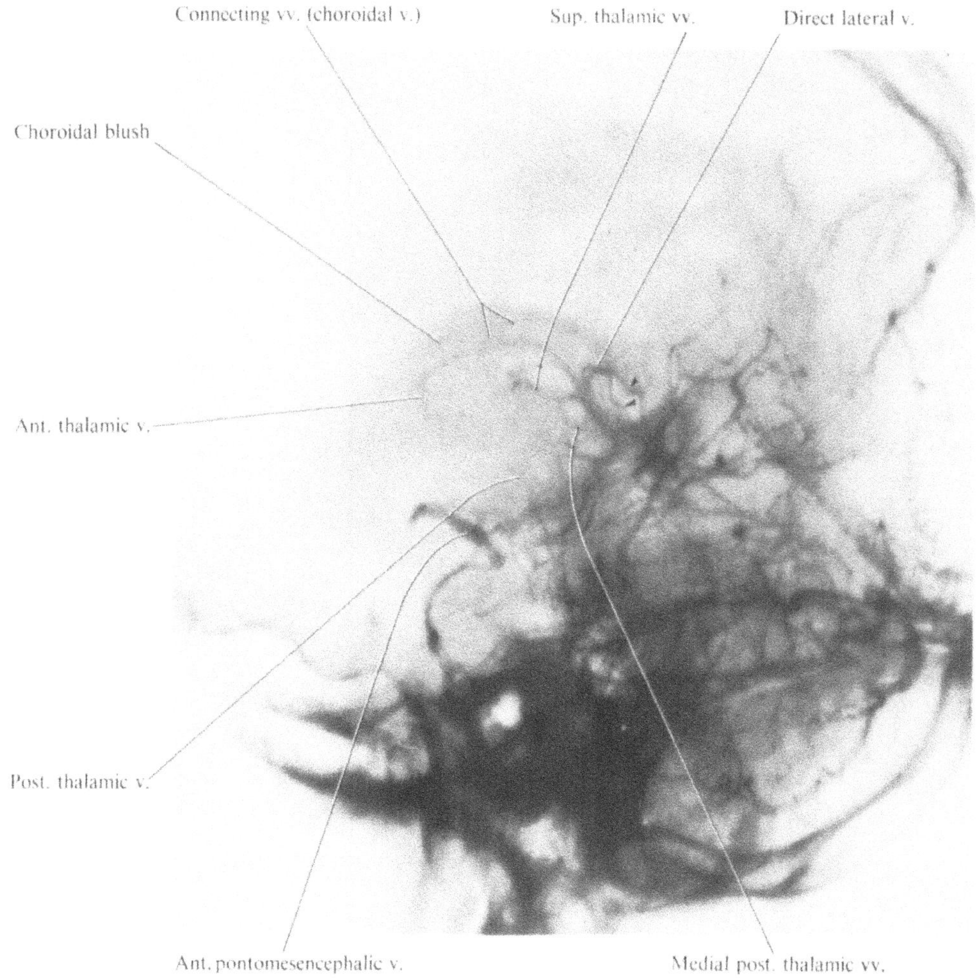

Fig. 198. Thalamic veins. Vertebral angiogram, venous phase, lateral view

The anterior thalamic veins run downwards, forwards, upwards, and then backwards to join the internal cerebral vein. Two superior thalamic veins are seen, one running backwards to join the posterior portion of the internal cerebral vein, the other opening into its midportion. The medial posterior thalamic vein is seen on each side. One drains backwards to join the posterior part of the internal cerebral vein and the other runs backwards and downwards to join the posterior part of the posterior mesencephalic vein. Inferior thalamic veins emerge from the interpeduncular fossa to join the mesencephalic segment of the anterior pontomesencephalic vein. Some of the posterior thalamic veins are prominent and drain downwards to join the posterior mesencephalic vein. The choroidal blush, numerous fine choroidal veins within the blush and fine connecting veins draining into the internal cerebral vein, are noted. Note the prominent, tortuous, middle choroidal veins (arrowheads) joining the stem of the direct lateral vein

PART 3

POSTERIOR FOSSA

Chapter 1

Fourth Ventricle and Cisterns of the Posterior Fossa

Introduction

Knowledge of the radiologic anatomy of the posterior fossa has certainly benefited from recent investigations into the arterial supply and venous drainage of its structures, and from studies of the anatomy of the fourth ventricle and cisterns of the posterior fossa.
We shall describe successively the anatomy and radiology of the ventricles and cisterns, the arteries of vertebrobasilar origin and the veins which drain the posterior fossa.
As in the previous chapters, the radiologic anatomy will be closely correlated with the gross anatomy, so that during interpretation the maximum information can be extracted from the radiographs. The latter therefore constitute a veritable "dissection *in vivo*".

I. Anatomic Study of the Fourth Ventricle

The fourth ventricle is a midline cavity located between the brainstem and the cerebellum. The floor is formed by the posterior part of the pons and medulla and its roof is formed by the anterior surface of the cerebellum.
Opposite the pontomedullary junction, the fourth ventricle has two pairs of symmetrical recesses. The two anterolateral recesses pass around the upper portion of the medulla. The two posterolateral recesses are located near the roof, one above each cerebellar tonsil on either side of the nodule. The anatomy of these recesses has been known since 1850 through the works of BOCHDALEK and RETZIUS.

1. Floor of the Fourth Ventricle
(Figs. 199, 203, 207)

The floor of the fourth ventricle is rhomboidal in configuration. Its length is 35 mm and its width 16 mm. A midline sulcus marks its major longitudinal axis. At the level of the medulla and pons it contains the sensory and motor nuclei of the lower cranial nerves (V–XII). The lateral limits of the floor of the fourth ventricle are as follows:

(1) Superiorly: the superior cerebellar peduncles (brachium conjunctivum).

(2) Midportion: the inferior cerebellar peduncles (restiform bodies). These also form the anterior limits of the anterolateral recesses, which open into the cavity of the fourth ventricle at this level.

(3) Inferiorly: the ligula (toenia), a flat square of white matter which passes from the obex to the inferior cerebellar peduncles.

The most superior limit of the floor of the fourth ventricle corresponds to the termination of the aqueduct of Sylvius. The most inferior limit is formed by the obex.

2. Roof of the Fourth Ventricle
(Figs. 199, 204, 206, 208)

The shape of the roof of the fourth ventricle is classically described as that of a tent. Its composition differs according to the level under consideration: the superior or pontine portion, or the inferior or medullary portion.
In its superior portion, the roof of the fourth ventricle is formed by two laminae of nervous tissue: anteriorly, by the anterior medullary velum, which is white matter; more posteriorly, by the lingula, which is grey matter.
In its inferior portion, the roof of the fourth ventricle is formed by two structures, the membrana tectoria and more posteriorly the tela choroidea of the fourth ventricle. The membrana tectoria inserts superiorly on the nodule and on the free edges of the posterior medullarly vela (which are more appropriately described later with the posterolateral recesses). Laterally, it lies between the inferior cerebellar peduncles which are reinforced at this level by the ligula. Its inferior insertion is at the obex. The membrana tectoria is continuous with the ependymal lining of the fourth ventricle. More posteriorly, the tela choroidea of the fourth ventricle also covers the anterior surface of the cerebellum and the posterior surface of

the medulla. The tela choroidea is formed by the coalescence of two sheets of pia mater. It thickens on either side of the midline to form the choroid plexus of the fourth ventricle.

Inferiorly, the membrana tectoria and the tela choroidea present a midline orifice, the foramen of Magendie. Its diameter is 5 mm.

The apex of the roof of the fourth ventricle forms the fastigium, which is situated superiorly to the nodule.

3. Posterolateral Recesses

(Figs. 200, 202, 204, 206)

The posterior medullary vela are two semilunar bands of white matter located above the cerebellar tonsils. Their anterior borders are continuous with the membrana tectoria to help form the roof of the fourth ventricle in its inferior portion. Their medial borders insert on the uvula and the nodule and posteriorly they are continuous with the white matter of the cerebellum. Laterally they are related to the floccular peduncles.

The posterolateral recesses are the spaces located on either side of the nodule, between the posterior medullary vela which form their floors and the white matter of the cerebellum which forms their roofs. The dentate nuclei make impressions on the lateral walls of these recesses. Consequently, the posterolateral recesses project behind the fastigium, on lateral pneumoencephalograms, and on either side of the midline.

4. Anterolateral Recesses

(Figs. 201, 202, 204, 206)

The anterolateral recesses result from the incomplete union of the roof and floor at the lateral angle of the fourth ventricle. They extend from the lateral angles of the fourth ventricle to the cerebellopontine angles on either side. The lateral limit of each recess is the flocculus and the medial limit is the inferior cerebellar peduncle and the ninth, tenth, and eleventh cranial nerves. Each recess terminates at the foramen of Luschka and has a curvilinear shape with a medial concavity, around the pontomedullary junction.

II. Anatomic Study of the Posterior Fossa Cisterns

The cisterns of the posterior fossa, like those of the tentorial incisura or the sellar region, have been the subject of many works, which has resulted in various classifications [Key and Retzius (1875) and Duret (1874)]. The development of fractional pneumoencephalography placed additional emphasis on the anatomy of these fluid-filled spaces [Robertson (1951), Liliequist (1959)].

The cisterns of the posterior fossa can be arranged in four groups, according to their location:

1. Anterior to the brainstem
2. Posterior to the medulla and below the inferior vermis
3. Posterior to the tectum and superior to the cerebellum
4. Around the cerebral peduncles

The medullary and pontine cisterns are situated anteriorly to the brainstem. Their lateral extensions contribute to form the cisterns of the cerebellopontine angles. At the level of the foramen magnum, posterior to the medulla and below the inferior vermis, lies the cisterna magna, communicating anteriorly, around the brainstem, with the medullary cistern and inferiorly with the spinal subarachnoid space. The cisterns located posteriorly to the quadrigeminal plate, anteriorly to the culmen and inferiorly to the splenium of the corpus callosum, join to form the cistern of the vein of Galen. Posteriorly to this cistern is the superior cerebellar cistern.

The circumpeduncular or ambient cisterns, because of their wide communication with the cisterns anteriorly to the brainstem and with those posteriorly to the tectum, are best included with the cisterns of the posterior fossa. Their two lateral extensions, the ambient wing cisterns or retropulvinar cisterns, cover the posterior aspects of the pulvinar regions of the thalamus.

1. Cisterns Anterior to the Brainstem

Medullary cistern (Figs. 209, 212, 216)
Pontine cistern (Figs. 209, 211, 214, 218)
Cerebellopontine angle cistern (Figs. 211, 213, 217)

The boundaries and relationships of each cistern have been studied by means of sagittal, horizontal and frontal sections. Frozen skulls and their contents have been sectioned in these planes and radiographs of the specimens taken. This technique permits the radiographic study of the morphology of the cisterns which can be related to tomographic cuts made during fractional pneumoencephalography. This technique has proved to be more satisfactory than filling the cisterns with a radiopaque contrast medium.

a) Medullary Cistern
(Figs. 209, 212, 216)

The medullary cistern is located anteriorly to the medulla and extends from the foramen magnum to the pontomedullary junction. Its posterior limit is the anterior surface of the medulla and its anterior limit is the clivus with its dural covering. The lateral limit of the medullary cistern on each side is an angle formed anteriorly by the occipital condyle and posteriorly by the anterior surface of the cerebellar tonsil.
On each side of the midline, two lateral protrusions of the medullary cistern are present, corresponding to the hypoglossal canal medially and more laterally to the jugular foramen. The medullary cistern communicates posteriorly around the brainstem with the cisterna magna, inferiorly with the spinal subarachnoid space and superiorly with the pontine cistern. The lateral angles of the medullary cistern are continuous superiorly with the cisterns of the cerebellopontine angles.
The medullary cistern is crossed obliquely by the two vertebral arteries, which join near the midline to form the basilar trunk at the level of the pontomedullary junction. More laterally, the cistern is crossed by the ninth, tenth and eleventh cranial nerves passing towards the jugular foramen, and by the twelfth cranial nerve which passes forwards the hypoglossal canal.

b) Pontine Cistern
(Figs. 209, 211, 214, 218)

The pontine cistern is continous inferiorly with the medullary cistern. Quite narrow in its midsagittal portion due to the bulging of the pons, it continues superiorly into the interpeduncular cistern. The boundaries of the pontine cistern are, therefore, the clivus anteriorly and the anterior surface of the pons posteriorly. Laterally it communicates with the cerebellopontine angle cisterns, the course of the fifth cranial nerve marking the boundary between the two on each side. Usually there is a further extension of this cistern into Meckel's cave. The sixth cranial nerves have a long course in front of the pons, through this cistern.

c) Cerebellopontine Angle Cistern
(Figs. 211, 213, 217)

The cerebellopontine angle cisterns are triangular in shape. The anterior limit of each is constituted by the posterior aspect of the petrous portion of the temporal bone, and by that portion of petrous ridge medial to the porus acousticus. More laterally, the anterior limit corresponds to the porus itself. The medial limit of this cistern is the lateral surface of the pons and the pontomedullary junction. Its posterior limit is made up of the cerebellar flocculus and the closely related seventh and eighth cranial nerves, which traverse the cistern, passing laterally towards the internal auditory meatus. The internal auditory artery, a branch of the anterior inferior cerebellar artery, is also found at this level in the cistern.
Thus, the cisternal space anterior to the brainstem is formed by the medullary and pontine cisterns, containing the fifth and sixth cranial nerves. Likewise, the angle formed between the petrous bone, the occipital condyle and the brainstem consists of, from inferiorly to superiorly, the lateral angle of the medullary cistern, which contains the ninth, tenth and eleventh cranial nerves, and the cerebellopontine angle cistern, which contains the seventh and eighth cranial nerves.

2. Cistern Posterior to the Medulla and Below the Inferior Vermis-Cisterna Magna
(Figs. 209, 211)

In sagittal section, the anterior limit of the cisterna magna is formed by the medulla which is covered at this level by the tela choroidea of the fourth ventricle. The superior limit is formed by the inferior vermis, while the posterior and inferior limits are made up of the occipital bone and the ligaments which join the posterior aspect of the foramen magnum with the posterior arch of the atlas.
In horizontal section, the shape of the cisterna magna is more complex. Its anterior margin lies against the posterior medulla, is straight and tapers laterally. Superiorly, the anterior aspect of the cisterna magna communicates with the vallecula, which lies between the two cerebellar tonsils. More posteriorly, the cisterna magna enlarges and is related, not only to the inferior surface of the vermis, but also to the inferior surfaces of the cerebellar hemispheres. Its superolateral extent, posterior to the vermis and the cerebellar hemispheres, is quite variable (Liliequist, 1959).
The cisterna magna communicates anteriorly with the medullary cistern, to which it is connected by a space between the posterolateral surface of the medulla and the anterior surfaces of the cerebellar tonsils. Inferiorly, it communicates with the spinal subarachnoid space. Finally, by means of its extension posteriorly and superiorly to the vermis and the cerebellar hemispheres, it can also communicate with the superior cerebellar cistern.

3. Cisterns Posterior to the Tectum and Superior to the Cerebellum

Cistern of the vein of Galen or quadrigeminal cistern (Figs. 199, 209, 211, 215, 219)
Superior cerebellar cistern (Figs. 209, 211)
Cistern of the velum interpositum (Figs. 209, 211)
Precentral cerebellar cistern (Figs. 210)
Posterior pericallosal cistern (Figs. 211)

Posteriorly to the quadrigeminal plate and inferiorly to the pineal body and the splenium of the corpus callosum, lies a cisternal space, the quadrigeminal cistern or cistern of the vein of Galen. The boundaries of this cistern are as follows: the roof is formed, from anteriorly to posteriorly by the pineal body, the splenium of the corpus callosum, the inferomedial surfaces of the occipital lobes and the tentorium of the cerebellum. The anterior margin of the cistern is formed, from superiorly to inferiorly, by the superior and inferior colliculi and the anterior medullary velum. The postero-inferior surface corresponds to the superior vermis (lingula, central lobule and culmen). However, at this level, in the angle formed between the culmen and the tentorium, it is more convenient to name this cistern the superior cerebellar cistern. The cistern of the vein of Galen, thus represents a confluence of cisterns along the posterior aspect of the mesencephalon.
The cistern of the vein of Galen contains the vein of Galen and its tributaries, including the posterior portions of the internal cerebral and basal veins, and also the posterior choroidal arteries, the arteries to the tectum and the quadrigeminal segments of the posterior cerebral arteries. This cistern communicates on either side with the circumpeduncular or ambient cisterns. Posteriorly, it can extend as far back as the cisterna magna when the latter is well developed. Superiorly it joins the cistern of the velum interpositum (or the cistern of the roof of the third ventricle), and also the pericallosal cistern.
A cisternal space, the precentral cerebellar cistern, arises from the postero-inferior part of the cistern of the vein of Galen between the lingula and central lobule. The precentral cerebellar vein runs in this cistern. There is likewise a cisternal space between each lobule of the vermis, which permits separation of these structures on sagittal tomography.

4. Cisterns Around the Cerebral Peduncles

Circumpeduncular or ambient cisterns (Figs. 211, 215, 219, 220)
Ambient wing cisterns (Figs. 211, 220)

The examination of frontal and horizontal sections of the brain, passing through the mesencephalic region, permits the best understanding of the distribution and relationships of the circumpeduncular or ambient cisterns. Two different portions of the ambient cisterns can be distinguished: supratentorial and infratentorial (Liliequist, 1959).
The supratentorial portions of the ambient cisterns encircle the cerebral peduncles, between the lateral surfaces of the peduncles and the internal aspects of the temporal lobes. They communicate anteriorly with the crural cisterns, on the anterior surfaces of the peduncles, and posteriorly with the cistern of the vein of Galen. On either side of the midline, lateral extensions of the ambient cisterns, the ambient wing cisterns or retropulvinar cisterns, cap the posterior aspects of the pulvinar regions of the thalamus. Several nervous and vascular structures pass through these portions of the ambient cisterns. They are the posterior cerebral arteries, the mesencephalic arteries, the posteromedial and posterolateral choroidal arteries, the basal veins, the lateral mesencephalic veins and the fourth cranial nerves. The optic tract and medial and lateral geniculate bodies form the superolateral boundary of this cistern, while the roof corresponds to the lateral part of the choroidal fissure.
The infratentorial portions of the ambient cisterns are located between the brainstem and the cerebellum, and encircle the lateral walls of the pons and the superior and middle cerebellar peduncles. They communicate anteriorly with the pontine cistern and posteriorly with the anterior part of the superior cerebellar cistern. These portions of the ambient cisterns contain the superior cerebellar arteries and the posterior mesencephalic and basal veins.

III. Radiologic Study of Posterior Fossa, Fourth Ventricle and Cisterns of the Posterior Fossa

Although the radiologic anatomy of the fourth ventricle was well outlined in the classical treatises, recent interest has been rekindled by the works of Corrales and Greitz (1972), who studied the fourth ventricle, and its deformation and displacement by tumors of the posterior fossa.
To study the fourth ventricle and its recesses, the usual technique of pneumoencephalography must be slightly modified. The head must be flexed more sharply forward

than usual, to prevent the escape of air through the aqueduct and thus enhance filling of the fourth ventricle and posterior fossa cisterns. An alternative method is to opacify this structure with a water-soluble contrast medium (CORRALES and GREITZ, 1972).

Lateral radiographs visualize the floor of the fourth ventricle, its superior limit, which is continuous with the aqueduct, and its inferior limit or obex (Figs. 221, 222). The roof of the fourth ventricle is formed superiorly by the anterior medullary velum and the lingula. Its summit corresponds to the fastigium.

In lateral tomograms, the faint tonal image posterior to the fastigium is caused by the posterolateral recesses of the fourth ventricle (Figs. 222, 223). Bounded by the cerebellum above and extending laterally on each side of the nodule, the posterolateral recesses project on either side of the midline, behind the fastigium.

The inferior portion of the roof of the fourth ventricle is more difficult to discern. It is formed by the tela choroidea and the membrana tectoria.

The fourth ventricle communicates with the cisterna magna via the foramen of Magendie.

The anterolateral recesses of the fourth ventricle create tonal images perpendicular to its main axis, best seen in the frontal projection (Fig. 228A and B).

Examination of the fourth ventricle in the frontal projection must not be performed only by standard radiographs, but also by tomography (Fig. 230), (CORRALLES, GREITZ, 1972). Tomography, especially in the hypocycloidal mode, imparts a high degree of precision to the examination. Structures which lie parallel to the plane of section, such as the anterior medullary velum, fastigium and posterolateral recesses, are not well seen in this projection, but structures perpendicular to the floor of the fourth ventricle are clearly identified. The median sulcus in the floor of the ventricle can be followed from its bulbar portion to its termination at the obex. More anteriorly details of the pontine portion of the floor can also be studied.

On both sides of the fourth ventricle, frontal tomograms reveal the lyre-shaped image of the anterolateral recesses (Fig. 228A and B). Their external aspects are marked by the imprints of the dentate nuclei. Their internal aspects enclose the pontomedullary junction. The peduncle of the flocculus forms the lateral boundary of each anterolateral recess while the inferior cerebellar peduncle (restiform body) marks its medial extent. Both of these recesses open anteriorly through the foramina of Luschka. The embryologic development explains the configuration of these recesses (HUANG and WOLF, 1967).

The localization of the fourth ventricle can be accomplished by using TWINNING's line. The midpoint of this line, from the tuberculum to the torcular, should fall within the ventricular cavity close to its floor, (Fig. 155B).

The height of the fourth ventricle and the dimensions of its floor were the subject of measurements by DAVIDOFF and DYKE (1951), EPSTEIN (1950), TAVERAS and WOOD (1964), and OBERSON (1969). These measurements correspond with those found anatomically:

length of the floor – 35 mm,
width of the floor – 16 mm.

The examination of the cisterns of the posterior fossa has benefited from the works of LILIEQUIST (1959). In our laboratory we have studied the anatomy of these cisterns by means of sections of the head, which are subsequently radiographed and photographed. These radiographs correspond quite closely to the images obtained with hypocycloidal tomography of this region. The matching photographs provide an unparalleled radiologic anatomic correlation, not only of the posterior fossa cisterns, but also of the tentorial incisure.

The examination of the cisterns of the posterior fossa is accomplished during pneumoencephalography, while the patient is seated. Recently, investigation of small tumors of the eighth nerve has been enhanced by opacification of the cerebellopontine angle cistern with iodinated contrast media.

Tomographic exploration of the posterior fossa cisterns demonstrates their limits with precision. The initial studies of this nature were reported by WACKENHEIM *et al.* (1970). Midsagittal tomograms demonstrate the brainstem and, anteriorly to it, the medullary, pontine and interpeduncular cisterns (Figs. 222, 223). However, it must be realized that these three confluent cisterns extend laterally, and are also well visualized in frontal tomograms.

Behind the brainstem lateral tomograms demonstrate the cisterna magna, limited posteriorly by the occipital bone and anteriorly by the cerebellum. A wide range of variations are possible in the size and configuration of this cistern. The portion of the cisterna magna which extends between the cerebellar hemispheres, to lie on the inferior vermis, is the vallecula.

Finally, lateral tomograms permit the investigation of the cistern of the vein of Galen, bounded by the splenium of the corpus callosum, the quadrigeminal plate and the culmen of the cerebellum. Three prolongations of the cistern of the vein of Galen are commonly identified. These include; (1) the precentral cistern, between the lingula and the central lobule; (2) the superior cerebellar cistern, between the tentorium, the superior vermis and the cerebellum; and (3) the cistern of the velum interpositum extending into the space of the tela choroidea, above the third ventricle.

Frontal tomograms which are perpendicular to or slightly oblique to the long axis of the brainstem demonstrate well the cisterns which extend laterally from those in front of the brainstem, as well as those cisterns at the level of the tentorial incisure (Figs. 225–229). Progressing from posteriorly to anteriorly these tomograms demonstrate first the medullary cistern, with its lateral extensions containing the nerves which pass through the jugular foramen and the condyloid canal (Figs. 228, 229). The image of the medulla in this frontal projection, is recognized not only by its shape but also by the presence of the occipital condyles lying laterally to this cistern.

Further anteriorly, the sections show the pons and the fourth ventricle (Figs. 227, 228). The pontine cistern is situated anteriorly to the belly of the pons. Laterally to the pontine cisterns are the cerebellopontine angle cisterns, each one being bounded by the petrous pyramid, the pons and the cerebellar hemisphere including the flocculus. Each cistern is traversed by the eighth and seventh cranial nerves (Fig. 227E).

Slightly anteriorly to the plane of the cerebellopontine angles, linear collections of air, lateral to the fourth ventricle, outline the infratentorial portions of the circumpeduncular cisterns. In conjunction with the air in the fourth ventricle, these cisterns delineate the brachia conjunctiva or superior cerebellar peduncles.

A small triangular image situated in the midline and above the superior vermis is due to the cistern of the vein of Galen. Cuts taken further anteriorly demonstrate the upper pontine region (Fig. 227A–C). In this region the image of the fourth ventricle fades.

The pontine cistern extends laterally as far as the trigeminal nerve. The extension into Meckel's cave is usually not visible at pneumoencephalography. The superior part of the pontine cistern, at the level of the trigeminal nerve, including the part extending into Meckel's cave, which usually fills during cisternography with water-soluble contrast medium (GREPE, 1974), may be called the trigeminal cistern.

The circumpeduncular (ambient) cisterns define the posterolateral walls of the cerebral peduncles. Posteriorly they unite with the cistern of the vein of Galen. Each has an extension behind the pulvinar region of the thalamus, known as the retropulvinar (or ambient wing) cistern.

Tomograms obtained anteriorly to this plane demonstrate the triangular image of the interpeduncular cistern. On both sides of the midline air also outlines the crural cisterns, lying anterolaterally to the cerebral peduncles (Fig. 226).

Examination of these cisterns may be accomplished by standard radiographs in the lateral and semiaxial projections (Fig. 224). The lateral projection demonstrates the cisterns in front of the brainstem (especially the pontine and interpeduncular cisterns) and the cistern of the vein of Galen. The ambient cisterns and retropulvinar cisterns are also seen as fine curvilinear collections of gas, concave anterior, which superimpose upon each other.

Routine frontal projections also exhibit superimposition of the infratentorial and supratentorial circumpeduncular cisterns upon each other, as described by LILIEQUIST (1959). The latter cistern is the larger and possesses lateral extensions, the retropulvinar cisterns (Fig. 231). Likewise, in the region of the internal auditory meatus the trigeminal and cerebellopontine angle cisterns overlap.

The use of opaque contrast media is merited in the search for small tumors of the eighth nerve [REESE and BULL (1967), HASTINGS-JAMES (1969), BAKER (1972)], as well as for the exact localization and delineation of these tumors (GREPE, 1974). It allows the diagnosis of very small intracanalicular tumors. It can be considered negative only if the contrast medium extends from the cerebellopontine angle to fill the whole internal auditory canal.

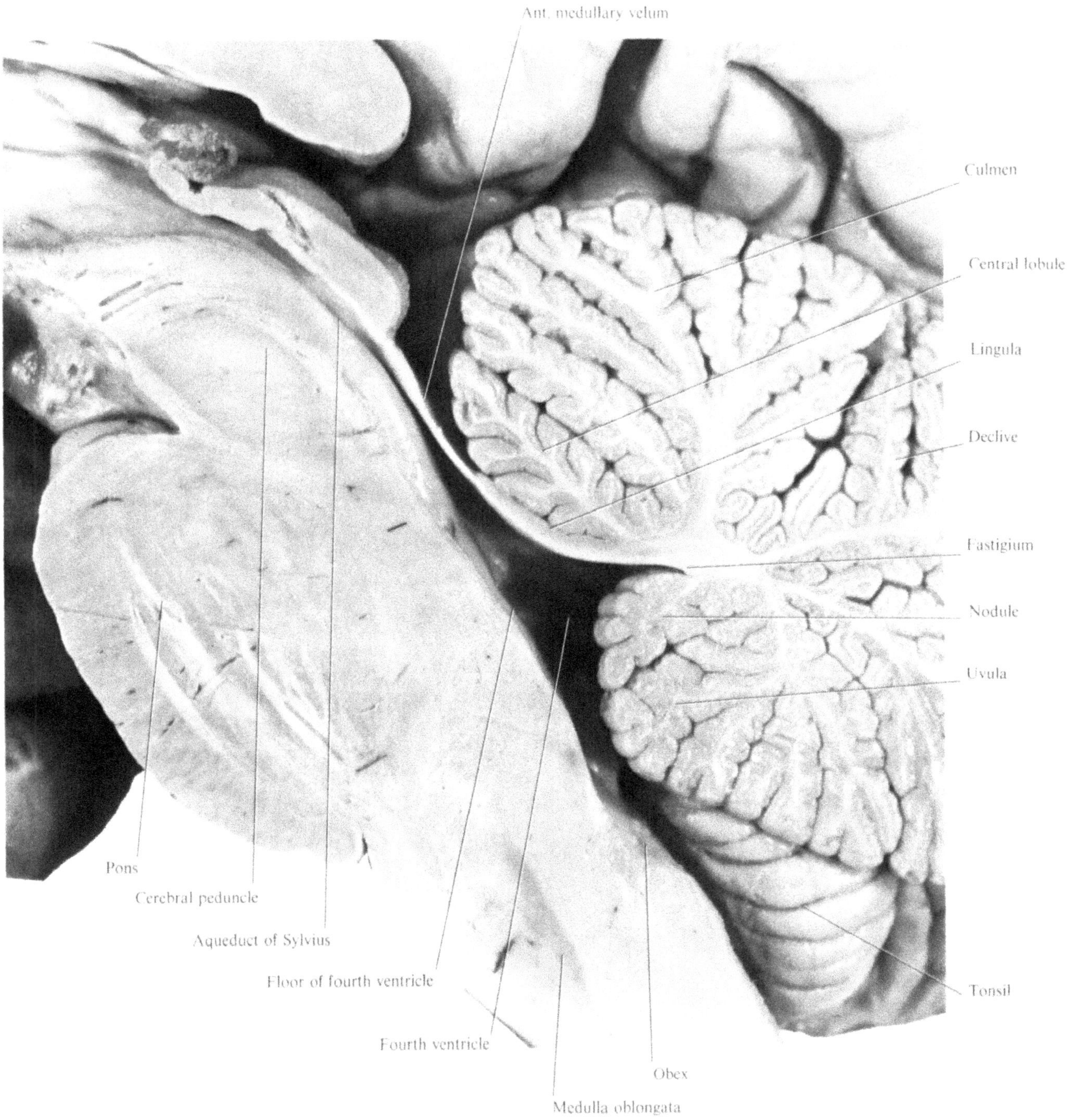

Fig. 199. Sagittal section through the fourth ventricle

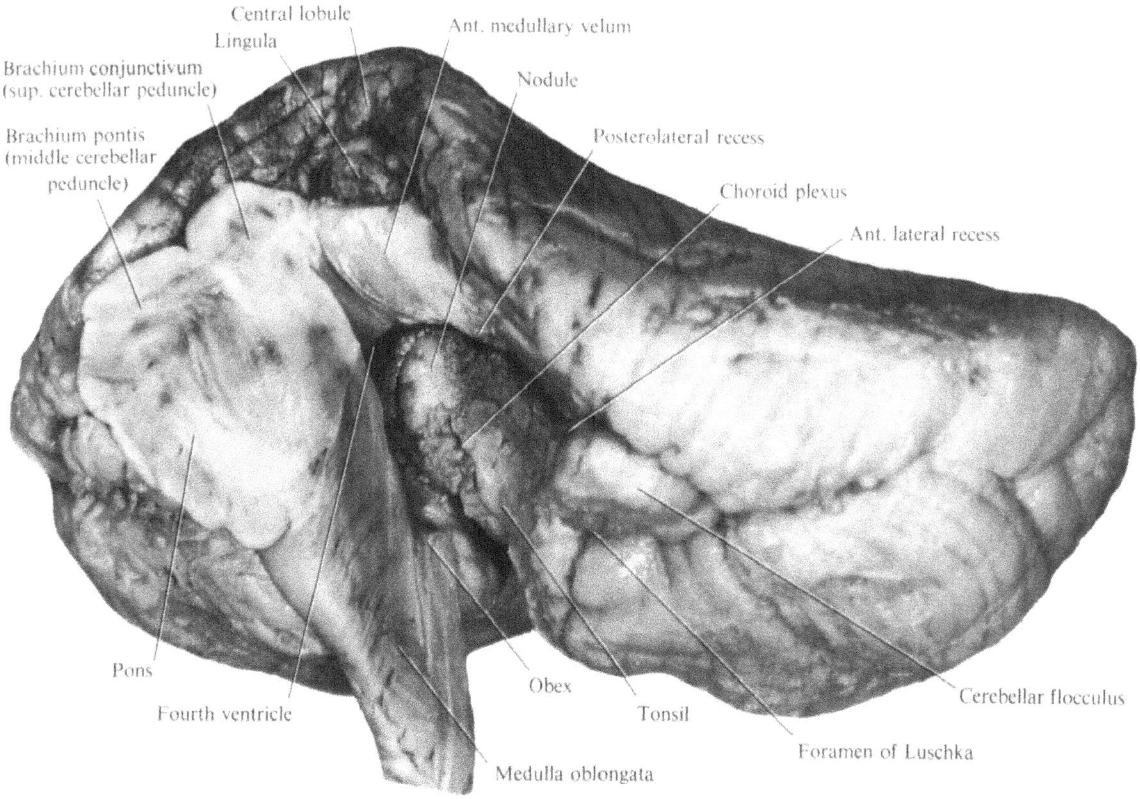

Fig. 200

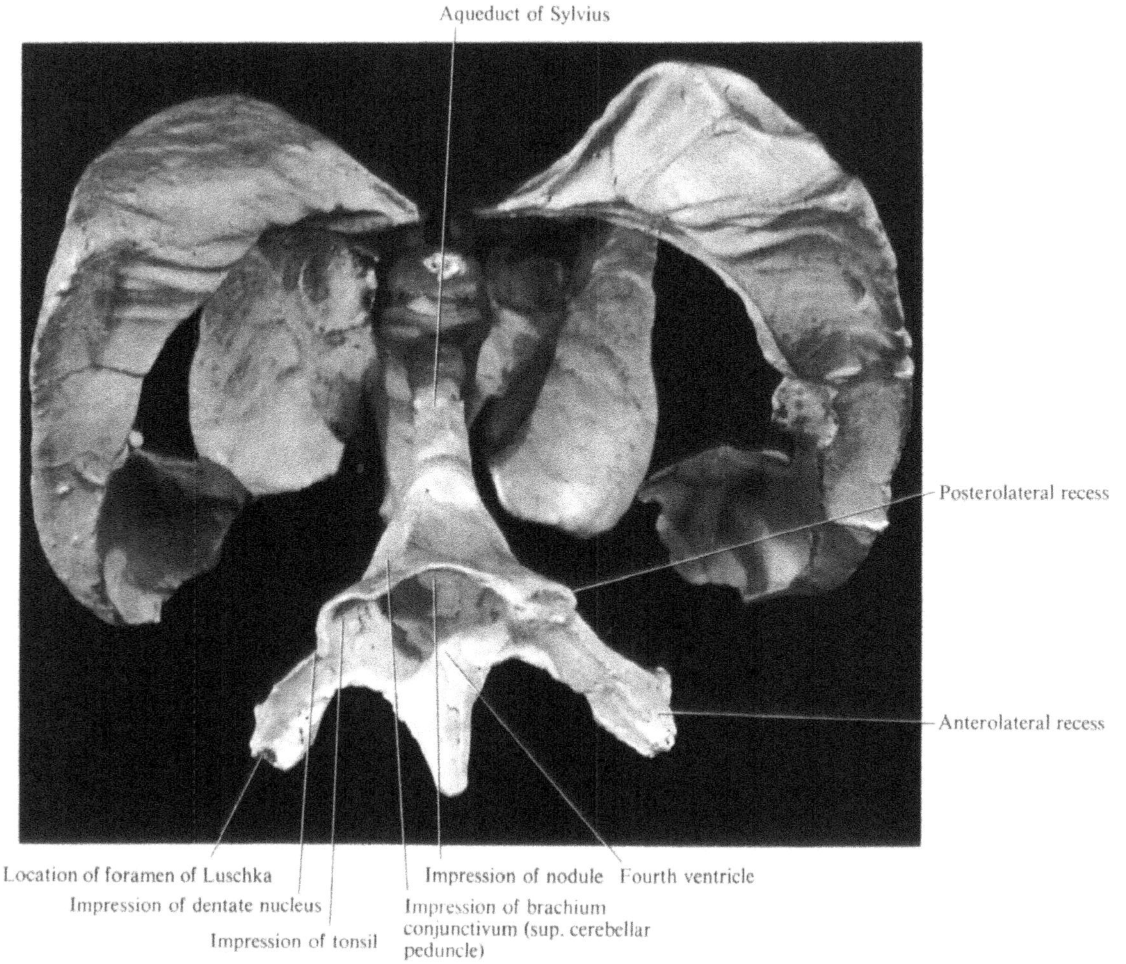

Fig. 201

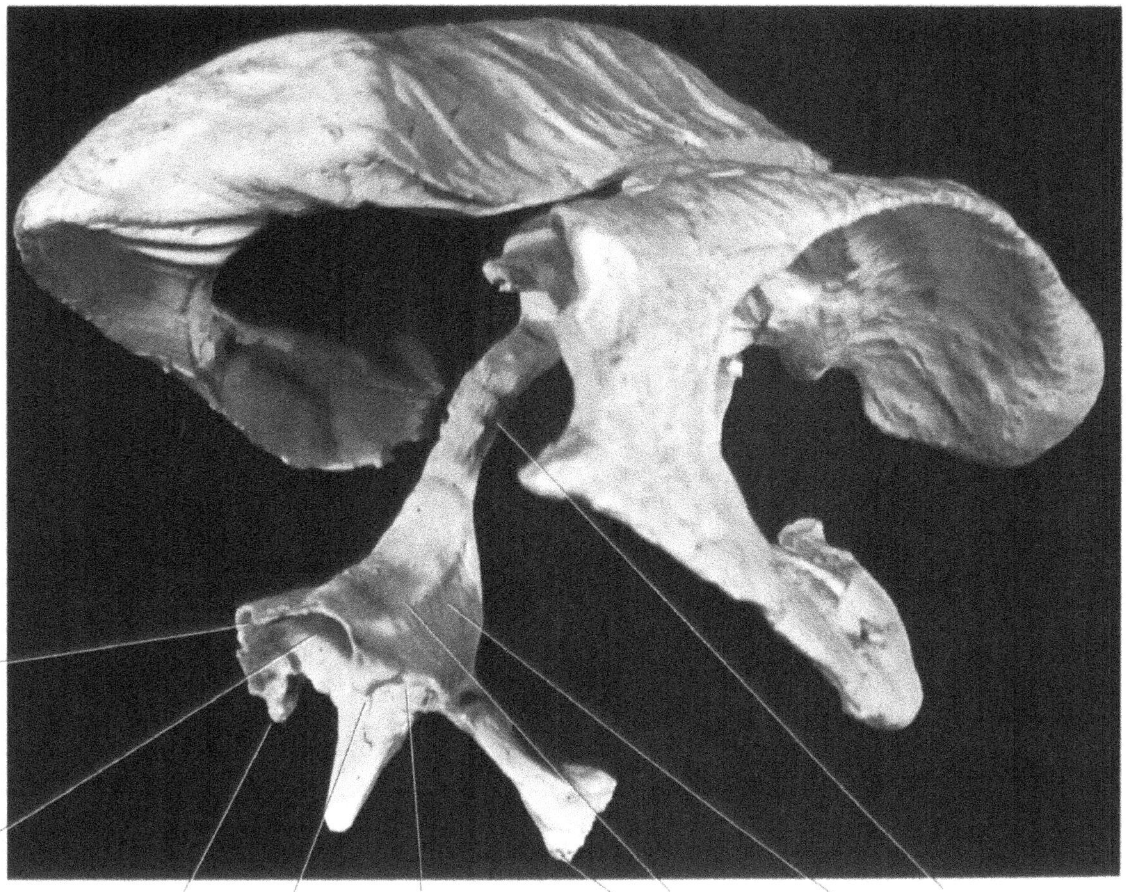

Fig. 202. Cast of the ventricular system, posterolateral view

◁

Fig. 200. Anterolateral view into the fourth ventricle (the entire left half of the brainstem has been removed)

Fig. 201. Cast of the ventricular system, posterior view

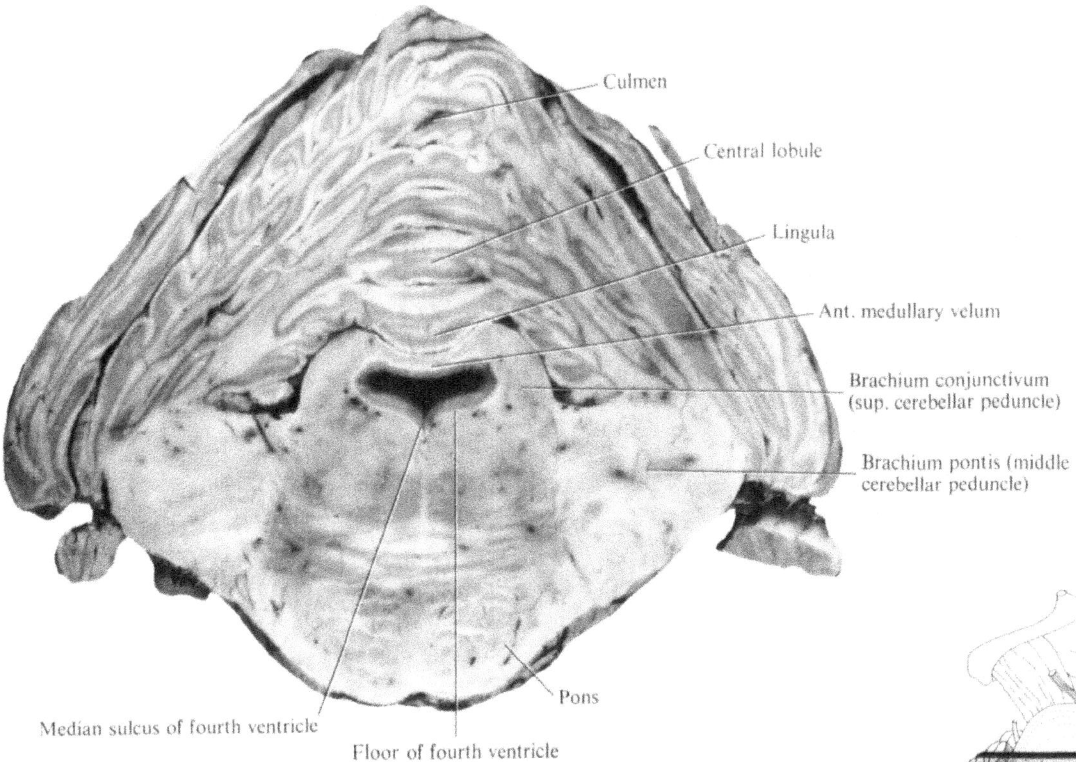

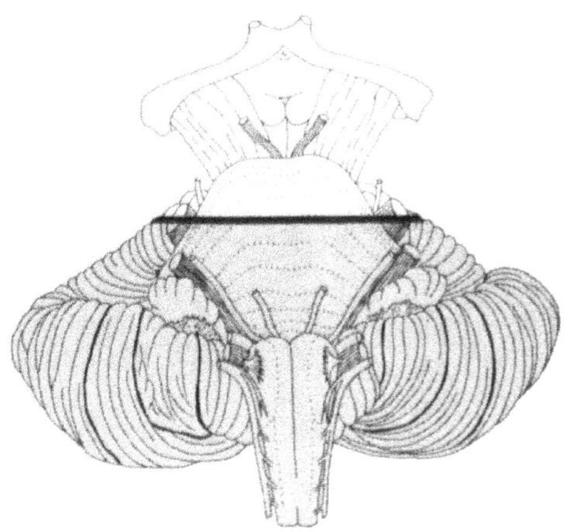

Fig. 203. Section perpendicular to the axis of the brainstem, passing through the superior part of the fourth ventricle

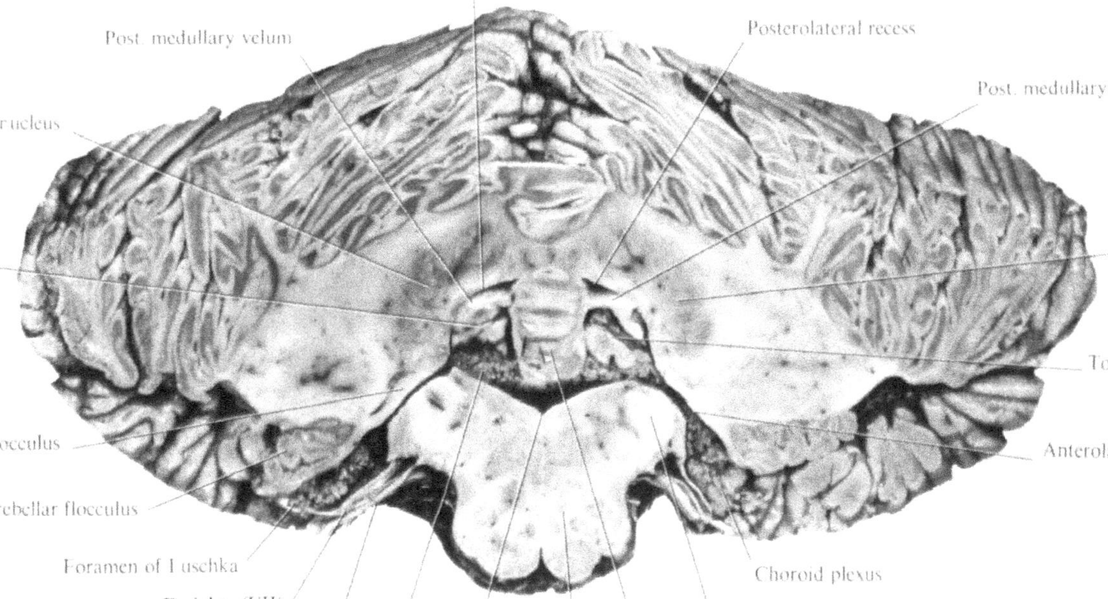

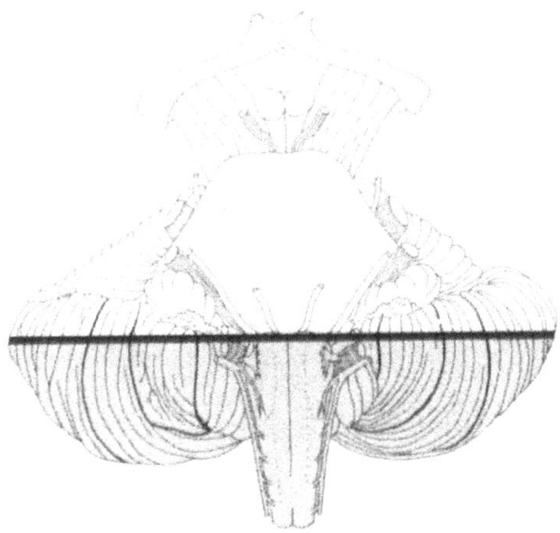

Fig. 204. Section perpendicular to the axis of the brainstem, passing through the antero- and posterolateral recesses of the fourth ventricle

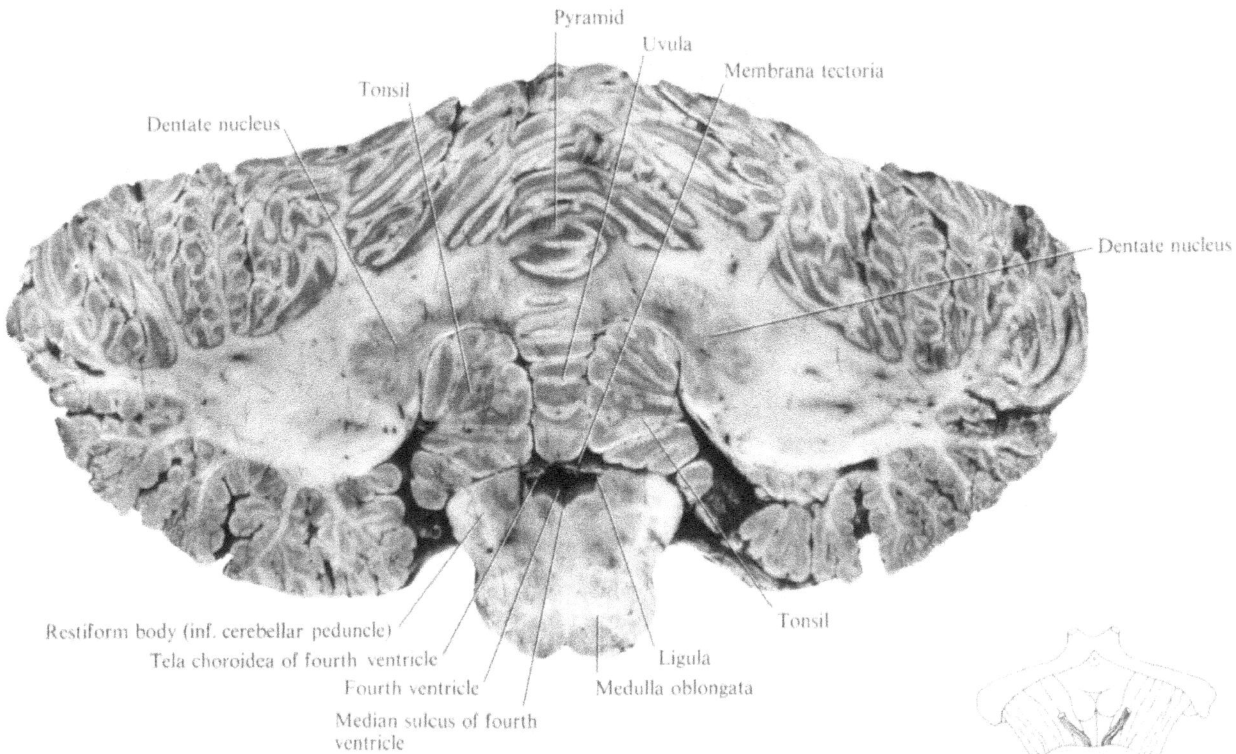

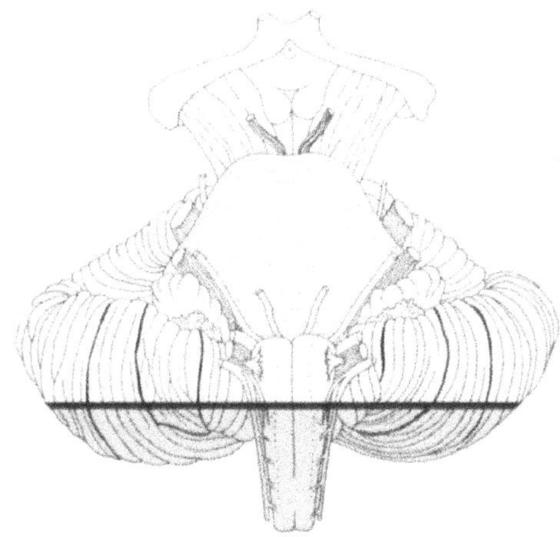

Fig. 205. Section perpendicular to the axis of the brainstem, passing through the inferior part of the fourth ventricle

▷

Fig. 206 A. Drawing of the fourth ventricle, viewed slightly off lateral projection; (the cerebellum has been divided in the midline but the brainstem is intact)

Fig. 206 B. Superimposition of the cast of the fourth ventricle on the drawing in Fig. 206 A

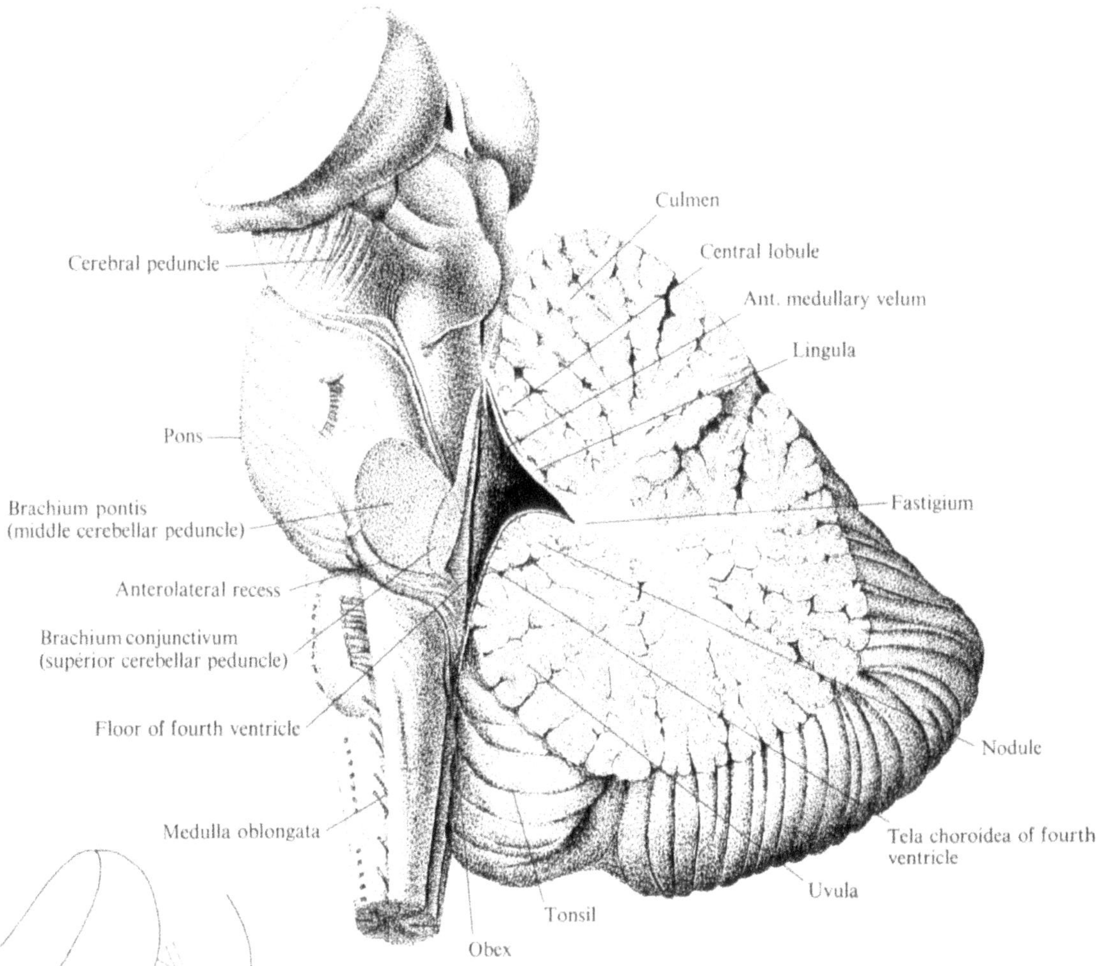

Fig. 206 A

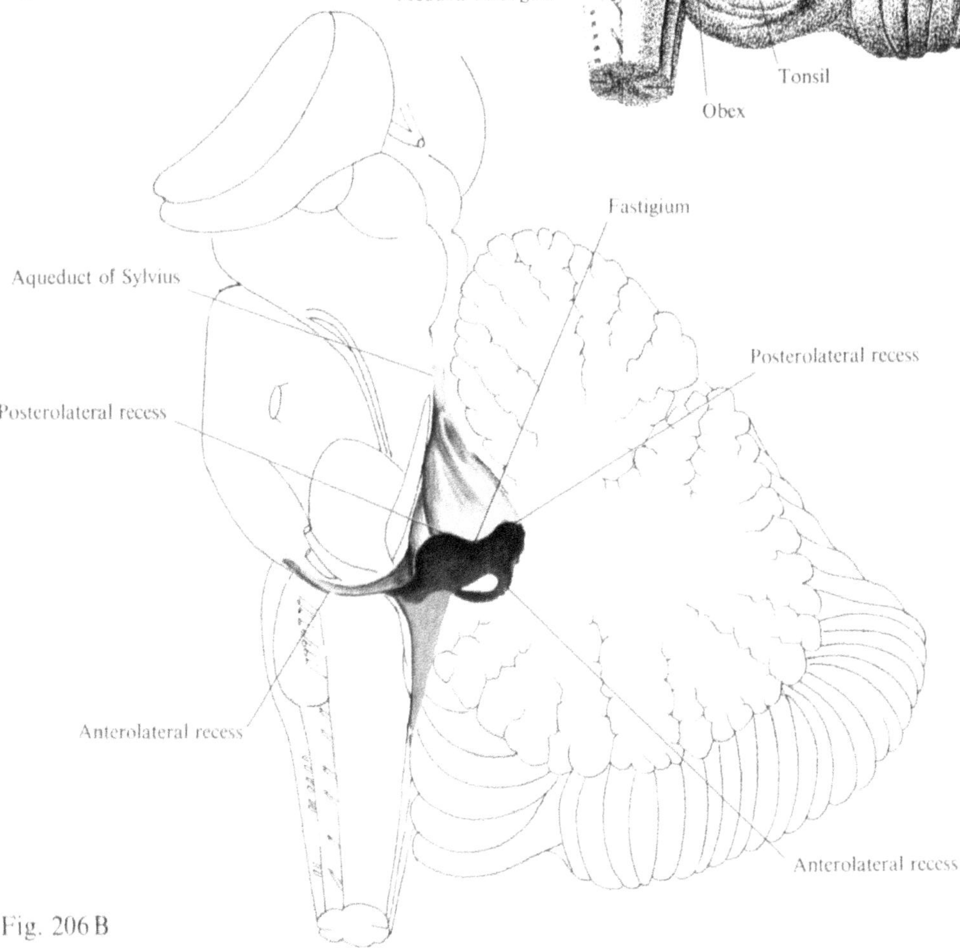

Fig. 206 B

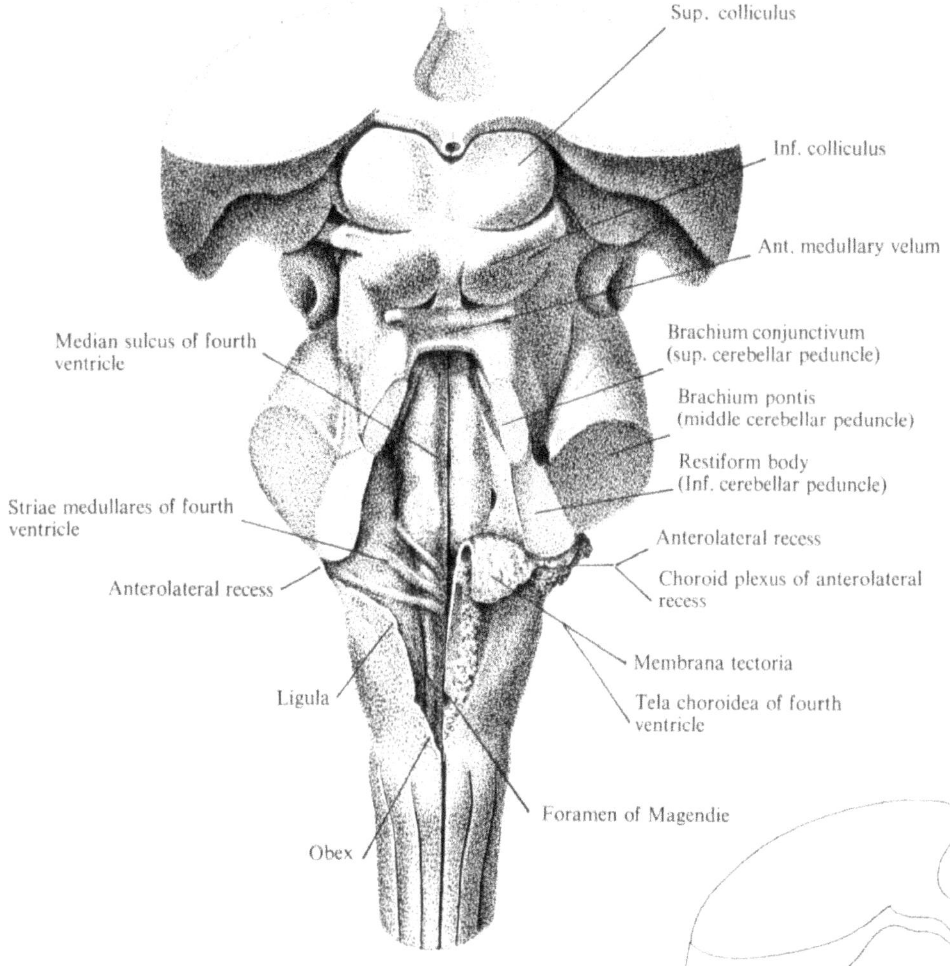

Fig. 207A. Posterior view of the brainstem; drawing of the floor of the fourth ventricle

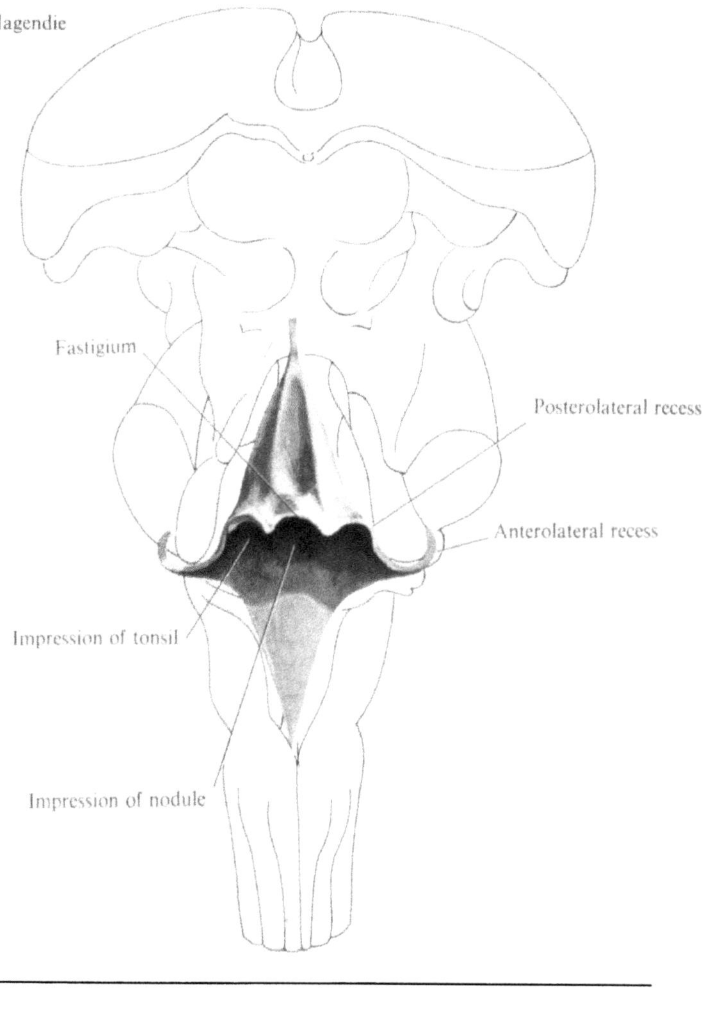

▷

Fig. 207B. Superimposition of the cast of the fourth ventricle on the drawing in Fig. 207A

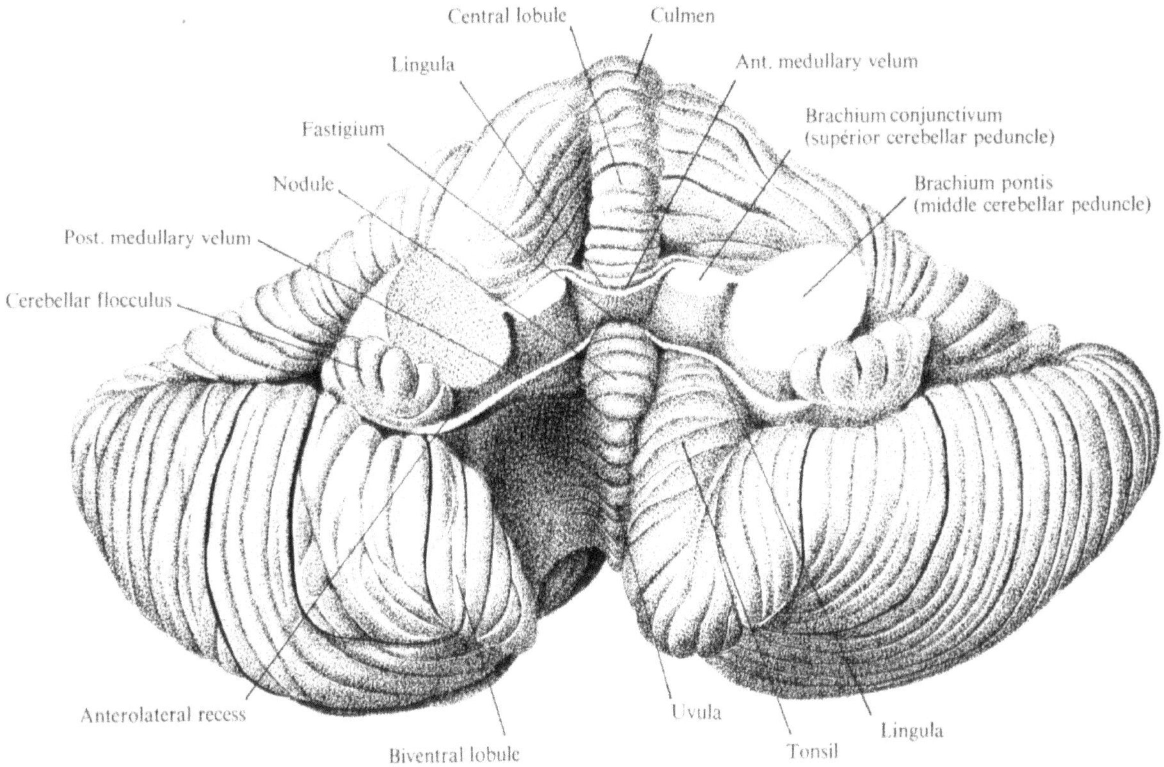

Fig. 208 A. Anterior view of the cerebellum; drawing of the roof of the fourth ventricle
Note that the right tonsil has been removed

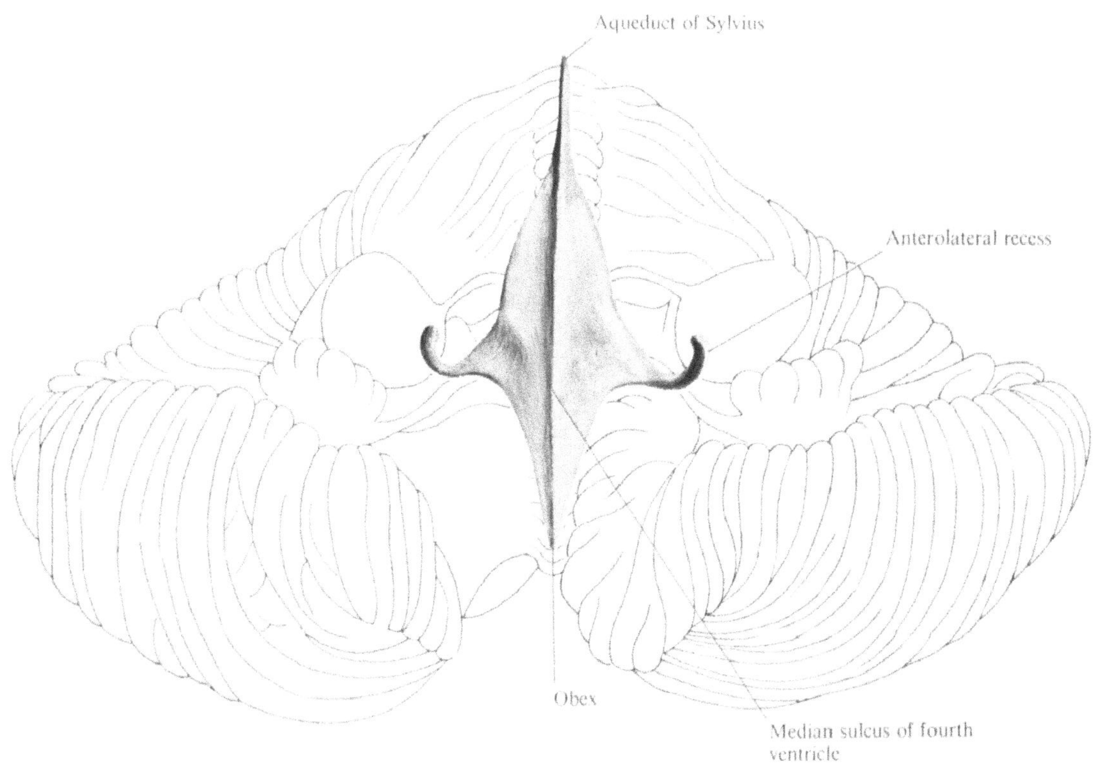

Fig. 208 B. Superimposition of the cast of the fourth ventricle on the drawing in Fig. 208 A

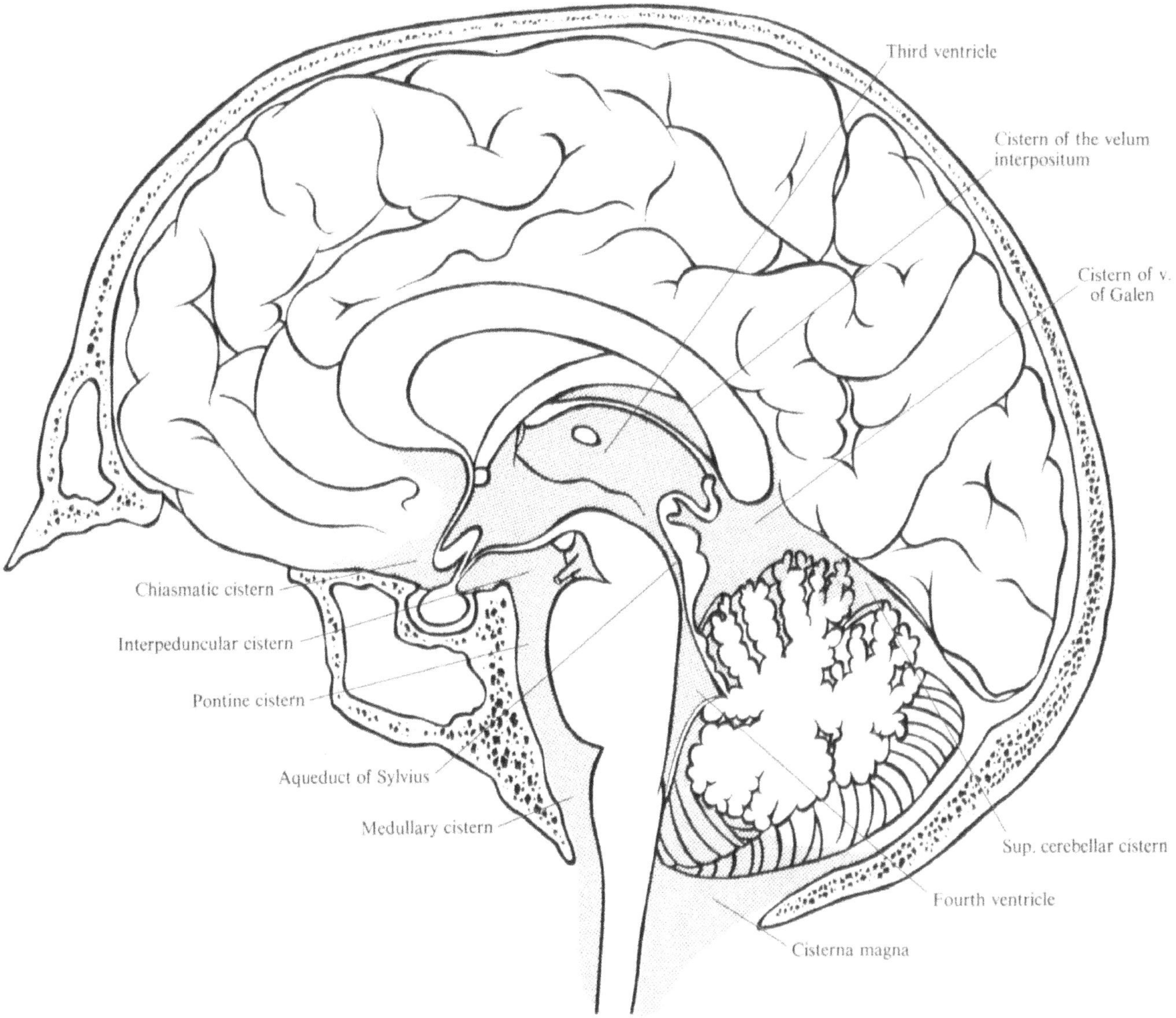

Fig. 209. Schematic drawing showing the cisterns of the posterior fossa, lateral view

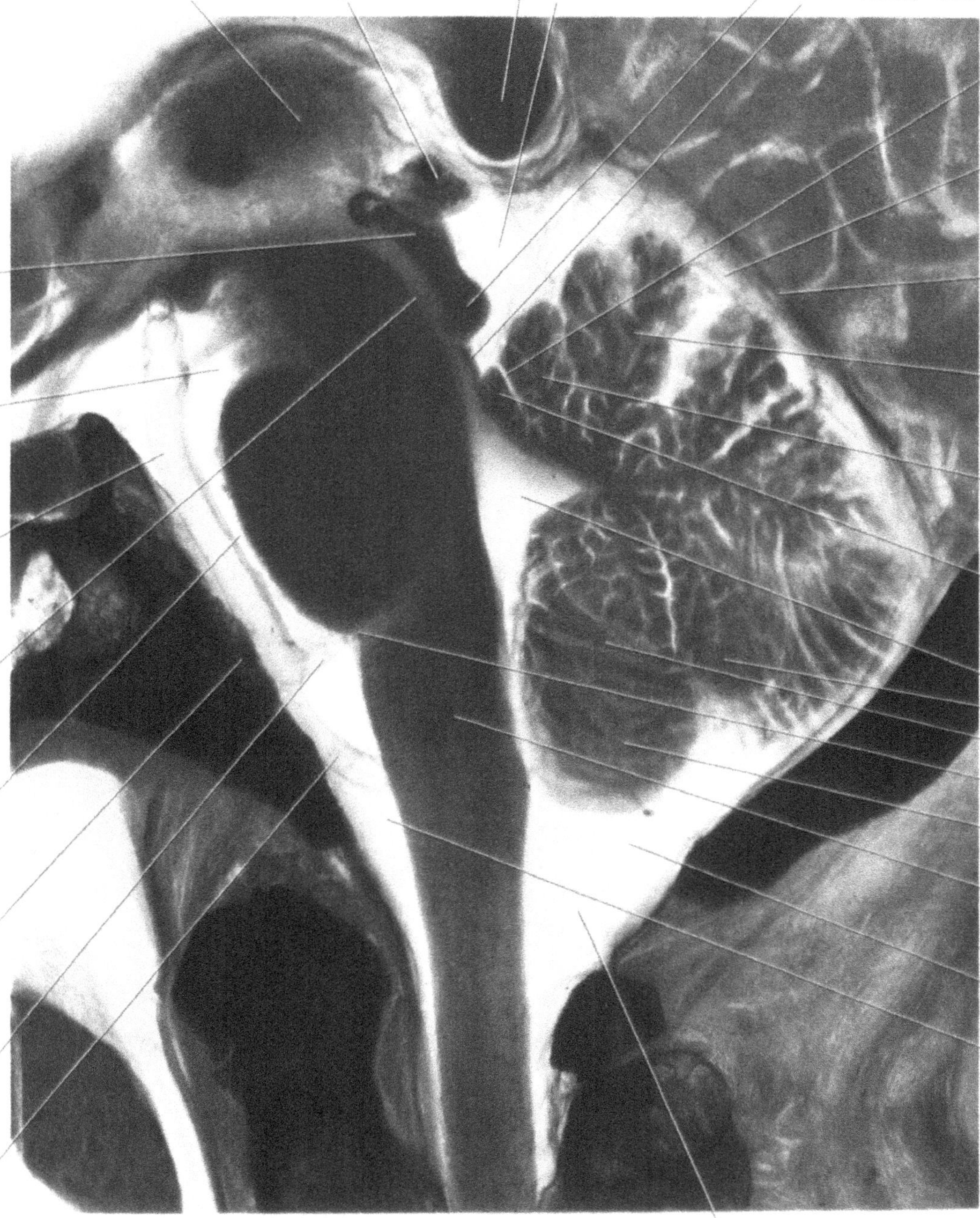

Fig. 210. Radiograph of a specimen, 1 cm thick, cut sagittally

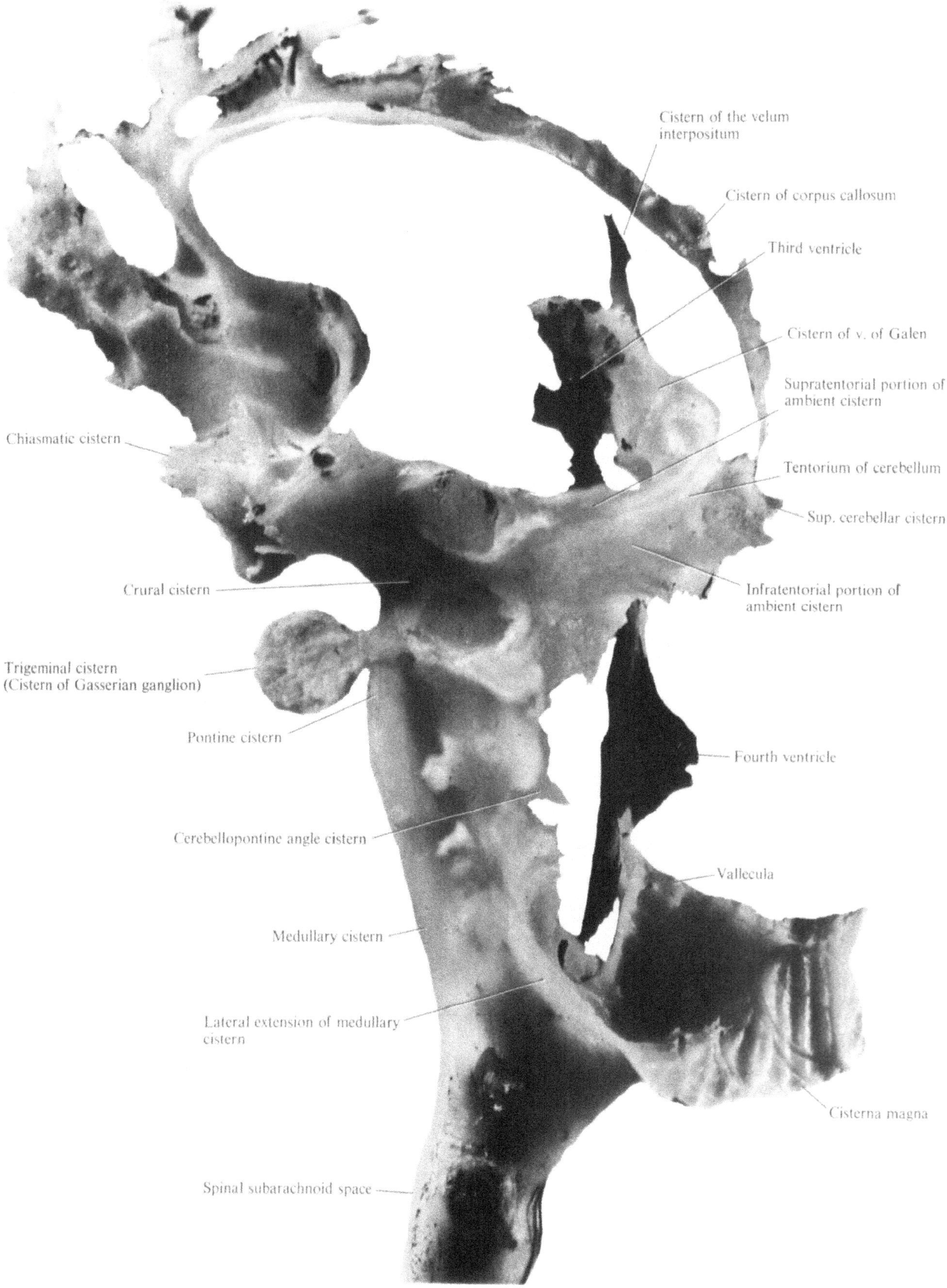

Fig. 211. Cast of the cisterns of the posterior fossa and of the fourth ventricle, lateral view

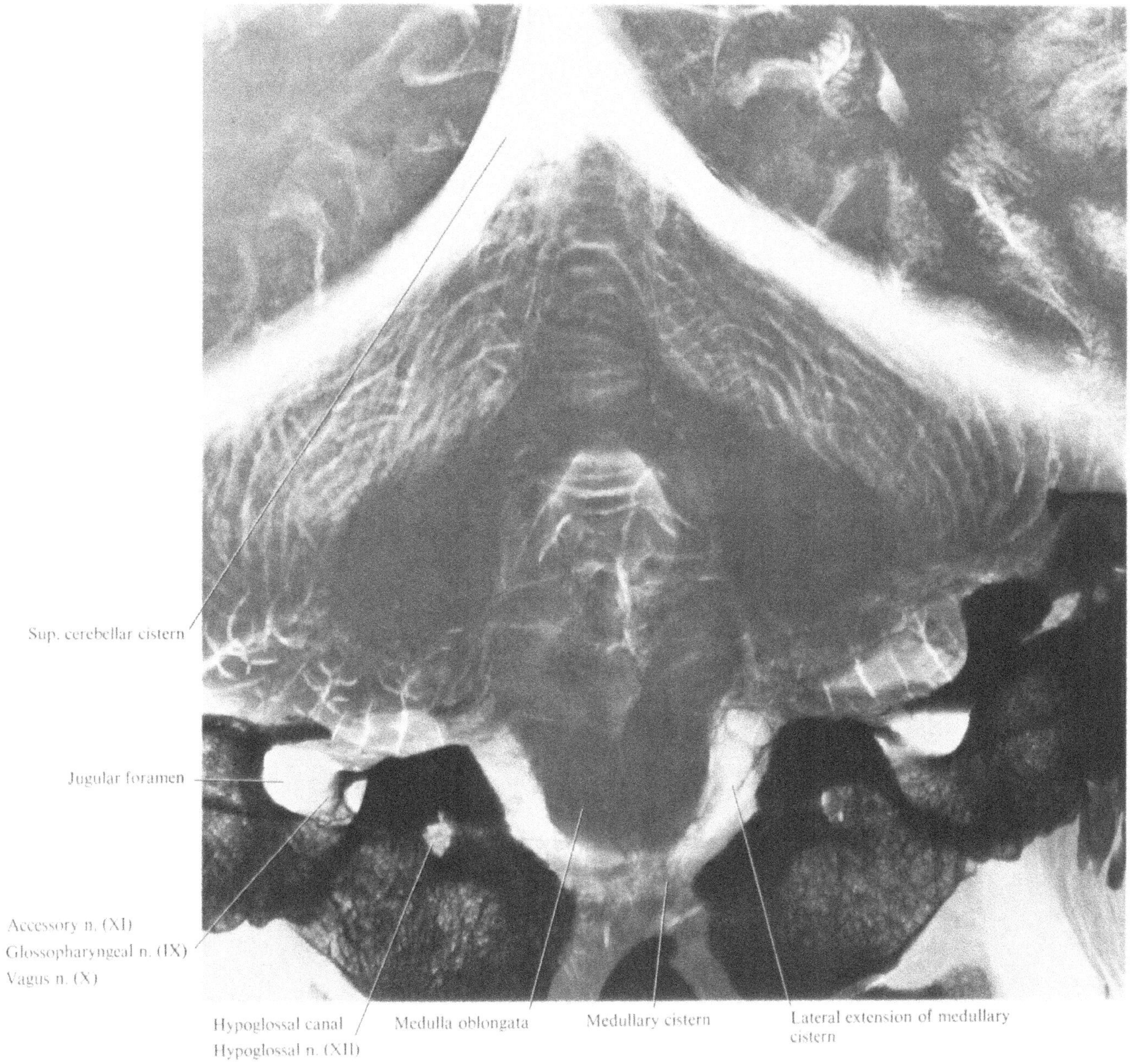

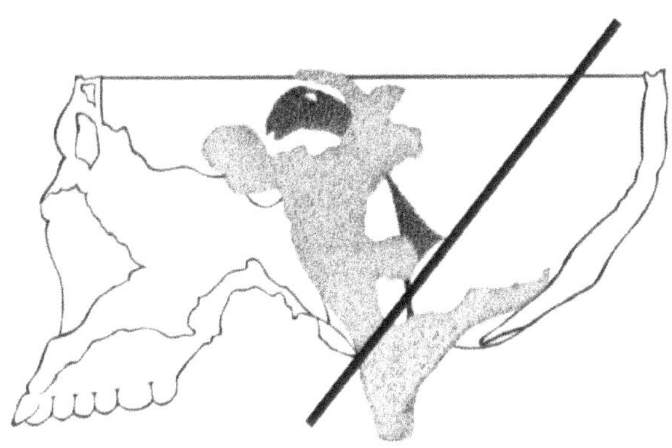

Fig. 212. Radiograph of a specimen, 1 cm thick, passing through the medullary cistern, frontal projection

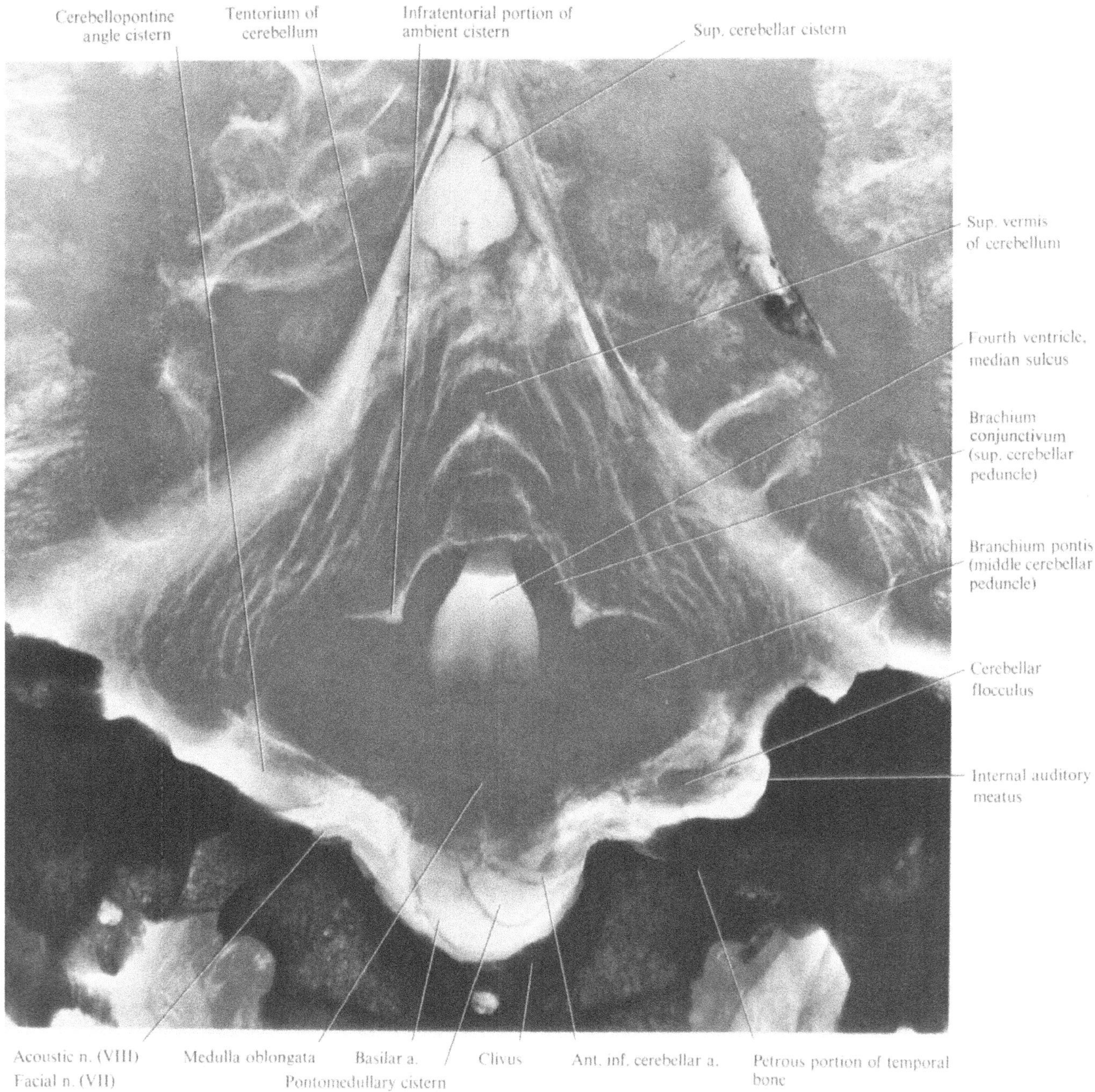

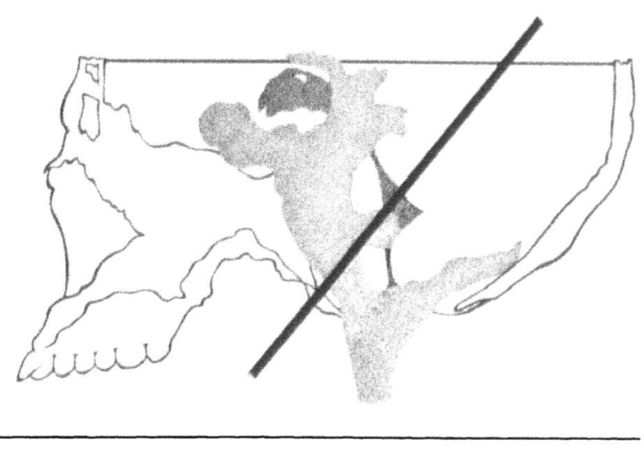

Fig. 213. Radiograph of a specimen, 1 cm thick, passing through the cerebellopontine angles, frontal projection

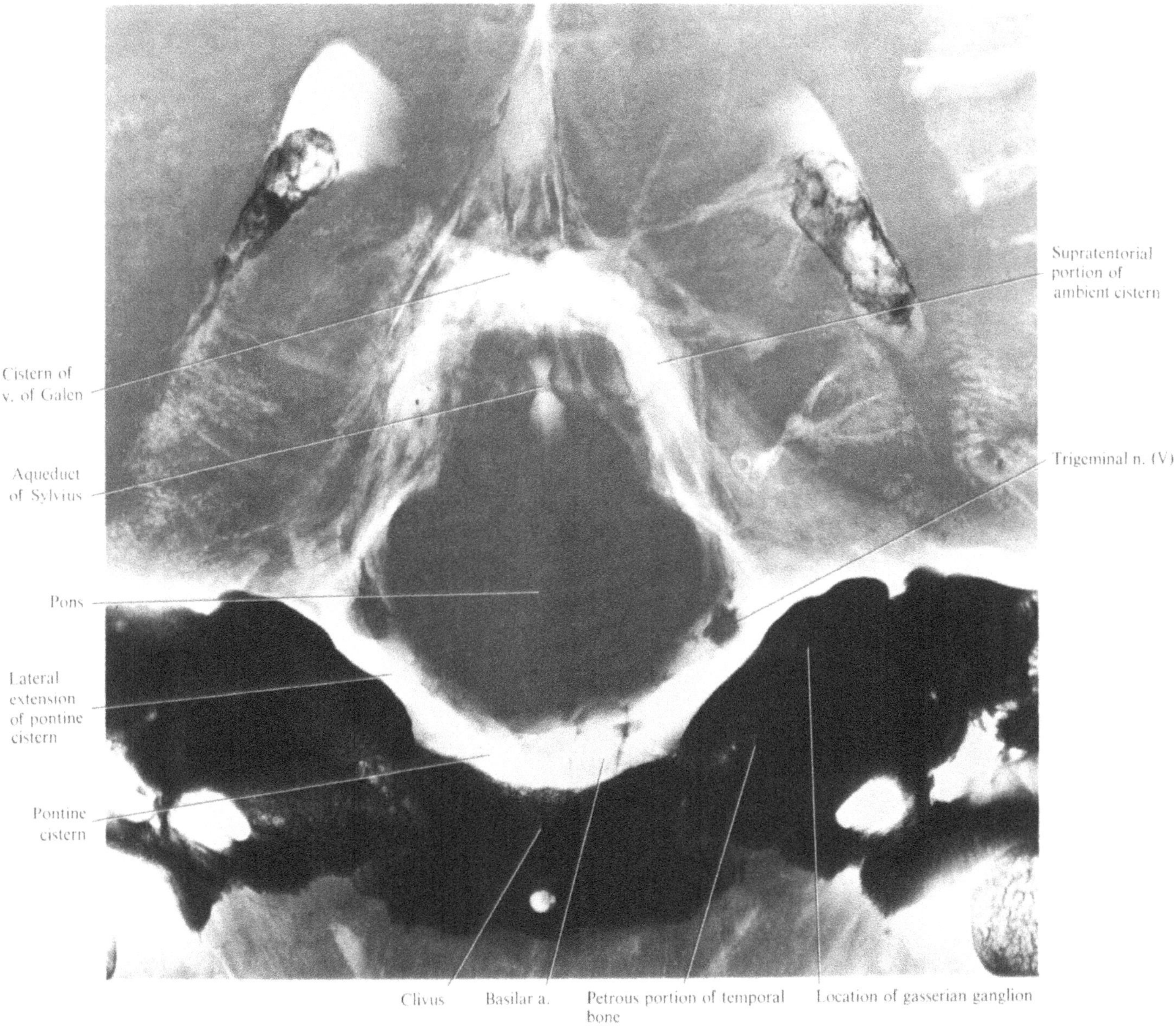

Supratentorial portion of ambient cistern
Cistern of v. of Galen
Aqueduct of Sylvius
Trigeminal n. (V)
Pons
Lateral extension of pontine cistern
Pontine cistern
Clivus
Basilar a.
Petrous portion of temporal bone
Location of gasserian ganglion

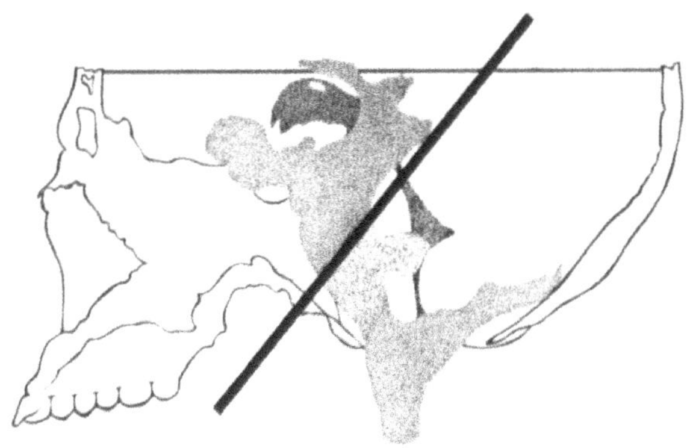

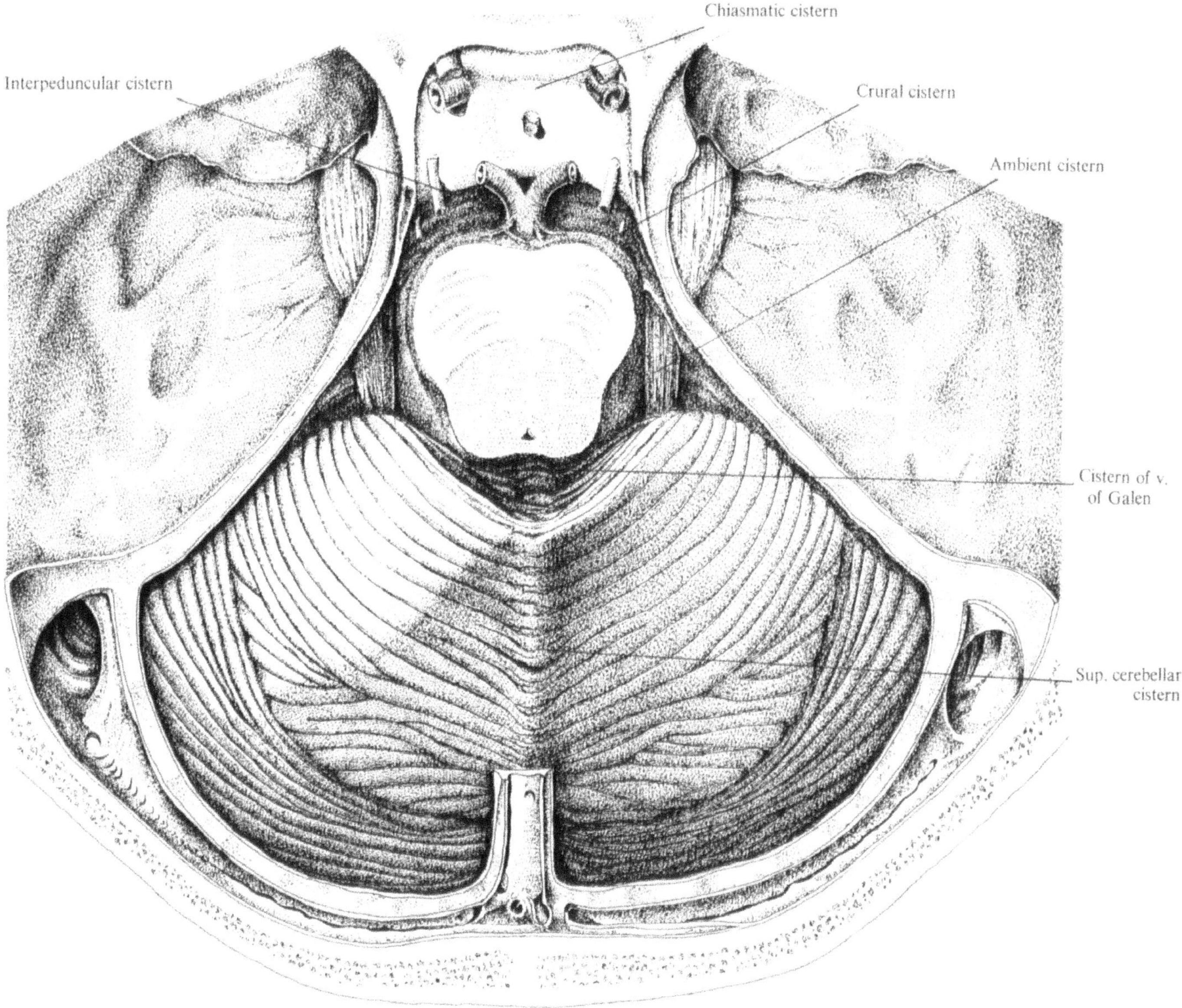

Fig. 215. Drawing of the cisterns at the tentorial incisura, superior view

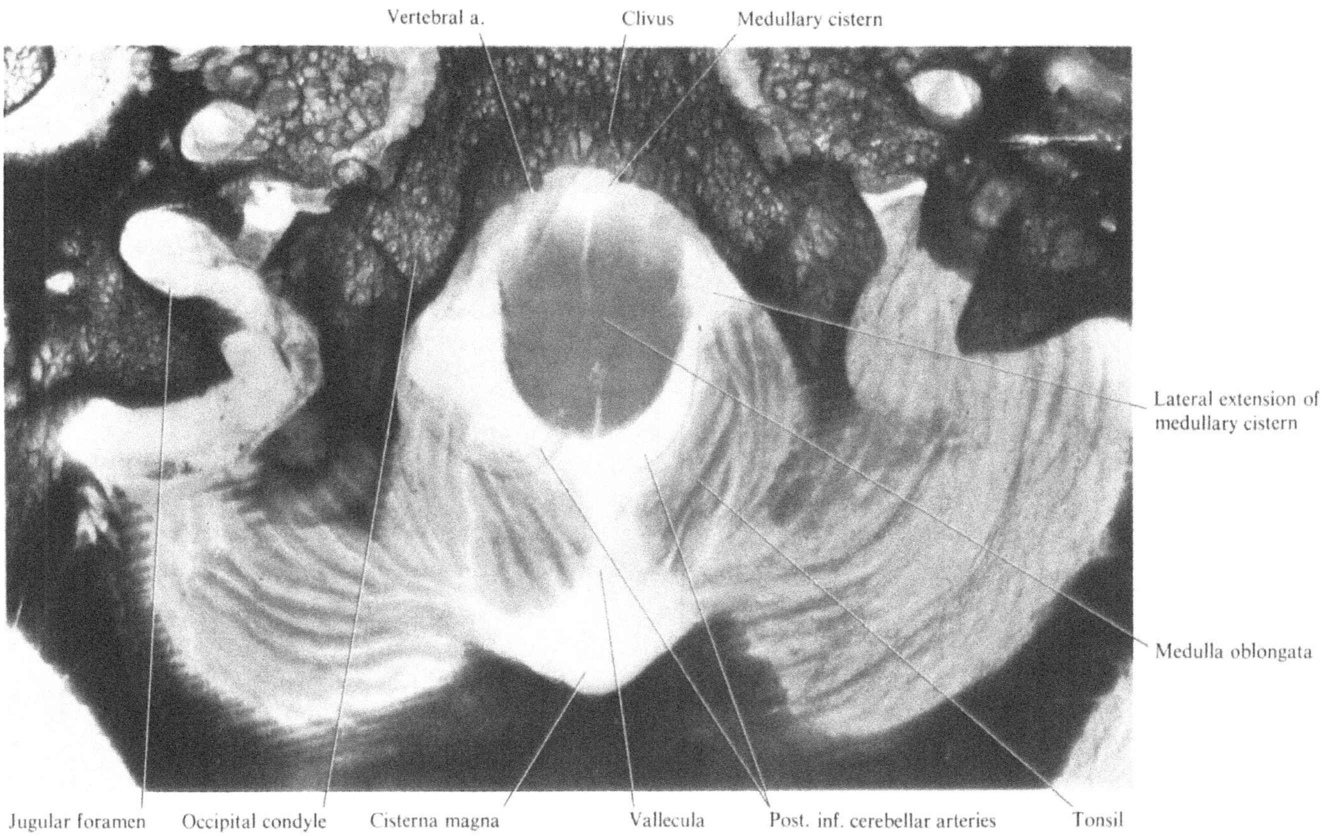

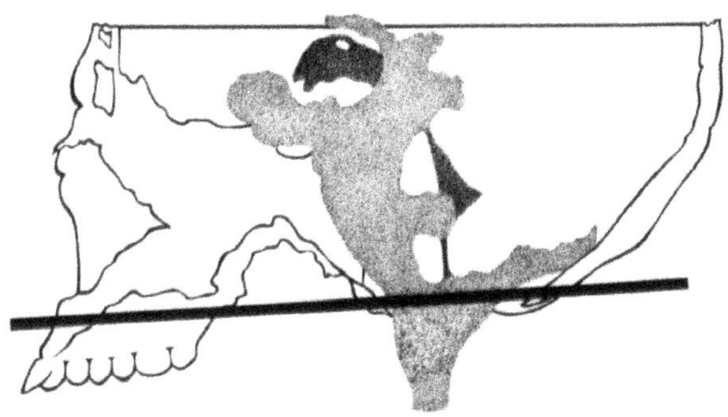

Fig. 216. Radiograph of a specimen, 1 cm thick, passing through the jugular foramina and the hypoglossal canals

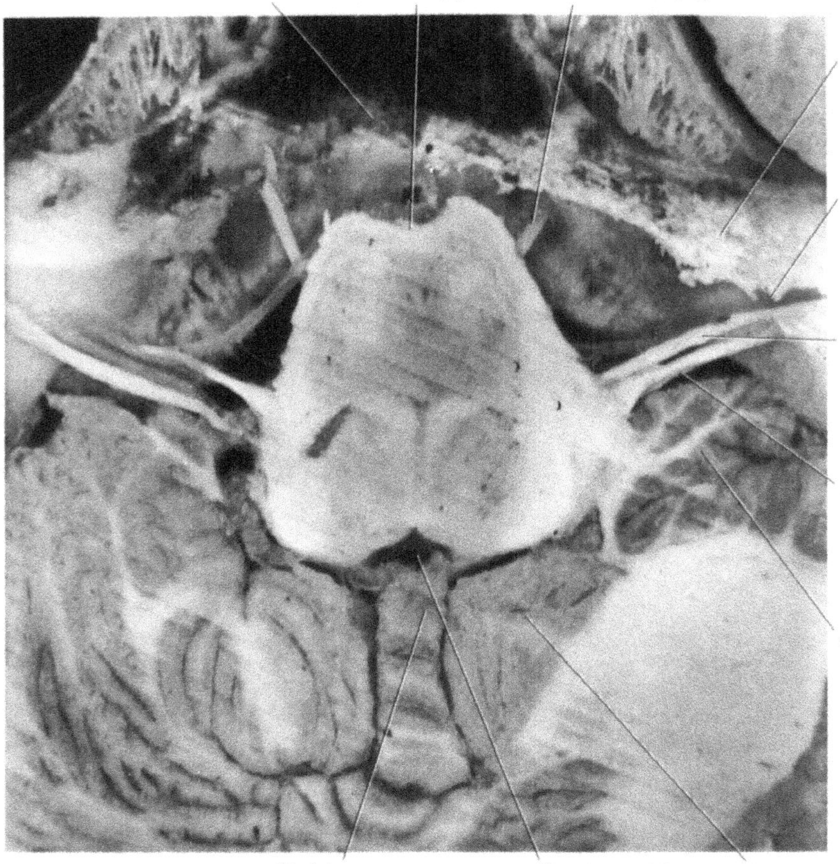

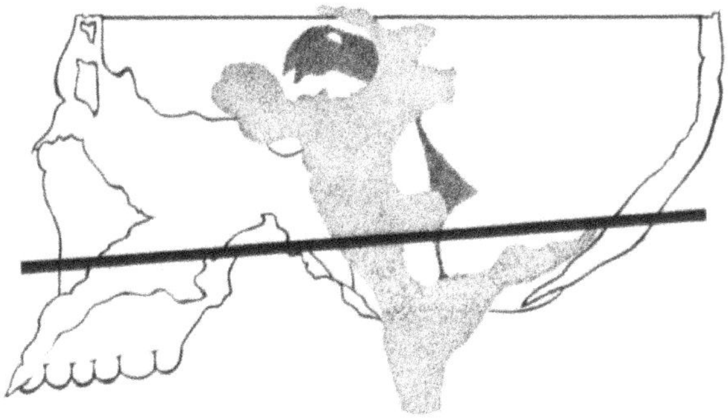

Fig. 217. Photograph of a horizontal section passing through the cerebellopontine angles

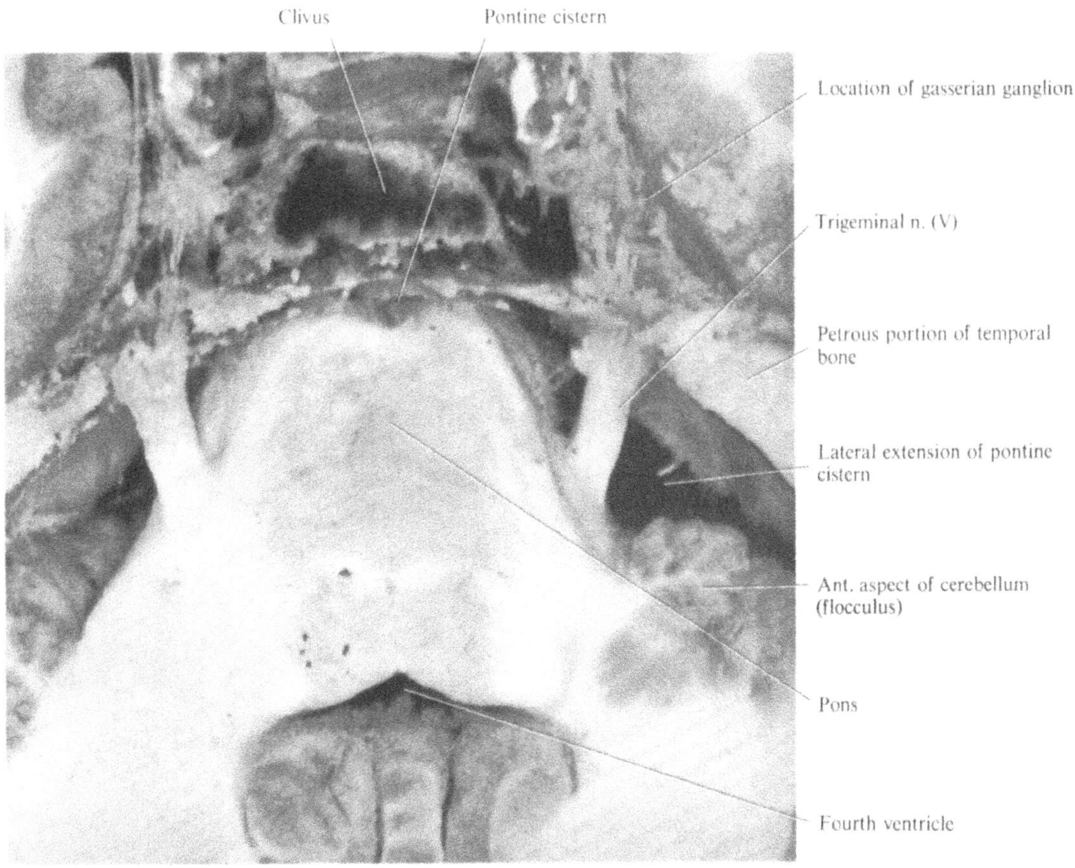

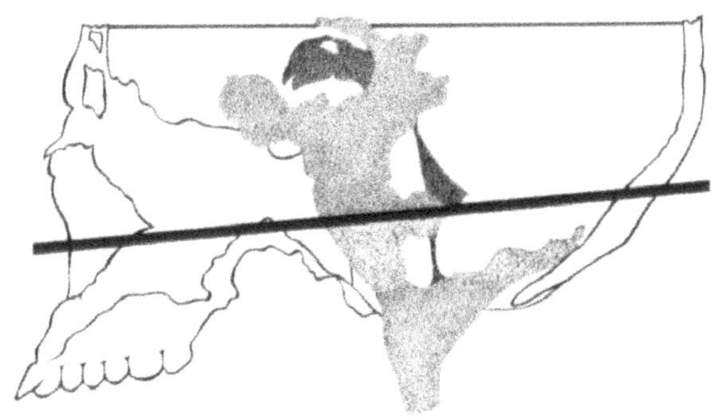

Fig. 218. Photograph of a horizontal section passing through the pontine cistern

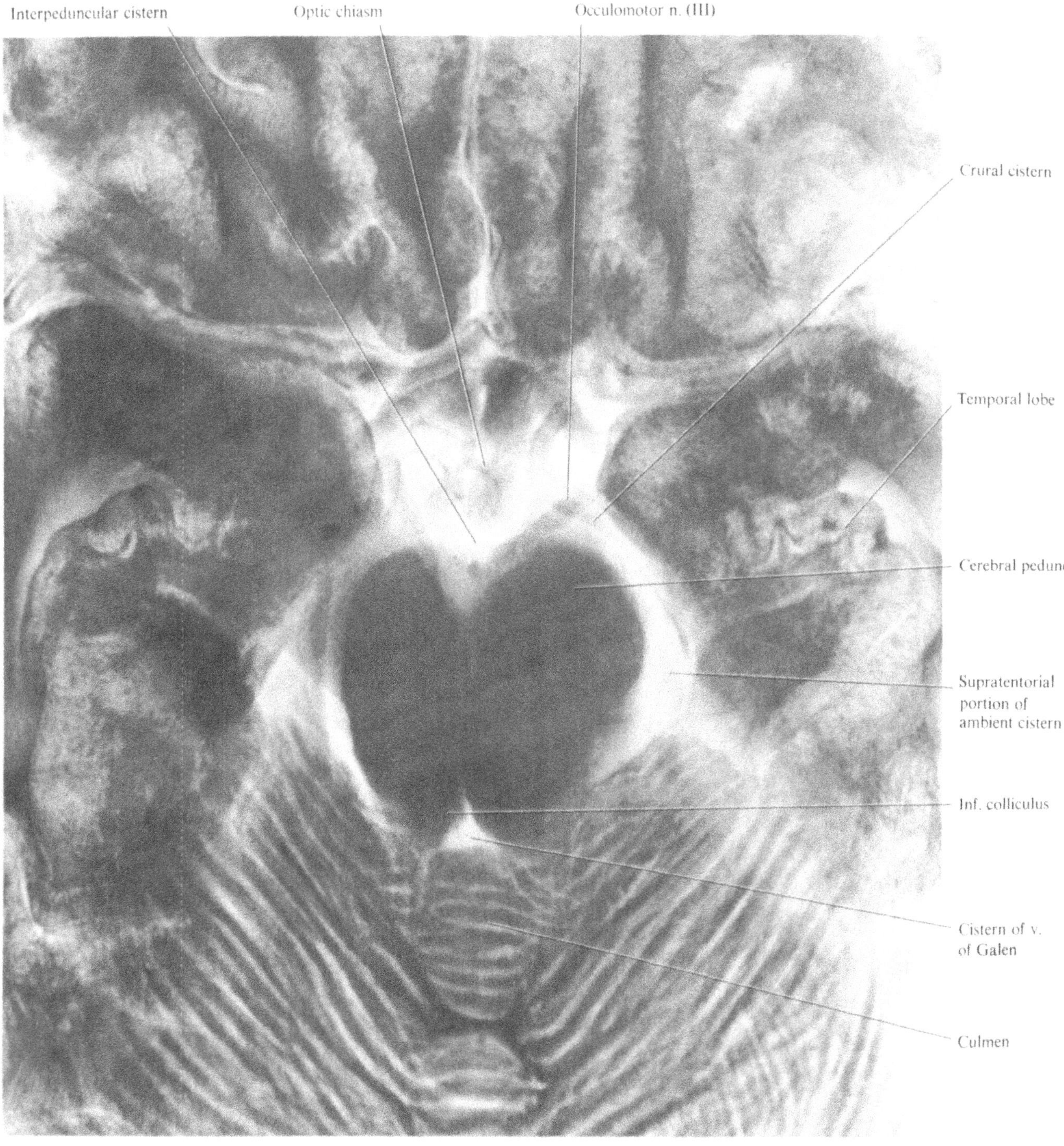

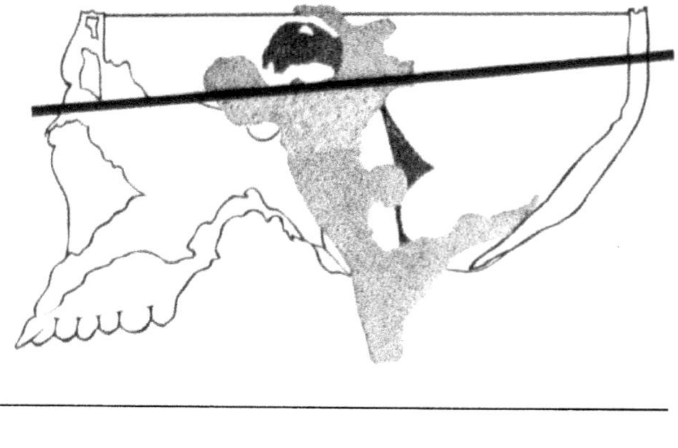

Fig. 219. Radiograph of a horizontal section, 1 cm thick, passing through the cistern of the vein of Galen and the interpeduncular cistern

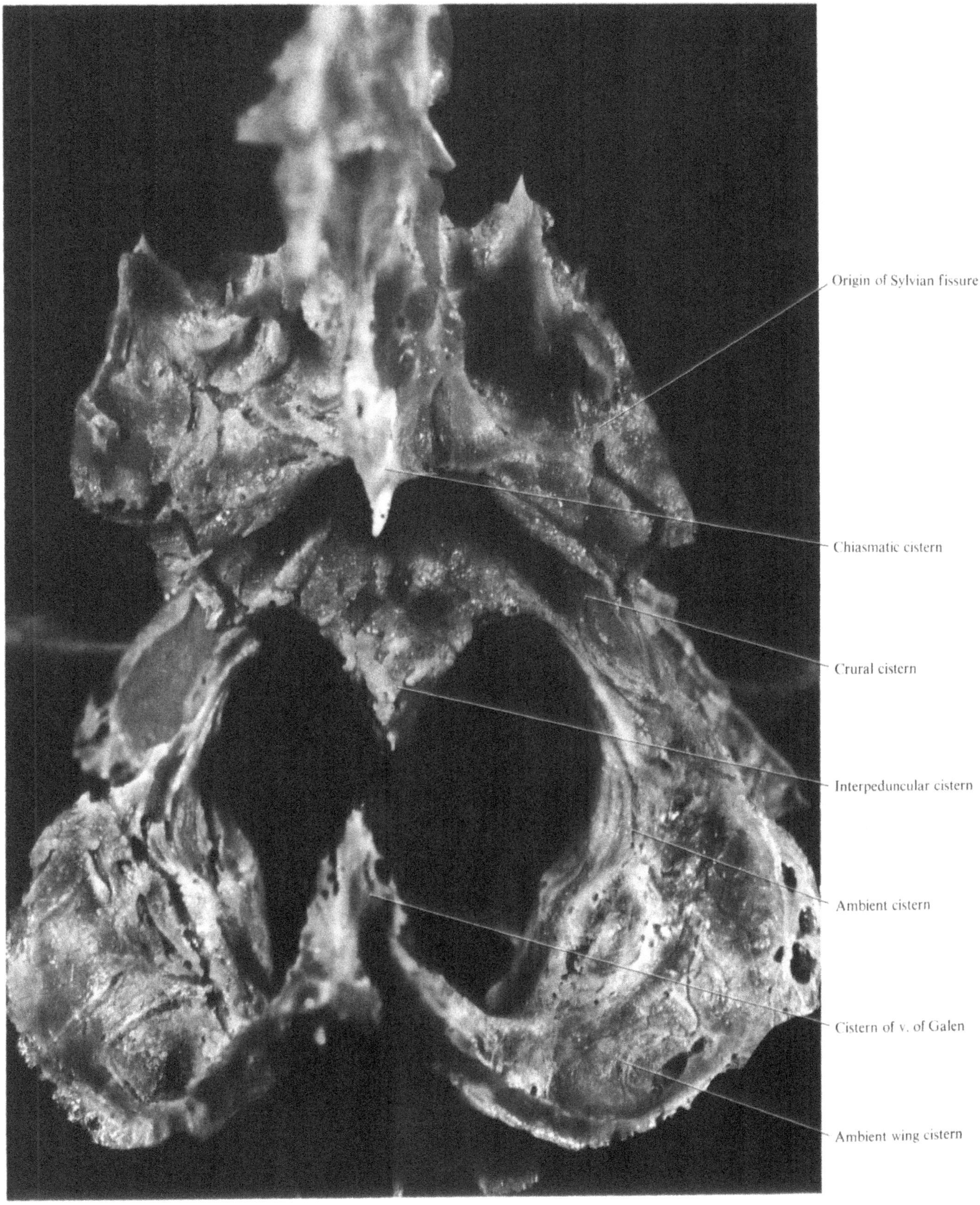

Fig. 220. Cast of the cisterns at the tentorial incisura

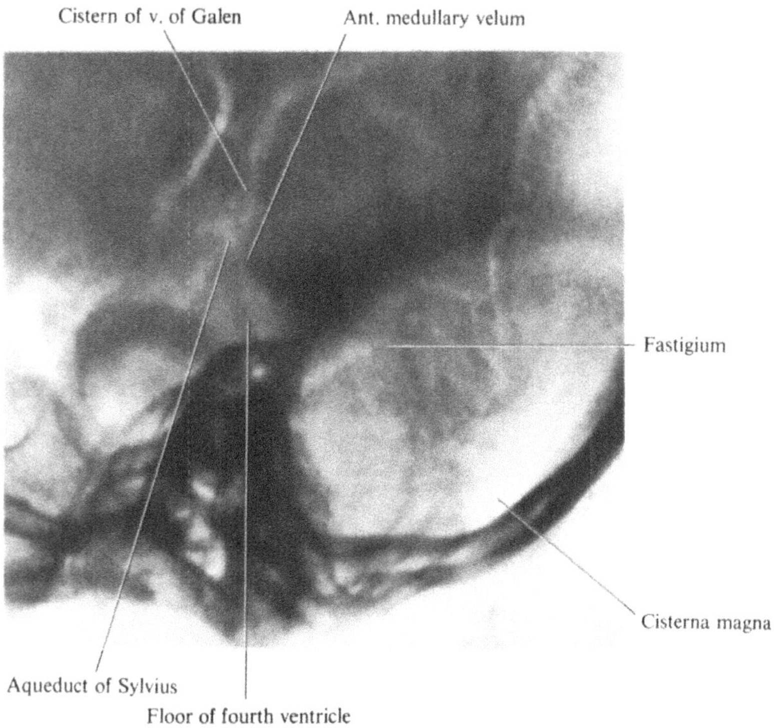

Fig. 221 A

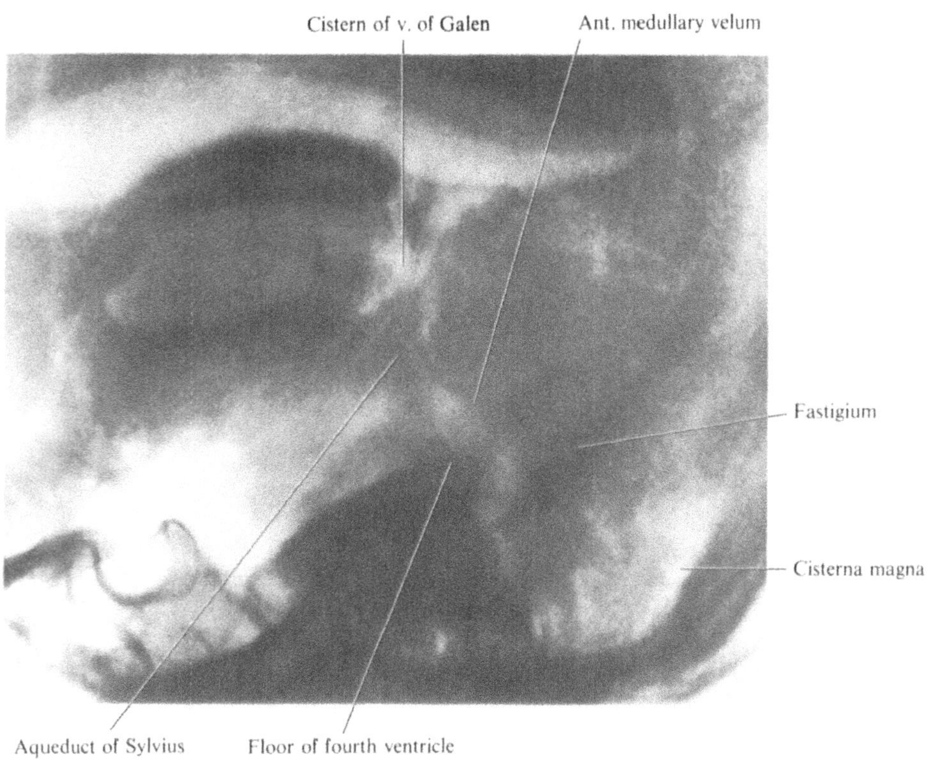

Fig. 221 B

Fig. 221 A–B. Pneumoencephalograms, lateral views ▷

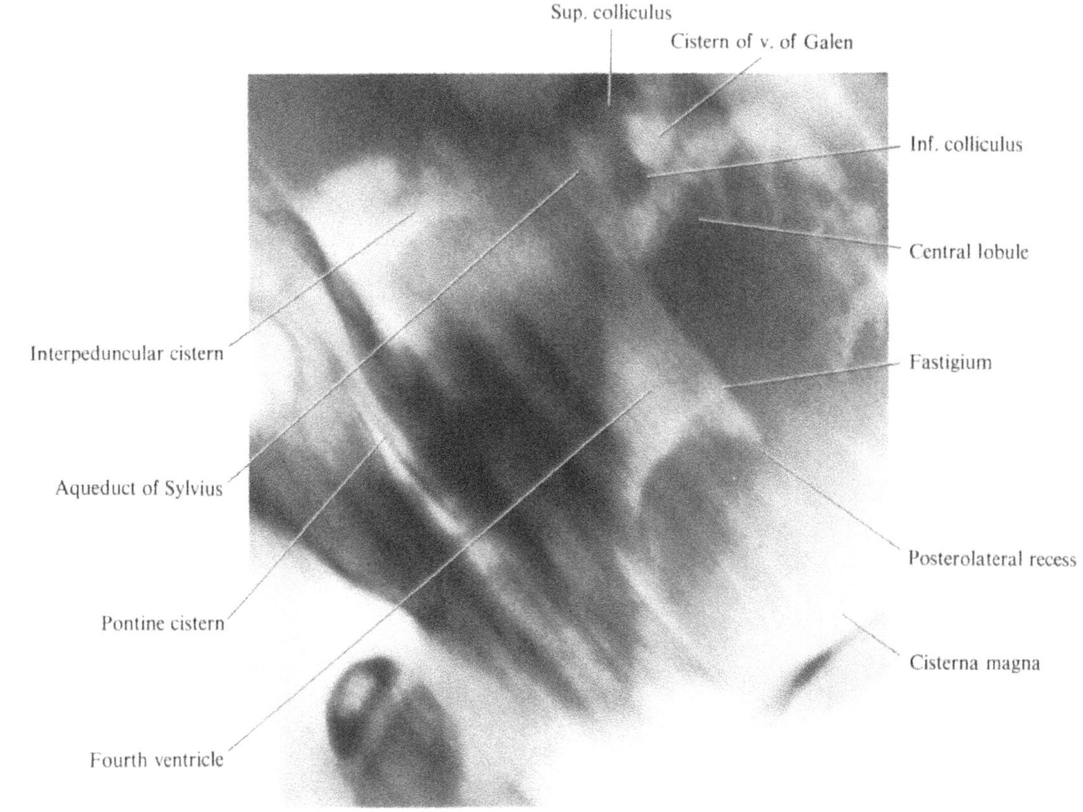

Fig. 222 A

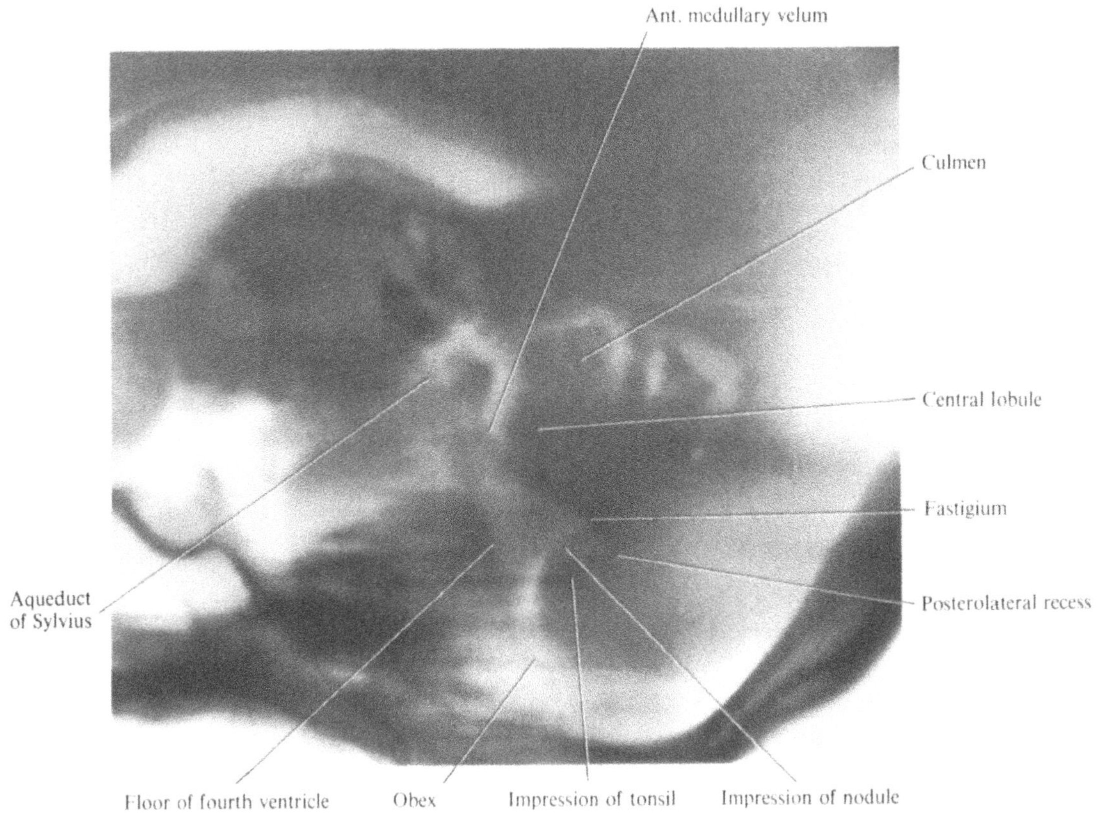

Fig. 222 B

Fig. 222 A–D. Pneumoencephalograms, sagittal tomograms ▷

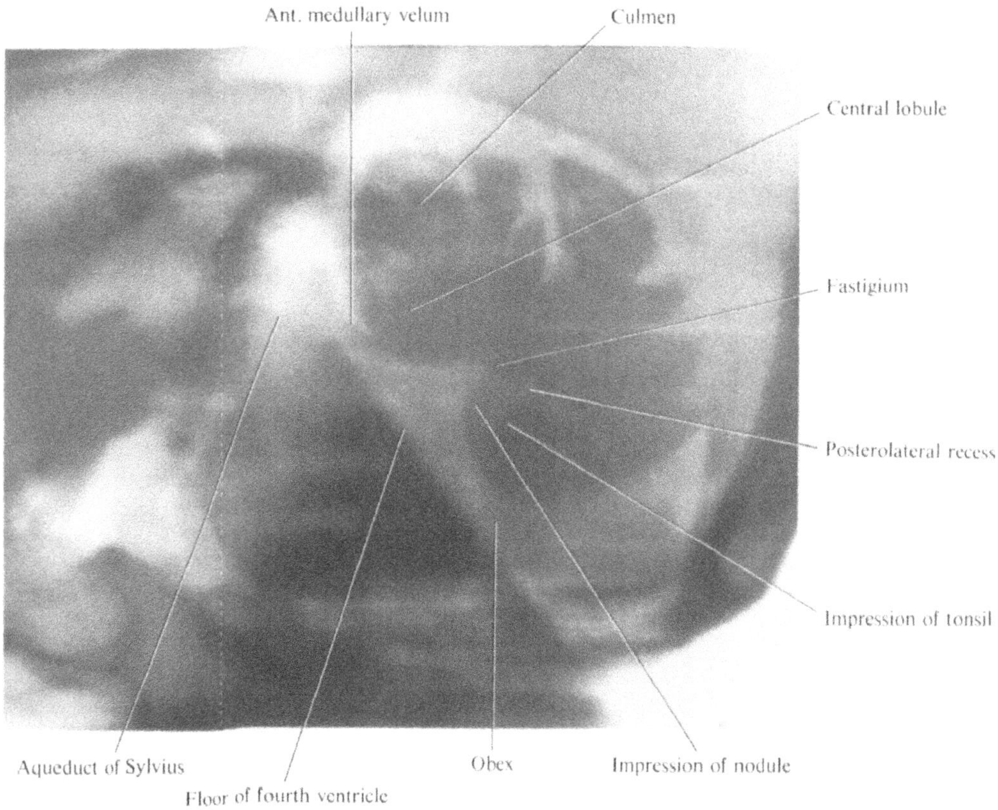

Fig. 222C

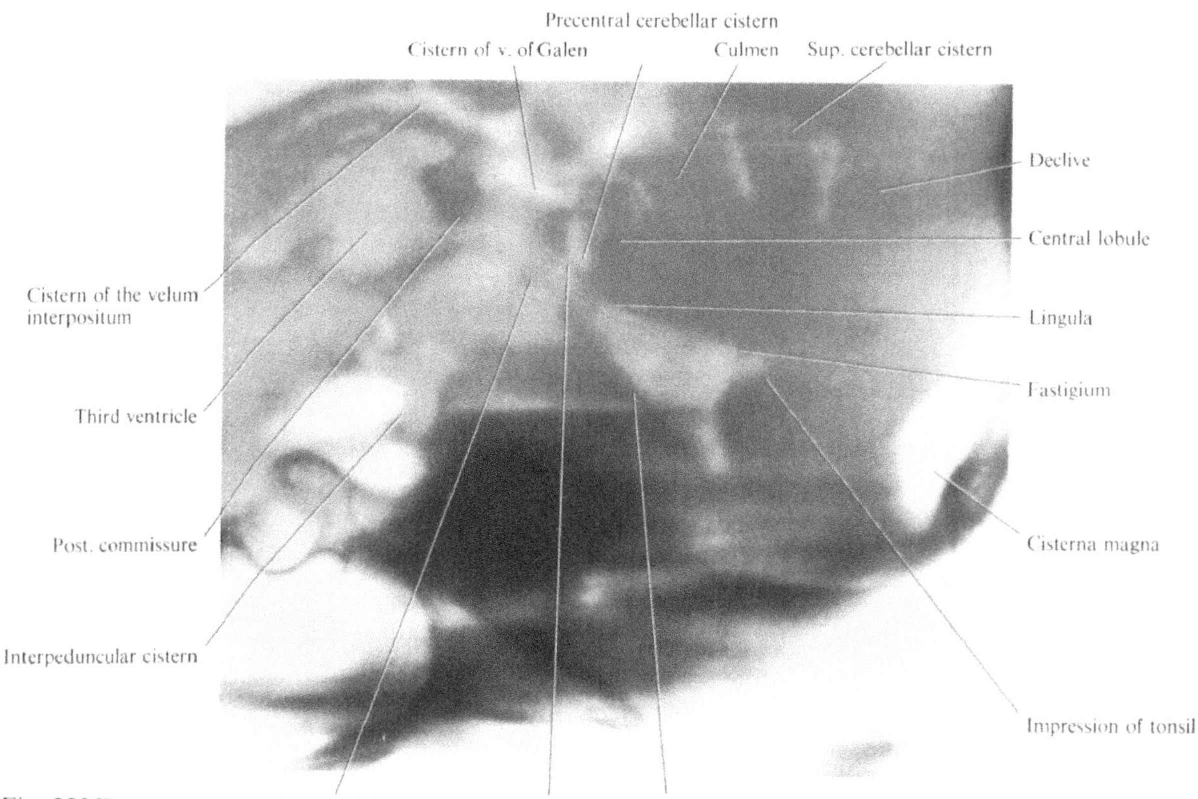

Fig. 222D

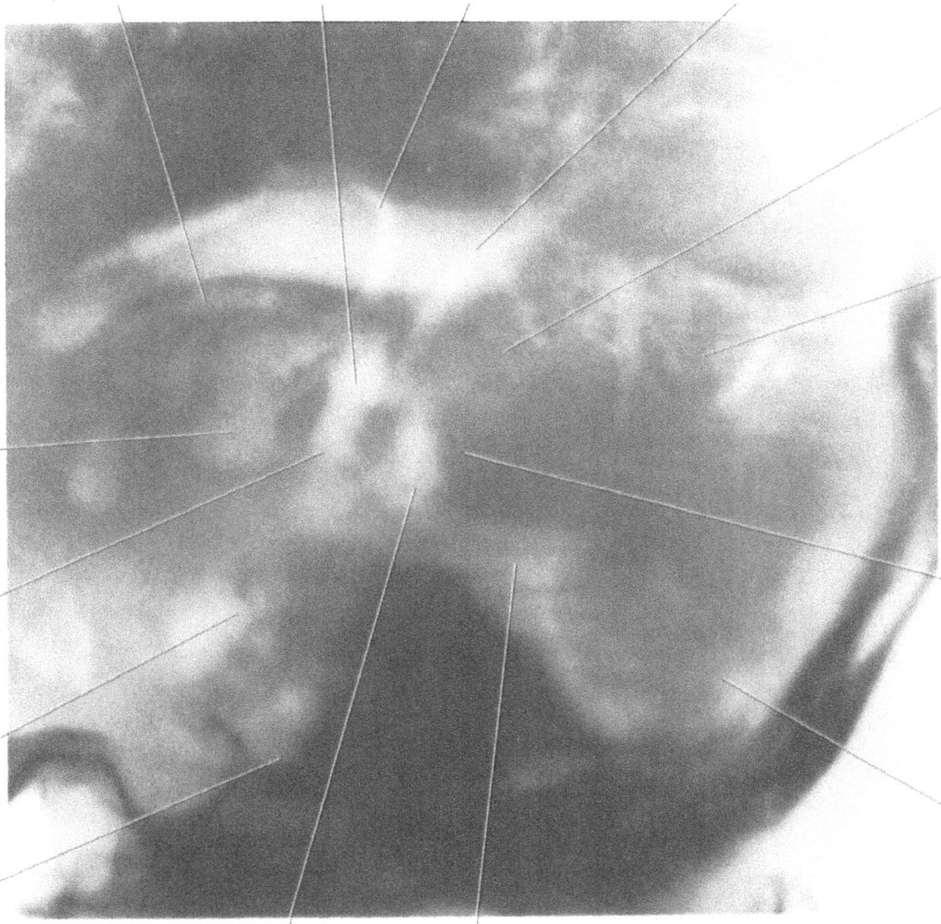

Fig. 223A

Fig. 223A–B. Pneumoencephalograms, sagittal tomograms ▷

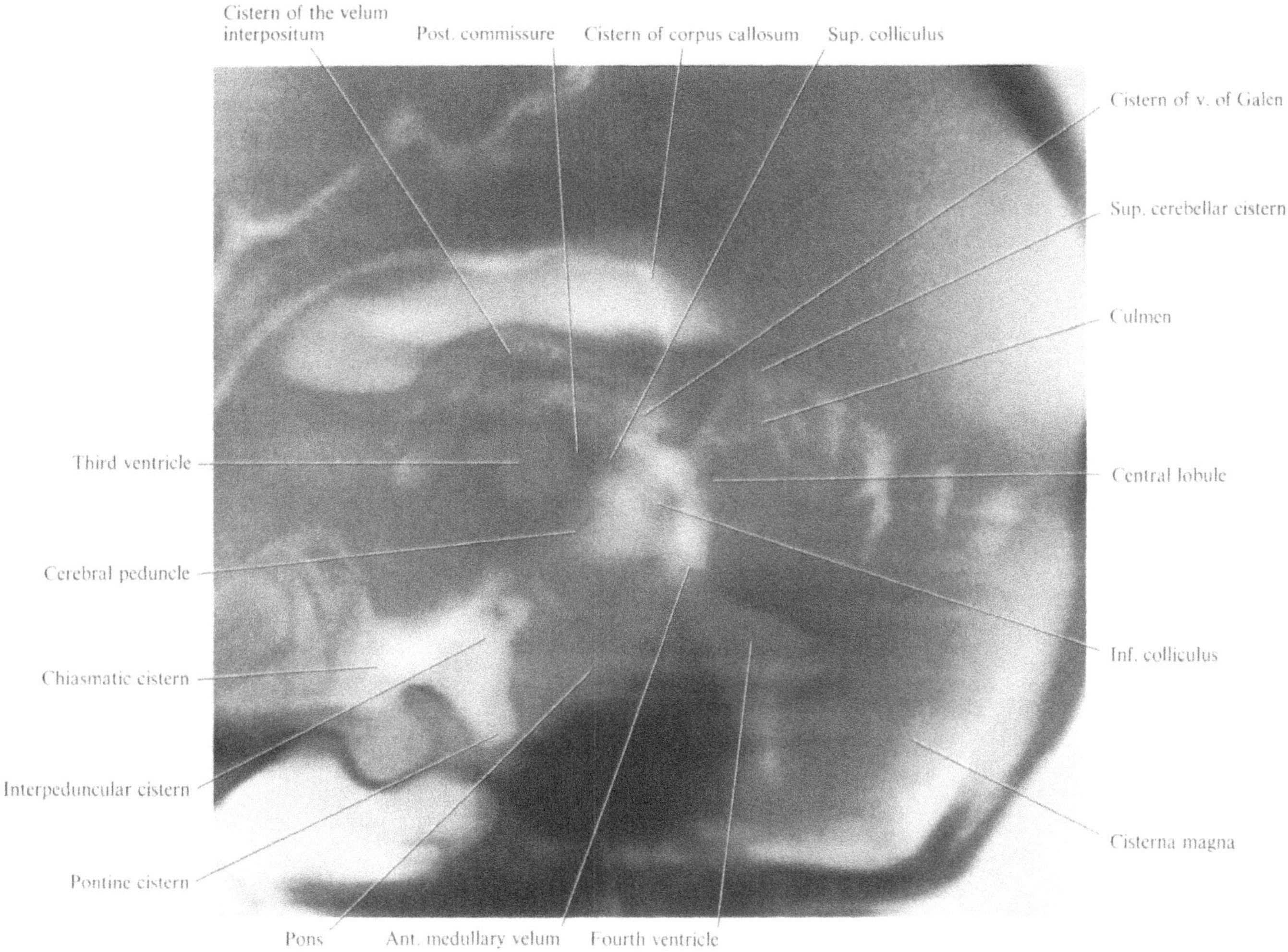

Fig. 223 B. Pneumoencephalogram, sagittal tomogram

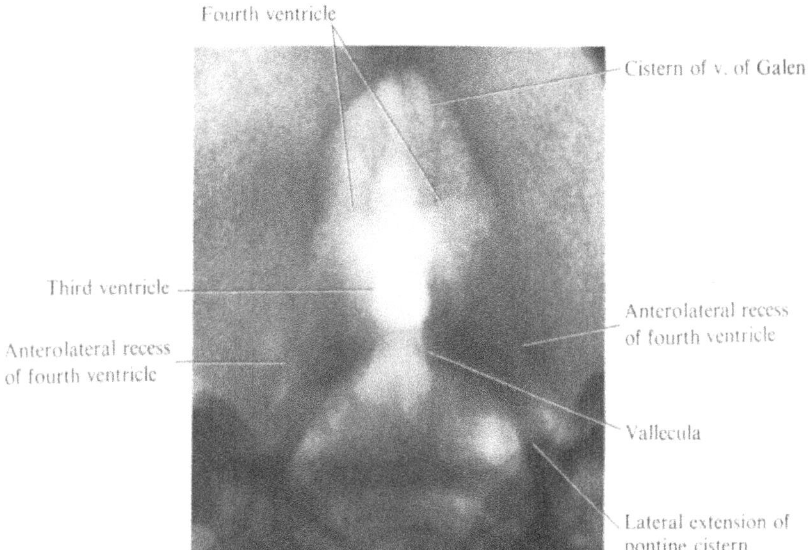

◁
Fig. 224 A

▷
Fig. 224 A–B. Pneumoencephalograms, frontal projections

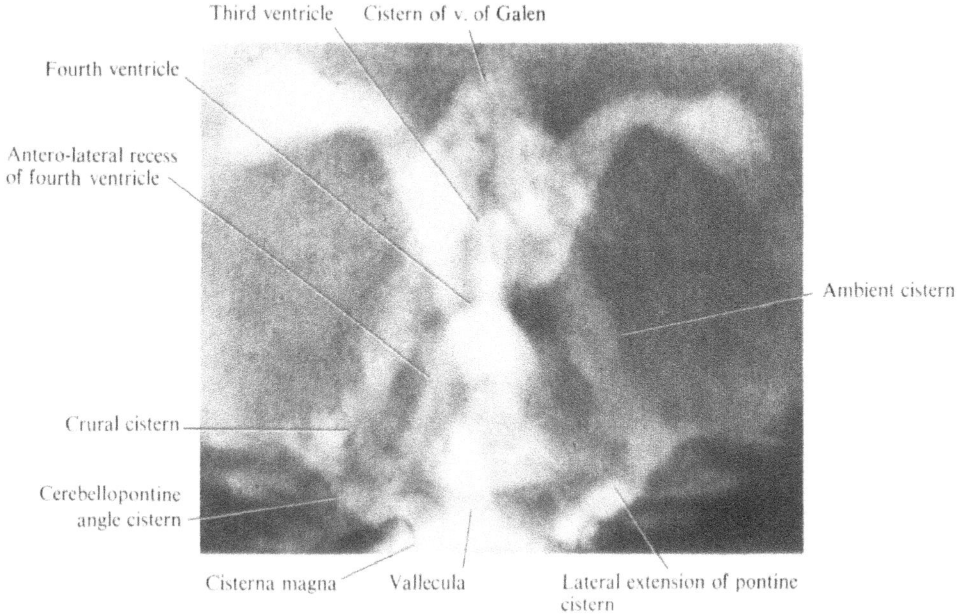

Fig. 224 B

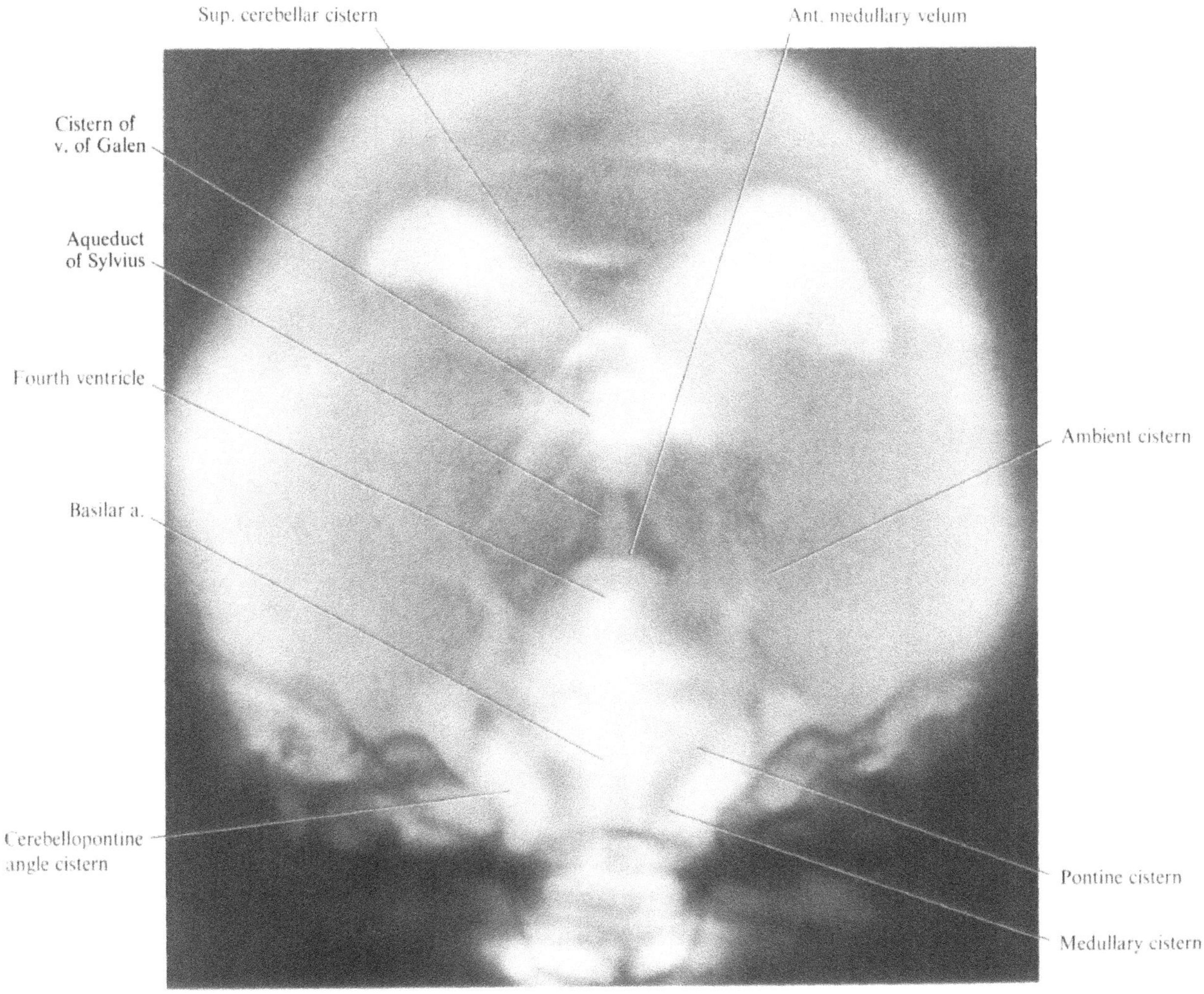

Fig. 225. Pneumoencephalogram, half-axial projection

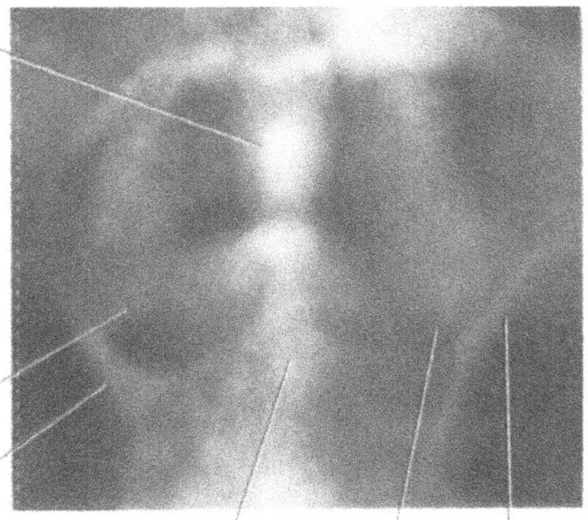

Fig. 226 A

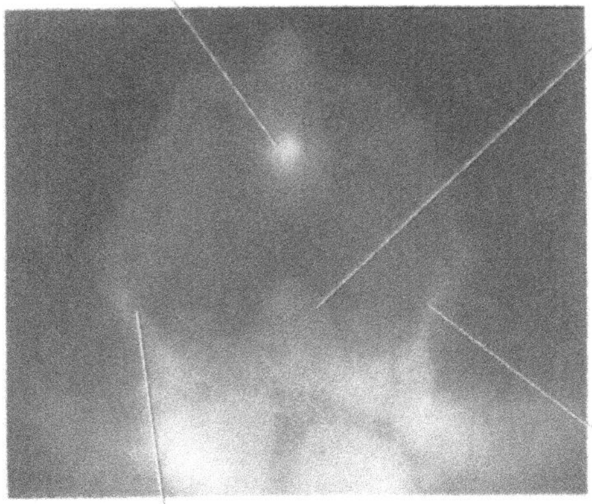

Fig. 226 B

Fig. 226 A–B. Pneumoencephalograms, frontal tomograms passing through the interpeduncular and crural cisterns

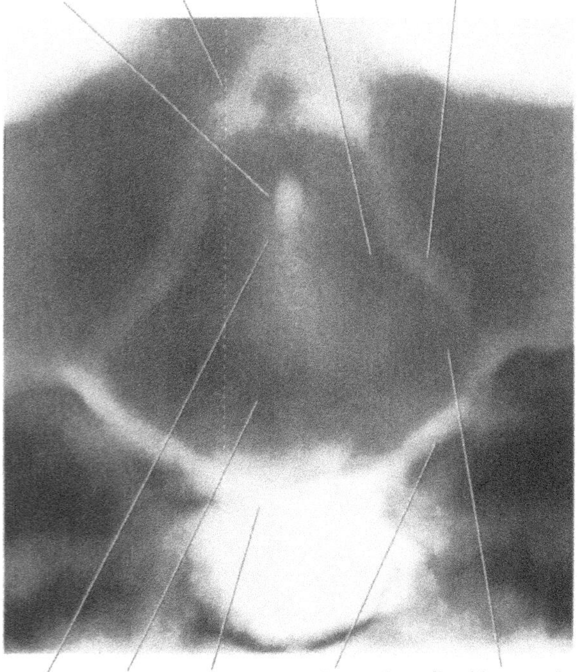

Fig. 227 A

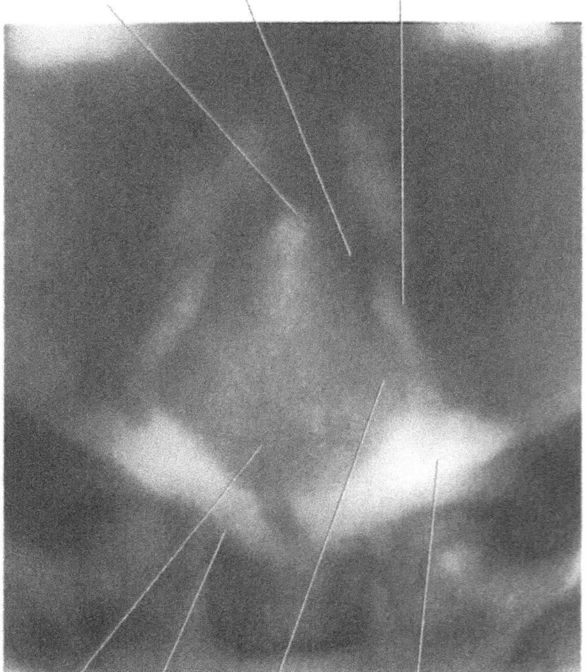

Fig. 227 B

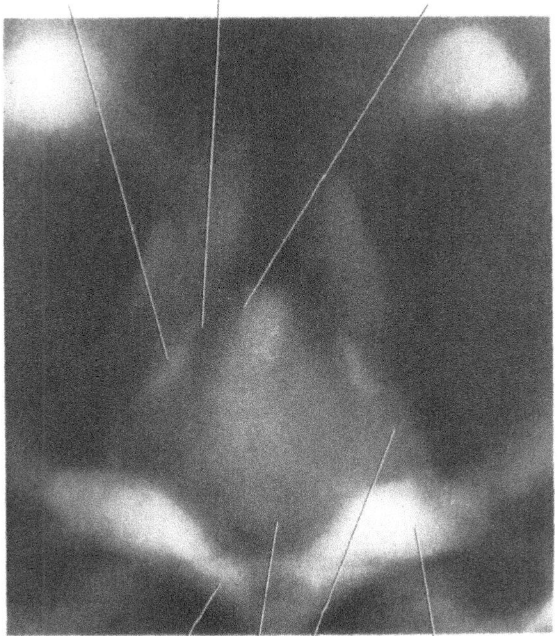

Fig. 227C

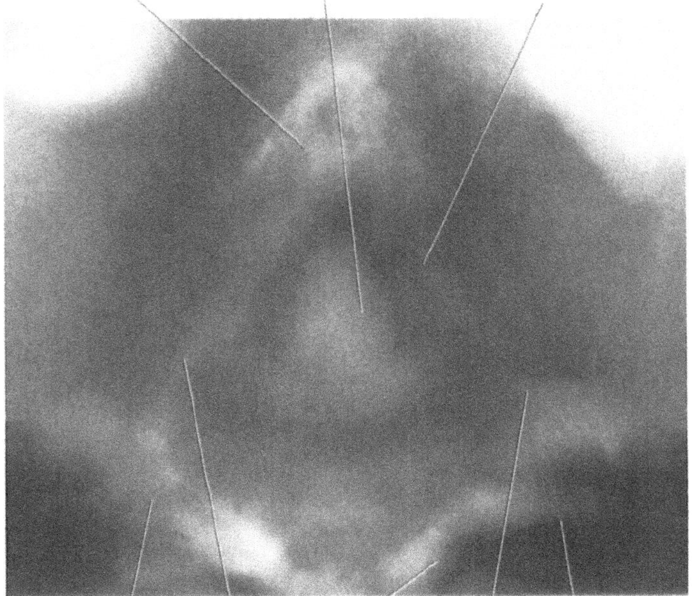

Fig. 227D

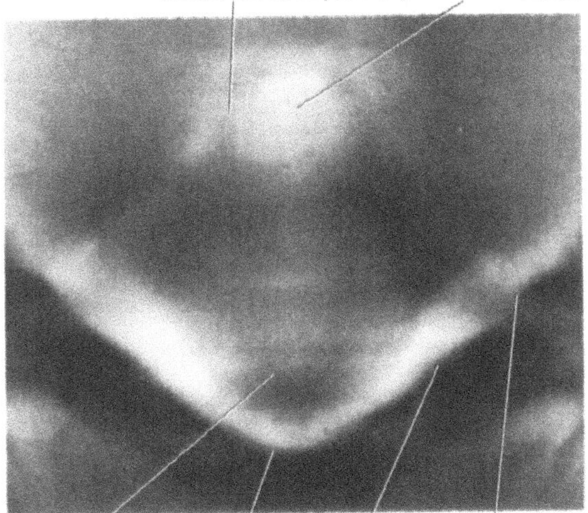

Fig. 227E

Fig. 227A–E. Pneumoencephalograms, frontal tomograms, passing through the pontine cistern

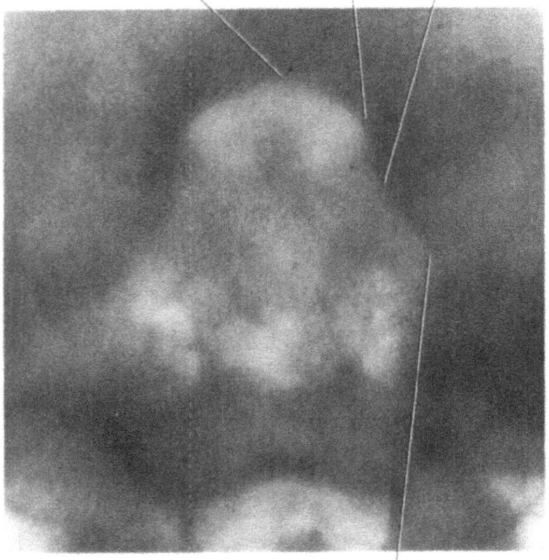

Fig. 228A

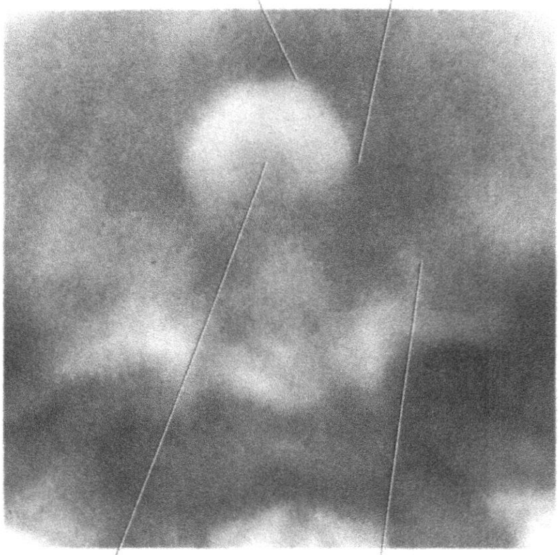

Fig. 228B

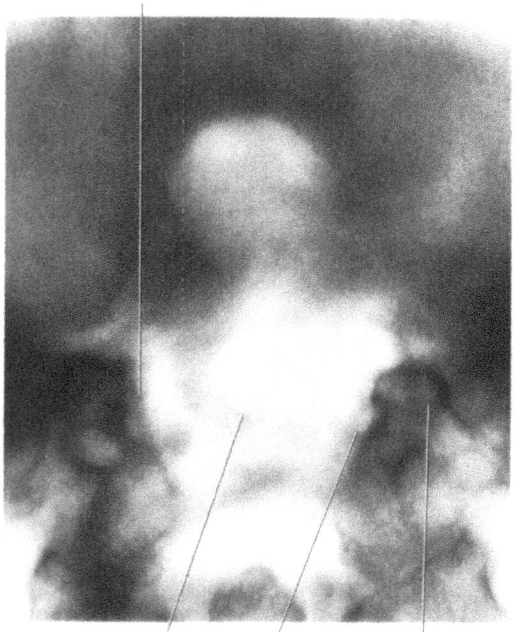

Fig. 228C

Fig. 228A–C. Pneumoencephalograms, frontal tomograms through the fourth ventricle

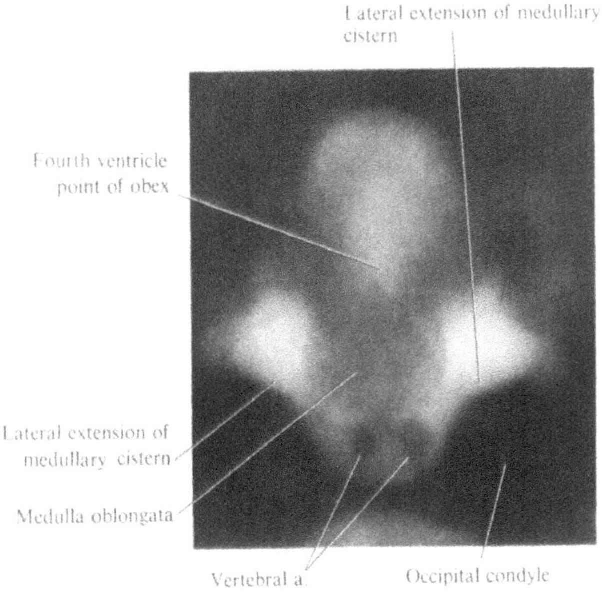

Fig. 229 A

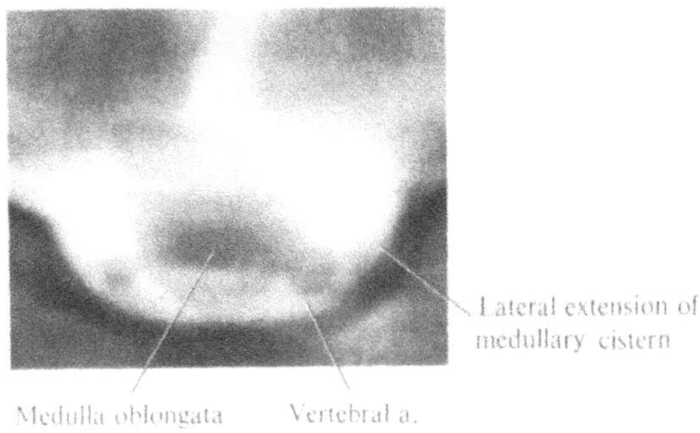

Fig. 229 B

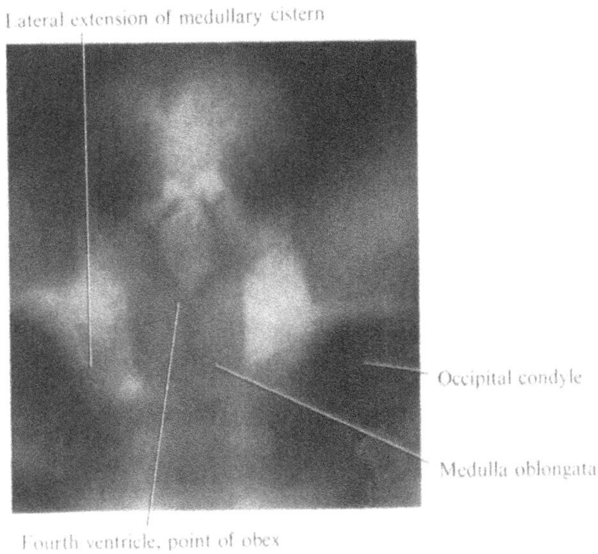

Fig. 229 C

Fig. 229 A–C. Pneumoencephalograms, frontal tomograms, passing through the medullary cistern

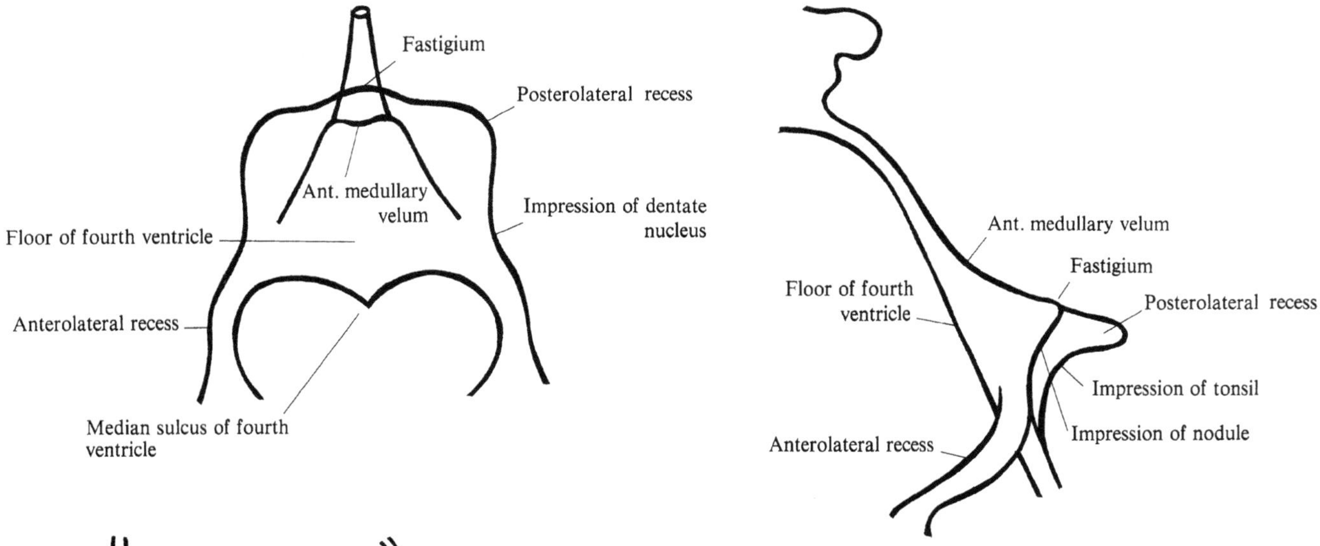

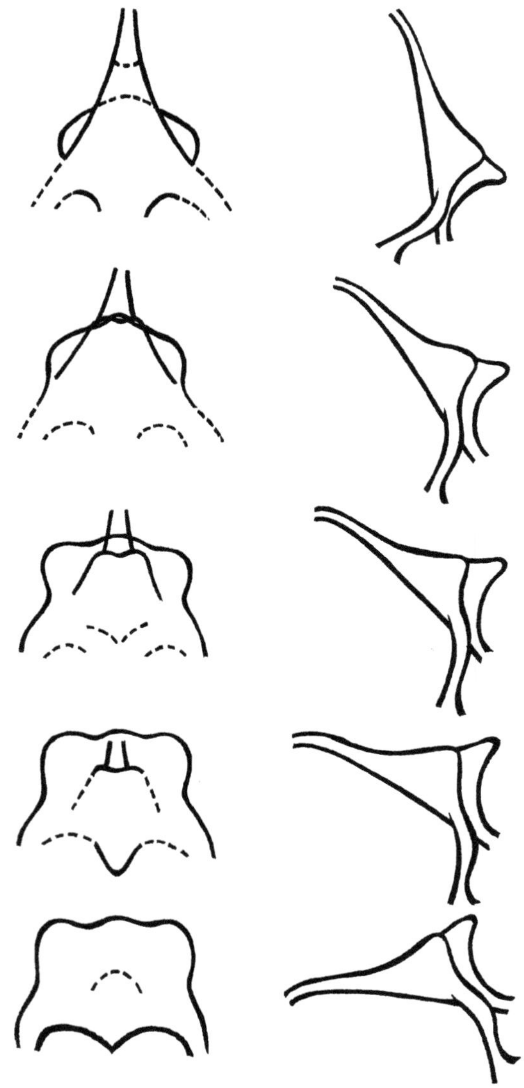

Fig. 230. Schematic representation of the fourth ventricle in frontal and lateral projections, according to CORALLES and GREITZ (1972)

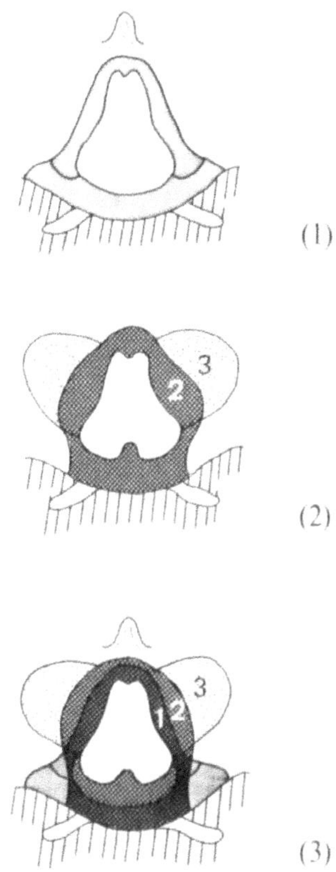

Fig. 231. Schematic representation of the cisterns of the posterior fossa as seen in the semiaxial projection during pneumoencephalography (after LILIEQUIST, 1959)

(1) Infratentorial portion of the circumpeduncular cistern
(2) Supratentorial portion of the circumpeduncular cistern
(3) Ambient wing (retropulvinar) cistern

Chapter 2

Arteries of the Vertebrobasilar System

I. Anatomic Study of the Arteries of the Vertebrobasilar System*

The vertebral arteries, basilar trunk and their branches provide the vascular supply to the brainstem and cerebellum. The anatomy of these arteries has been studied by STOPFORD (1917), FOIX and HILLEMAND (1925) and LAZORTHES, POULHES and ESPAGNO (1950).
In our laboratory, we have studied 45 specimens in which the vertebrobasilar system was selectively injected (SCIALFA, RAYBAUD, MICHOTEY and BANK, 1976). Despite their fixed territories of vascular supply, numerous variations in the origins and courses of these vessels hamper their anatomic study. For this reason we have included percentage values for the incidences of the various origins, numbers, courses and vascular territories of each major vessel.

This study is divided into the following sections:
Intracranial vertebral artery
Basilar trunk
Branches to the brainstem
Branches to the cerebellum

1. Intracranial Segment of the Vertebral Artery
(Figs. 232, 233, 238, 239, 240, 244)

After traversing the transverse foramina of the upper six cervical vertebrae, the vertebral artery loops posteriorly behind the atlanto-occipital joint and perforates the atlanto-occipital membrane. It then enters the cranial cavity via the foramen magnum. Once inside the skull, the artery remains paramedian in position lying along the lateral aspect of the brainstem. At the level of the pontomedullary junction it passes in front of the brainstem, to unite with the opposite vertebral artery to form the basilar trunk.
Asymmetry between the intracranial vertebral arteries (95%) is very common. It usually occurs in the calibers of these vessels (81%) but atresia is frequently seen (19%). Not infrequently, one vertebral artery terminates as a large posterior inferior cerebellar artery (13%) with only a fine branch continuing cephalad to show the beginning of the basilar trunk. In a few cases, fusion of the two vertebral arteries is incomplete and fenestration results (6.5%). (Variations in the level of termination of the vertebral arteries are discussed under the origin of the basilar trunk.)
Beside the branches to the central nervous system, the vertebral artery provides two branches to the meninges. The anterior meningeal artery usually arises in the distal extracranial segment of the vertebral artery and supplies the dura in front of the foramen magnum. The posterior meningeal artery also arises from the extracranial segment of the vertebral artery. It vascularizes the dura of the medial portions of the posterior fossa, the falx cerebelli, and sometimes the falx cerebri and adjacent tentorium.
Vertebral artery branches to the spinal cord include the anterior and posterolateral spinal arteries. The anterior spinal artery can be single (37%) or double (60%). Occasionally it cannot be identified (3%). Although this artery usually defines the midline of the cord, it can also be paramedian (13%).
The most important branch of the vertebral artery is the posterior inferior cerebellar artery, which will be described with the other branches to the cerebellum.

2. Basilar Trunk
(Figs. 232, 233, 238, 239, 240, 245)

Arising from the union of the two vertebral arteries, this trunk lies between the two sixth cranial nerves, on the anterior surface of the brainstem. Although it normally extends from the pontomedullary sulcus to the pontopeduncular sulcus, variations do occur. The usual origin of the basilar trunk is at the middle of the pontomedullary sulcus (54%) or a few millimeters above or below it (15%). A lateral origin can also occur at this level (31%).

* Except for the posterior cerebral arteries, which have been previously described in Part 1, Chap. 3, p. 108, and the posterior choroidal and thalamoperforate arteries in Part 2, Chap. 3, p. 196.

The basilar trunk normally runs cephalad on the middle of the anterior surface of the pons (53%). In these cases it measures about 3 cm in length. Its course can also demonstrate a single wide curve, concave to the right or left (33%), or a double curve in the shape of an "S" (14%). Rarely, fenestration of the basilar trunk is present with the consequent appearance of a buttonhole (6%).
The basilar trunk terminates in the midline at the level of the pontopeduncular sulcus (93%). Only occasionally is this termination situated laterally (7%), and then only slightly.
Innumerable fine perforating arteries anchor the basilar trunk to the anterior surface of the pons. The slight indentation of the pons caused by this artery is called the basilar sulcus.
Numerous lateral branches arise from the basilar trunk. These include the arteries to the lateral medullary fossa, the internal auditory artery, and the superior and anterior inferior cerebellar arteries.

3. Arteries of the Brainstem
(Figs. 232–234, 241–243)

Classically these arteries are divided into those which supply the medulla, the pons and the cerebral peduncles [Foix and Hillemand (1925), Lazorthes *et al.* (1950)]. At each level, it is possible to divide the arteries into three groups: paramedian, short circumferential and long circumferential.

a) Arteries of the Medulla
(Figs. 232–234, 243)

Multiple branches to the medulla arise from the terminal segments of both vertebral arteries and from the proximal segment of the basilar trunk. Other branches arise from the anterior spinal artery and the posterior inferior cerebellar artery.
The branches arising from the vertebral, basilar and anterior spinal arteries are destined for the anterior surface of the medulla and form the paramedian group of arteries (Foix and Hillemand, 1925).
The arteries to the lateral medullary fossa (rarely a solitary branch) constitute the short circumferential arteries. They can usually be identified bilaterally (90%), less frequently on only one side (7%), and occasionally are not seen at all (3%). Characteristically, two, three or four branches arise from the basilar trunk, the vertebral artery, the anterior inferior cerebellar artery, or the posterior inferior cerebellar artery.
The internal auditory artery is also a short circumferential artery. One can identify this branch in 80% of cases. It may arise from the anterior inferior cerebellar artery (89%) or the basilar trunk (11%).
The long circumferential arteries supply the vascularization of the cerebellum and are represented by the posterior inferior cerebellar arteries.

b) Arteries of the Pons
(Figs. 232–234, 242)

The paramedian arteries to the pons arise directly from the basilar trunk. These numerous branches constitute a rich network of vessels as they penetrate the belly of the pons.
The short circumferential arteries to the pons arise from the lateral aspects of the basilar trunk and divide into fine branches which penetrate the pons. They number five or six on each side, frequently being asymmetrical. The most important of these branches is the artery to the trigeminal nerve. It can be identified in 80% of cases and usually arises directly from the basilar trunk.

c) Arteries of the Cerebral Peduncles
(Figs. 232–234, 241)

These arteries arise from the basilar trunk, the posterior cerebral arteries and the superior cerebellar arteries. The posteromedial and posterolateral choroidal arteries also participate in the vascularization of the posterior aspect of the mesencephalon.
The paramedian arteries to the cerebral peduncles arise from the posterior cerebral arteries. These are the thalamoperforate arteries of Foix and Hillemand (1925), or the arteries to the inferior surface of the thalamus of Lazorthes *et al.* (1950). They penetrate the cerebral peduncles in the interpeduncular fossa.
The short circumferential arteries to the cerebral peduncles arise as branches of the posterior cerebral arteries. The long circumferential arteries include the posterior cerebral artery itself, the posteromedial and posterolateral choroidal arteries and the quadrigeminal artery.

4. Arteries of the Cerebellum

Basically three major arteries supply each side of the cerebellum:
Superior cerebellar artery
Anterior inferior cerebellar artery
Posterior inferior cerebellar artery

a) Superior Cerebellar Artery – SCA
(Figs. 232–235, 238–240, 246, 247, 251 A)

This artery arises from the basilar trunk just proximal to its terminal bifurcation. It passes around the cerebral peduncles, describing a curve which is concave medially, posteriorly and superiorly. It passes between the trigeminal and oculomotor nerves and then into the sulcus between the mesencephalon and cerebellum. Here it divides into its terminal branches.

Frequently, this artery arises as a branch of the posterior cerebral artery (22%). The presence of two superior cerebellar arteries on one side is also not uncommon (20%). Asymmetry between the two sides is generally seen (76%). Terminal branches may arise early (30%) or late (70%). They run in the sulcus between the cerebral peduncle and the pons (62%) or meander slightly below this level (38%).

The superior cerebellar artery terminates as the vermian and hemispheric branches. The vermian artery is usually identified (82%), being solitary (29%), double (47%), or triple (6%). Its course is usually midline (63%) but it may be paramedian (37%). It terminates at the level of the declive near the postclival sulcus.

The hemispheric branches of the superior cerebellar artery are more variable. Four major branches can usually be identified: the internal (95%), the middle (91%), the external (80%), and the marginal (62%). The latter, when present, marks the boundary between the anterior and inferior surfaces of the cerebellum.

The hemispheric branches frequently change course or present loops as they cross the preclival and postclival (superior semilunar) sulci. They generally terminate within the posterior superior lobule.

The superior cerebellar arteries possess a characteristic morphology. They are markedly sinuous, while the arteries on the inferior surface of the cerebellum tend to be rectilinear.

b) Anterior Inferior Cerebellar Artery – AICA
(Figs. 232–234, 238–240, 248)

The AICA arises from the inferior third of the basilar trunk and courses towards the flocculus. It then changes direction, passing obliquely laterally and inferiorly. It travels beneath the fifth cranial nerve, at a varying distance from the sixth cranial nerve and then crosses the acoustic-facial bundle from front to back.

The AICA may be solitary bilaterally (60%), paired on one side and solitary on the other (25%), or bilaterally paired (11%). Infrequently, the AICA is paired on one side with three distinct arteries on the other (2%), or a solitary artery is present on one side with none on the other (2%).

While an origin of the AICA from the inferior third of the basilar artery is most common (93%), it may arise from the upper third of this artery (4%), its middle third (2%), or as a branch of the posterior inferior cerebellar artery (1%).

The length of the AICA falls into one of three categories: short, terminating at the flocculus (41%); intermediate, supplying the flocculus and continuing to the biventer and quadrilateral (crescentic) lobules (35%); or long (24%). In the latter case, the AICA supplies its usual territory as well as part or all of the territory of the posterior inferior cerebellar artery (PICA). When the AICA participates in the supply of the territory of the PICA, three branches are usually seen:

External hemispheric branch – 42%
Middle hemispheric branch – 30%
Internal hemispheric branch – 28%

The AICA also supplies the choroid plexus of the fourth ventricle near the foramen of Luschka.

c) Posterior Inferior Cerebellar Artery – PICA
(Figs. 232–234, 236, 240, 249, 251 B)

The AICA also supplies the choroid plexus of the fourth cerebellum. Usually arising from the preterminal part of the vertebral artery, it can be unilaterally absent in 26% of cases and bilaterally absent in 2%. The PICA can be hypoplastic (16%) or so well developed that the vertebral artery on one side terminates in it (13%). The relationship between the origin of the PICA and the medulla varies. In general it lies in the region of the olive (92%), but may be below (5%) or above (3%) this region.

The PICA courses posteriorly, lateral to the medulla, past the lower cranial nerve origins and then onto the posterior surface of the medulla medial to the cerebellar tonsil. Collateral branches supply the medulla and tela choroidea.

Generally the PICA divides on the inferior aspect of the cerebellar hemisphere into vermian and hemispheric branches. These branches may also arise before the PICA reaches the tonsil, or at the level of the tonsil.

At the level of the vermis, there may be a single vermian artery (32%) or two arteries (57%). Occasionally, no vermian branches can be identified (11%).

Hemispheric branches from the PICA may be demonstrable bilaterally (54%) or unilaterally (37%); sometimes there are none at all (9%). Usually three hemispheric branches can be identified: internal (91%), middle (86%), and external (56%). The internal branch usually defines the border of the pyramidal lobule. The middle and external branches each present a characteristic loop at the level of the postpyramidal sulcus, between the biventral and gracile lobules. These branches generally terminate at the level of the posterior inferior (inferior semilunar) lobule, in or near the great horizontal fissure.

II. Radiologic Study of the Arteries of the Vertebrobasilar System

Vertebral angiography has been the subject of numerous works. The technique of LINDGREN (1950) (direct puncture), and the more recent femoral aproach, have made the exploration of this region an everyday occurrence. BORIES (1958) devoted a monograph to vertebral angiography, as did HAUGE (1924) and YASARGIL (1962). The theses of LEIFER (1967) and MEGRET (1972) were devoted to this subject as well.

GREITZ and SJOGREN (1963) studied the anatomic relationships and the angiographic variations of the posterior inferior cerebellar artery (PICA). WOLF, NEWMAN and KILHANI (1962) studied methods of localizing the choroidal segment of the PICA. The cerebellar arteries were also the theme of the publication of LEMAN, COHADON and LEIFER (1967).

The semeiologic value of the superior cerebellar arteries was evaluated by ECONOMOS and PROSALENTIS (1963). The meningeal supply of the posterior fossa was detailed by SALAMON *et al.* (1967). Magnification has become a routine technique in vertebral angiography and for many authors, the analysis of the posterior fossa vessels is facilitated by stereoradiography.

One factor is constant: the full value of vertebral angiography is unobtainable without a firm foundation in the anatomy of the posterior fossa and the possible vascular variations.

The vertebral arteries (Figs. 252–258) exhibit asymmetry in their origin, course, caliber, and level of termination. This must be constantly borne in mind. Filling of only one vertebral artery is also frequently seen, but this is often purely technical. In these cases both arteries must be injected separately.

In the frontal projection, the union of the two vertebral arteries marks the approximate location of the pontomedullary junction. Atresia or a markedly reduced caliber is frequently present on one side. Termination of one vertebral artery as a PICA, although a rare variant, does not necessarily imply occlusion of the basilar trunk.

The most commonly seen of the small branches of the vertebral artery are the posterior meningeal artery and the anterior and posterolateral spinal arteries. These vessels have been studied by DJINDJIAN (1970) and by SCHECHTER and ZINGESSER (1966).

The largest branch of the vertebral artery is ***the posterior inferior cerebellar artery – PICA*** (Figs. 252, 254, 256, 260). It is important to carefully analyze the course of this artery in both frontal and lateral projections. This provides invaluable information on the position of the cerebellar tonsils and the choroid plexus of the fourth ventricle.

A frequent error is to fail to note, on the frontal projection that the PICA arises from the basilar trunk, which accounts for its bizarre appearance on the lateral projection. It is therefore an anterior inferior cerebellar artery (AICA) and the PICA is atretic on that side. (Contrary to GREITZ and SJOGREN (1963), we do not feel that a true PICA ever arises from the basilar trunk). This idea is extremely important. If one attempts to locate the choroid plexus of the fourth ventricle by following the course of an AICA, the cranial loop corresponds to the level of the flocculus, not the tonsil. (This is readily understood if one reviews the anatomic course of the AICA.)

The PICA can be divided schematically into several segments on the frontal projection. The first segment is situated in the region of the medulla. Frequently a loop convex inferiorly (called the caudal loop) occurs as the artery lies along the lateral wall of the medulla. It then reverses its course in a curve convex superiorly, called the cranial loop. The peak of this curve (or choroidal point) is the most medial part of the artery as viewed in the frontal projection and the closest to the roof of the fourth ventricle in the lateral projection. The arteries to the choroid plexus of the fourth ventricle originate in this region, and permit the identification of displacements of the fourth ventricle [WOLF *et al.* (1955), MEGRET (1972), LEIFER (1967)].

The vermian and hemispheric branches of the PICA may arise above, below or beside the cerebellar tonsil. The vermian branch is not always midline and not always present. Thus, calling it the "anterior cerebral artery of the posterior fossa" is not justified. The vermian artery presents a bump as it passes the postpyramidal sulcus and terminates at the level of the tuber. When visualized in the lateral projection, the vermian artery identifies the location of the inferior vermis.

The hemispheric branches of the PICA are usually three in number. The most medial of these corresponds to the lateral border of the pyramid and terminates at the level of the great horizontal fissure. The tonsillar branches are very fine and usually originate after the caudal loop of the PICA.

1. Basilar Trunk and Its Branches (Figs. 252–258)

The diameter, point of origin and course of the basilar artery are subject to many variations, if one accepts the premise that the normal basilar artery is situated in the midline on the belly of the pons, extending from the pontomedullary sulcus to the pontopeduncular sulcus. The variations include an angulated course towards one side or the other, a curved course, or an S-shaped course. In like manner, variations are also noted in the proximity of the basilar artery to the clivus in the lateral projection (LINDGREN, 1957). The point of termination of the basilar artery, as studied by GREITZ and LOFSTEDT (1954) is also variable. The anterior inferior cerebellar and superior cerebellar arteries arise from the basilar trunk, as do the short circumferential arteries such as the trigeminal, internal auditory and certain pontine arteries.

2. Anterior Inferior Cerebellar Artery – AICA (Figs. 253–258)

This artery is extremely variable and symmetry between the two sides rarely exists. It usually arises from the inferior third of the basilar trunk, as viewed in the frontal projection. The AICA travels laterally towards the flocculus, which can be localized angiographically by a loop which usually occurs in this region.

Occasionally the AICA does not reach the flocculus and is, in fact, hardly visible. At other times it is quite large, passes the flocculus and descends between the medulla and tonsil, to supply the territory of an atretic or absent posterior inferior cerebellar artery.

Some of the small arteries to the lateral medullary fossa originate from the AICA, being similar to the others which arise from the vertebral arteries or the posterior inferior cerebellar arteries. Angiography rarely provides diagnostic information in this region, not only because of the superimposition of paired structures in the lateral projection, but also because of the mass of the overlying petrous pyramids which obscures their origins despite the quality of substraction films.

3. Superior Cerebellar Artery – SCA (Figs. 252–258)

This artery usually arises from the basilar trunk but occasionally arises from the posterior cerebral artery on the same side. Its caliber is smaller than that of the posterior cerebral artery. The initial course is circumpeduncular, within the sulcus which separates the pons from the cerebral peduncle.

The SCA divides into vermian and hemispheric branches. In the lateral projection the vermian branches define the location of the superior vermis.

The hemispheric branches of the SCA may vary in number from being non-existent to being especially prominent on one side. The distances separating the hemispheric branches on one side may be markedly different from those separating them on the other side, since there may be only 2 on one side and 4 on the other.

The most anterior hemispheric branch of the SCA marks the anterior aspect of the cerebellar hemisphere. The other branches exhibit loops at the level of the preclival and postclival sulci. They terminate within the posterior superior lobule.

A choroidal artery and several tectal arteries may arise from the SCA, as well as from the short circumferential arteries.

Other basilar branches. In addition to the previously described and more commonly recognized branches, several small but important branches may arise from the basilar trunk. Of these, the most important are the internal auditory artery (which may also arise from the SCA) and the trigeminal artery. Four or five short circumferential arteries are occasionally visible in the frontal projection on one or both sides.

In the lateral projection, vertebral angiography identifies the anterior surface of the pons, the cerebral peduncles, the lateral aspect of the medulla, the location of the choroid plexus of the fourth ventricle, the tonsils, the vermis and the region of the tectum. The image of the hemispheres in this projection is admittedly imprecise, but it is possible to localize the great horizontal fissure, and the preclival and postclival sulci.

In the frontal projection, certain vessels are more easily followed in the anteroposterior projection and others are better visualized in the semiaxial projection. The medulla corresponds to the space that separates the caudal loops of the two PICAs. The pons is identified by the curve of the basilar trunk.

The origin of the basilar trunk approximately locates the two sixth cranial nerves, while its termination locates the two third cranial nerves. The width of the pons is occasionally marked by the course of a short circumferential artery.

The pontopeduncular junction and the anterior and lateral aspects of the cerebral peduncles are shown by the courses of the two superior cerebellar arteries.

The hemispheric branches of the PICA and the AICA may identify the positions of the great horizontal fissure and postclival sulcus, and thus localize the corresponding hemispheric lobules.

The anterior hemispheric branch of the superior cerebellar artery localizes the anterior surface of the cerebellum, just as the AICA identifies the flocculus, by a characteristic loop. Finally, the vermian branches of the superior cerebellar artery and the PICA indirectly localize the vermis.

Comparison of the arterial and venous phases of the vertebral angiogram with a knowledge of posterior fossa anatomy, allows the extraction of a large amount of information, provided one bears in mind the numerous important variations.

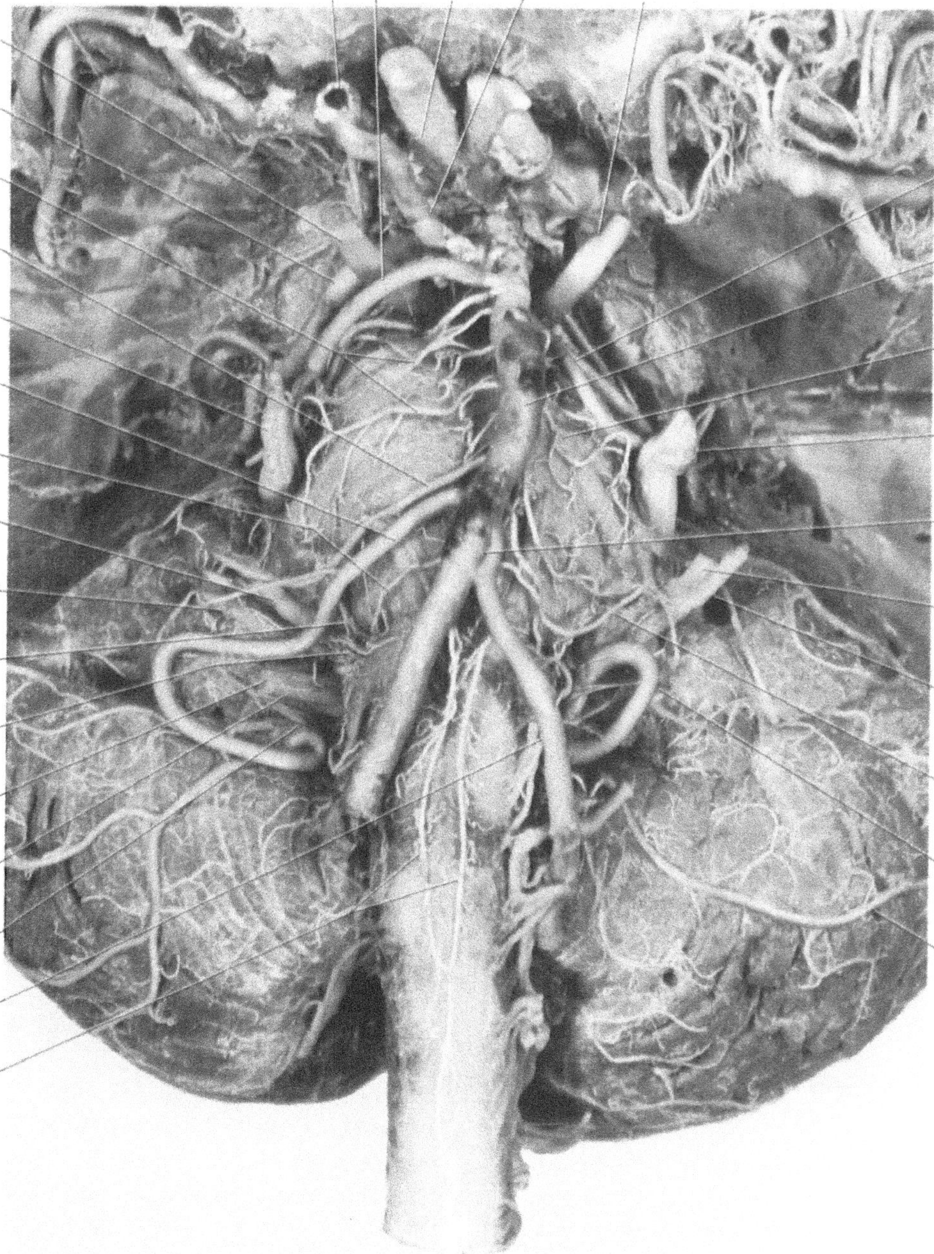

Fig. 232. Dissection of the brainstem and cerebellum after injection of the arteries, inferior view

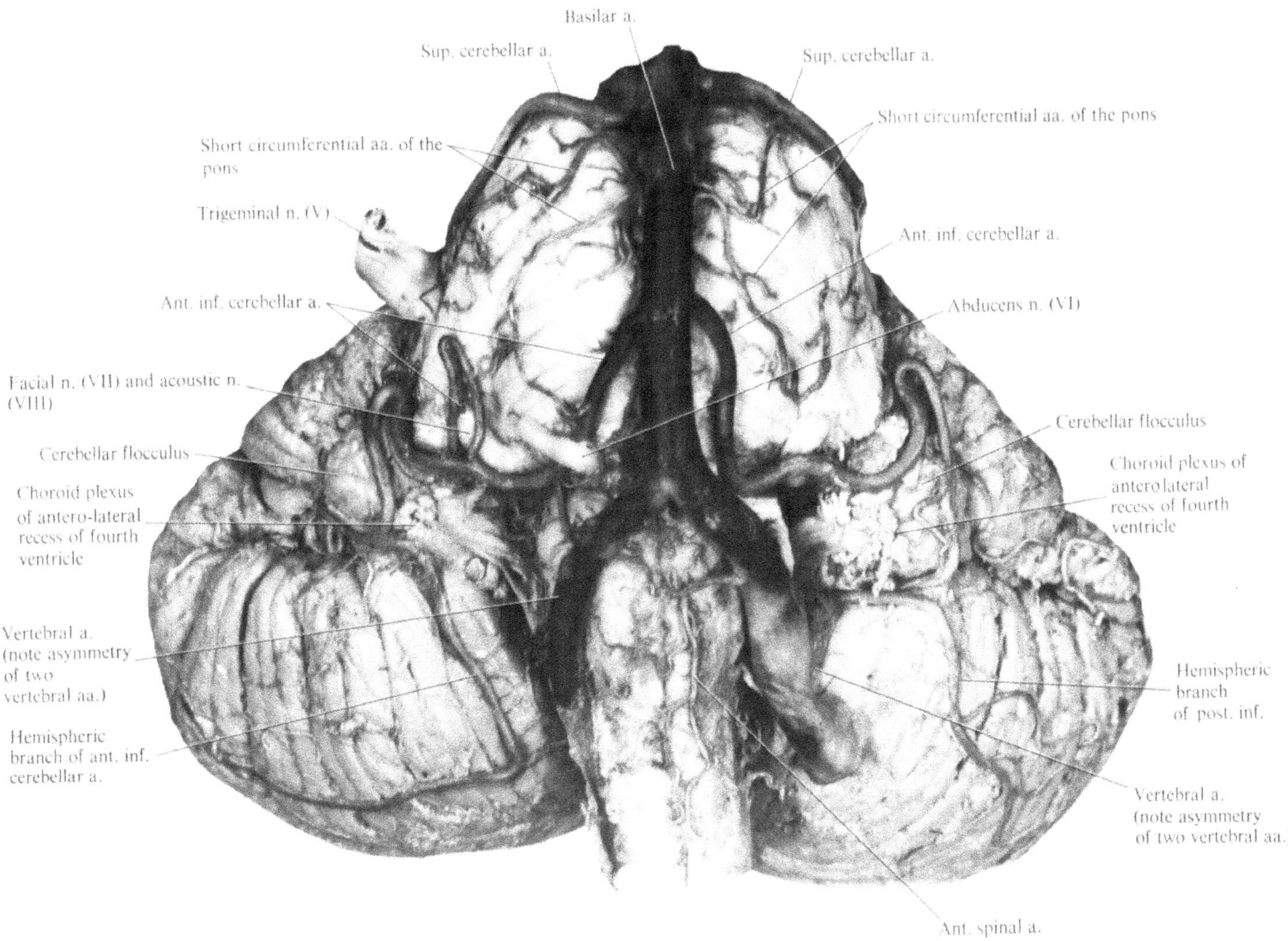

Fig. 233. Dissection of the brainstem and cerebellum after injection of the arteries of the vertebrobasilar system, inferior view

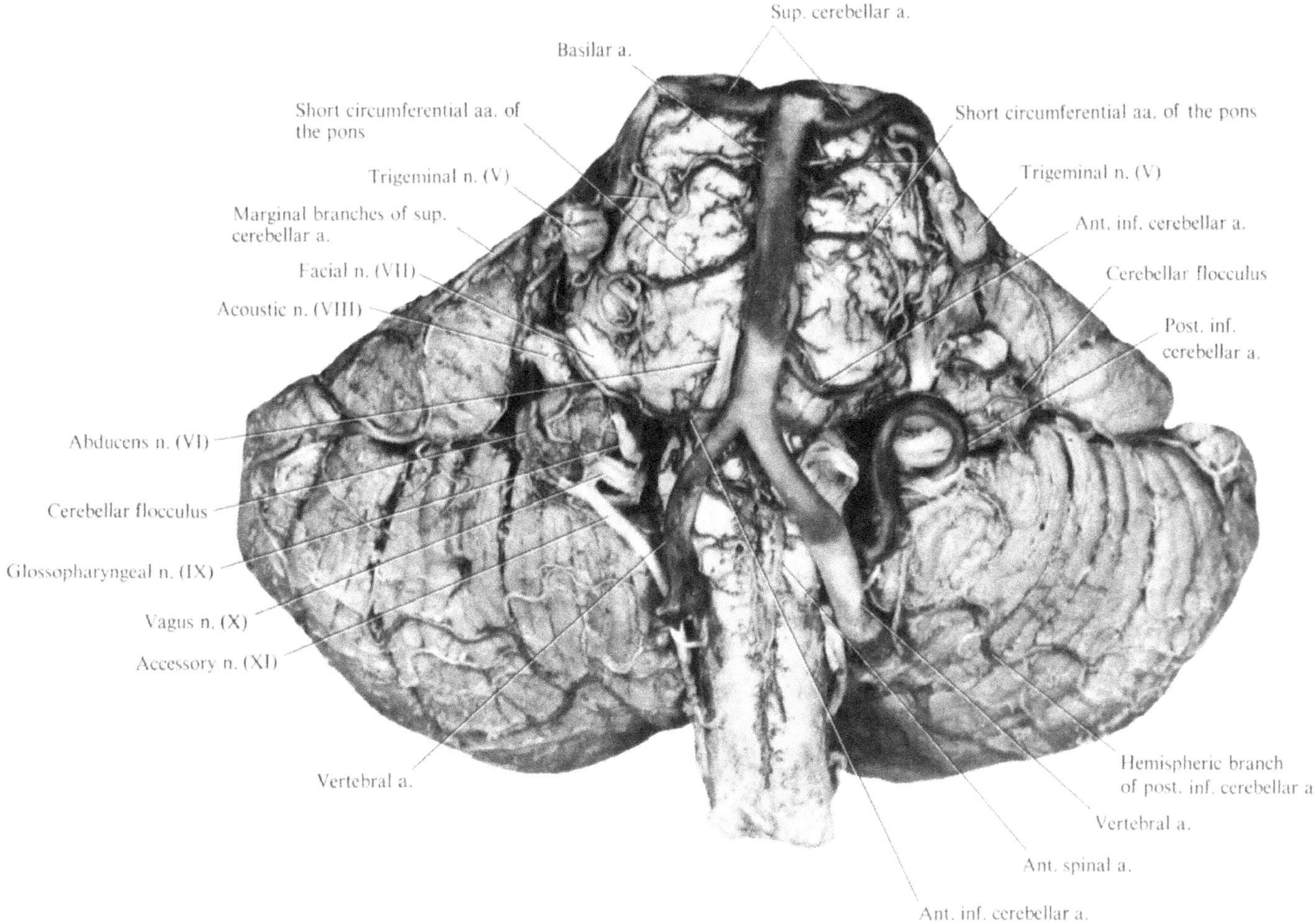

Fig. 234. Dissection of the brainstem and cerebellum after injection of the arteries of the vertebrobasilar system, inferior view

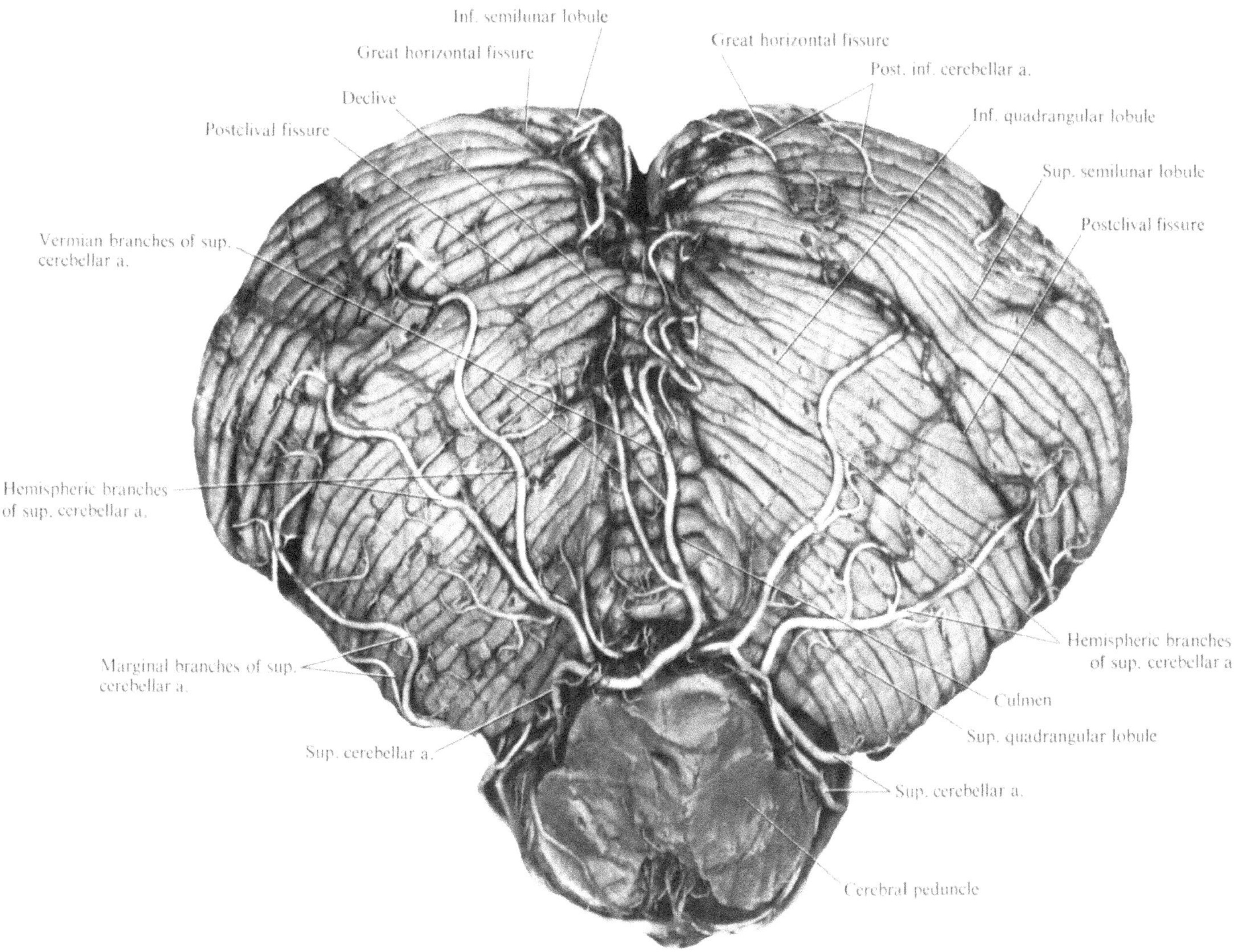

Fig. 235. Dissection of the brainstem and cerebellum after injection of the arteries of the vertebrobasilar system, superior view

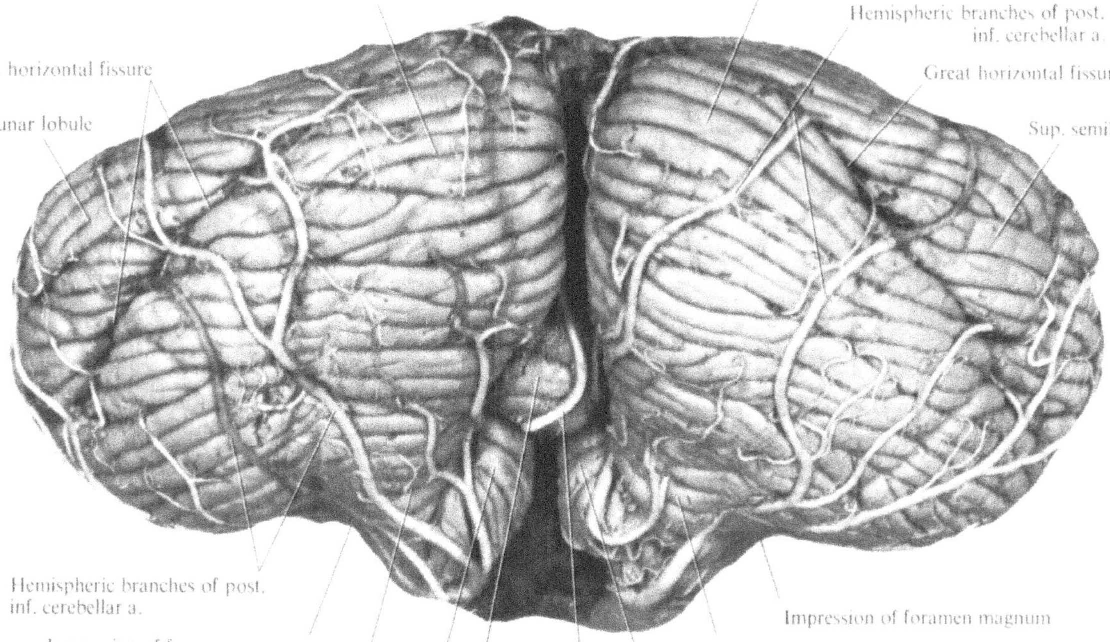

Fig. 236. Dissection of the brainstem and cerebellum after injection of the arteries of the vertebrobasilar system, postero-inferior view

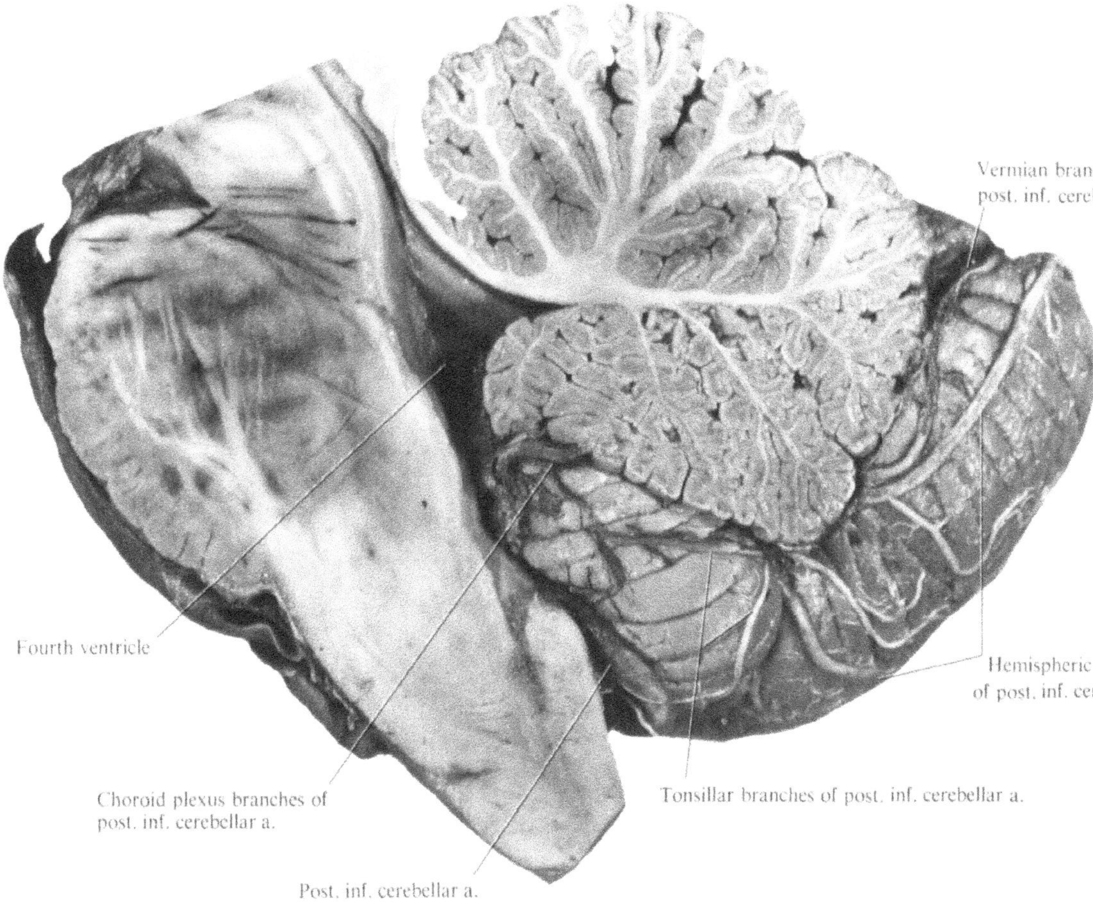

Fig. 237. Photograph after injection of the arteries of the vertebrobasilar system the lateral view

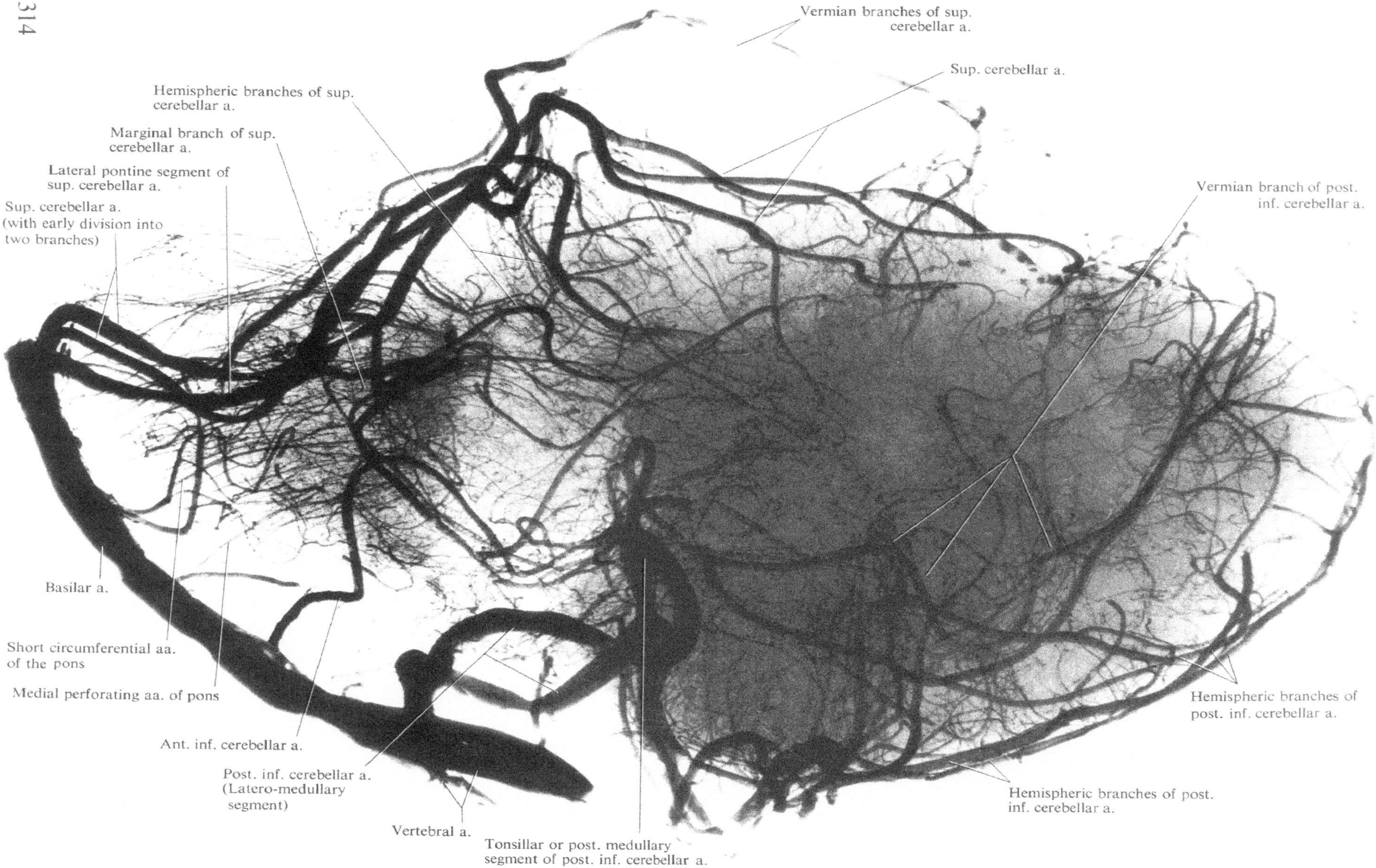

Fig. 238. Radiograph after injection of the arteries of the vertebrobasilar system, lateral view

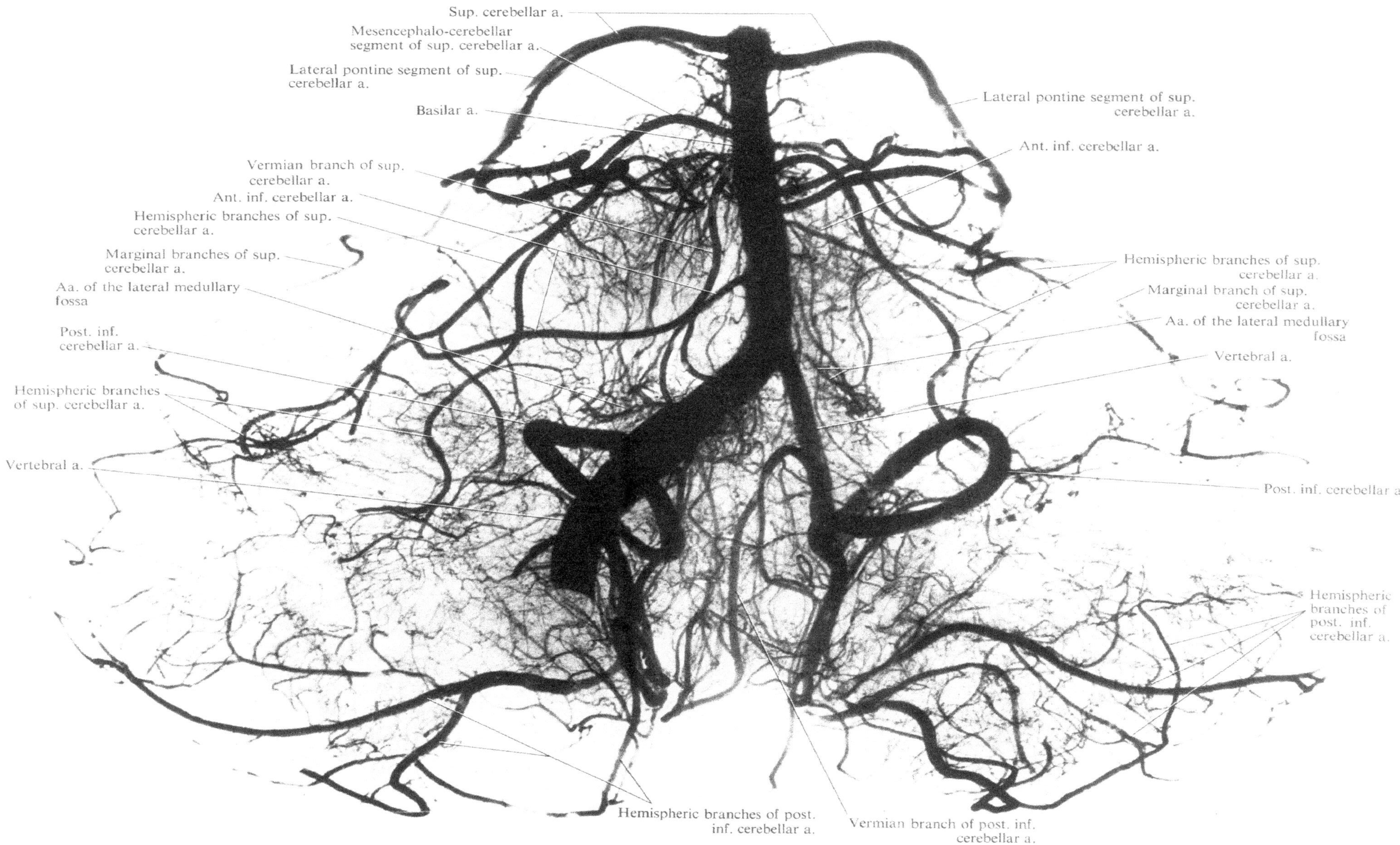

Fig. 239. Radiograph after injection of the arteries of the vertebrobasilar system, inferior view

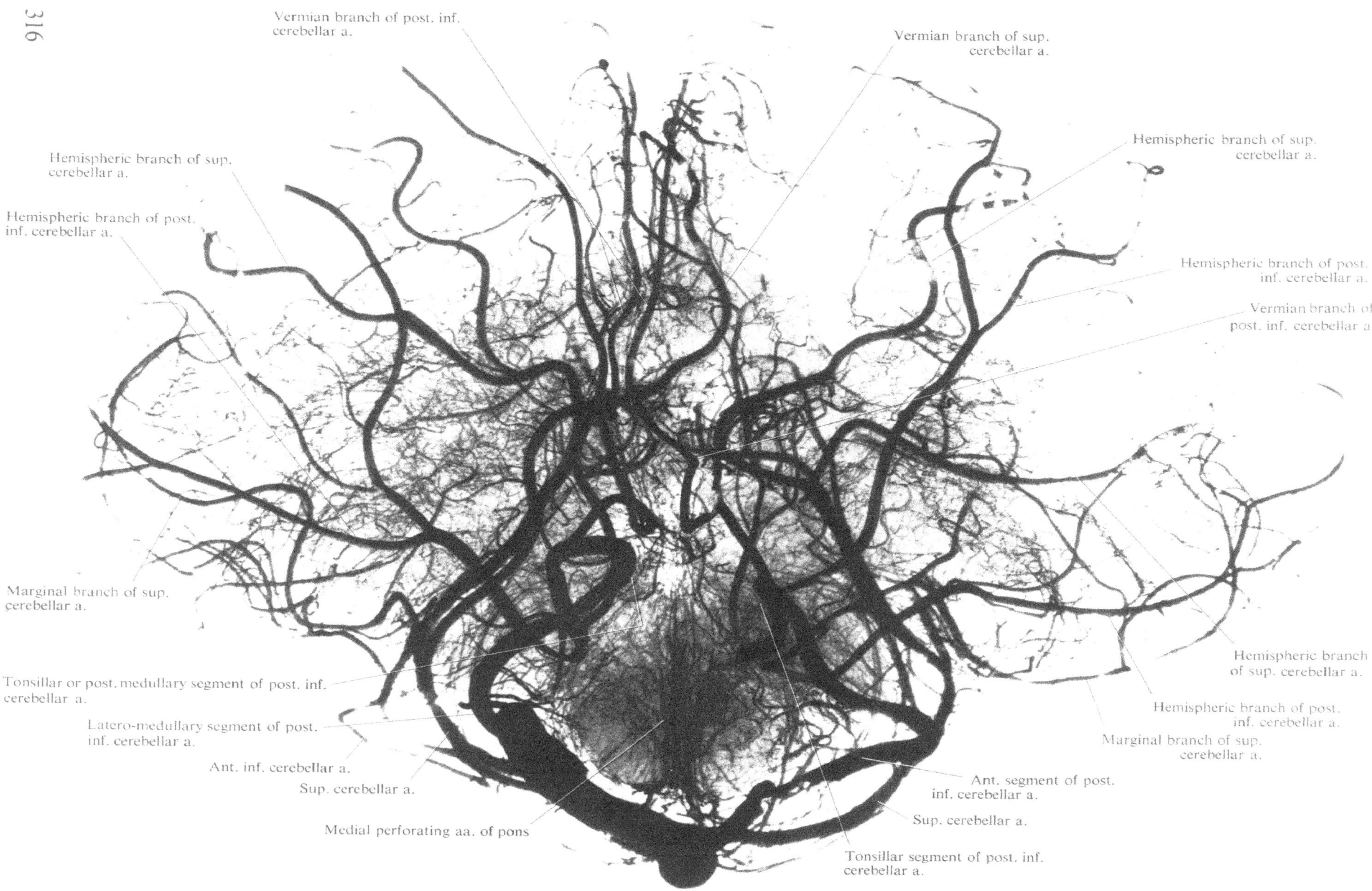

Fig. 240. Radiograph after injection of the arteries of the vertebrobasilar system, half-axial view

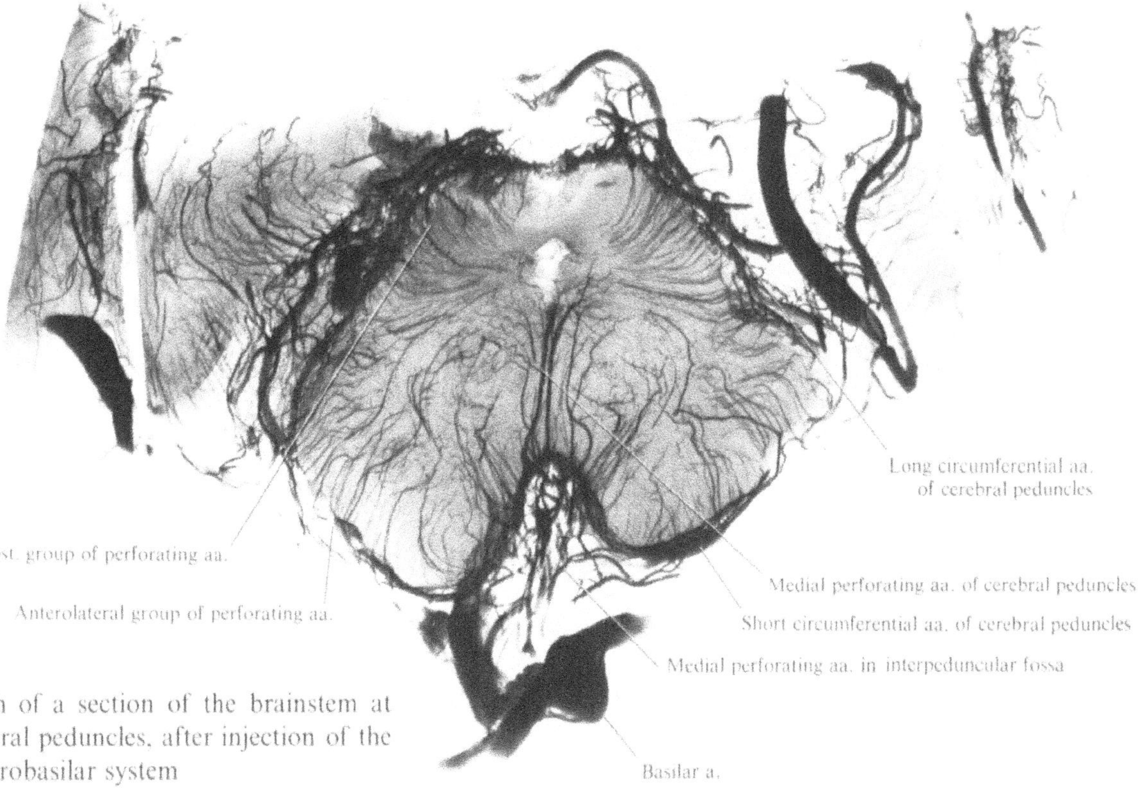

Fig. 241. Radiograph of a section of the brainstem at the level of the cerebral peduncles, after injection of the arteries of the vertebrobasilar system

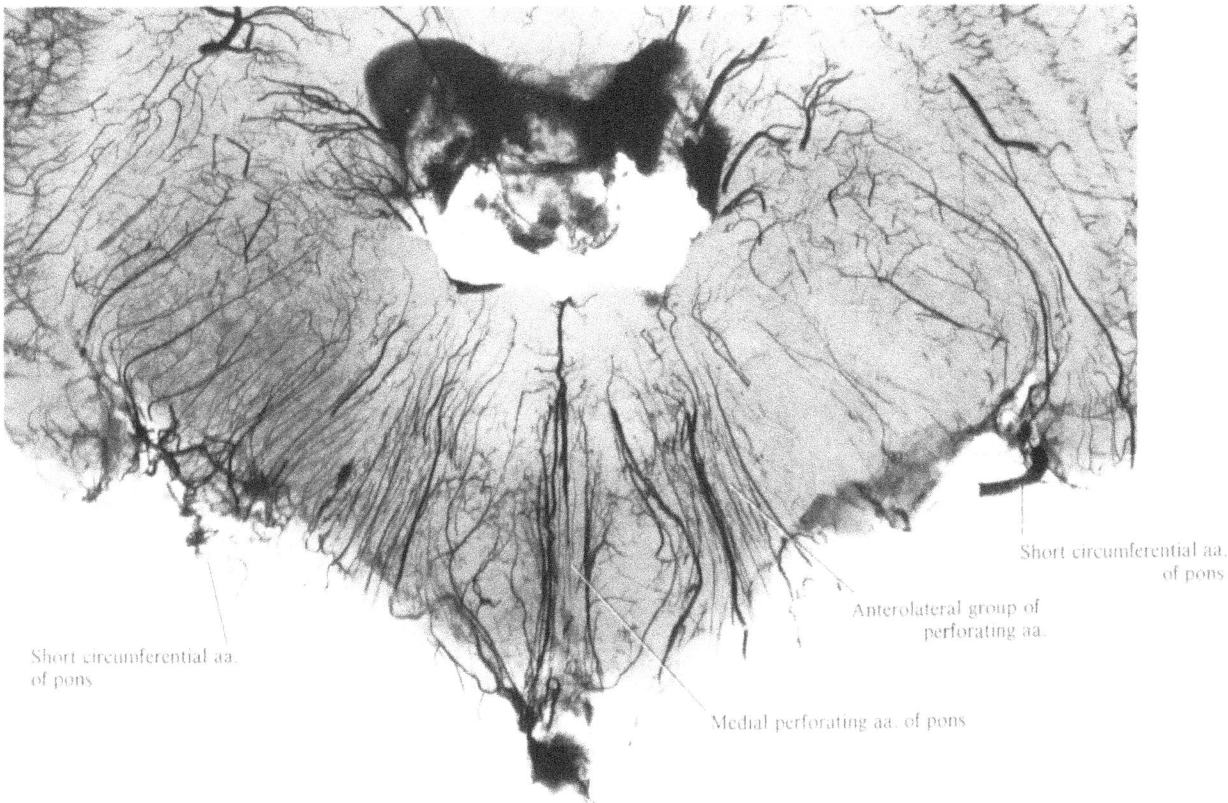

Fig. 242. Radiograph of a section of the brainstem at the level of the mid-pons, after injection of the arteries of the vertebrobasilar system

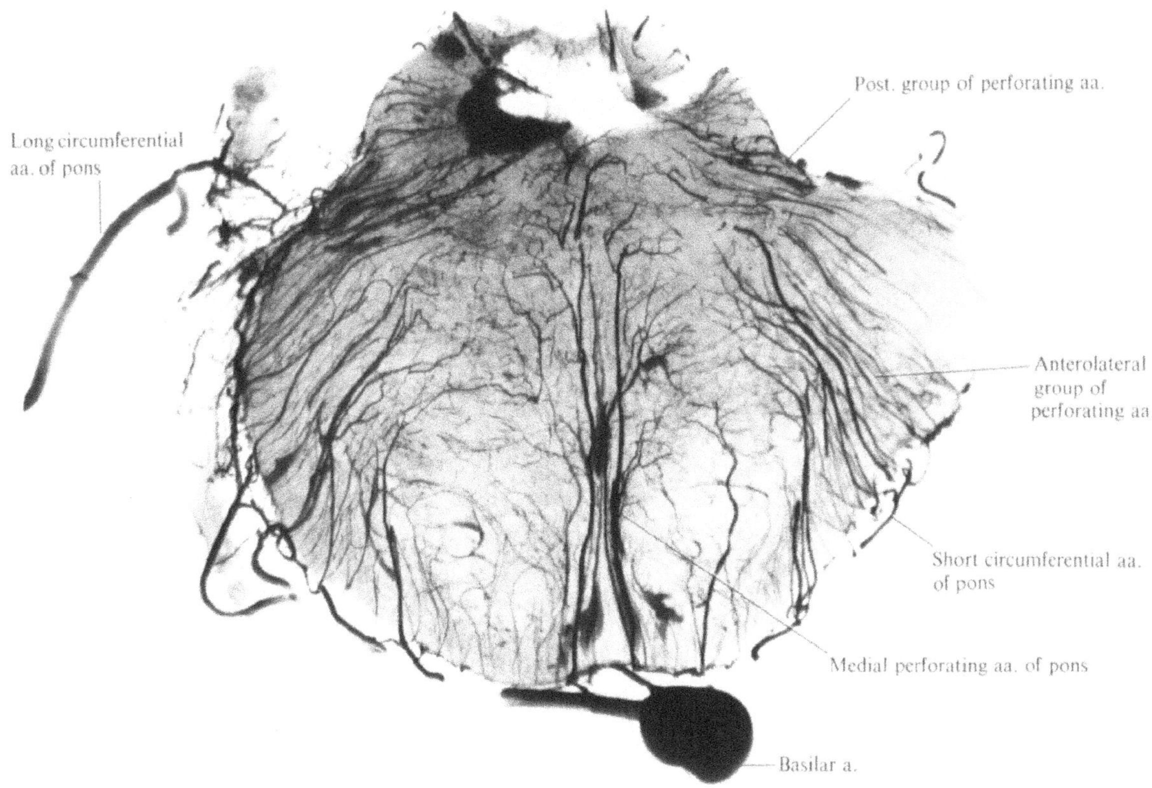

Fig. 243. Radiograph of a section of the brainstem at the level of the lower pons, after injection of the arteries of the vertebrobasilar system

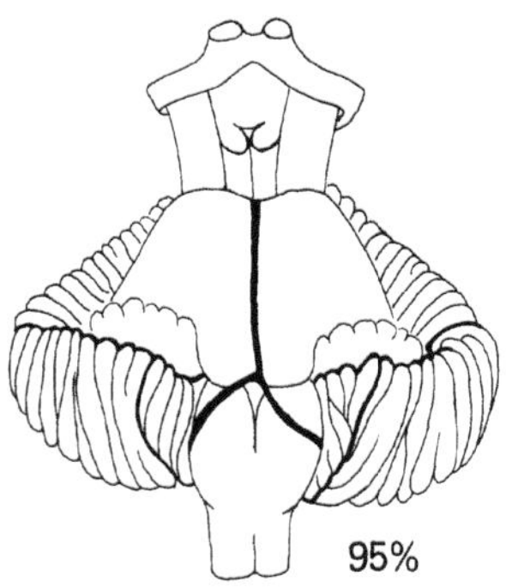

A. Asymmetry of course

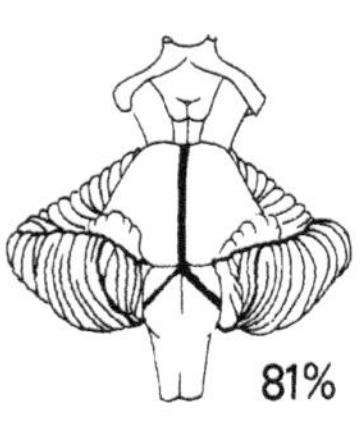

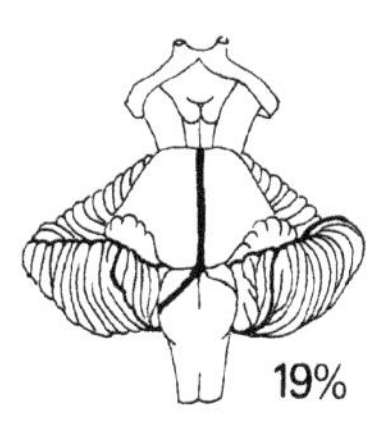

B. Asymmetry of caliber C. Unilateral vertebral atresia

Fig. 244 A–C. Vertebral artery. Schematic representation of the variations of the vertebral artery

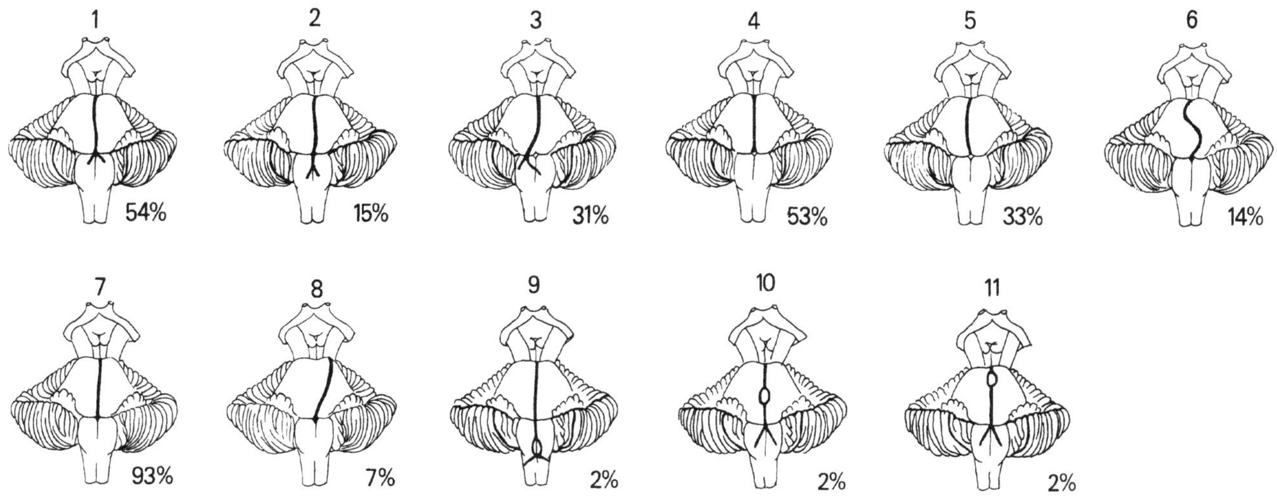

Fig. 245. Basilar trunk. Schematic representation of the variations of origin (1–3), course (4–6), termination (7–8), and morphology (9–11) of the basilar trunk

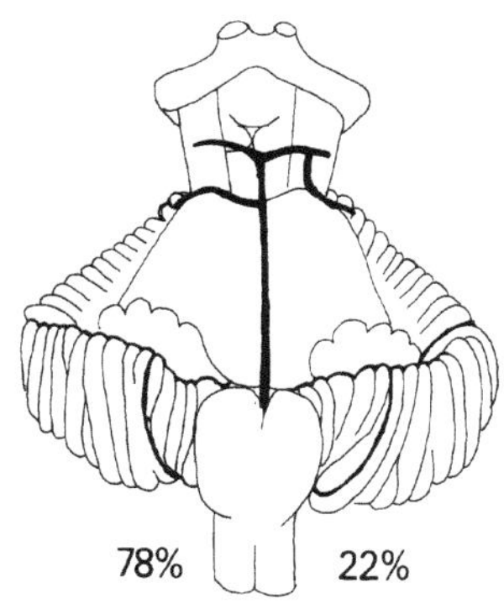

A. Origin of the SCA (on the right, origin from the posterior cerebral artery)

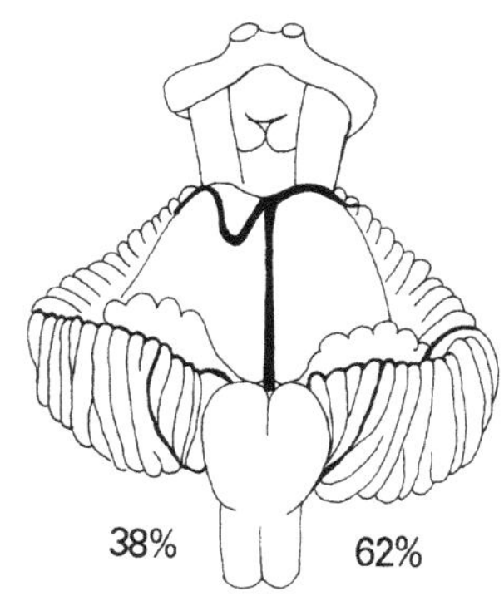

B. Variations in course of the SCA

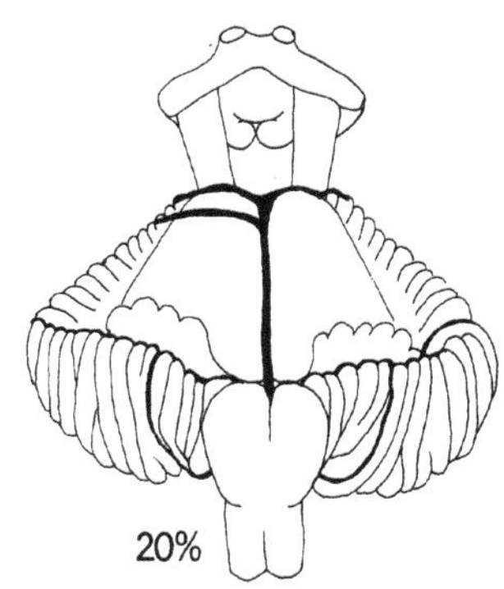

C. Appearance of single and double SCA

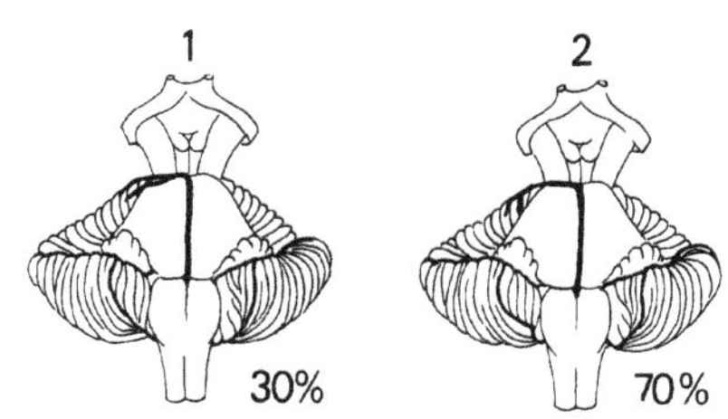

D (1, 2). Patterns of branching (early or late)

Fig. 246 A–D. Superior cerebellar artery (SCA). Schematic representation of the origin, course, and pattern of division of the SCA

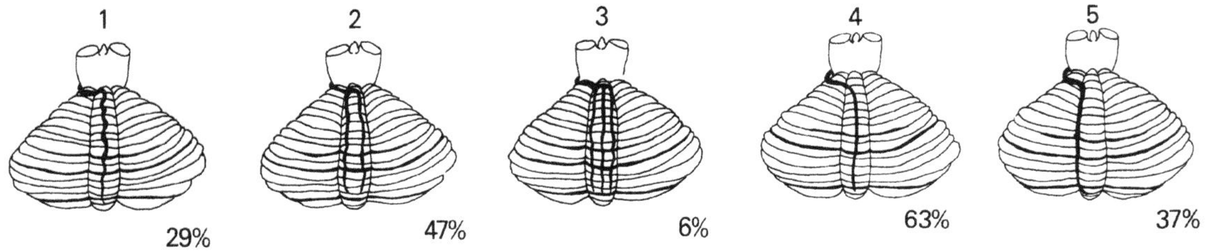

(1, 2, 3) Single, double and triple vermian arteries

(4, 5) Median and paramedian course of the vermian branches of the SCA

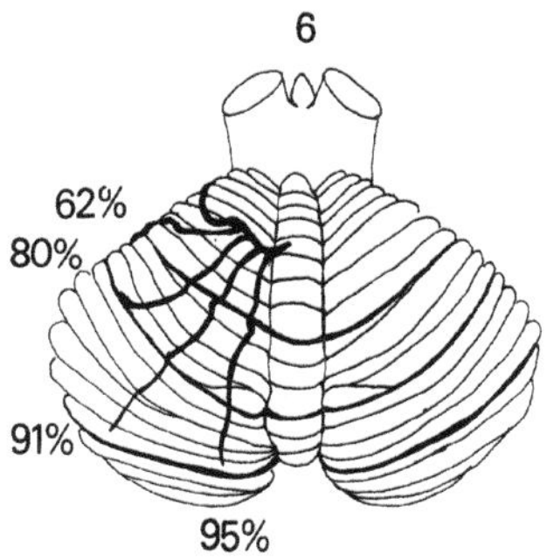

(6) Percentage incidence of the hemispheric branches of the SCA (marginal, external, intermediate and internal)

Fig. 247. Superior cerebellar artery (SCA). Schematic representation of the number of vermian branches and their course, and the number and incidence of the hemisphere branches arising from the SCA

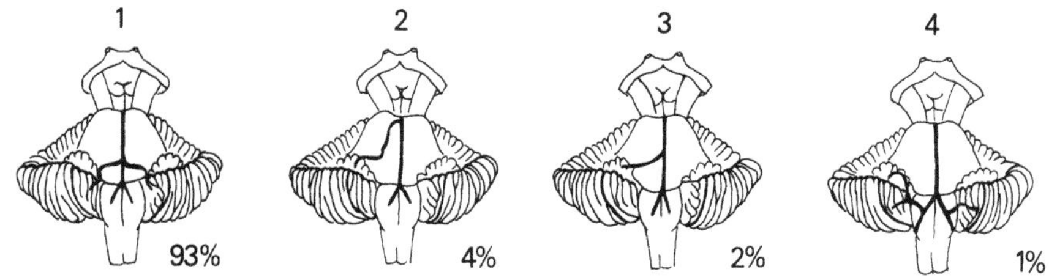

(1–4) Levels of origin

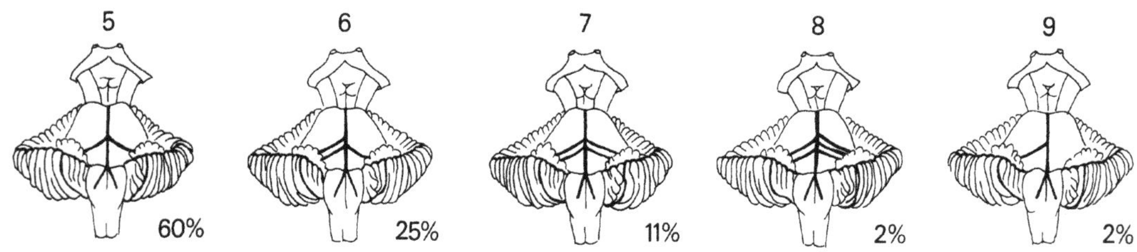

(5–9) Numbers

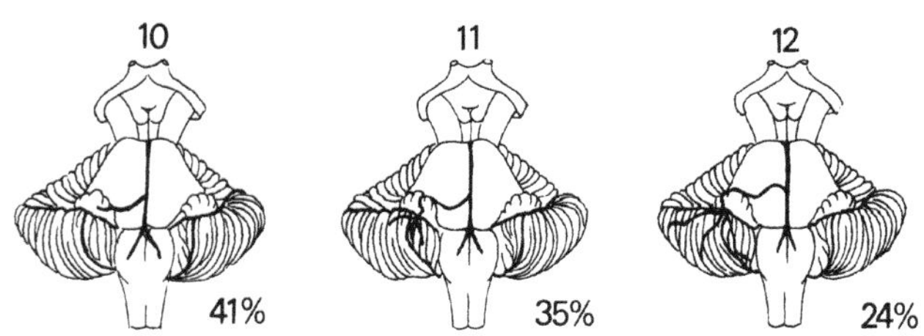

(10–12) Variations: short, intermediate and long

Fig. 248. Anterior inferior cerebellar artery (AICA). Schematic representation of the levels of origin, numbers and variations of the AICA

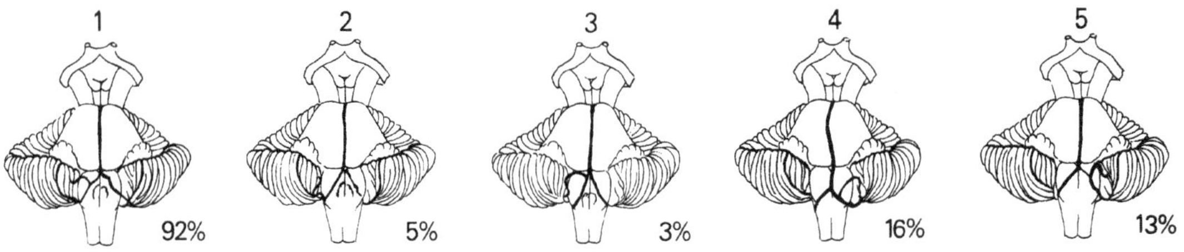

(1, 2, 3) Levels of origin: normal, low or high origin from the vertebral artery (relationship at the olive)

(4, 5) Variations: atresia or termination of one vertebral artery as a PICA

Fig. 249. Posterior inferior cerebellar artery (PICA). Schematic representation of the origins and variations of PICA

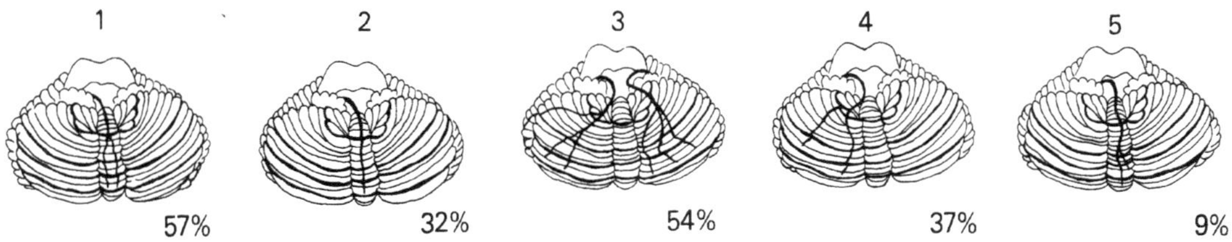

(1, 2) Double and single vermian arteries

(3, 4, 5) Hemispheric branches bilaterally, unilaterally, and absent

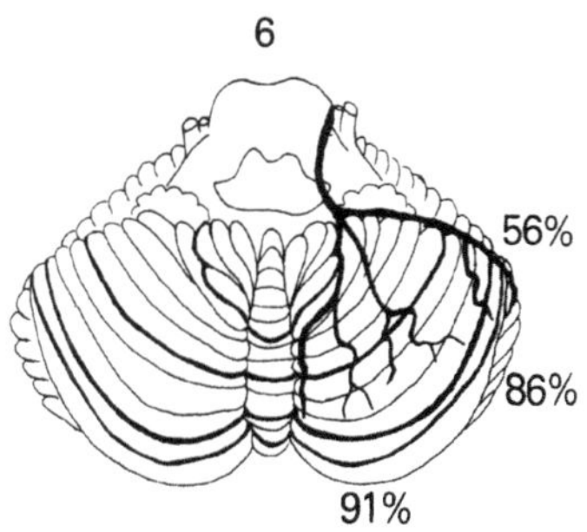

(6) Percentage incidence of the internal, middle and external hemispheric branches

Fig. 250. Posterior inferior cerebellar artery (PICA). Schematic representation of the variations in the vermian and hemispheric branches of the PICA

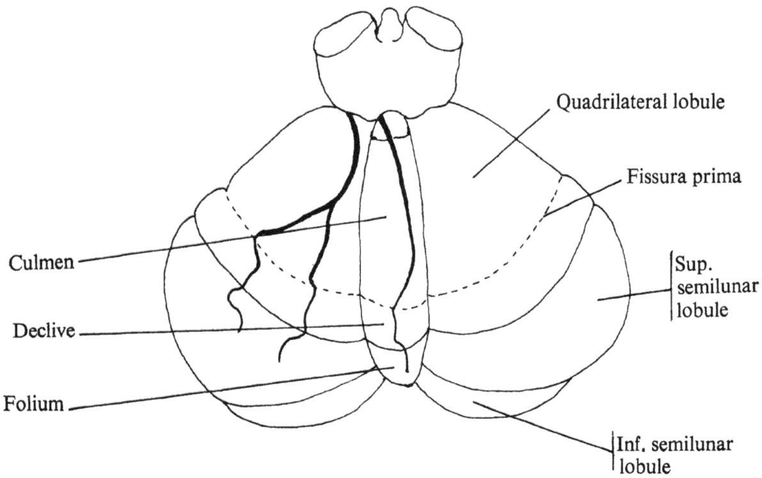

A. Superior surface of the cerebellum (SCA)

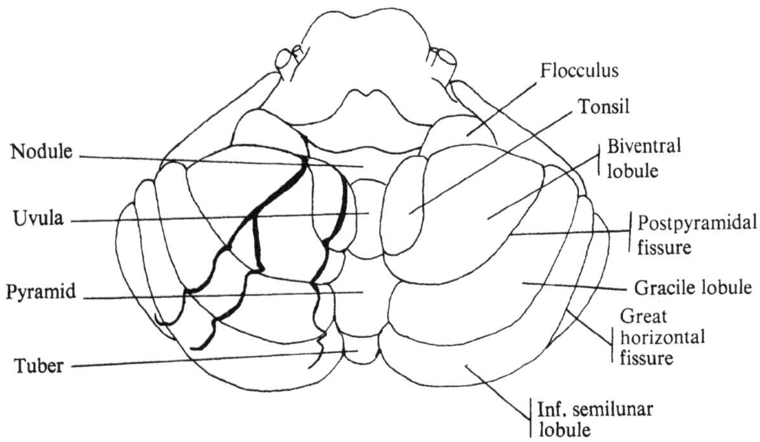

B. Inferior surface of the cerebellum (PICA)

Fig. 251 A–B. Localization of the cerebellar sulci by the course of the branches of the SCA and PICA on the surface of the cerebellar hemispheres

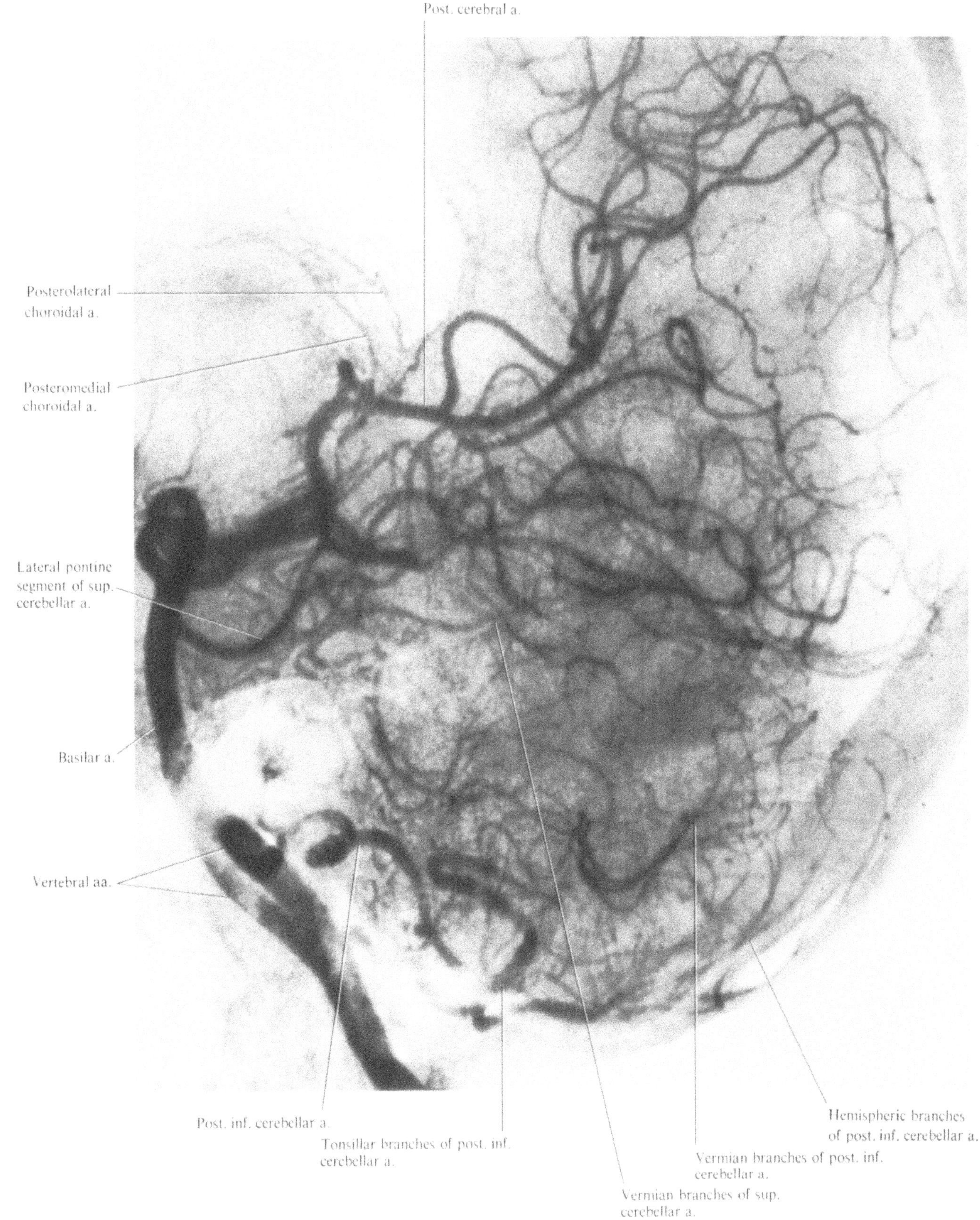

Fig. 252. Vertebral angiogram, lateral projection (× 2.5 magnification)

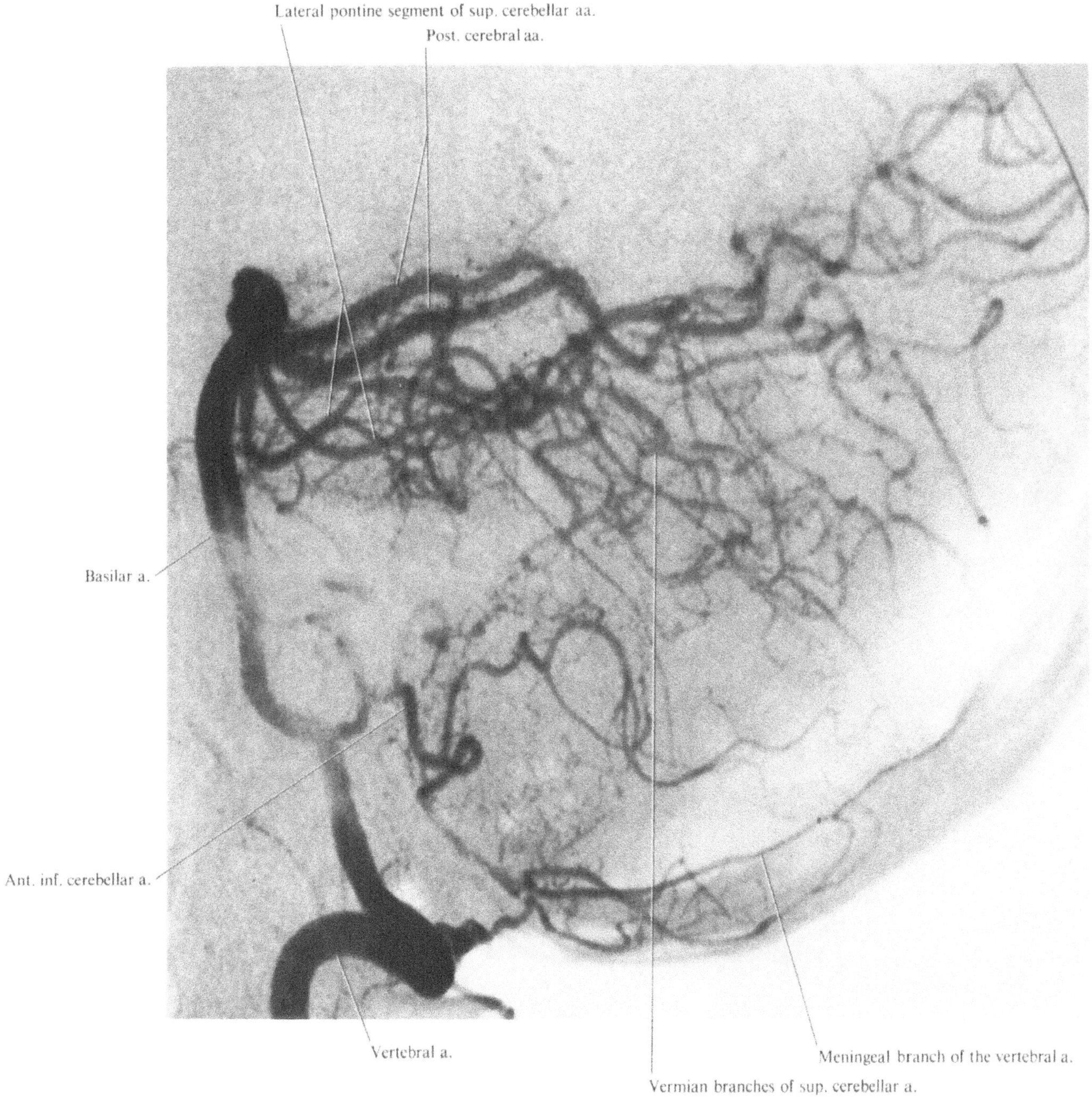

Fig. 253. Vertebral angiogram, lateral projection (×2.5 magnification)

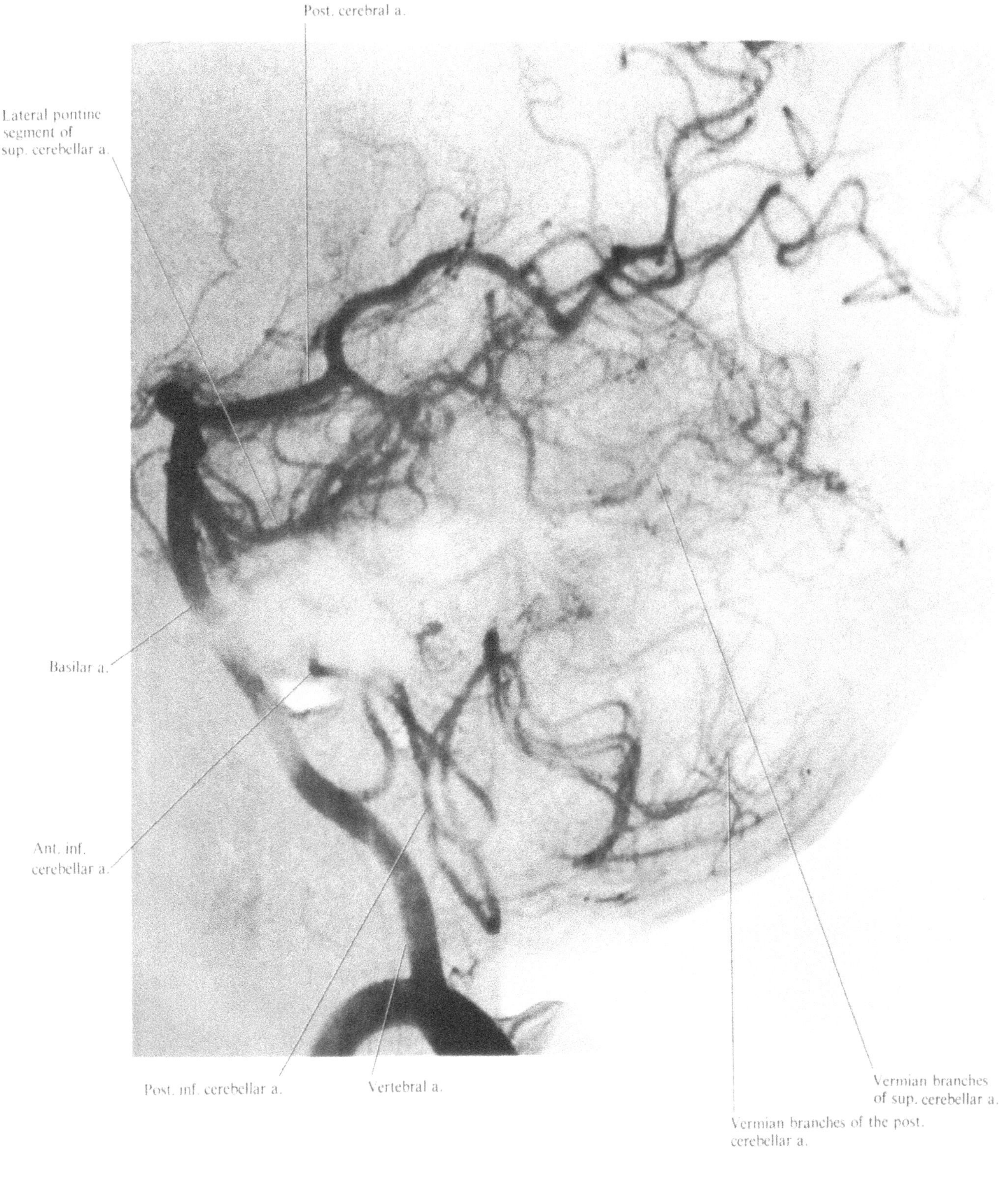

Fig. 254. Vertebral angiogram, lateral projection (×2.5 magnification)

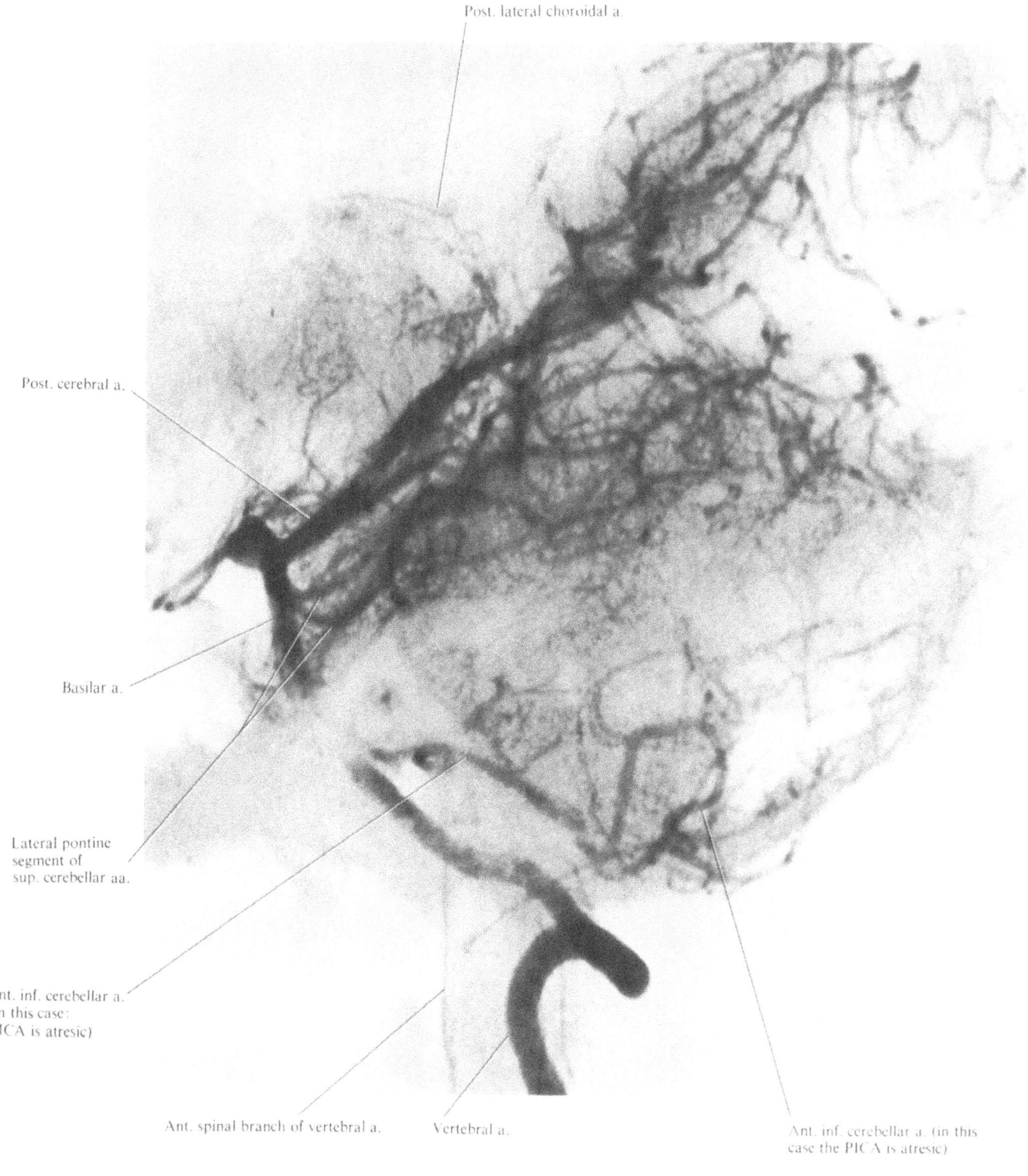

Fig. 255. Vertebral angiogram, lateral projection (×2.5 magnification)

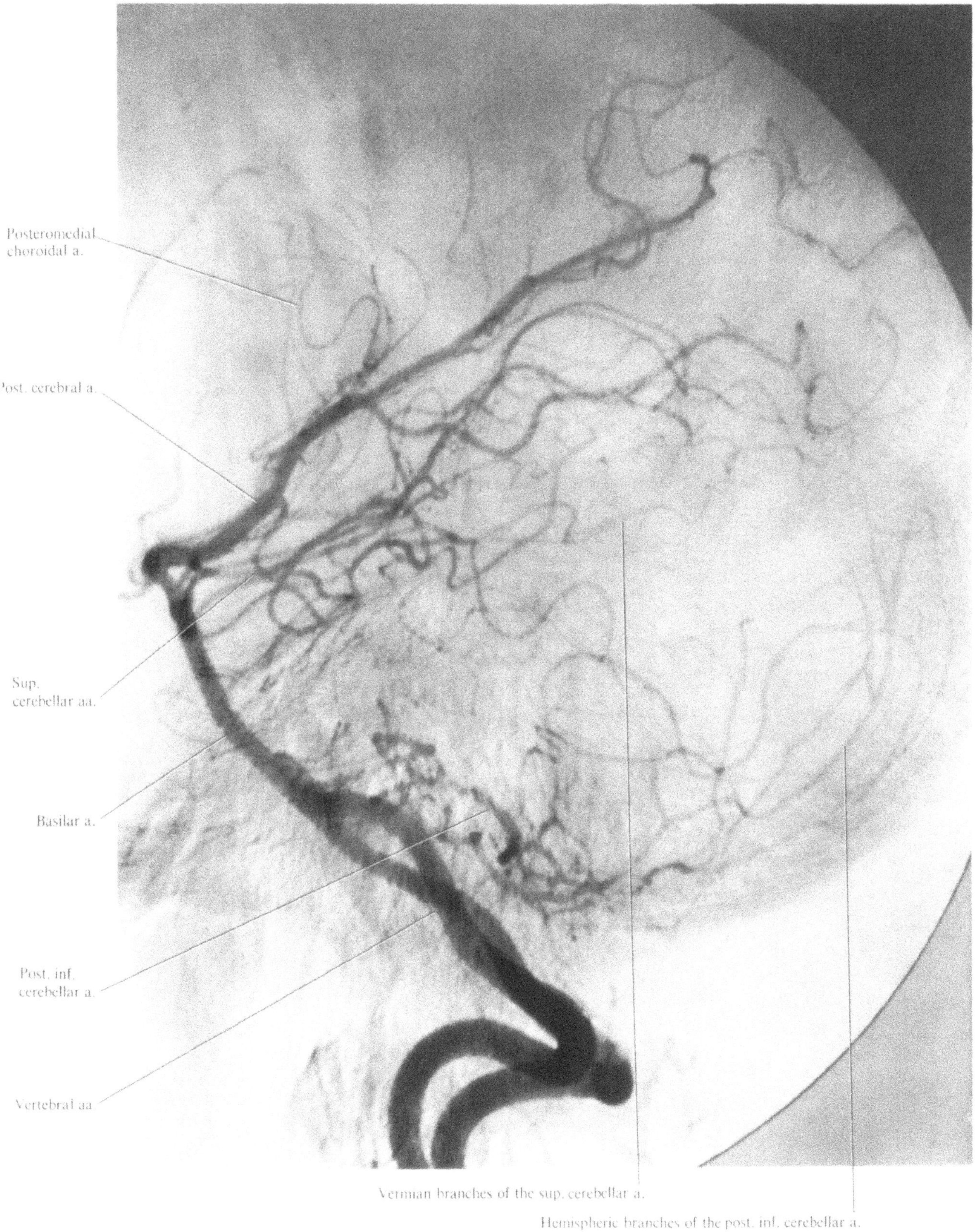

Fig. 256. Vertebral angiogram, lateral projection (×2.5 magnification)

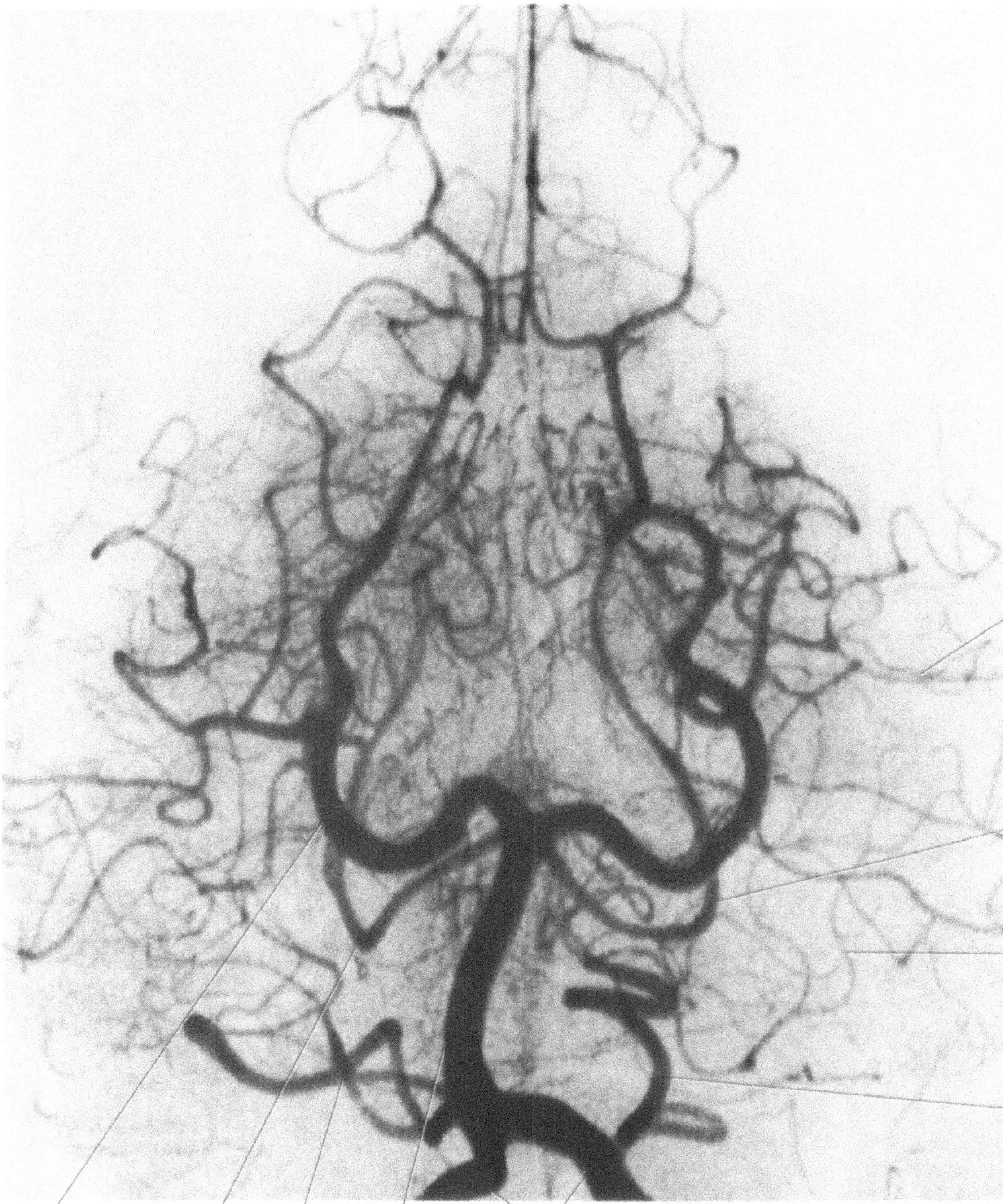

Fig. 257. Vertebral angiogram, half axial projection (×2.5 magnification)

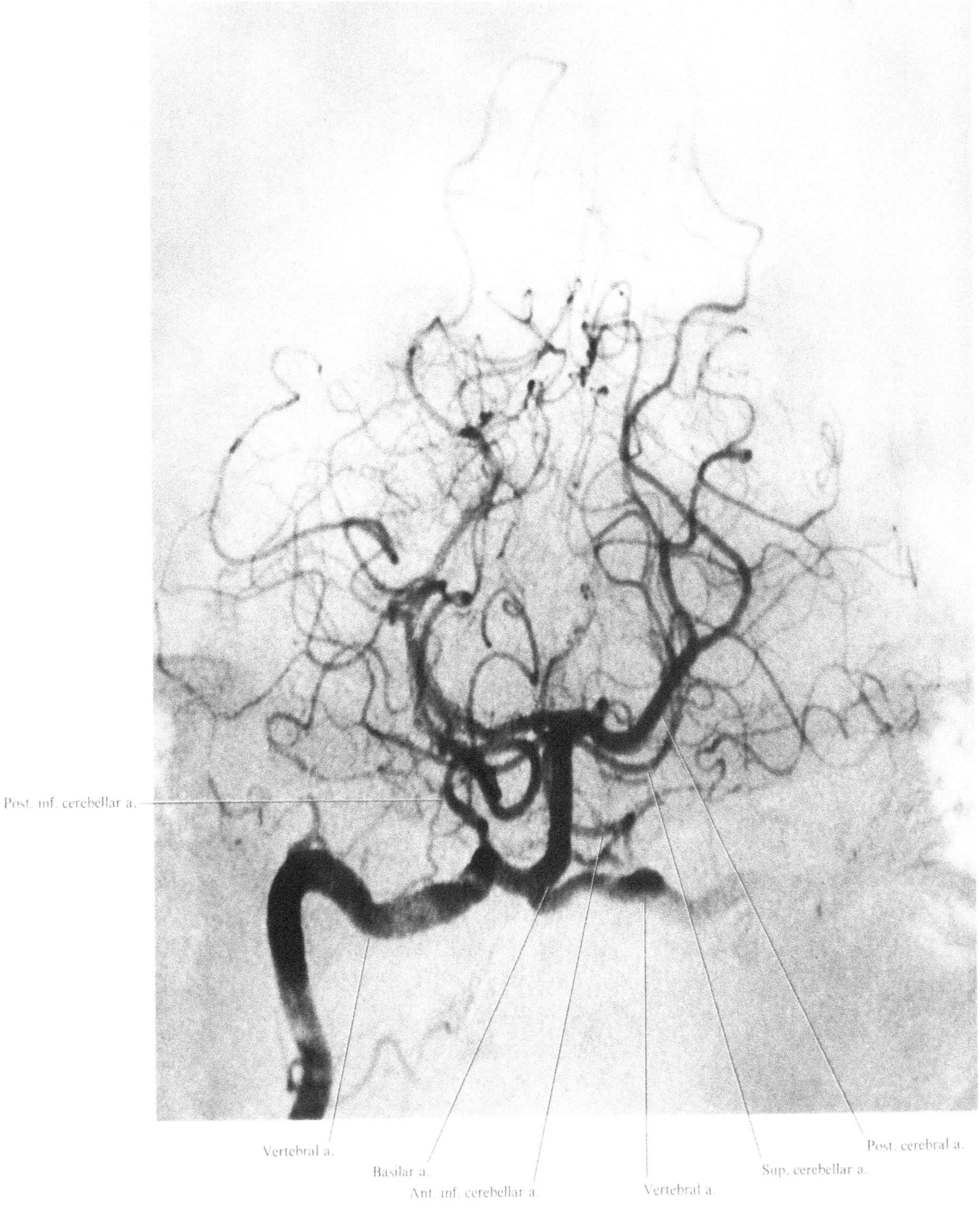

Fig. 258. Vertebral angiogram, half axial projection (×2.5 magnification)

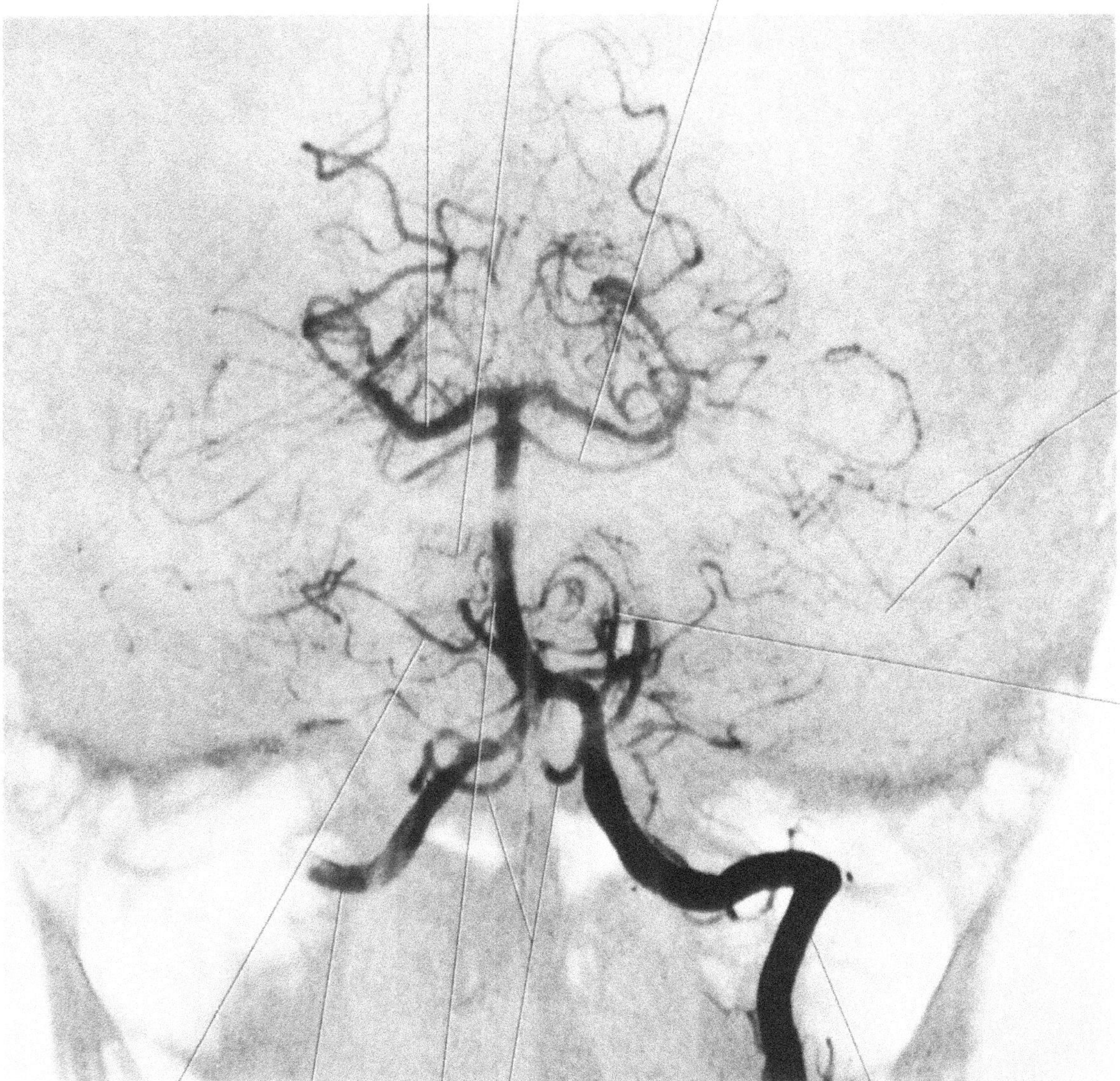

Fig. 259. Vertebral angiogram, frontal projection (×2.5 magnification)

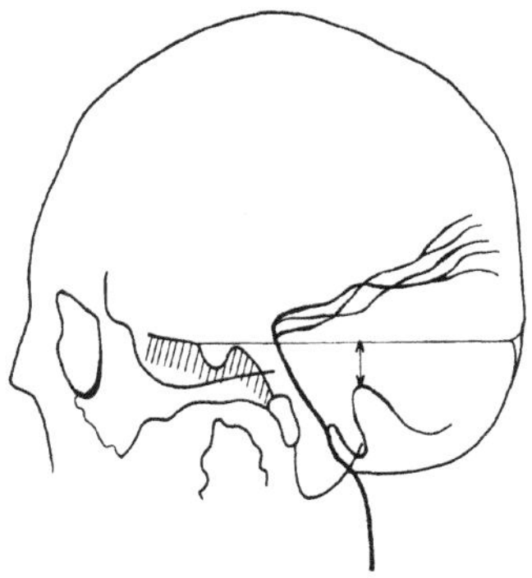

A. Wolf *et al.* (1955). The choroidal branch of the PICA is localized in relationship to Twinning's line (tuberculum to torcular)

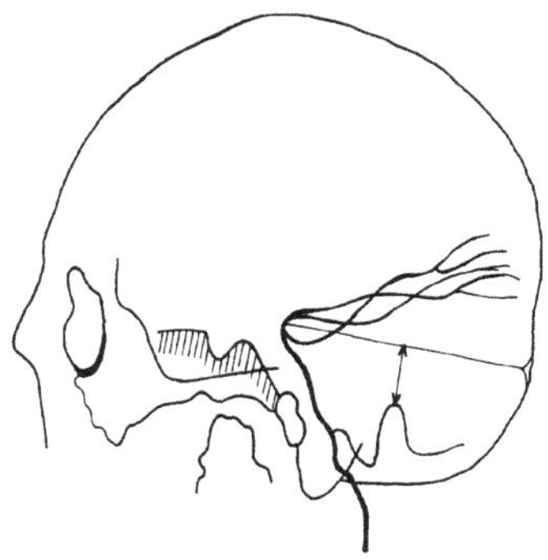

B. Megret (1952). The choroidal branch of the PICA is localized by a line uniting the superior tip of the basilar artery with the internal occipital protruberance

Fig. 260A–B. Localization of the choroid point and choroidal branch of the PICA, using the methods of Wolf *et al.* (1955) and Megret (1972)
Note that the frontal projection is important to exclude the possibility of an AICA supplying the territory of an atretic PICA, since their appearance on lateral projections is similar. When these methods are applied to a prominent AICA they localize the flocculus, not the choroidal branch to the fourth ventricle!

Chapter 3

Veins of the Posterior Fossa

During the development of the embryo, the first vein to appear in the posterior fossa is, according to PADGET (1956), the primitive ventral metencephalic vein since, at this stage, the cerebellar hemisphere is merely represented by a cerebellar plate. This ventral metencephalic vein, homologous to the trigeminal vein of lower vertebrates, will eventually become the petrosal vein. The proximal end of the ventral metencephalic vein becomes incorporated into the petrous crest to form the superior petrosal sinus. The primitive ventral myelencephalic vein, also called the vagal vein (PADGET, 1956), anastomoses superiorly with the ventral metencephalic vein and drains the medulla oblongata. The inferior petrosal sinus is derived from the proximal end of the ventral myelencephalic vein.

Unlike the ventral metencephalic vein, the dorsal metencephalic vein appears rather late in the development of the embryo and is relatively inconspicuous. With the development of the cerebellar hemispheres, the veins of the posterior group, derived from the dorsal metencephalic veins, become prominent and receive superior and inferior tributaries. Veins of the posterior group drain into the straight sinus either directly or indirectly, through the tentorial venous plexuses.

Although the veins of the posterior fossa can be divided into anterior and posterior draining groups, from the embryologic and phylogenetic viewpoint (PADGET, 1956), it seems more appropriate to divide the posterior fossa venous system into the following three groups, based on the direction in which they drain: (a) the superior or Galenic draining group, (b) the anterior or petrosal draining group and (c) the posterior or tentorial draining group (HUANG and WOLF, 1965; HUANG *et al.*, 1968).

I. Superior or Galenic Draining Group

The superior draining group (DUVERNOY, 1975; HUANG and WOLF, 1956; WACKENHEIM and BRAUN, 1970) may be further divided into (a) veins related to the mesencephalon (mesencephalic tributaries) and (b) veins related to the cerebellum (cerebellar tributaries) (Figs. 261–263 and 265–273) (HUANG and WOLF, 1975).

1. Mesencephalic Tributaries

Included in this group are (a) the median anterior pontomesencephalic vein, (b) the lateral anterior pontomesencephalic vein, (c) the lateral pontomesencephalic vein, (d) the lateral mesencephalic vein, (e) the posterior mesencephalic vein, (f) the peduncular (or interpeduncular) vein and (g) the quadrigeminal (or tectal) vein.

The ***median anterior pontomesencephalic vein*** runs vertically in the interpeduncular fossa, in or adjacent to the oculomotor sulcus, whereas the ***lateral anterior pantomesencephalic vein*** (HUANG and WOLF, 1974) lies longitudinally on the anterior aspect of the cerebral peduncle and on the anterolateral aspect of the pons (Fig. 268 A). These anterior pontomesencephalic veins may drain upwards to join the basal cerebral vein or its peduncular tributary. More often, however, they travel downwards to join one of the transverse pontine veins and open either into the petrosal veins or into the basilar plexus, through a bridging vein. Inferiorly, the median anterior pontomesencephalic vein frequently communicates with the median anterior medullary (or anterior medullary) vein.

The ***lateral pontomesencephalic vein,*** on the other hand, courses vertically on the lateral aspect of the cerebral peduncle and drains either superiorly or inferiorly (Figs. 279 A). Any vein running in or adjacent to the lateral mesencephalic sulcus may generically be called the ***lateral mesencephalic vein*** (Figs. 261, 262, 267–273, 275, 276, 279–281). This vein may drain either superiorly, to join the basal cerebral vein, or inferiorly into the brachial tributary of the petrosal vein. Quite frequently, the lateral mesencephalic vein is anastomotic in nature and connects the supratentorial basal cerebral vein to the infratentorial petrosal vein (WOLF *et al.*, 1963). The ***anastomotic lateral mesencephalic vein*** may be divided into three segments: supratentorial, mesencephalic and infratentorial (HUANG and WOLF, 1974). The supratentorial segment of the vein runs horizontally on the undersurface of the cerebral hemisphere, especially that of the geniculate bodies, whereas the mesencephalic segment lies vertically in, or adjacent to, the mesencephalic sulcus. The infratentorial segment travels anteroinferiorly and laterally over the superior and anterior surfaces of the brachium pontis and corresponds to the brachial tributary of the petrosal vein (to be described).

Since the longitudinally running mesencephalic veins frequently drain infratentorially into the petrosal vein, they may also be considered as part of the anterior or petrosal draining group.

Among the transversely running veins of the mesencephalon, the most constant venous channel is the ***peduncular*** (or ***interpeduncular***) ***vein***. It begins in the interpeduncular fossa by receiving the inferior thalamic (GIUDICELLI *et al.*, 1970) and central mesencephalic veins. The peduncular vein runs around the anterior aspect of the cerebral peduncle, at a variable level, and joins the basal cerebral or posterior mesencephalic vein (Figs. 261, 267B, 268B, 271B, 273, 275, 276A, 279A, 280A, 281B).

The ***posterior mesencephalic vein*** (HUANG and WOLF, 1965) is a variant of the second and third segments of the basal cerebral vein (HUANG and WOLF, 1974) (Figs. 261 C, 267, 268, 271 A, 272, 273 B, 274, 275, 277 A, 278, 279, 280 A, 281 A). The vein begins either in the interpeduncular fossa or on the anterior or lateral aspect of the mesencephalon, or, in rare instances, on the anterior aspect of the pons. It runs posteriorly around the brain stem to join the posterior portion of the internal cerebral vein or the great cerebral vein. The posterior mesencephalic vein may replace the posterior part of the basal cerebral vein or may be present in addition to the basal cerebral vein (***accessory basal cerebral vein*** or ***veins***). Rarely is the ***vein of the pontomesencephalic sulcus*** visualized in angiograms. When it is visualized, it courses either posteriorly to join the brachial tributary of the petrosal vein, or anteriorly to open into an anterior pontomesencephalic vein.

The ***quadrigeminal vein*** (HUANG and WOLF, 1965), also called the ***tectal vein***, begins in the midportion of the tectum by receiving the median superior and median inferior tectal veins, as well as a pair of intercollicular veins (DUVERNOY, 1975). They unite behind the tectum to form a single vein, the quadrigeminal vein, which flows backwards and upwards to join the second or third segment of the precentral cerebellar vein (to be described). It may, in some cases, open into the stem of the superior vermian vein, the internal cerebral vein or the great cerebral vein (Figs. 261, 262, 268 D, 271 B, 272, 276 B).

2. Cerebellar Tributaries

Included in this group are (a) the precentral cerebellar vein, (b) the superior vermian vein and its preculminate, intraculminate, and supraculminate tributaries.

The ***precentral cerebellar vein*** (HUANG and WOLF, 1966), a single midline vessel, runs upwards in front of the central lobule and culmen to join the great cerebral vein or the posterior portion of the internal cerebral vein. The precentral cerebellar vein may be said to be formed by two *brachial tributaries*. Each tributary begins in the wing of the precentral cerebellar fissure and travels medially, posteriorly, and superiorly, crossing the brachium pontis, interbrachial sulcus, and brachium conjunctivum to reach the vermian or central portion of the fissure. The brachial tributary is then joined by a similar tributary from the opposite side to form the precentral cerebellar vein. This vein then runs anterosuperiorly in the central portion of the precentral cerebellar fissure between the lingula and the central lobule (first or fissural segment). At the colliculocentral level, between the inferior margin of the inferior colliculi and the anterosuperior part of the central lobule, the vein turns posterosuperiorly to run in front of the culmen (second or anterior culminate segment).

Above the cerebellum, the vein follows its upward course in the cistern to join either the great cerebral vein or the posterior portion of the internal cerebral vein (third or terminal segment). The angle and its apex, formed by the first and second segments, are called the *colliculocentral angle* and the *colliculocentral point*, respectively. They are important angiographically, since they are closely related to the lower end of the aqueduct and the roof of the upper part of the fourth ventricle. The point of union of the two brachial tributaries, however, varies from deep in the fissure to well above it. When two brachial tributaries unite high above the fissure, the term *split precentral cerebellar vein* is more applicable (Figs. 270 B, 273 B, 281 B).

Other tributaries that join the precentral cerebellar vein are the parenchymal, tectal and superior hemispheric. Although the number of parenchymal tributaries varies, usually one fine vein is seen on each side. It drains the dentate nucleus and the adjacent medullary body of the cerebellar hemisphere, running anterosuperiorly with the brachium conjunctivum to join the brachial tributary in the superior paravermian sulcus. Not infrequently, the parenchymal tributaries are prominent and, together with the first segment of the vein, they outline more clearly the roof of the upper fourth ventricle (Figs. 261 B, 265, 269 A). In its fully developed form, the quadrigeminal or tectal vein, which is formed by the union of the median superior tectal, median inferior tectal, and occasionally the intercollicular tributaries, may join the precentral cerebellar vein or the internal cerebral vein (Figs. 261, 262, 268 D, 271 B, 272, 276 B). Often a *superior hemispheric tributary* of the precentral cerebellar vein runs medially, anteriorly, and superiorly on the superior surface of the cerebellar hemisphere. Upon reaching the anterior superior margin of the cerebellar hemisphere, the vein dips down into the precentral cerebellar fissure before it turns upwards to join the precentral cerebellar vein or its brachial tributary (Figs. 273 B and 280 B).

The superior aspect of the superior vermis and the adjacent part of the cerebellar hemisphere are drained by a group of vessels known as the ***superior vermian vein*** and its various ***culminate tributaries.*** In its typical form, the superior vermian vein begins as a midline *supraculminate vein* that travels upwards and forwards over the culmen to reach the apex of the cerebellum. The vein then dips down to run on the anterior aspect of the culmen and is joined by the other culminate tributaries (Fig. 261 B). The supraculminate vein frequently receives a superior hemispheric vein on each side. More commonly, however, the midline supraculminate vein is replaced by *superior hemispheric veins,* one in each cerebellar hemisphere, which take a tortuous course anterosuperiorly and medially over the quadrangular lobules. Upon reaching the anteriosuperior margin of the cerebellar hemisphere, the veins dip down into the upper part of the precentral cerebellar fissure and unite with the other culminate tributaries (Fig. 271 B). These tributaries include small veins from the preculminate fissure, lying between the central lobule and the culmen *(preculminate vein)*, and from the intraculminate fissures *(intraculminate veins)*. The pre-, intra- and supraculminate veins then unite at some distance anteriorly to the apex of the cerebellum to form the superior vermian vein, which turns backwards and upwards to join the anterior portion of the great cerebral vein. When the precentral cerebellar vein and the superior vermian vein unite to form a single trunk, it may more appropriately be called the ***superior cerebellar vein*** (HUANG and WOLFF, 1974) (Figs. 261 A, 265 A, 267 A, 269, 272, 279, 280 B).

II. Anterior or Petrosal Draining Group

Included in this group are tributaries related to (a) the anterior aspect of the brain stem, (b) the wing of the precentral cerebellar fissure, (c) the posterolateral fissure, (d) the cerebellomedullary fissure and (e) the cerebellar hemisphere. These tributaries converge towards the anterior angle of the cerebellar hemisphere to form a single stem, the petrosal vein. This vein, in turn, courses anterolaterally to run into the superior petrosal sinus immediately above the internal auditory meatus. This petrosal vein has also been called the ***superior petrosal vein*** *of Dandy* (DANDY, 1929) to distinguish it from the inferior petrosal vein, formed by the convergence of veins at the cerebellopontomedullary angle (BULL and KAZLOWSKI, 1970; DUVERNOY, 1975; HUANG and WOLF, 1967; HUANG *et al.*, 1968; TAKAHASHI *et al.*, 1967).

1. Tributaries Related to the Anterior Aspect of the Brain Stem

Veins lying on the anterior aspect of the mesencephalon – the median and lateral anterior pontomesencephalic veins, the lateral pontomesencephalic vein, the peduncular vein and the vein of the pontomesencephalic sulcus – have been briefly described. Although coarse networks of veins are frequently seen on the anterior aspect of the pons, the most important diagnostically and the most prominent are the median anterior pontomesencephalic and the transverse pontine veins.

The ***median anterior pontomesencephalic vein*** may be said to begin in the region of the anterior perforated substance or the lateral perforated substance, lateral to the mammillary body. It runs posteriorly and medially on the undersurface of the cerebral hemisphere to reach the roof of the interpeduncular fossa *(hypothalamic* or *roof segment)*. The vein then runs downwards on the posterior wall of the interpeduncular fossa to reach the superior foramen caecum *(mesencephalic* or *interpeduncular segment)*. It then travels forwards on the superior aspect and then downwards on the anterior aspect of the belly of the pons, in or adjacent to the midline (pontine segment) (Figs. 261, 267 A, 268 B, 271 B, 272, 276, 279 B). Inferiorly, the vein communicates with the median anterior medullary vein and the vein of the pontomedullary sulcus, in the inferior foramen caecum (HASSLER, 1967) (Figs. 261, 264, 275). When the vein originates from the posterior perforated substance, the hypothalamic segment may be absent.

The more laterally located ***lateral anterior pontomesencephalic vein*** runs on the anterior aspect of the cerebral peduncle and on the anterolateral aspect of the pons (Figs. 268 A, 276 A). It may replace the median anterior pontomesencephalic vein when the latter is hypoplastic. The lateral anterior pontomesencephalic vein, however, rarely extends below the level of the midpons (Fig. 264). At this level, it usually deviates either medially to join the median anterior pontomesencephalic vein or laterally, to open into the petrosal vein through a transverse pontine vein. There are two or three ***transverse pontine veins*** (superior, middle and inferior transverse pontine veins) on the anterior aspect of the pons on each side (Figs. 262 and 264). The most prominent one is usually located at the level of the midpons and connects the median anterior pontomesencephalic vein with the petrosal vein.

In lateral venograms, the hypothalamic, mesencephalic and pontine segments of the median anterior pontomesencephalic vein outline the roof of the chiasmatic and interpeduncular cisterns, and also the posterior wall of the interpeduncular and pontine cisterns. In the semiaxial view, in the venous phase, the transverse pontine veins outline the posterior wall of the pontine cistern and its lateral extensions (Figs. 266, 267 B, 273 B, 275, 278). The ***median anterior medullary vein,*** running in the median anterior medullary sulcus, is occasionally seen in the angiograms. It joins the median anterior pontine vein in the inferior foramen caecum (Figs. 264, 275, 281 A).

2. Tributaries Related to the Wing of the Precentral Cerebellar Fissure

These tributaries are generically called the ***brachial veins,*** since they are related to the brachium pontis and the brachium conjunctivum (Figs. 261, 267, 268 B and D, 269, 270, 271 A, 272–276, 277 B, 278–280). They run anterolaterally and inferiorly on the superior and then anterior aspects of the brachium pontis, to join the petrosal vein in the region of the anterior angle of the cerebellum.

Posteromedially and superiorly, the brachial tributary of the petrosal vein communicates with the brachial tributary of the precentral cerebellar vein. At the level of the lateral mesencephalic sulcus, the brachial vein frequently anastomoses with the basal cerebral vein or posterior mesencephalic vein via the anastomotic lateral mesencephalic vein. Together with the brachial tributaries of the precentral cerebellar vein, the brachial tributaries of the petrosal vein outline the inverted "V"-shaped anterior cerebellar notch, in the semiaxial projection (Figs. 261, 269 B, 270, 273 A, 274 B, 275, 277 B).

3. Tributaries Related to the Posterolateral Fissure

The posterolateral fissure (HUANG and WOLF, 1967) has been divided into the floccular portion (fissure below the flocculus), peduncular portion (fissure parallel and immediately inferior to the anterolateral recess of the fourth ventricle), supratonsillar portion (fissure above the superior pole of the cerebellar tonsil), and nodulo-uvular portion (fissure between the nodulus and the uvula).

The ***vein of the lateral recess of the fourth ventricle*** may be said to be formed by the union of the transverse and lateral supratonsillar tributaries at the dentate impression of the cerebellar tonsil. The *transverse supratonsillar tributary* receives veins from the nodulo-uvular fissure, from the superior surface of the nodulus, from the medial surface of the cerebellar tonsil, and from the inferior paravermian sulcus. Frequently, the transverse supratonsillar vein communicates with a similar vein on the opposite side through veins related to the nodulus *(transverse nodular* and *nodulo-uvular veins)* (Fig. 266). The *lateral supratonsillar tributary* lies above the lateral border of the superior pole of the tonsil, parallel and inferior to the lateral margin of the posterolateral recess. It receives the parenchymal veins *(dentate veins)* and a tiny vein from the roof of the fourth ventricle *(subependymal vein)*.

The first segment of the vein of the lateral recess, which is formed by the union of the lateral and transverse supratonsillar veins, runs anterolaterally and inferiorly to the tonsillar incisura. It continues in the peduncular portion of the posterolateral fissure inferior and parallel to the anterolateral recess of the fourth ventricle, to reach the cerebellopontomedullary angle (the first or peduncular segment). The vein of the lateral recess makes an obtuse lateral turn at the cerebellopontomedullary angle and continues laterally in the floccular portion of the posterolateral fissure, below the flocculus (the second or floccular segment). At the lateral border of the flocculus, the vein turns superiorly and medially to travel in the suprafloccular portion of the great horizontal fissure, to reach the anterior angle of the cerebellum (the third or suprafloccular segment), where it opens into the stem of the petrosal vein.

The course of the first segment of the vein is quite constant; however, that of the second and third segments, particularly the latter, is variable (Figs. 261 C, 266, 267, 269 B, 270 B, 272, 273 A, 274, 275, 276 B, 278). Frequently, the third segment of the vein joins the petrosal vein, not at the anterior angle of the cerebellum but near its junction with the superior petrosal sinus. The petrosal vein and its tributaries may also join a tentorial sinus (Fig. 275). Not infrequently, the vein, after emerging from the cerebellopontomedullary angle, continues anterolaterally and inferiorly in the cistern of the cerebellopontine angle, and finally joins the inferior portion of the inferior petrosal sinus, the medial portion of the sigmoid sinus, or the circular sinus. In these cases, the second and third segments of the vein are replaced by the cisternal segment (HUANG and WOLF, 1967) (Fig. 261 C).

Since the vein of the lateral recess of the fourth ventricle runs in various segments of the posterolateral fissure, it could have been called the *vein of the posterolateral fissure*. However, to emphasize its close relationship to the anterolateral and posterolateral recesses of the fourth ventricle, it has been designated the vein of the lateral recess of the fourth ventricle (HUANG and WOLF, 1967).

4. Tributaries Related to the Cerebellomedullary Fissure

The ***retro-olivary vein*** is a most diagnostically useful vein (DUVERNOY, 1975; HUANG *et al.*, 1968). It runs upwards in the retro-olivary sulcus between the olive and the restiform eminence, joining the *vein of the pontomedullary sulcus* superiorly. Inferiorly, it is continuous with the *lateral medullary vein* (Figs. 261, 264, 266, 274 B, 275). The *vein of the restiform eminence*, located laterally to the retro-olivary vein, is continuous inferomedially and posteriorly with the *vein of the restiform body* (HEDON, 1888; HUANG *et al.*, 1968). The latter vein lies on the posterior aspect of the medulla oblongata adjacent to the lateral margin of the lower part of the fourth ventricle (Fig. 266). The *vein of the restiform body* is, in turn, continuous inferomedially with the *median posterior medullary vein*, which is the superior extension of the median posterior spinal vein.

Connections are frequently observed between the retro-olivary vein and the vein of the restiform eminence at the level of the IXth and Xth cranial nerves. Similar multiple anastomoses are noted between the retro- and preolivary veins and between the preolivary and the median anterior medullary veins (Fig. 264). The vein of the pontomedullary sulcus, the pre- and retro-olivary veins, and the vein of the restiform eminence often unite to form a single trunk that flows into the lateral pontine vein, along with the vein of the lateral recess of the fourth ventricle. Less frequently, the single trunk runs with the vagal nerve and flows into the inferior petrosal, sigmoid or circular sinus. For this reason, it may be called the ***vagal vein*** or ***inferior petrosal vein.*** In some cases, the single trunk may travel with the glossopharyngeal or accessory nerve. Since the retro-olivary vein, one of the tributaries of the single trunk, marks the lateral border of the medulla oblongata, except in its upper part (the medullary eminence), it is important angiographically. In the semiaxial projection the distance between the lateral margin of the foramen magnum and the retro-olivary vein indicates the size of the lateral medullary cistern (Figs. 274 B, 275).

5. Tributaries Related to the Cerebellar Hemisphere

Veins located within the great horizontal fissure may generically be designated ***veins of the great horizontal fissure.*** Most often, the posterior portion of this fissure is drained by numerous veins that are tributaries of the inferior hemispheric veins of the posterior draining group (Figs. 265, 268 A, 274 A, 275). Anteriorly, the vein of the great horizontal fissure lies on the petrosal aspect and receives superior and inferior hemispheric tributaries (Fig. 266). The ***superior hemispheric tributaries*** drain forwards and downwards on the superior surface of the cerebellar hemisphere, while the ***inferior hemispheric tributaries*** drain forwards and upwards on the occipital and petrosal surfaces of the cerebellar hemisphere.

In rare cases, the vein of the great horizontal fissure begins posteriorly, in the depths of the fissure. It runs anterolaterally and then anteromedially as a continuous venous channel to reach the anterior aspect of the brachium pontis. It then runs above the flocculus to join the stem of the petrosal vein, usually in the region of the anterior angle of the cerebellum (Fig. 270 B). In some cases, the vein of the great horizontal fissure may run in the reverse direction, i.e., posteromedially and superiorly, to drain into the stem of the inferior vermian vein or the lateral sinus (Fig. 263).

Some of the superior and inferior hemispheric tributaries may drain independently into the ***anterior lateral marginal vein*** or into the superior petrosal, inferior petrosal, sigmoid or lateral sinus.

The vein of the great horizontal fissure, the transverse pontine vein, the brachial vein, the vein of the lateral recess of the fourth ventricle, and the lateral pontine vein usually converge towards the anterior angle of the cerebellum where they form a single stem, the ***petrosal vein.*** This vein runs anterolaterally and opens into the superior petrosal sinus, usually above the internal auditory meatus (Figs. 261, 264, 266, 269, 270, 274, 275). In some cases, the tributaries of the petrosal vein may form several stems that drain into the superior petrosal sinus at different points. As described above, occasionally a small vein, the inferior petrosal or vagal vein, originating from the cerebellopontomedullary angle, joins the lower end of the inferior petrosal or the sigmoid sinus.

III. Posterior or Tentorial Draining Group

Included in this group are the inferior vermian vein and the superior and inferior hemispheric veins (HUANG *et al.*, 1969; HUANG *et al.*, 1975). Diagnostically, the most important vein in this group is the ***inferior vermian vein*** and its ***superior and inferior retrotonsillar tributaries.*** This vein may be said to be formed by the union of the superior and inferior retrotonsillar tributaries, behind the cerebellar tonsil. The combined vein then runs posterosuperiorly in the inferior paravermian sulcus, receives the suprapyramidal, hemispheric and declival veins, and joins the straight or lateral sinus directly or indirectly through a tentorial sinus (Figs. 261, 263, 265, 267, 268 A–C, 269–272, 275, 276, 278, 279 A, 280).

The medial, lateral, and occasionally the apical tributaries unite in the supratonsillar portion of the posterolateral fissure, behind the superior pole of the cerebellar tonsil, to form the ***superior retrotonsillar vein.*** This vein travels downwards in the retrotonsillar fissure. After it emerges from the tonsillobiventral notch, it makes a rather sharp posterosuperior turn, running around the anterior and inferior aspects of the copula pyramidis (ANGEVINE *et al.*, 1961) to join the inferior vermian vein.

The configuration and location of the curve formed by the inferior vermian and superior retrotonsillar veins, as seen in the lateral venous phase in posterior fossa angiography, are therefore important (Figs. 267 A, 268 and C, 269 A, 272, 276 B). The most antero-inferior point of the curve has been designated the *copular point.* As measured on angiograms from 30 presumably normal adults, this point is situated within a circle of 6 mm in diameter, with its center located 4 mm posterior and 4 mm inferior to the midpoint of a line connecting the anterior rim of the foramen magnum to the torcular. Similarly, in the semiaxial projection, the inferior vermian and superior retrotonsillar veins form a typical acute angle pointing inferiorly. Its apex marks the antero-inferior margin of the copula pyramidis (Figs. 267 B, 269 B, 270 B, 275, 277, 278).
The *lateral supratonsillar tributary* lies below and parallel to the lateral margin of the posterolateral recess of the fourth ventricle and above the attachment of the cerebellar tonsil to the cerebellar hemisphere. It receives veinlets from the dentate nucleus and the neighboring medullary body of the cerebellum *(dentate veins).* The *medial and apical supratonsillar tributaries* are situated on the medial and apical aspects, respectively, of the superior pole of the cerebellar tonsil. They frequently communicate anteriorly with the corresponding supratonsillar tributaries of the vein of the lateral recess of the fourth ventricle. When the supratonsillar tributaries of the superior retrotonsillar vein are prominent, it is likely that the supratonsillar tributaries of the vein of the lateral recess of the fourth ventricle are small. On the other hand, when the supratonsillar tributaries of the inferior vermian vein are hypoplastic, the supratonsillar tributaries of the vein of the lateral recess are often prominent.

The ***inferior retrotonsillar vein,*** which originates on the undersurface of the biventral lobule, travels medially and superiorly. It receives tributaries from the other parts of the biventral lobule *(biventral tributaries)* and from the medial, lateral and occasionally the posterior aspects of the cerebellar tonsil *(medial, lateral and posterior tonsillar tributaries).* Behind the midportion of the cerebellar tonsil, the inferior and superior retrotonsillar tributaries unite to form the inferior vermian vein.
Other tributaries that flow into the inferior vermian vein include the suprapyramidal, declival, and hemispheric veins. The ***suprapyramidal vein*** begins in the suprapyramidal fissure between the tuber above and the pyramid below. It runs postero-inferiorly and joins the inferior vermian vein, either immediately after it leaves the fissure or after it follows a short upward course, behind the tuber. The pyramid, therefore, may be outlined by the superior retrotonsillar and suprapyramidal veins in both the lateral and semiaxial projections (Figs. 261, 265, 268 B and C, 269 A, 276 B, 277 A). The ***declival vein*** usually emerges as the ***vein of the primary fissure,*** between the culmen and the declive monticuli (Figs. 261, 263, 265, 268 B, 269 A, 276 A, 280 A). Usually there is one vein on each side but sometimes there are more, and their sizes are variable. It runs downwards and backwards, in or adjacent to the declival sulcus, and flows into the stem of the inferior vermian vein, near its junction with the straight sinus. Not infrequently, the vein originates more laterally, from the hemispheric portion of the primary fissure or from the neighboring sulcus. It runs posteromedially and inferiorly towards the upper end of the posterior cerebellar notch, where it joins the inferior vermian vein. In these cases, these ***paradeclival veins*** take a more horizontal course in the lateral venogram (Fig. 276 A). Not infrequently one or two ***hemispheric tributaries,*** originating from the inferior surface of the cerebellar hemisphere, run medially to join the inferior vermian vein.
Variations in the course of the inferior vermian vein are not uncommon. The vein may not lie in the depths of the inferior paravermian sulcus, but some distance behind it. Or, it may leave the posterior cerebellar notch entirely and run superolaterally on the inferior surface of the cerebellar hemisphere, to open into the lateral sinus (Figs. 261, 269 A, 274 B, 280 B). The inferior vermian vein may be quite tortuous and form a loop in the posterior cerebellar notch (Fig. 267 A). Finally, it may drain into the lateral sinus or torcular, after crossing the posterior cerebellar notch, to travel along the hemisphere of the opposite side (Fig. 277 B).
Other hemispheric veins of the posterior group often drain into the lateral sinus (HAGUE, 1954). The ***superior hemispheric veins*** run posteriorly and inferiorly on the superior surface of the cerebellar hemisphere and open into the transverse sinus. The ***inferior hemispheric veins,*** on the other hand, run superiorly on the inferior aspect of the cerebellar hemisphere and flow into the transverse

sinus, directly or indirectly, through a tentorial sinus. Quite frequently, some of the inferior hemispheric veins run upwards on the inferior surface, cross the posterior lateral margin, and travel superomedially on the superior surface of the cerebellar hemisphere, where they open into a tentorial sinus, with a superior hemispheric vein or veins (Figs. 269, 273 A, 274).

Although the number of tentorial sinuses (Bouchet *et al.*, 1963–1964; Huang *et al.*, 1975) varies from 0 to 6, usually only one or two can be seen on each side in the posterior fossa angiograms. They run either posteromedially to join the torcular or adjacent sinuses, or flow posterolaterally to open into the lateral sinus near its junction with the sigmoid sinus (Figs. 275, 278).

IV. Intercommunications Among the Superior, Anterior and Posterior Draining Groups and Between the Supra- and Infratentorial Veins

As described above, there are frequently communications between the superior and anterior draining groups via brachial tributaries of the precentral cerebellar and petrosal veins. A communication may take place at the bottom of the precentral cerebellar fissure (Figs. 266 A, 268 B, 270 B, 279 A), or along the anterior superior margin of the cerebellar hemisphere—anterior superior marginal vein (Fig. 280). There may be a linkage between superior hemispheric tributaries of the precentral cerebellar and petrosal veins (Fig. 261).

Anastomoses between veins of the anterior and posterior draining groups are usually via superior and inferior hemispheric tributaries, running respectively on the superior and inferior surfaces of the cerebellar hemisphere. Communications between the inferior vermian vein and the vein of the lateral recess of the fourth ventricle frequently occur through the medial tonsillar and supratonsillar tributaries (Figs. 261, 266, 274).

Connections between the superior and posterior draining groups are usually through the supraculminate and declival veins (Fig. 269 A), or through a hemispheric tributary connecting the precentral cerebellar vein and the lateral sinus (Figs. 268 B, 269 A, 280 B). Occasionally, the inferior vermian vein, originating from the retrotonsillar fissure, may drain into the galenic system by traversing the posterior aspect of the entire vermis to flow into the superior vermian or superior cerebellar vein (Fig. 279 A). An inferior hemispheric vein of the posterior group may rarely drain upwards, cross the posterolateral margin, and run onto the superior surface of the cerebellar hemisphere to drain into the superior vermian vein (Fig. 279 B). The tributaries of the petrosal vein may, in rare cases, drain into the great cerebral vein via the brachial, anastomotic lateral mesencephalic, and posterior mesencephalic veins with no connection with the superior petrosal sinus (Fig. 273 B). Another unusual connection between the posterior portion of the internal cerebral vein and the straight sinus is the ***galenovermorectal vein,*** which traverses the superior vermis (Figs. 276 A, 281). Rarely encountered is the ***precentrovermorectal vein.*** This vein begins in the precentral cerebellar fissure, runs superiorly and posteriorly over the culmen and declive, and flows into the posterior portion of the straight sinus (Figs. 271 A, 276 A).

Other communications between the supra- and infratentorial veins are frequently encountered. The basal cerebral and the petrosal veins are often connected via the ***anastomotic lateral mesencephalic vein*** (Wolf *et al.*, 1963). When the anterior portion of the basal cerebral vein is absent, the anastomotic lateral mesencephalic vein may bridge the posterior mesencephalic and petrosal veins. In these cases, it seems more appropriate to use the term ***galenopetrosal vein*** (Duvernoy, 1975). Communication between the basal cerebral vein and the petrosal vein via the peduncular, anterior pontomesencephalic and transverse pontine veins is described above, also encountered relatively often. Anastomoses through the lateral anterior pontomesencephalic and lateral pontomesencephalic veins are, however, relatively rare. It should be noted that supra- and infratentorial veins frequently open into the same tentorial sinus from both sides of the tentorium. Therefore, these veins may be said to be connected through the tentorial sinus (Figs. 273 A, 274, 278).

Drainage of the dural sinuses of the posterior fossa into the extracranial venous system may occur through the mastoid, anterior and posterior condyloid, and occipital emissary veins (Fig. 282). There may also be a connection between the circular sinus and the internal vertebral venous plexuses (Theron and Djindjian, 1973a; 1973b).

V. Circulation Times of Veins of the Posterior Fossa

The angiographic circulation times of the vessels within the posterior fossa (Greiz, 1969) were measured from the moment of maximal bilateral filling of the vertebral arteries, at the level of the first cervical vertebra, to the moment of maximal filling of each individual vein of the posterior fossa. These times were measured from rapid serial angiograms of 30 presumably normal adults (Huang *et al.*, 1975). Compared with the mean circulation time of supratentorial vessels on vertebral angiograms, that of the cerebellar tributaries of the anterior and posterior draining groups, in the same series of angiograms, is about 1 second longer, whereas that of the spinal and medullary tributaries is about 2 seconds longer. Although the angiographic circulation time of the mesencephalic and cerebellar tributaries of the superior draining group is shorter than that of the anterior or posterior draining groups, it is still roughly 0.5 seconds longer than that of the supratentorial tributaries.

Fig. 261. Anatomic diagrams showing the veins of the posterior fossa and related structures

A. Lateral view, B. midsagittal view, C. view from above and front, D. view from below, E. view from behind and below. Covered portions of vessels are shown in dashed fashion. Different arrangements of venous drainage are shown on the two sides.
In the superior draining group, the superior vermis and adjacent brain stem may be drained either by a single vessel, the superior cerebellar vein (Fig. A), or by two separate veins, the precentral cerebellar and superior vermian (Fig. B). In the anterior draining group, the vein of the lateral recess of the fourth ventricle on the left side is joined by the retro-olivary vein, the inferior hemispheric veins and the vein of the great horizontal fissure (Figs. A and C). Together with the brachial and transverse pontine veins, the combined stem drains into the petrosal vein. On the right side, the vein of the lateral recess of the fourth ventricle, after emerging from the cerebellopontomedullary angle, runs antero-inferiorly and laterally in the pontocerebellar cistern, before opening directly into the inferior end of the inferior petrosal sinus (Figs. B, C and D). In the posterior draining group, on the right side the retrotonsillar tributaries unite to form the inferior vermian vein, behind the midportion of the cerebellar tonsil. The inferior vermian vein then runs upwards and backwards in the inferior paravermian sulcus, to join the straight sinus together with the declival vein (Figs. B and E). On the other hand, the retrotonsillar tributaries on the left side unite to form a single stem that emerges from the posterior cerebellar notch to run superiorly and laterally on the inferior surface of the cerebellar hemisphere. This inferior hemispheric vein then crosses the posterolateral margin, to run upwards onto the superior surface of the cerebellar hemisphere and joins a tentorial sinus, together with other superior and inferior hemispheric tributaries (Figs. A and E).
Note anastomoses between the petrosal vein and the galenic venous system via the anterior pontomesencephalic, lateral mesencephalic and precentral cerebellar veins (Figs. A and C). A link between the superior and anterior groups via superior hemispheric tributaries is, however, not illustrated. Communications between the superior and posterior draining groups, via superior hemispheric tributaries, and between the anterior and posterior groups, via tributaries around the cerebellar tonsil, are also shown. Note possible anastomoses between the median posterior medullary vein and the vein of the lateral recess via a chain of veins—vein of the restiform body, vein of the restiform eminence, retro-olivary vein and lateral pontine vein (Figs. A and B). Also note likely connections between the median posterior medullary vein and the inferior vermian vein via the medial tonsillar and supratonsillar tributaries. The isthmus of the rhombencephalon is indicated by the distance between the lower end (↑) of the mesencephalic segment of the anterior pontomesencephalic vein and the colliculocentral point of the precentral cerebellar vein (Fig. B). The copular point—the most anteroinferior point in the course of the inferior vermian vein and its superior retrotonsillar tributary around the copular pyramidis—is labelled in Figs. B and E (Figs. 261 A, D and E from HUANG *et al.*, 1975)

Figs. 261 A–E see pp. 340–344 ▷

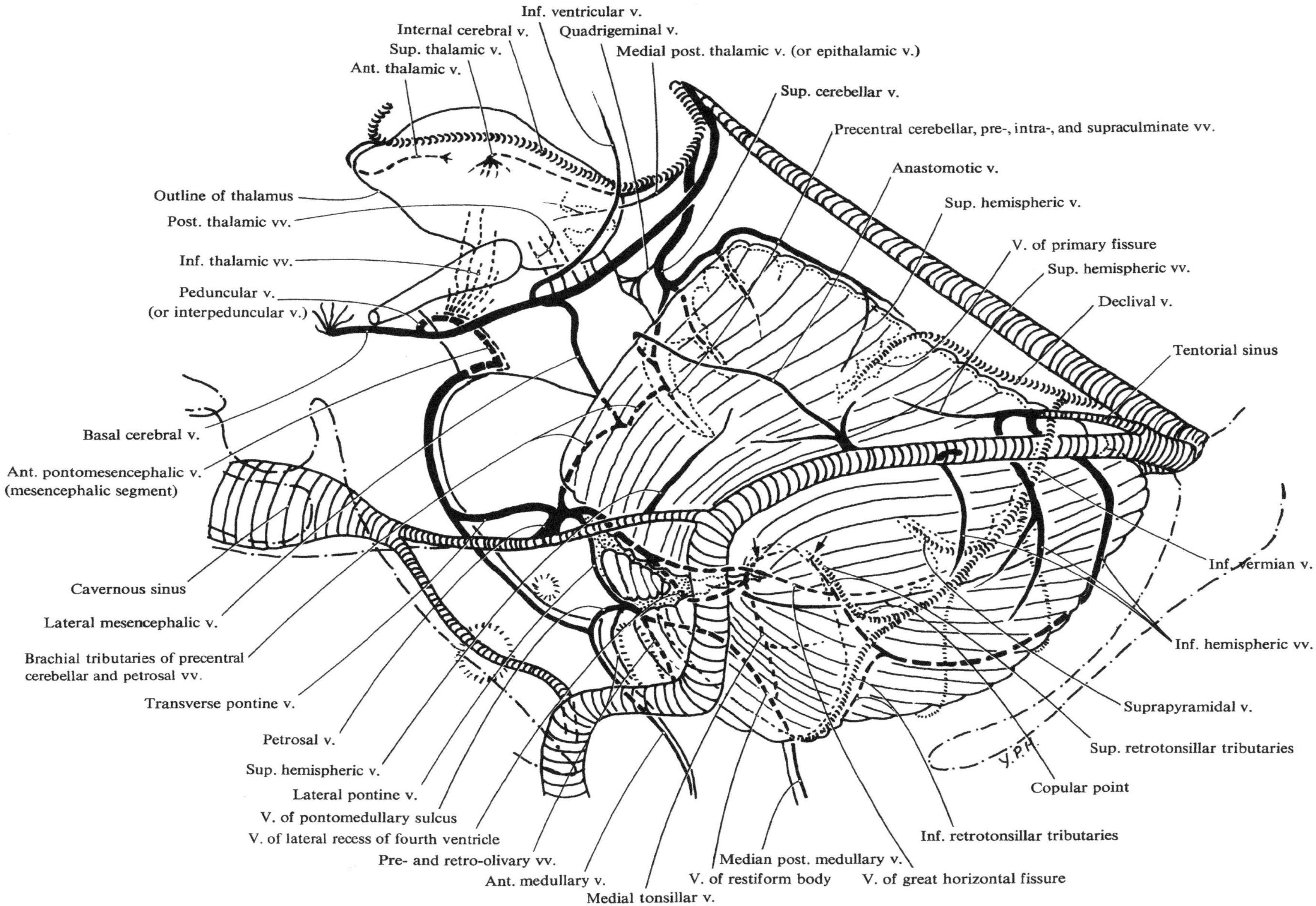

Fig. 261 A. Lateral view

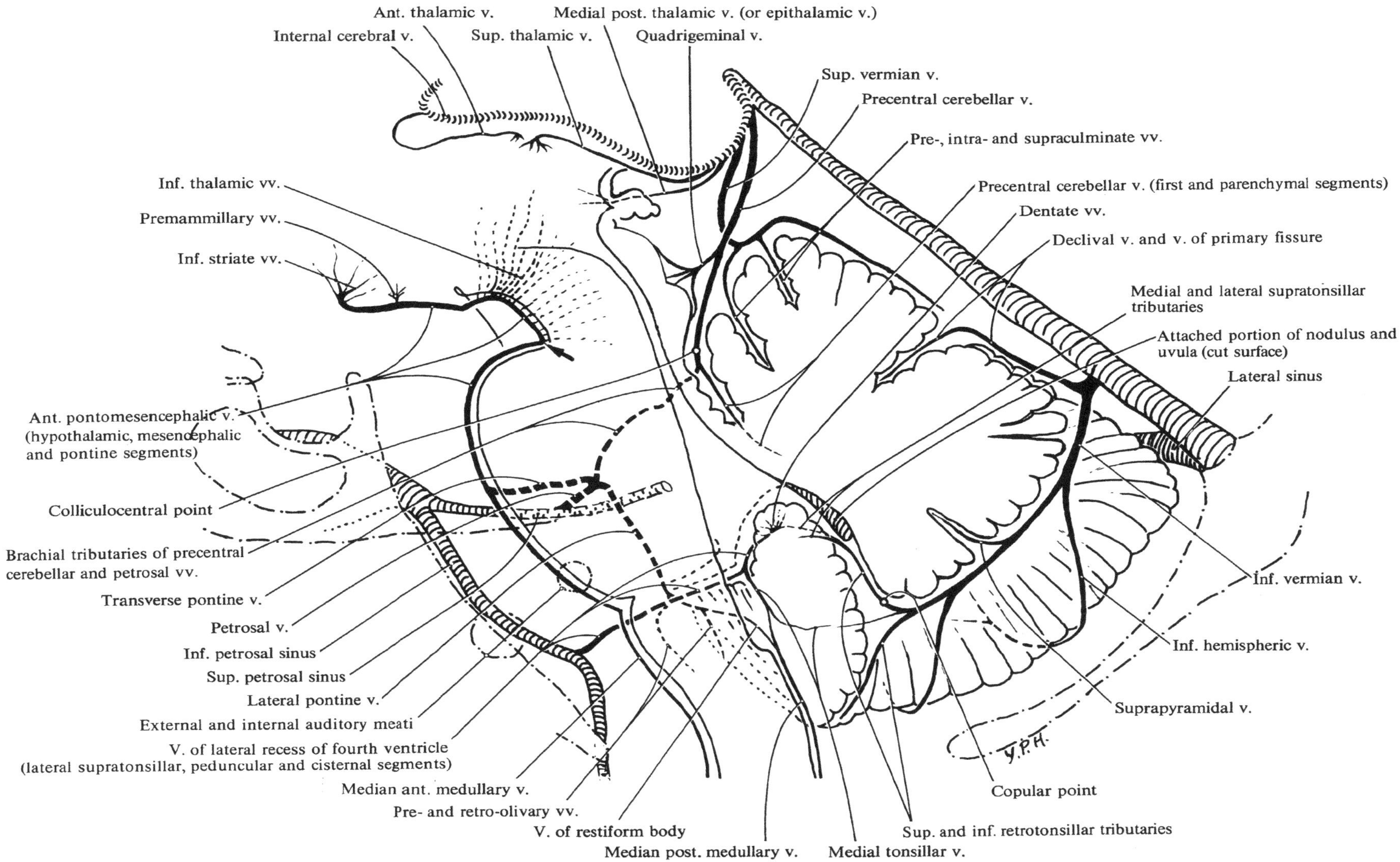

Fig. 261 B. Midsagittal view

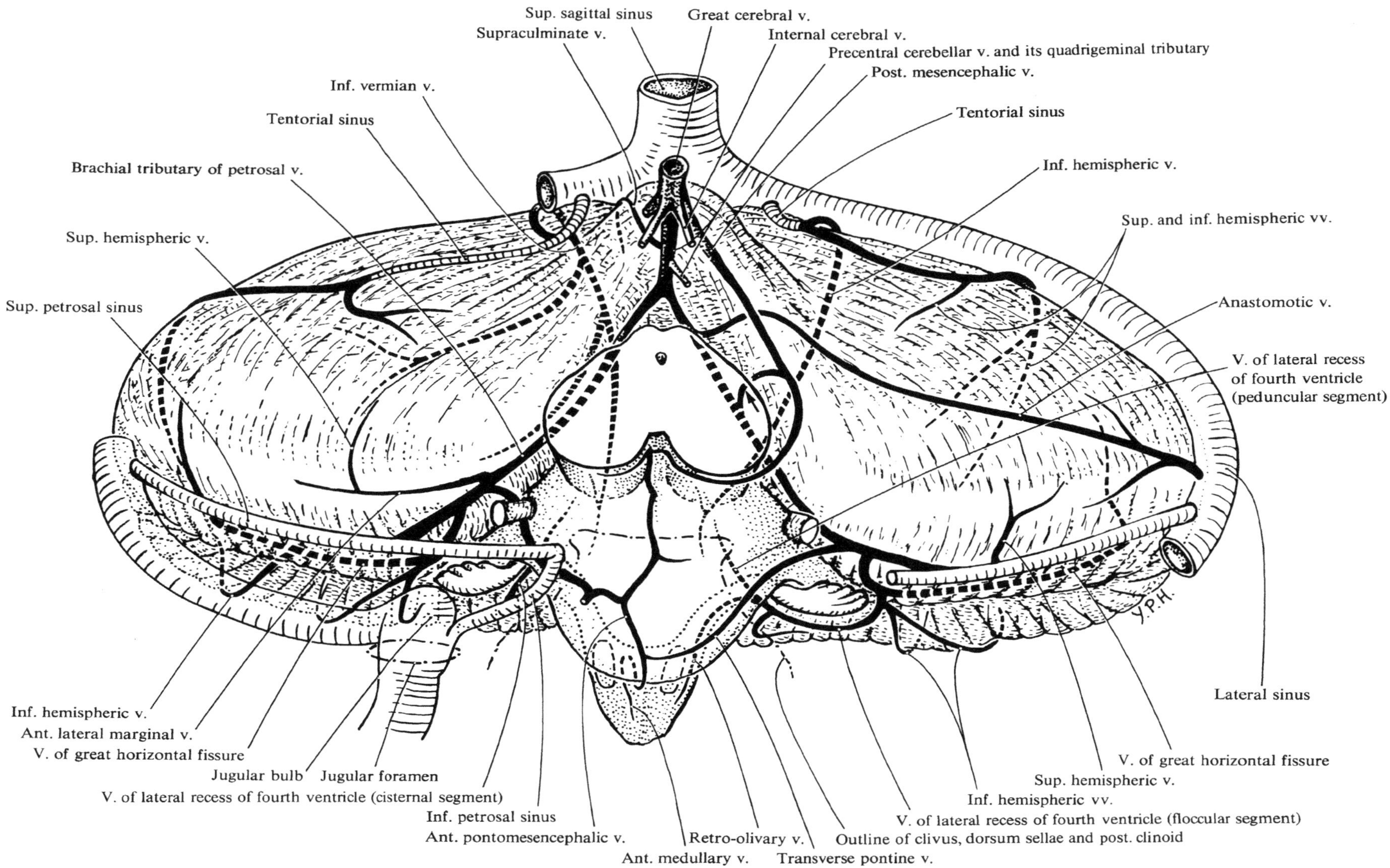

Fig. 261 C. View from above and front

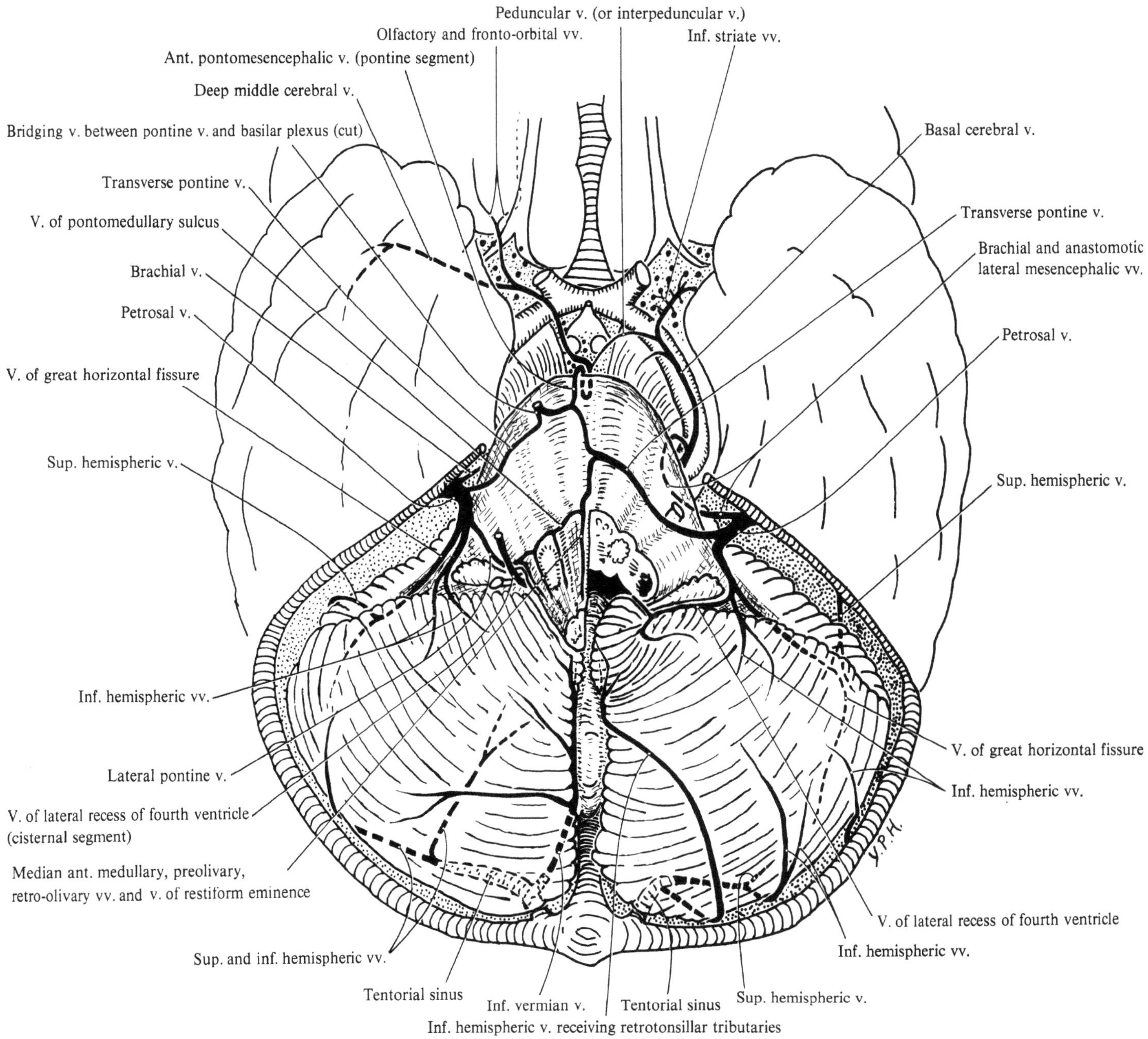

Fig. 261 D. View from below

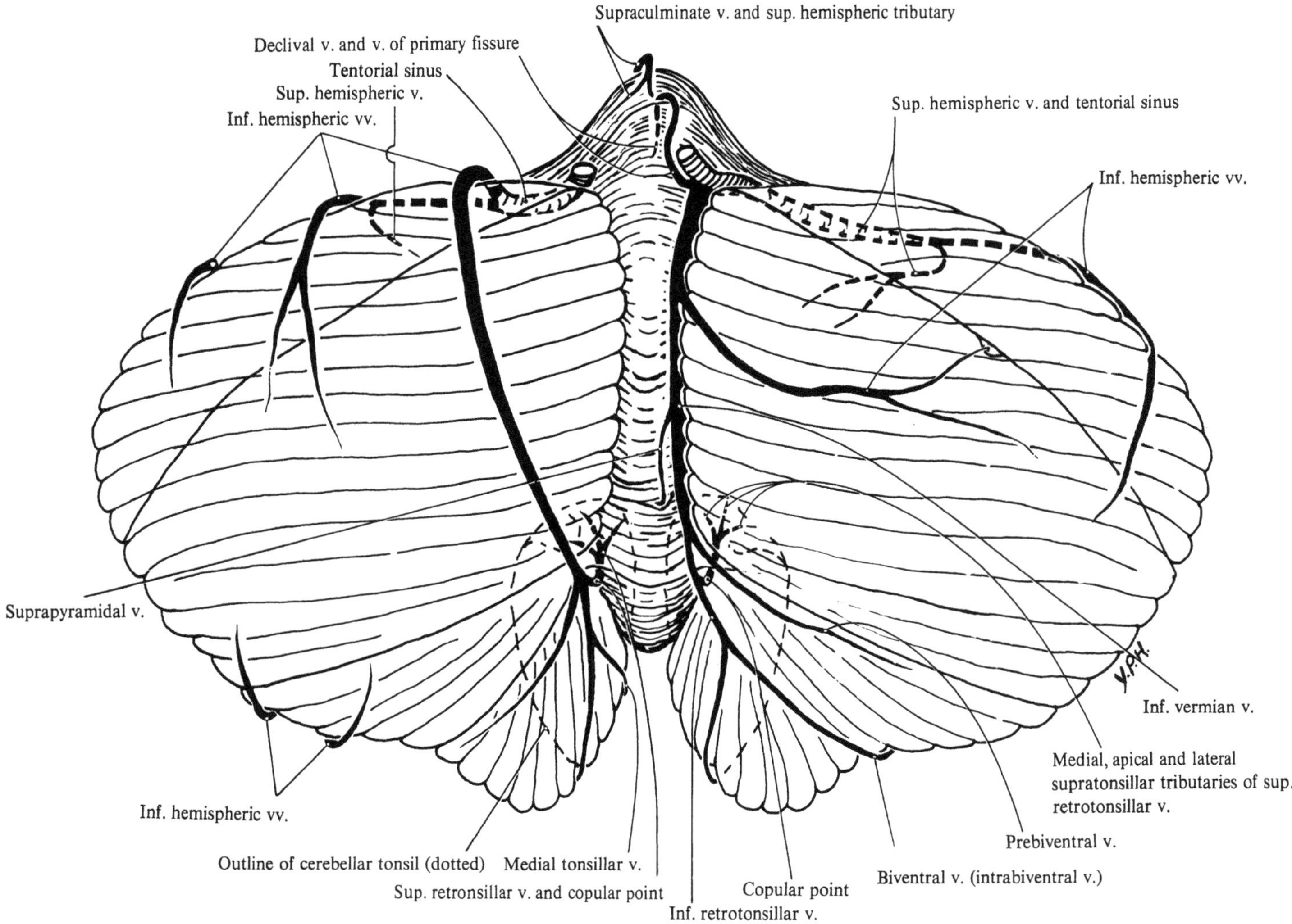

Fig. 261 E. View from behind and below

▷

Fig. 262. Photographs of an injected specimen showing the course of the precentral cerebellar vein, lateral mesencephalic veins, basal cerebral veins and related anatomical structures

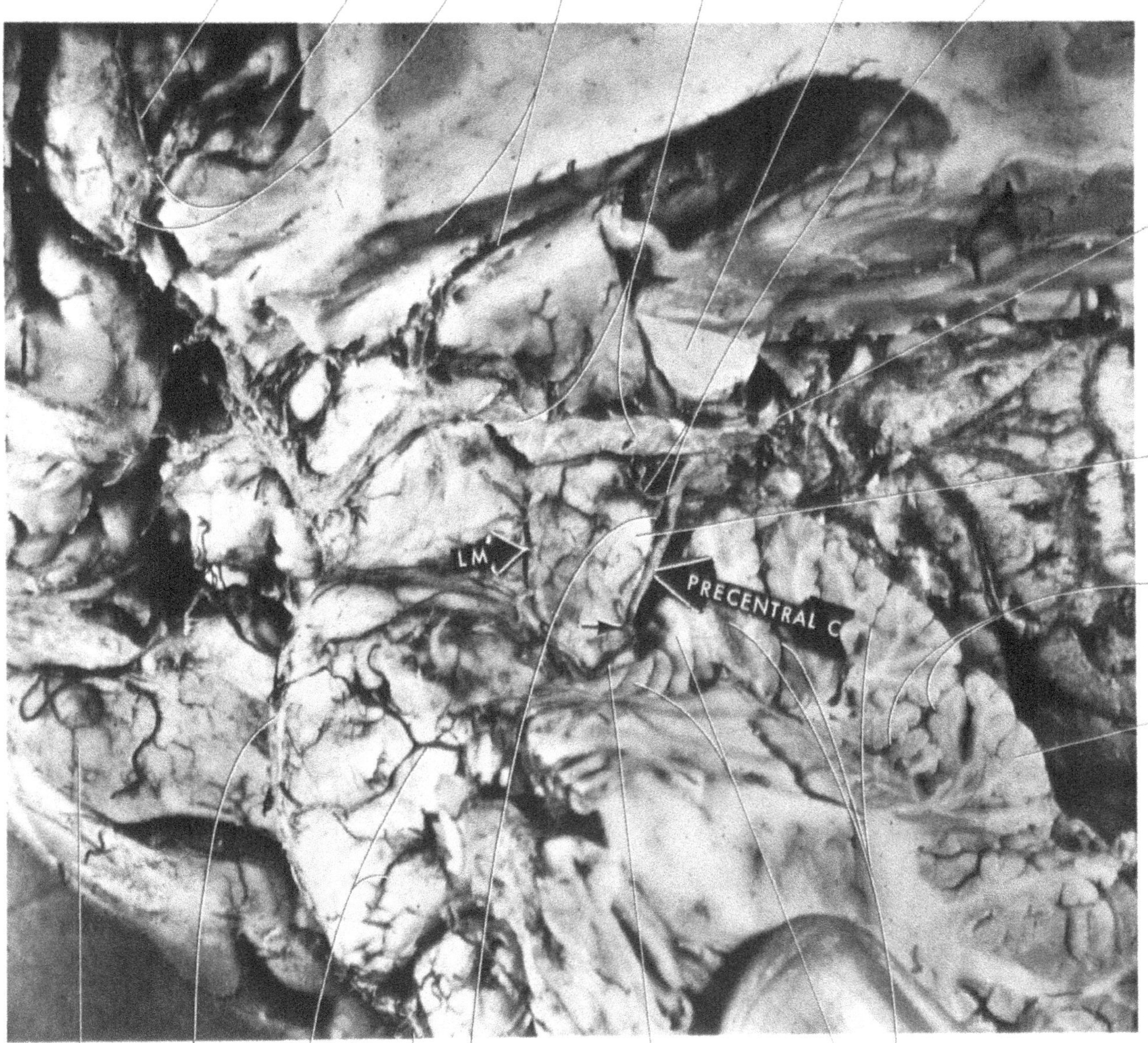

Fig. 262 A. Lateral view. Part of the temporal lobe and the lateral part of the cerebellar hemisphere have been removed on the left side, exposing the temporal horn, lateral aspect of the mesencephalon, central lobule and its wings, and the midsagittal plane of the culmen and declive. The colliculocentral point (unlabelled small arrow) of the precentral cerebellar vein (PRECENTRAL C) is located anteriorly to the upper part of the central lobule, immediately behind the lower ends of the inferior colliculi. Behind the tectum, the median superior and median inferior tectal veins unite to form a single stem, the tectal or quadrigeminal vein, which runs backwards and upwards to join the precentral cerebellar vein near its junction with the great cerebral vein. The brachial tributary of the precentral cerebellar vein runs over the brachium pontis and anastomoses with the lower end of the lateral mesencephalic vein and the brachial tributary of the petrosal vein (not labelled). The lateral mesencephalic vein (LM) drains upwards to join the basal cerebral vein—junction fractured in this specimen. The inferior ventricular vein, emerging from the inferior choroidal point (not labelled) to join the basal cerebral vein, is also seen

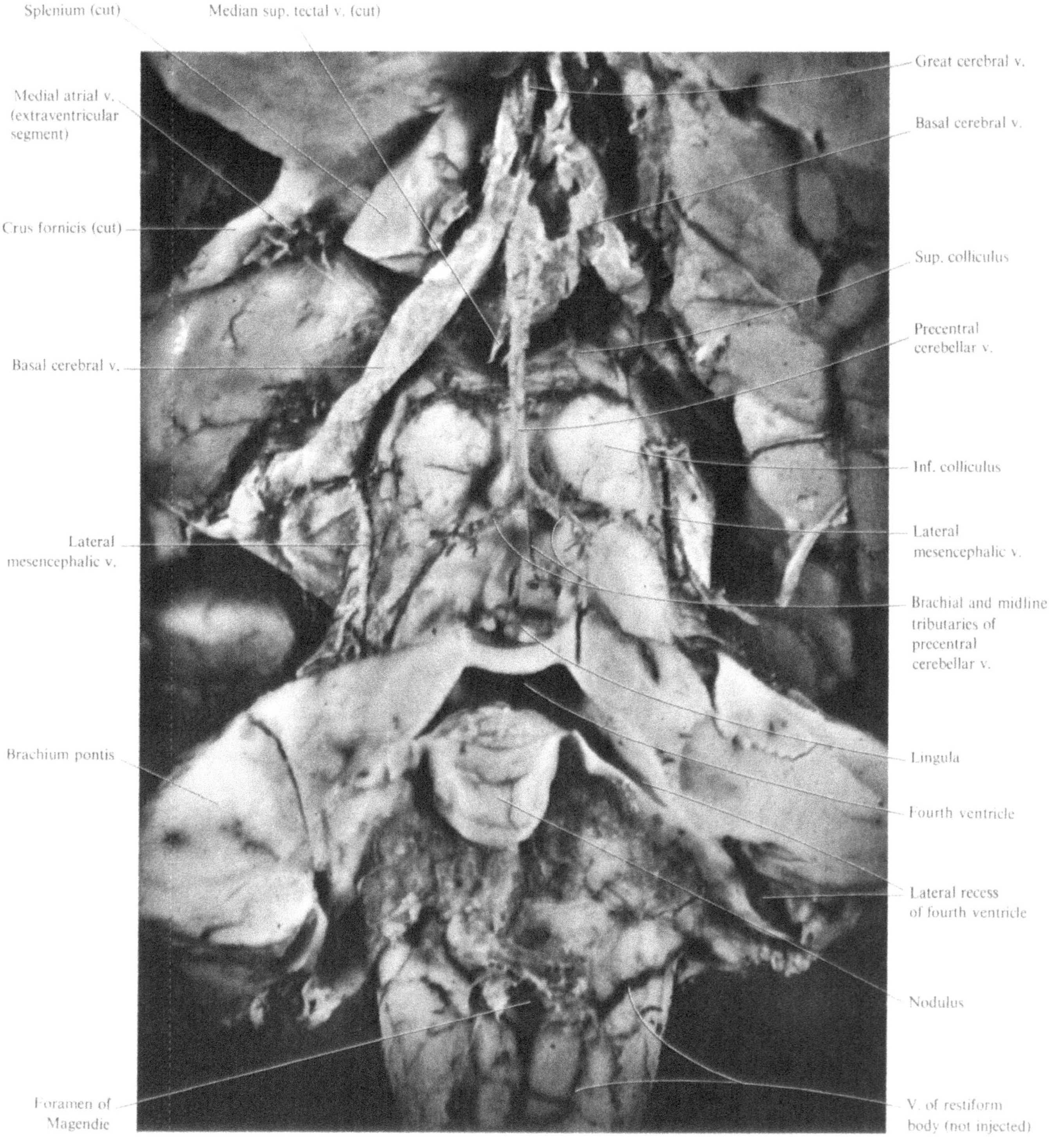

Fig. 262 B. Posterior view, same specimen. The cerebellum has been removed, exposing the posterior aspect of the mesencephalon, cut surface of the brachia conjunctiva, brachia pontis, restiform bodies, lingula, and nodulus. The fourth ventricle and parts of its lateral recesses are open. The precentral cerebellar vein and its brachial tributaries have a typical inverted "Y" configuration. A small midline tributary also joins the precentral cere-

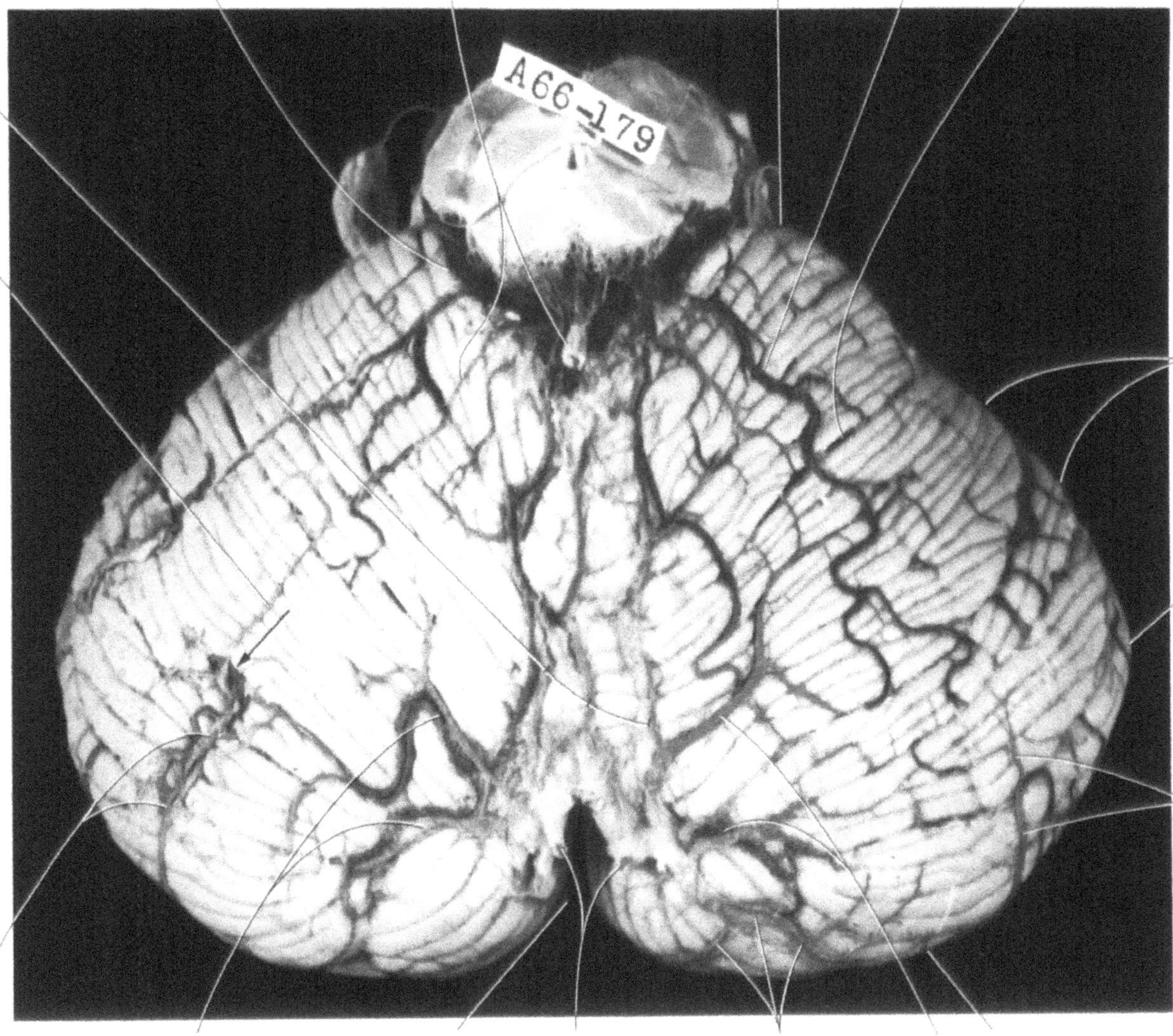

Fig. 263A. view from above

Fig. 263. Photographs of an injected specimen, showing the hemispheric tributaries of the superior and posterior draining groups of veins of the posterior fossa
A. View from above, B. view from below, C. view from behind, D. view from behind and below. Arteries are black, veins are grey. The precentral cerebellar vein is located in the fissure between the cerebellum and the brain stem, behind the lingula (Fig. A). Three declival veins join the stems of the inferior vermian veins, together with the inferior and superior hemispheric veins (Figs. A and C). On the right, one of the inferior hemispheric veins runs in and adjacent to the great horizontal fissure and, therefore, may be called the vein of the great horizontal fissure (Figs. C and D). This vein is, however, labelled as an inferior hemispheric vein. On the left, the superior and inferior hemispheric veins unite and eventually open into a dural sinus (arrow) within the tentorium (tentorium removed) (Figs. A and C)

Figs. 263A–D see pp. 348–350

◁
Fig. 262B (continued)
bellar vein. The lateral mesencephalic veins drain mainly upwards to flow into the basal cerebral vein on each side. The distance between the two lateral mesencephalic veins indicates the transverse width of the mesencephalon at the level of the corresponding sulci (Fig. 262 from Huang and Wolf, 1965)

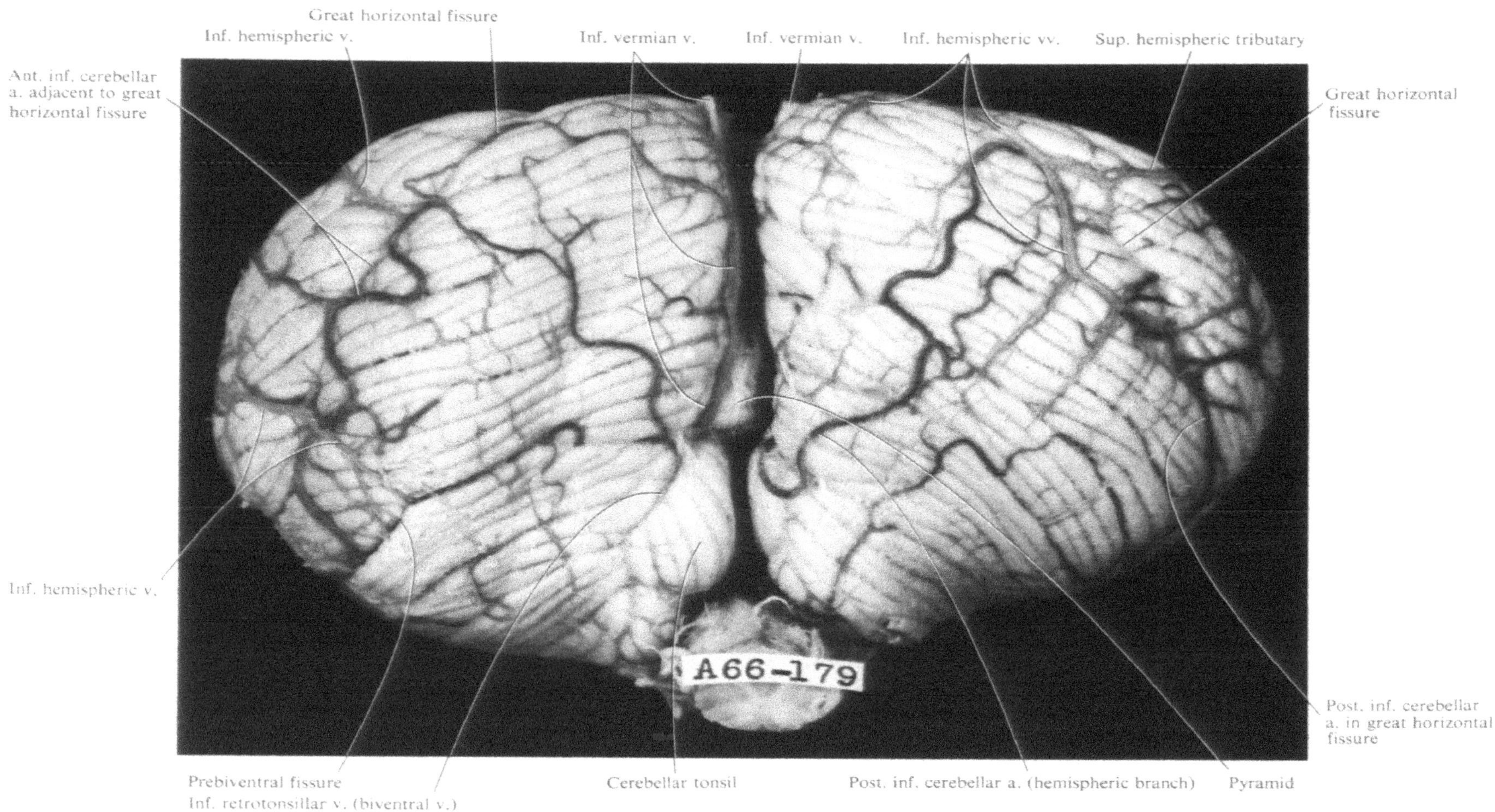

Fig. 263 B. View from below

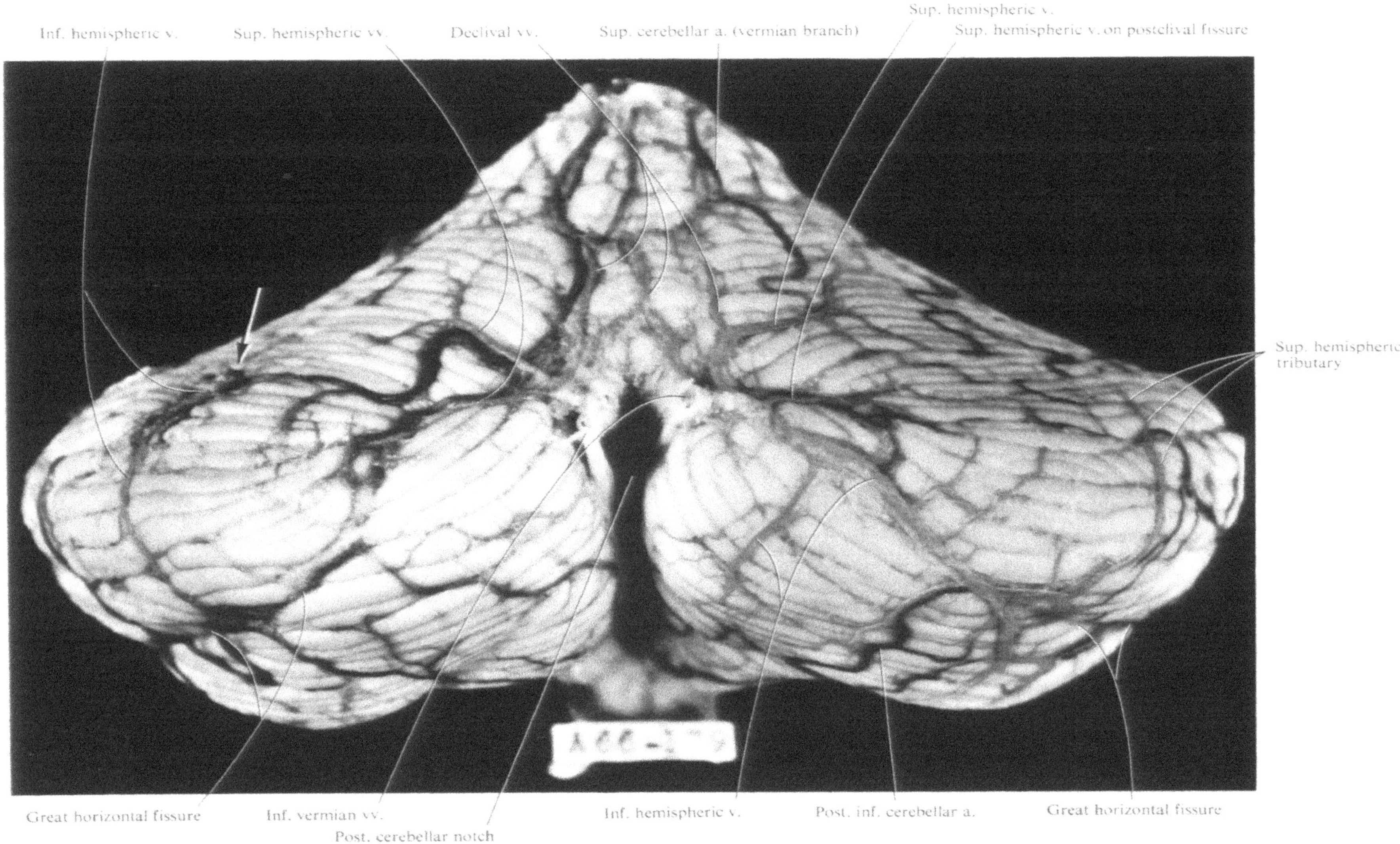

Fig. 263C. View from behind

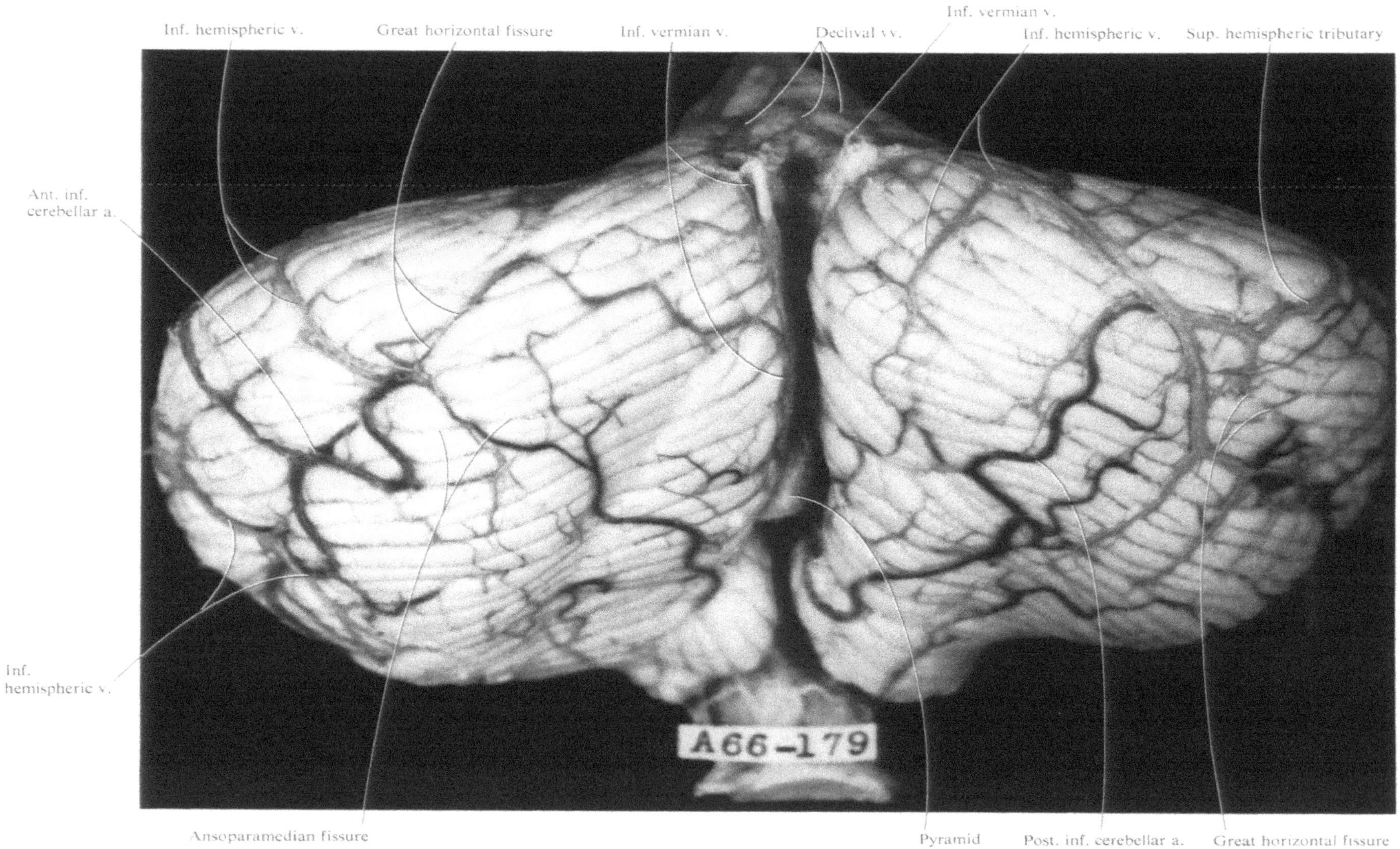

Fig. 263 D. View from behind and below

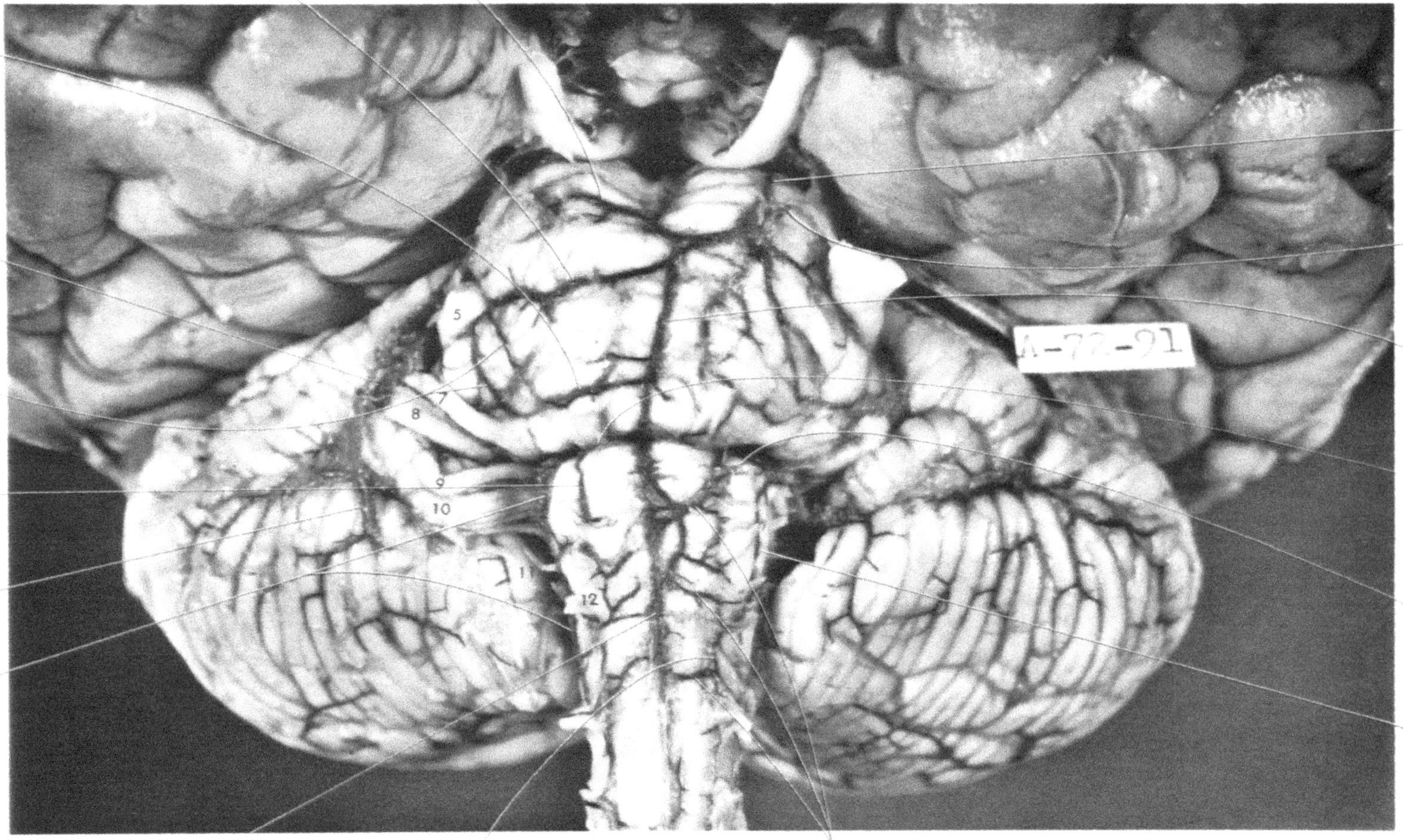

Fig. 264A. View from the front and below (Text see p. 352)

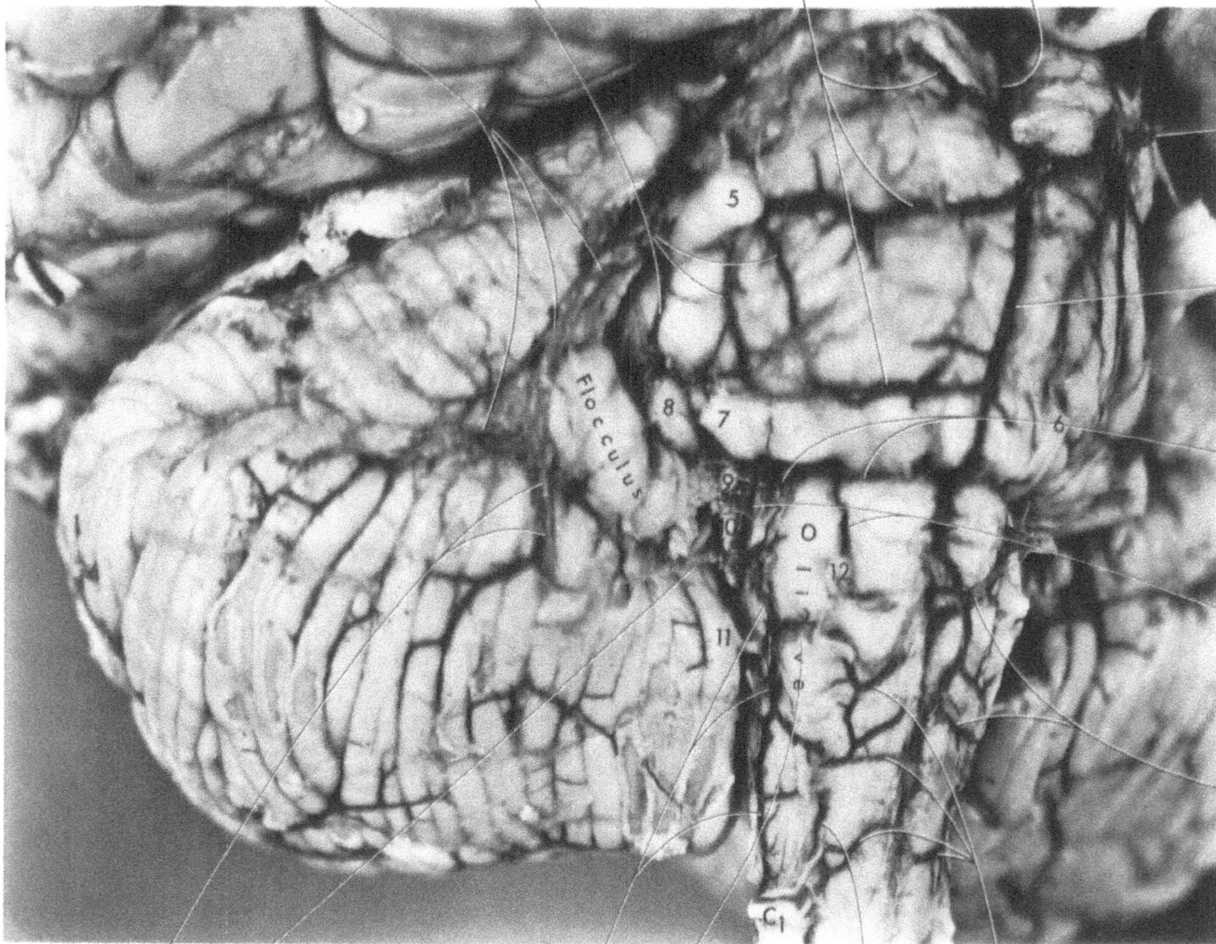

Fig. 264 B. View from the right, front and below

Fig. 264. Injected specimen showing the course of the anterior draining group of veins of the posterior fossa

A. View from the front and below, and B. view from the right, front and below. Arteries have been removed, leaving veins filled with colored radiopaque material (veins are black).

Apart from the median anterior pontine veins, other pontine veins are distributed asymmetrically between the two sides. On the right, the transversely running pontine veins (superior, middle and inferior transverse pontine veins) are prominent, whereas on the left, both vertically running (lateral anterior pontine veins) and transversely running veins (transverse pontine veins) can be identified. Veins on the anterior aspect of the medulla oblongata are orientated in the sagittal and parasagittal planes, running in the anterior medullary fissure (median anterior medullary vein or simply anterior medullary vein), in the pre-olivary sulcus (pre-olivary vein) or in the retro-olivary sulcus (retro-olivary vein or lateral medullary vein). The vagal vein (or inferior petrosal vein) runs forwards with the Xth nerve (to drain into the inferior end of the inferior petrosal sinus). Numerous transverse connections between the various longitudinally running medullary veins can be identified (transverse medullary veins)

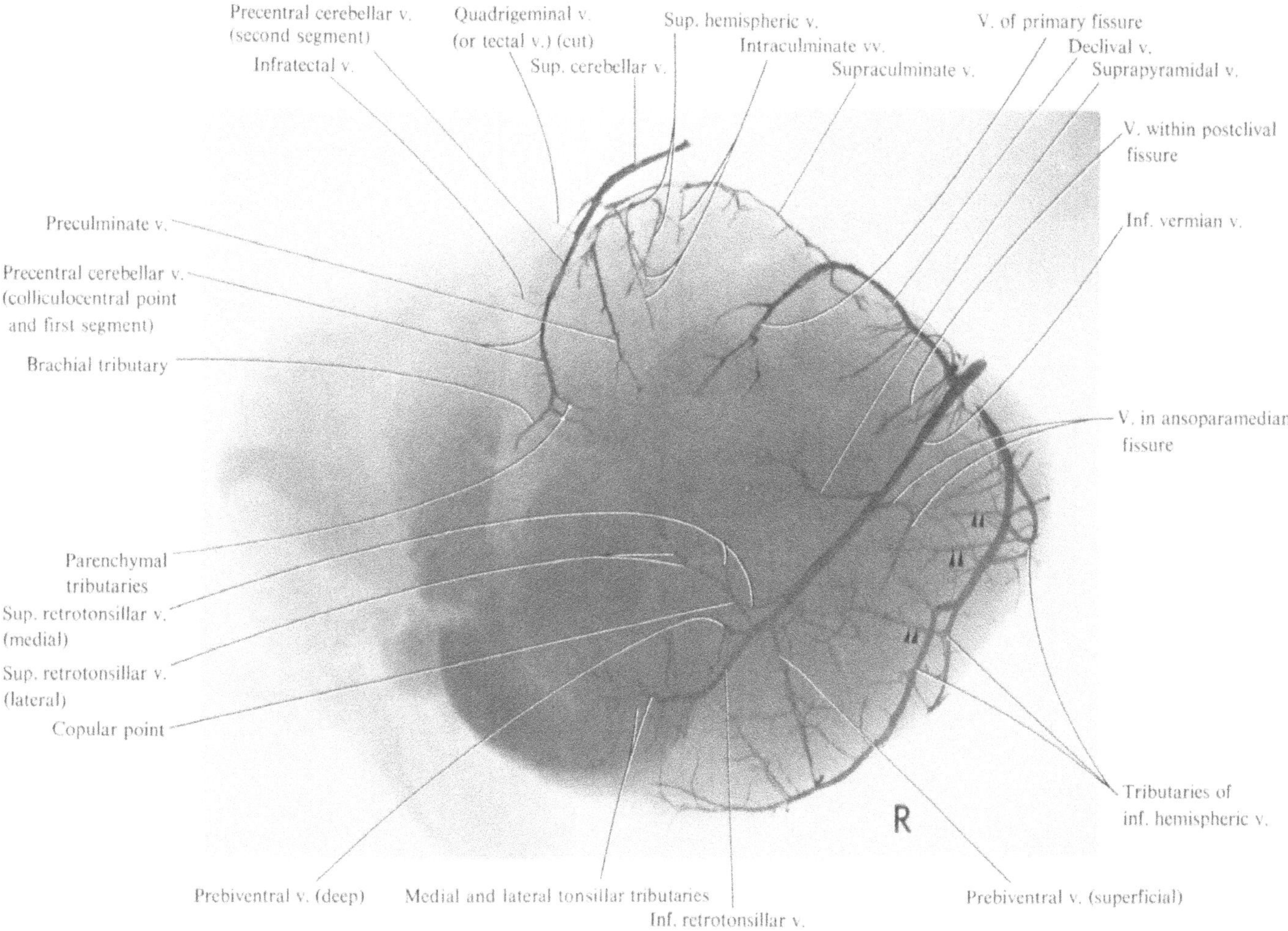

Fig. 265 A. Lateral view

Fig. 265. Radiographs of an injected specimen, showing the course of the superior and posterior draining groups of veins of the posterior fossa

A. Lateral view, B. submentovertical view, C. Towne or semiaxial view and D. anteroposterior view.
↑, split precentral cerebellar vein; ▲ ▲ veins within the great horizontal fissure; ▲, ⍏ connecting veins between two inferior vermian veins; △, copular point; △ △, preculminate vein. In the lateral radiograph, the right half of the brain stem and cerebellum is shown (Fig. A).
In the superior draining group, the superior vermian vein receives the supraculminate, intraculminate, preculminate and superior hemispheric tributaries. It is joined by the precentral cerebellar vein to form the superior cerebellar vein. The two brachial tributaries of the precentral cerebellar vein unite, not in the depths of the precentral cerebellar fissure but immediately below the inferior colliculi. In the posterior draining group, the right declival vein, which receives the vein of the primary fissure, is prominent and is located adjacent to the midline, whereas the left declival vein, which receives veins from the posterior part of the quadrangular lobule, lies adjacent to the left declival sulcus. The inferior vermian veins are connected by two anastomotic channels, one located near the distal ends (⍏) and the other near the midportions (▲) of the inferior vermian veins. A large number of veins, emerging from the great horizontal fissure (▲ ▲) and postclival fissure (Fig. D), can be identified. Two superior retrotonsillar veins are seen: the more medially located vein lies more posteriorly than the more laterally located one (Figs. A and B). On the right, the medial and lateral tonsillar veins outline the transverse width of the posterior part of the cerebellar tonsil (Figs. B, C and D)

Figs. 265 A–D see pp. 353–356 ▷

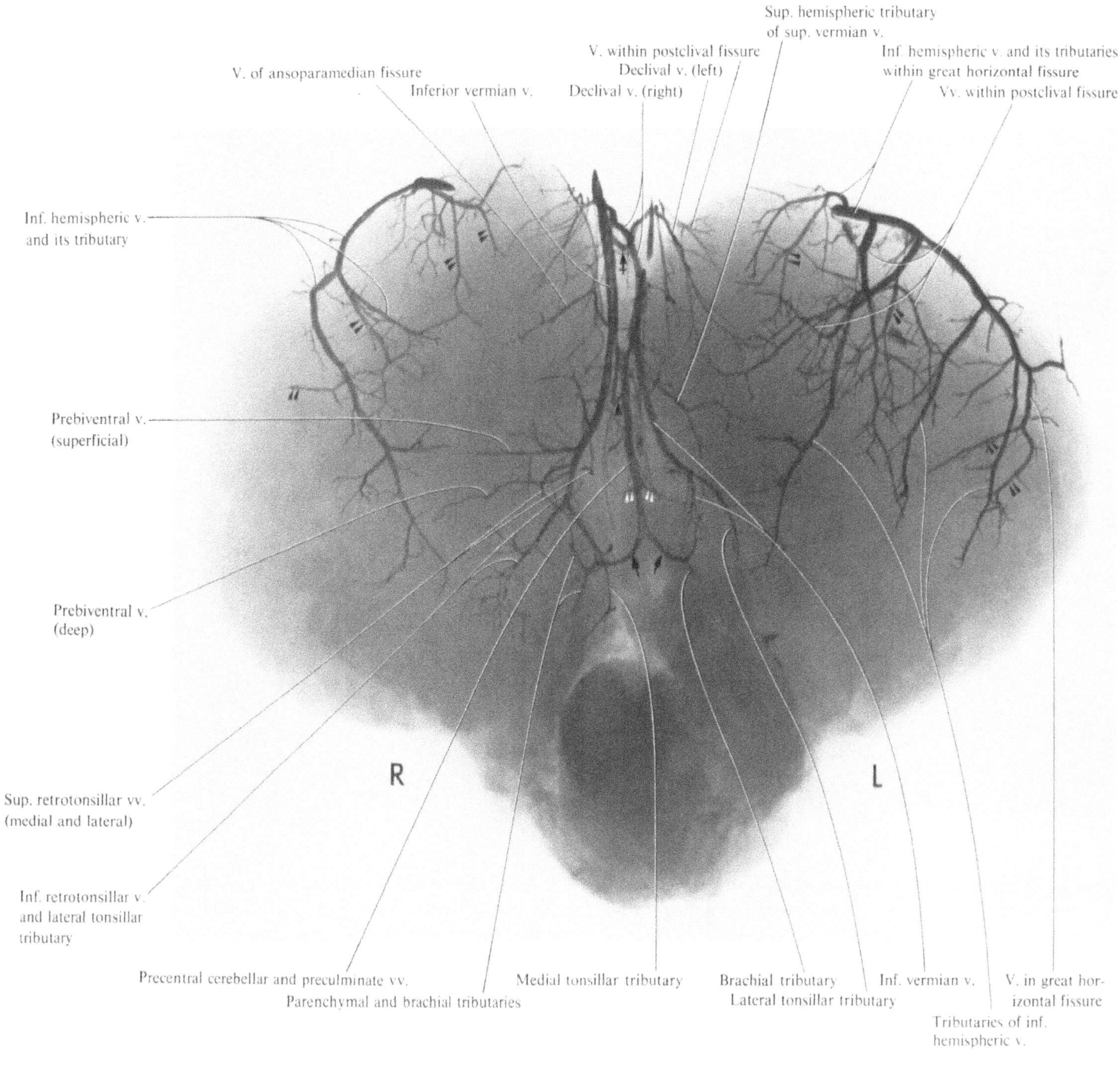

Fig. 265B. Submentovertical view

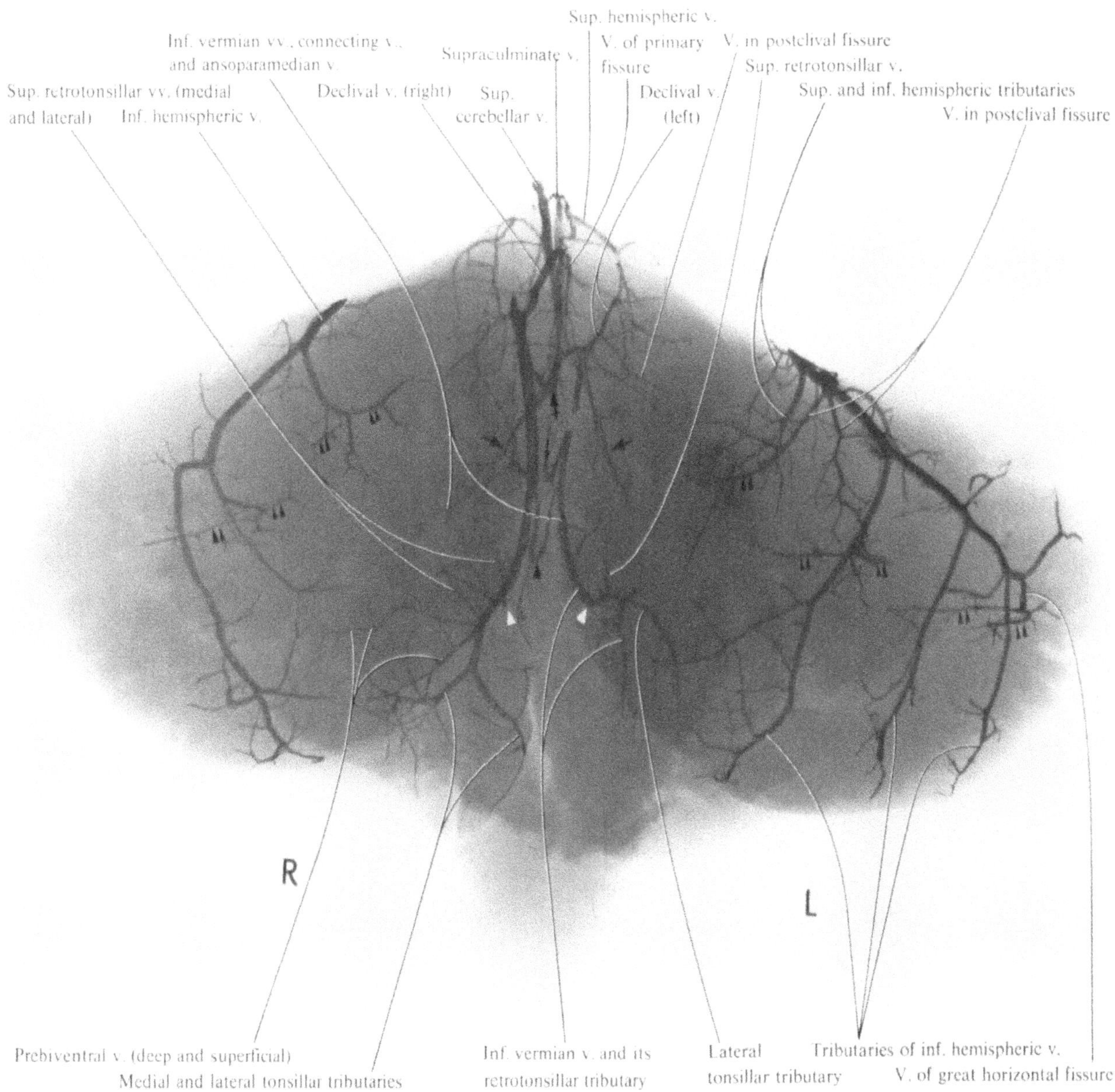

Fig. 265C. Towne or semiaxial view

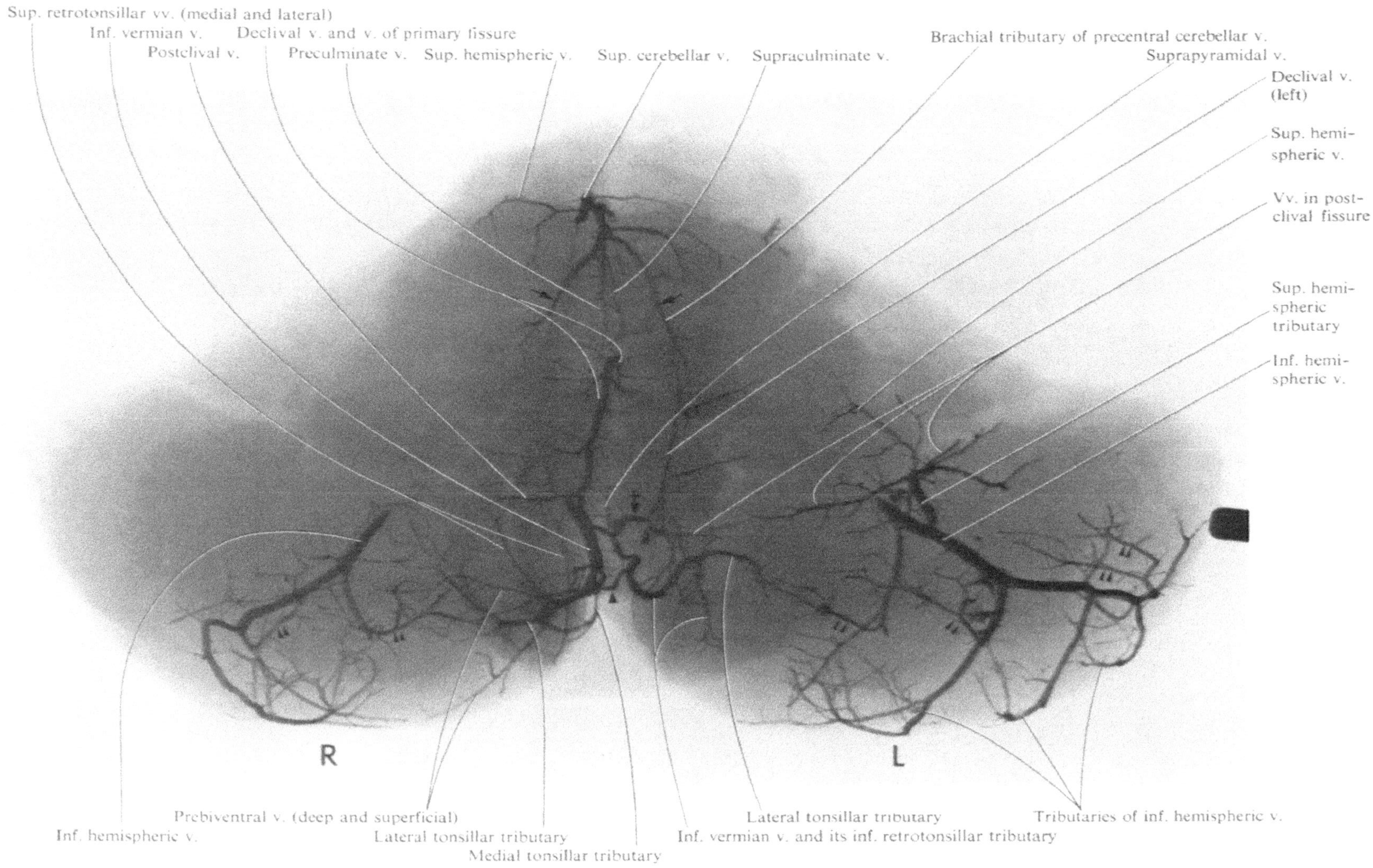

Fig. 265D. Anteroposterior view

Fig. 266. Radiographs of an injected specimen, showing the course of veins of the anterior draining group

A. Submentovertical view, B. axial view, C. semiaxial view and D. lateral view.
The petrosal vein receives the vein of the great horizontal fissure, the brachial vein, the transverse pontine vein, the lateral pontine vein and the vein of the lateral recess of the fourth ventricle (Fig. A). The flocculus (*F*) is outlined inferiorly by the vein of the lateral recess and laterally by the stem of the vein of the great horizontal fissure (Fig. A). The vein of the pontomedullary sulcus, the preolivary vein, the retro-olivary vein and the vein of the restiform eminence drain into the lateral pontine vein (Figs. A and B). The retro-olivary vein is continuous inferiorly with the lateral medullary vein (Fig. A), while the vein of the restiform eminence communicates postero-inferiorly with the vein of the restiform body and the median posterior medullary vein (Figs. A and D).
The floccular and peduncular segments, and the transverse supratonsillar tributary, of the vein of the lateral recess mark the location of the tonsillar incisura (⇕), the lateral recess of the fourth ventricle, and the cerebellopontomedullary angle (▲) (Fig. D). Numerous fine parenchymal veins, i.e., dentate veins (small opposing arrowheads), converge towards the tonsillar incisura and join the vein of the lateral recess. The transverse nodular vein receives the paramedian nodular and paramedian nodulo-uvular veins (small arrows). The transverse nodular vein, located superficially in the anterior part of the nodulo-uvular fissure, receives supratonsillar veins of the opposite side and drains into the transverse supratonsillar vein. The latter vein, in turn, opens into the vein of the lateral recess (Figs. B, C and D). A communication between the petrosal and precentral cerebellar veins through their brachial tributaries, and a connection between the partly filled inferior vermian vein and the vein of the lateral recess through their supratonsillar tributaries, can be identified

Figs. 266 A–D see pp. 358–361

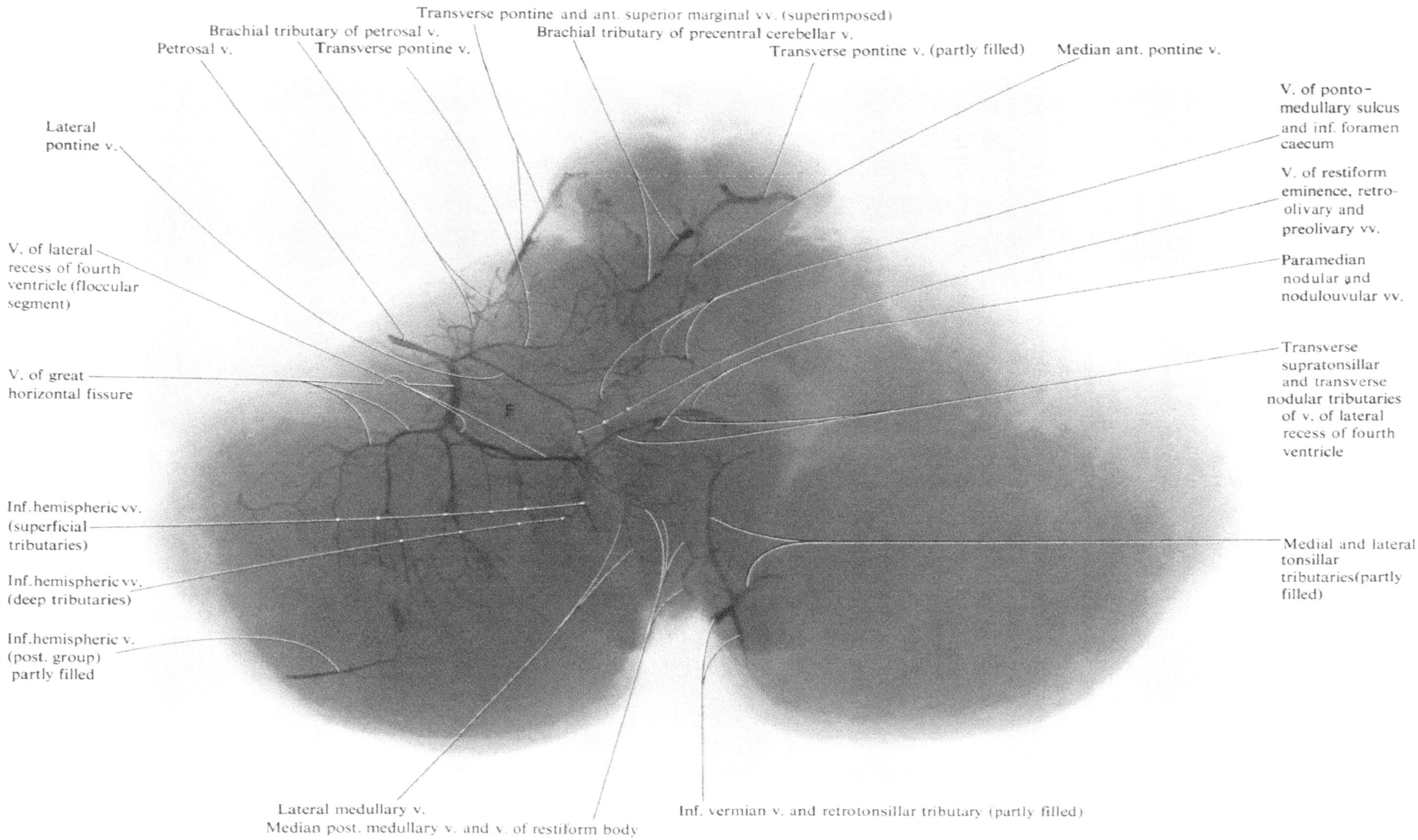

Fig. 266 A. Submentovertical view

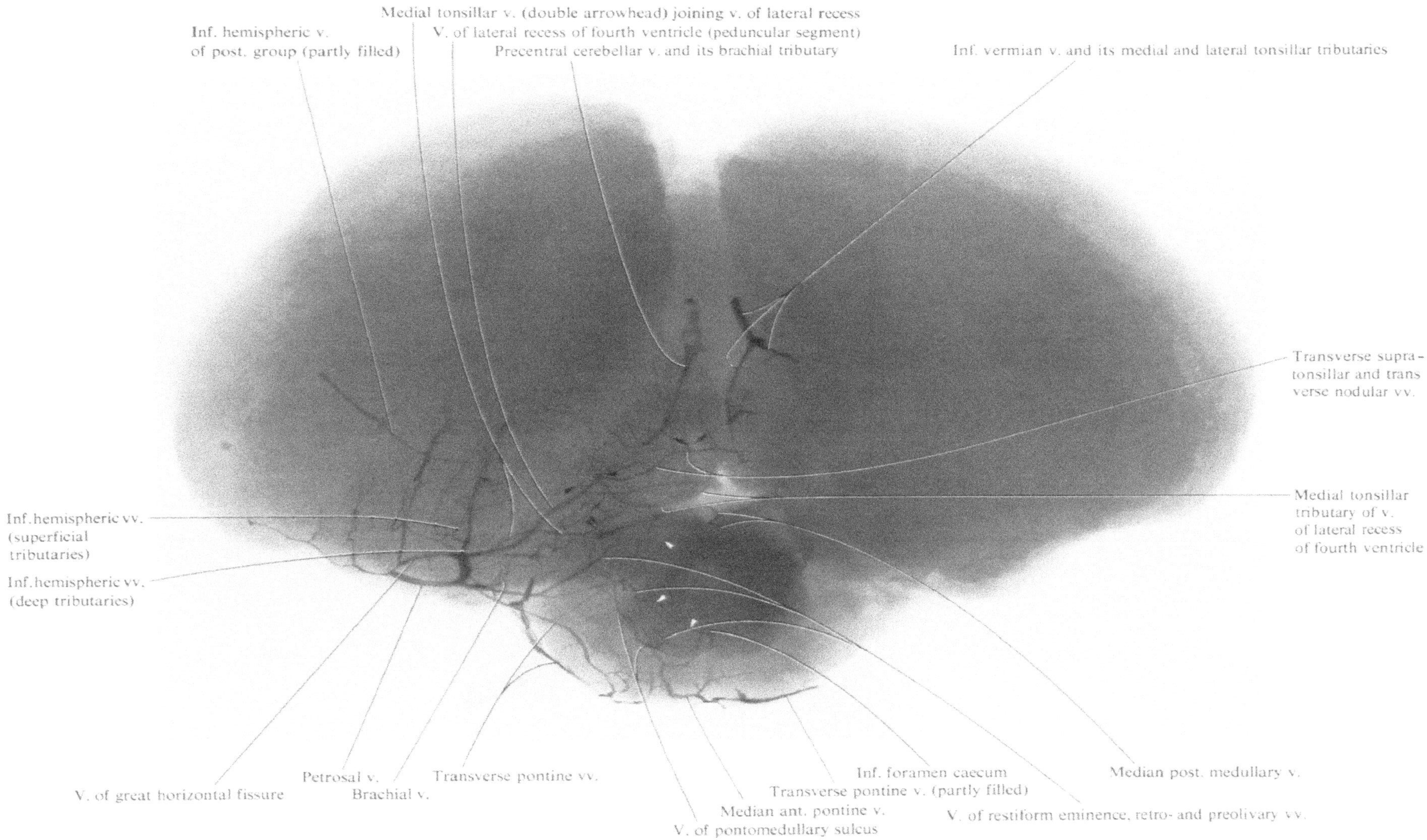

Fig. 266 B. Axial view

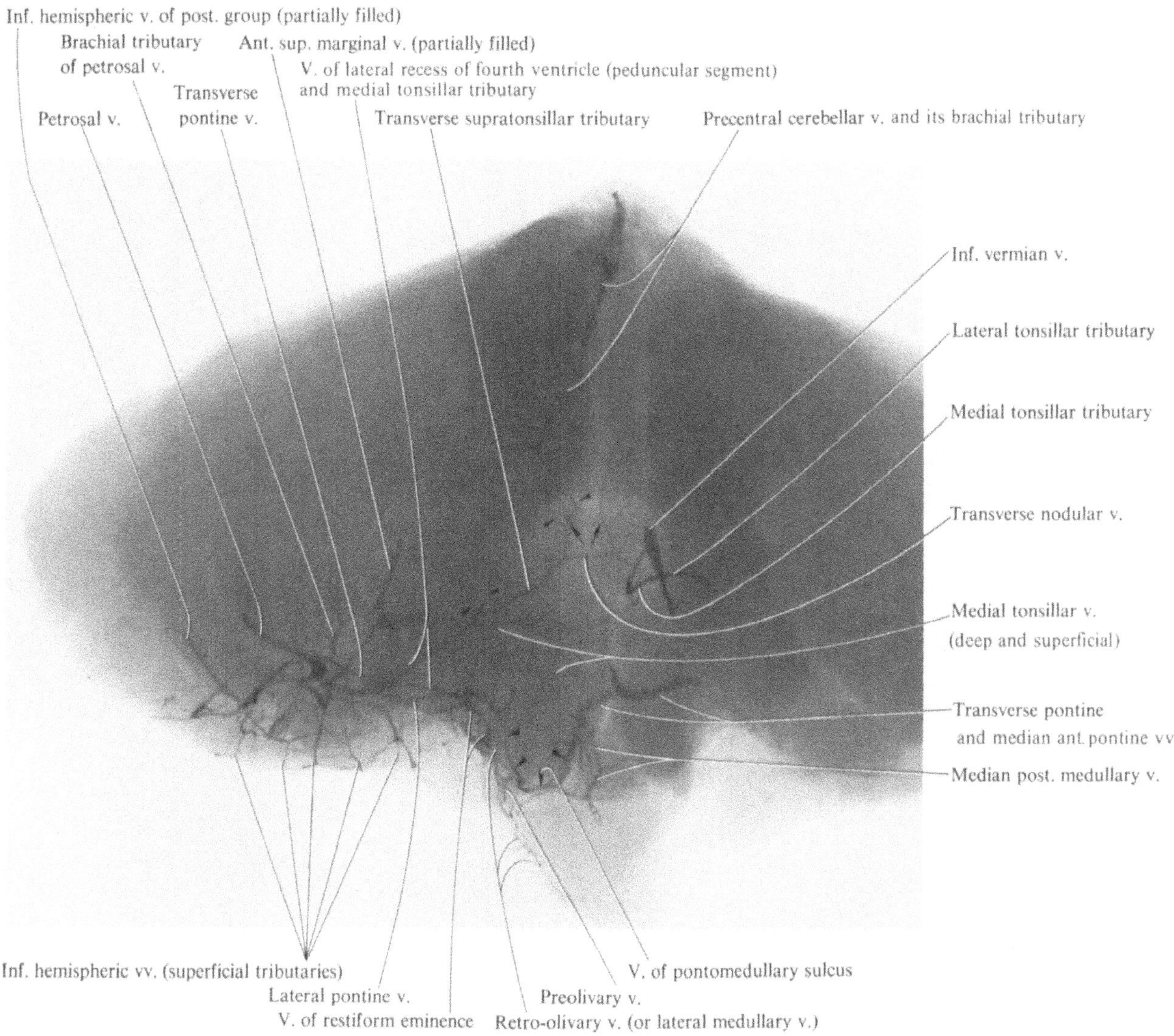

Fig. 266C. Semiaxial view

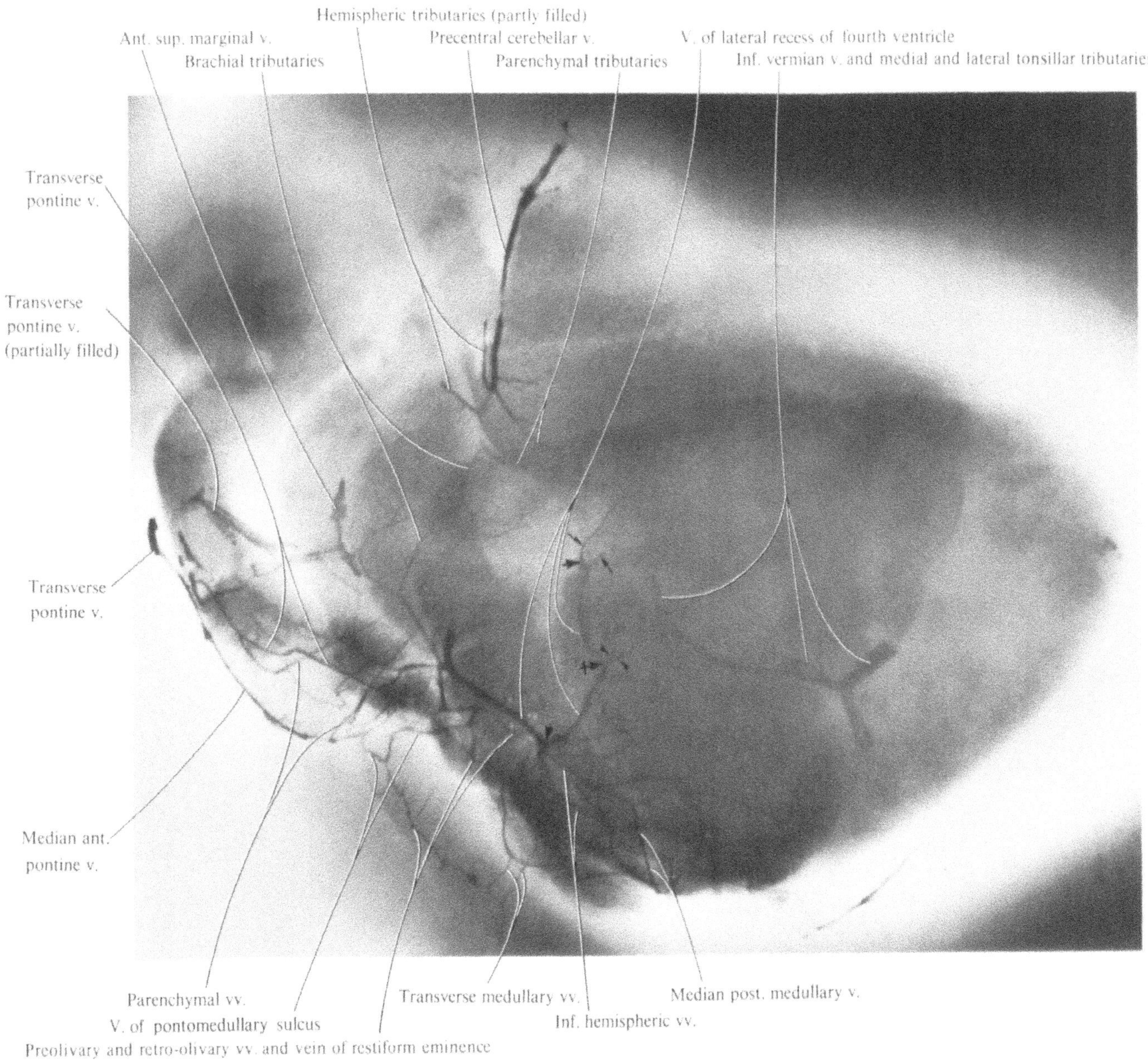

Fig. 266 D. Lateral view

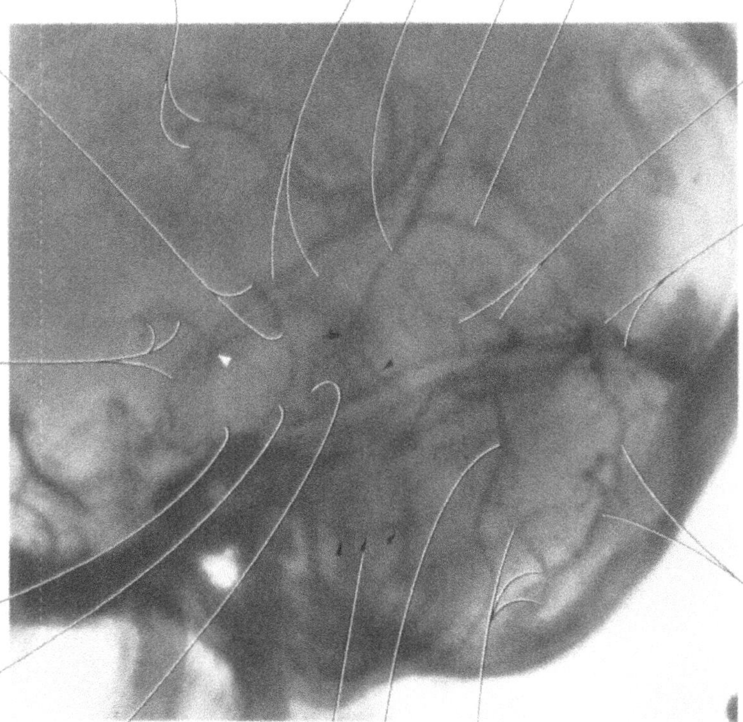

Fig. 267A

Fig. 267. Prominent superior draining group of the veins of the posterior fossa. Vertebral angiogram, venous phase

Fig. 267A. Lateral view. The anterior pontomesencephalic vein outlines the posterior wall of the interpeduncular and pontine cisterns. The colliculocentral point (↑) and the first segment (▲) of the precentral cerebellar vein mark the inferior border of the inferior colliculi and the precentral cerebellar fissure. This indirectly shows the position of the lower end of the aqueduct and the roof of the upper part of the fourth ventricle. The isthmus of the rhombencephalon is indicated by the inferior end (white arrowhead) of the mesencephalic segment of the anterior pontomesencephalic vein and by the colliculocentral point (↑). The supraculminate and precentral cerebellar veins outline the superior vermis. The location of the lateral recess of the fourth ventricle is revealed by the peduncular segment (row of arrowheads) of the vein of the lateral recess. The posterior margin of the cerebellar tonsil is outlined by the superior and inferior retrotonsillar tributaries of the inferior vermian vein

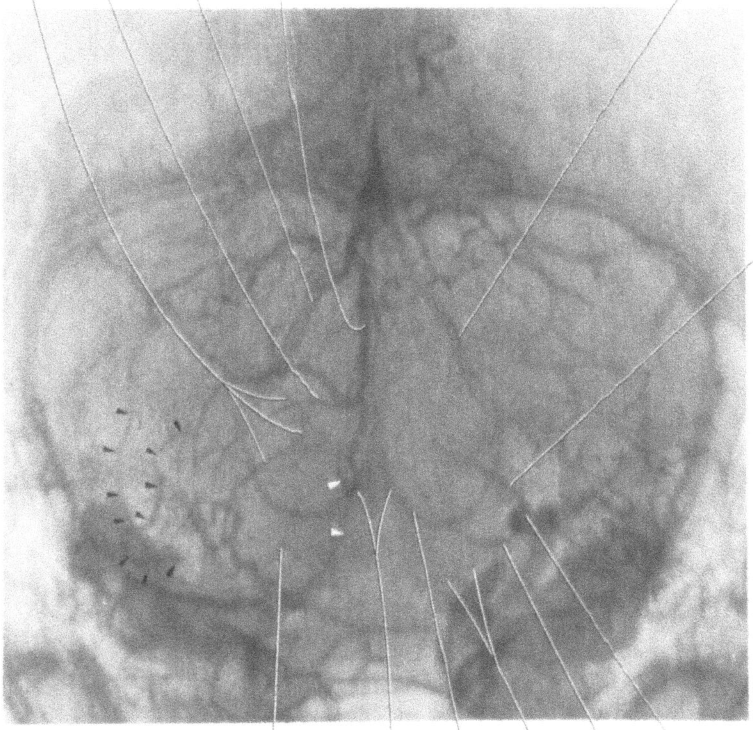

Fig. 267 B. Towne view. The posterior mesencephalic veins are prominent and outline the cerebral peduncles. The anastomotic lateral mesencephalic vein on the right marks the location of the lateral mesencephalic sulcus. Brachial tributaries of the petrosal veins mark the anterolateral portion of the wings of the precentral cerebellar fissure. The peduncular segment of the vein of the lateral recess of the fourth ventricle marks the location of the anterolateral recess and the cerebellopontomedullary angle on each side. The inferior vermian vein and its superior and inferior retrotonsillar tributaries (white arrowheads) reveal the location of the copular pyramidis, tonsillobiventral notch and the lateral wall of the cerebellar vallecula on each side. Some of the prominent hemispheric tributaries of the anterior draining group can also be identified (rows of black arrows)

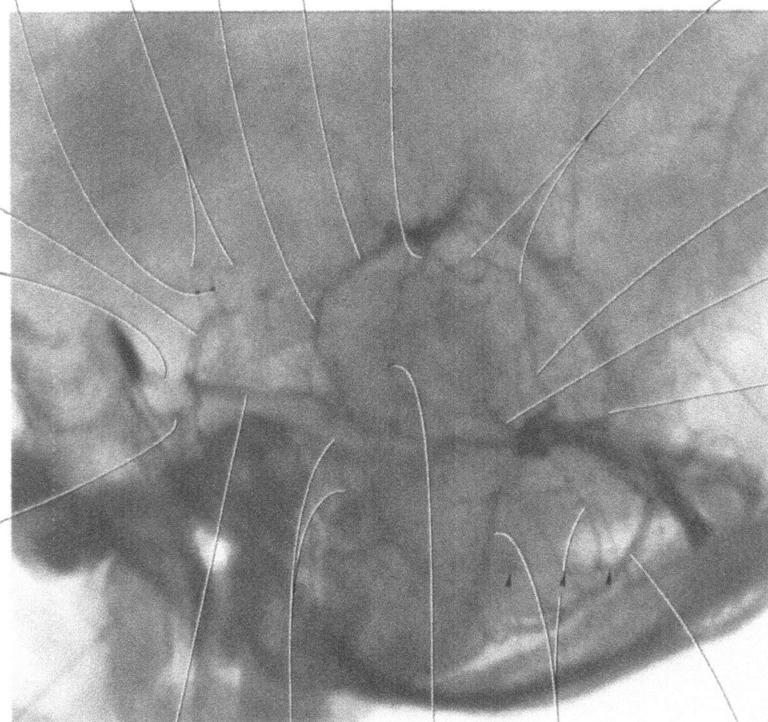

Fig. 268A

Fig. 268. Superior draining group of the veins of the posterior fossa. Vertebral angiogram, venous phase, lateral views, 4 cases

Fig. 268A. The lateral mesencephalic vein, which drains upwards into the posterior mesencephalic vein, mimics a displaced precentral cerebellar vein. The latter vein is small but normal in its position and course. The median anterior pontine and transverse pontine veins are unusually prominent. The great horizontal fissure is outlined anteriorly by a vein located above the flocculus, which joins the petrosal vein, and posteriorly by the tributaries of the inferior hemispheric veins, located within the fissure (arrowheads). Note a communication between the supraculminate vein and a superior hemispheric vein of the posterior draining group

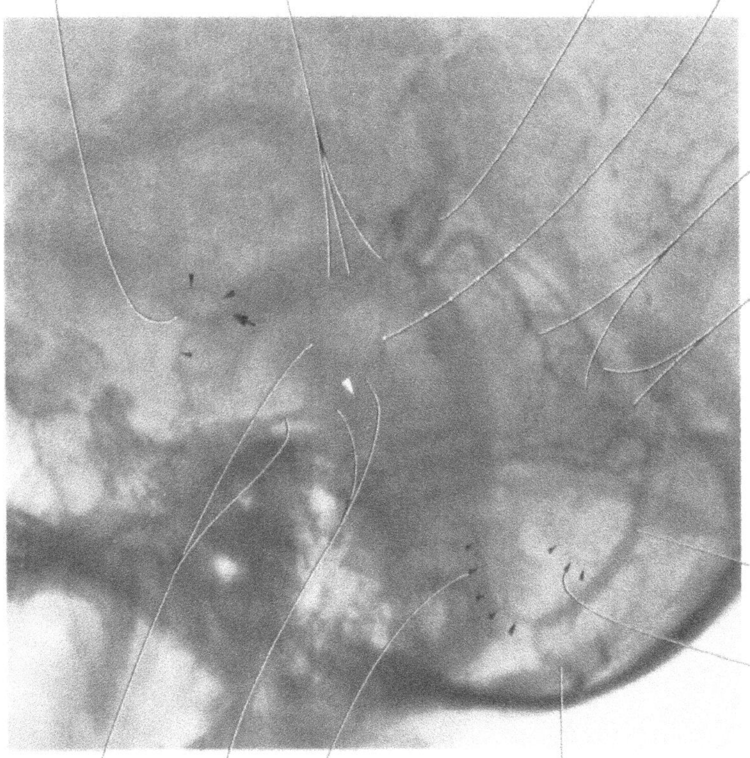

Fig. 268 B. Brachial tributaries. The lateral mesencephalic vein drains mainly downwards and forwards to join the petrosal vein. Another brachial vein, originating from the posterosuperior aspect of the brachium conjunctivum, runs downwards and forwards, crossing the interbrachial sulcus (white arrowhead) and traversing the dorsal aspect of the brachium pontis, to join the infratentorial segment of the lateral mesencephalic vein, which corresponds to the brachial tributary of the petrosal vein. A prominent superior hemispheric tributary of the superior vermian vein connects with a superior hemispheric tributary of the posterior draining group. Similarly, the supraculminate vein anastomoses with the declival vein. Anteriorly, the hypothalamic, mesencephalic and pontine segments (small black arrowheads) of the anterior pontomesencephalic vein outline the posterior wall of the interpeduncular and pontine cisterns and the superior foramen caecum (↑)

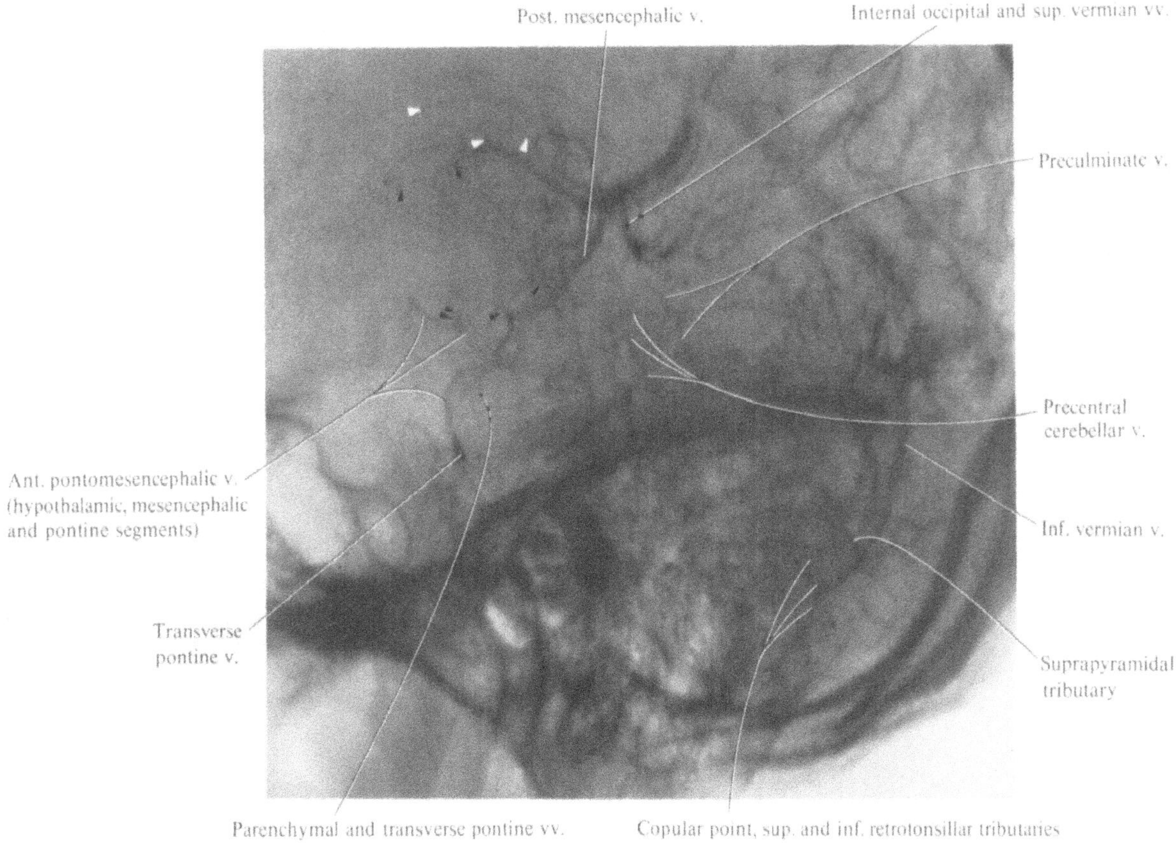

Fig. 268 C. Prominent inferior and posterior thalamic veins. Many thalamic veins (black arrowheads) are seen. Inferior thalamic veins (double black arrowheads) run forwards and downwards to join the mesencephalic segment of the anterior pontomesencephalic vein in the upper part of the interpeduncular fossa, while fine posterior thalamic veins drain downwards and backwards to join the posterior mesencephalic vein. The superior and anterior thalamic veins can also be identified. Several connecting veins (white arrowheads), originating from the choroid plexuses of the lateral ventricles, join the internal cerebral veins

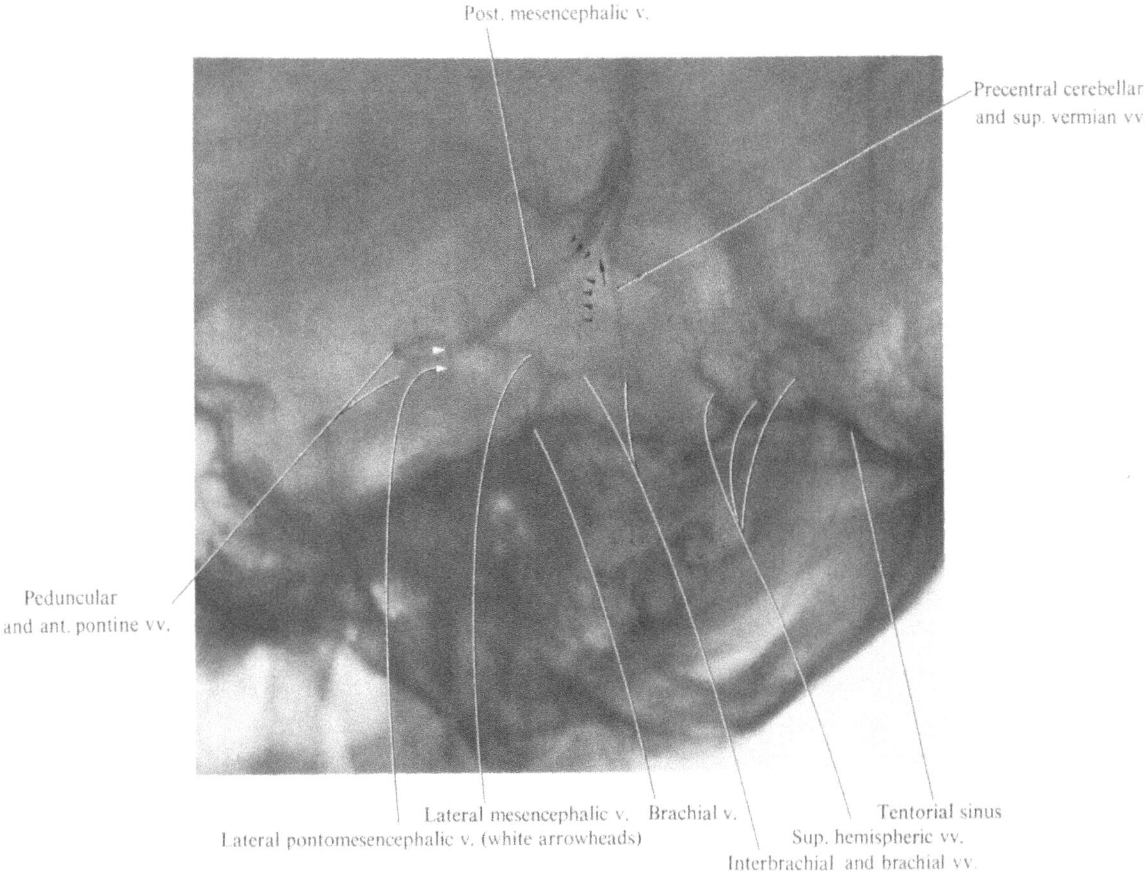

Fig. 268 D. Prominent quadrigeminal (or tectal) vein (rows of arrowheads). The median superior quadrigeminal vein (row of three arrowheads) runs downwards and backwards and is joined by the median inferior quadrigeminal vein (row of four arrowheads), to form a single stem (↑), the quadrigeminal vein, which, in turn, joins the stem of the superior cerebellar vein. The lateral pontomesencephalic vein (white arrowheads) runs upwards on the lateral aspect of the cerebral peduncule

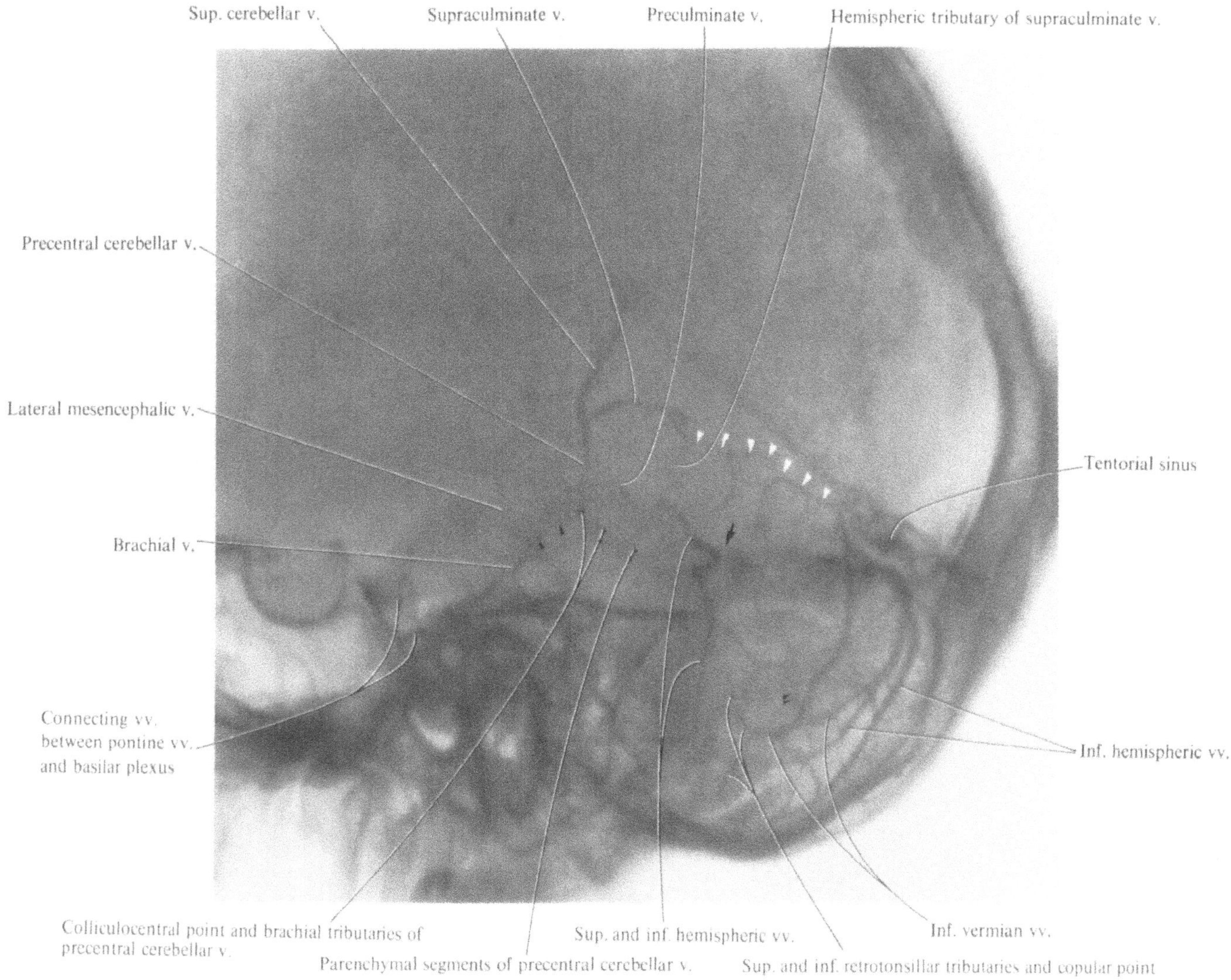

Fig. 269A. Lateral view

Fig. 269. Prominent superior cerebellar vein. Vertebral angiogram, venous phase

The prominent superior cerebellar vein receives the precentral cerebellar and superior vermian veins. The colliculocentral point and the brachial and parenchymal tributaries of the precentral cerebellar vein mark, indirectly, the position of the roof of the upper part of the fourth ventricle (Fig. A). The brachial tributary (single arrowhead) of the precentral cerebellar vein is seen on the right side (Fig. B). There is a connection between the supraculminate and the declival veins (row of white arrowheads) (Fig. A). In the posterior draining group, a superior and an inferior hemispheric vein unite to form a single trunk (arrow) before opening into a dural sinus (Fig. A). The right inferior vermian vein directly joins the straight sinus, whereas the left inferior vermian vein is joined by an inferior hemispheric vein and opens into the lateral sinus, following a short course within the tentorium (Fig. B). The copular point and superior retrotonsillar vein mark the anterior border of the pyramid, while the suprapyramidal veins (double arrowheads) indicate its posterior border in both lateral and semiaxial views. The flocculus (*F*) is outlined by the tributaries of the petrosal vein on each side. The inferior hemispheric tributaries of the petrosal veins outline the petrosal aspect of the cerebellar hemispheres (Fig. B)

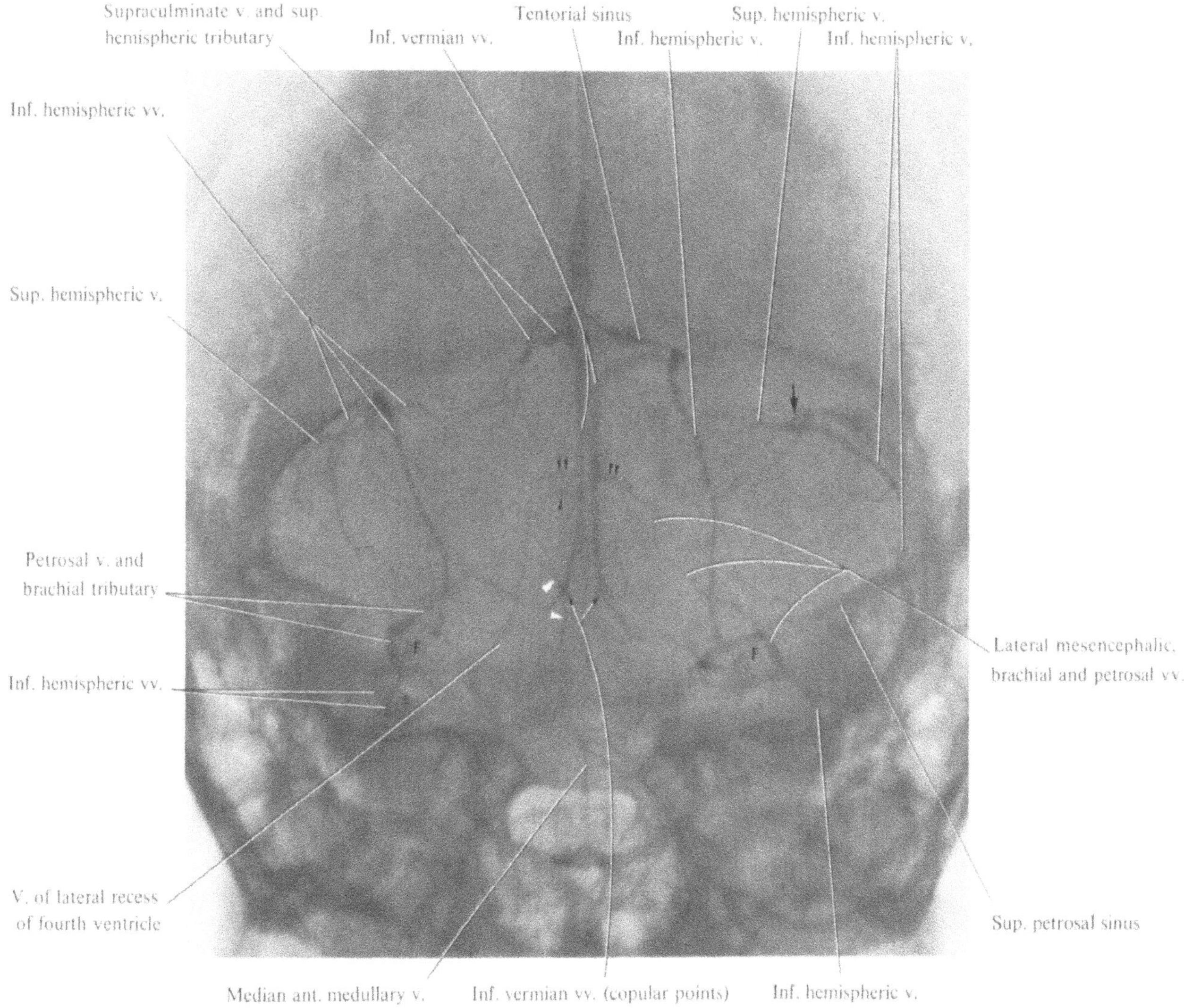

Fig. 269B. Semiaxial view

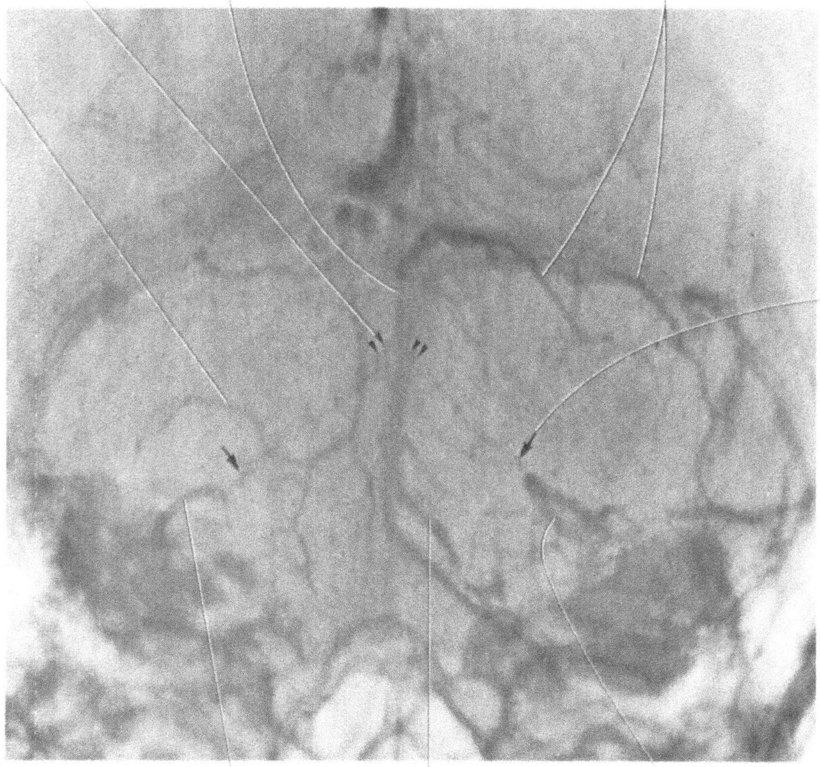

Fig. 270A

Fig. 270. Brachial veins. Vertebral angiogram, venous phase, semiaxial views, 2 cases

Fig. 270A. The precentral cerebellar vein and its brachial tributaries (double arrowheads) have a typical inverted "Y" configuration. Together with the brachial tributaries (arrows) of the petrosal veins, they outline the inverted "V" shaped anterior cerebellar notch

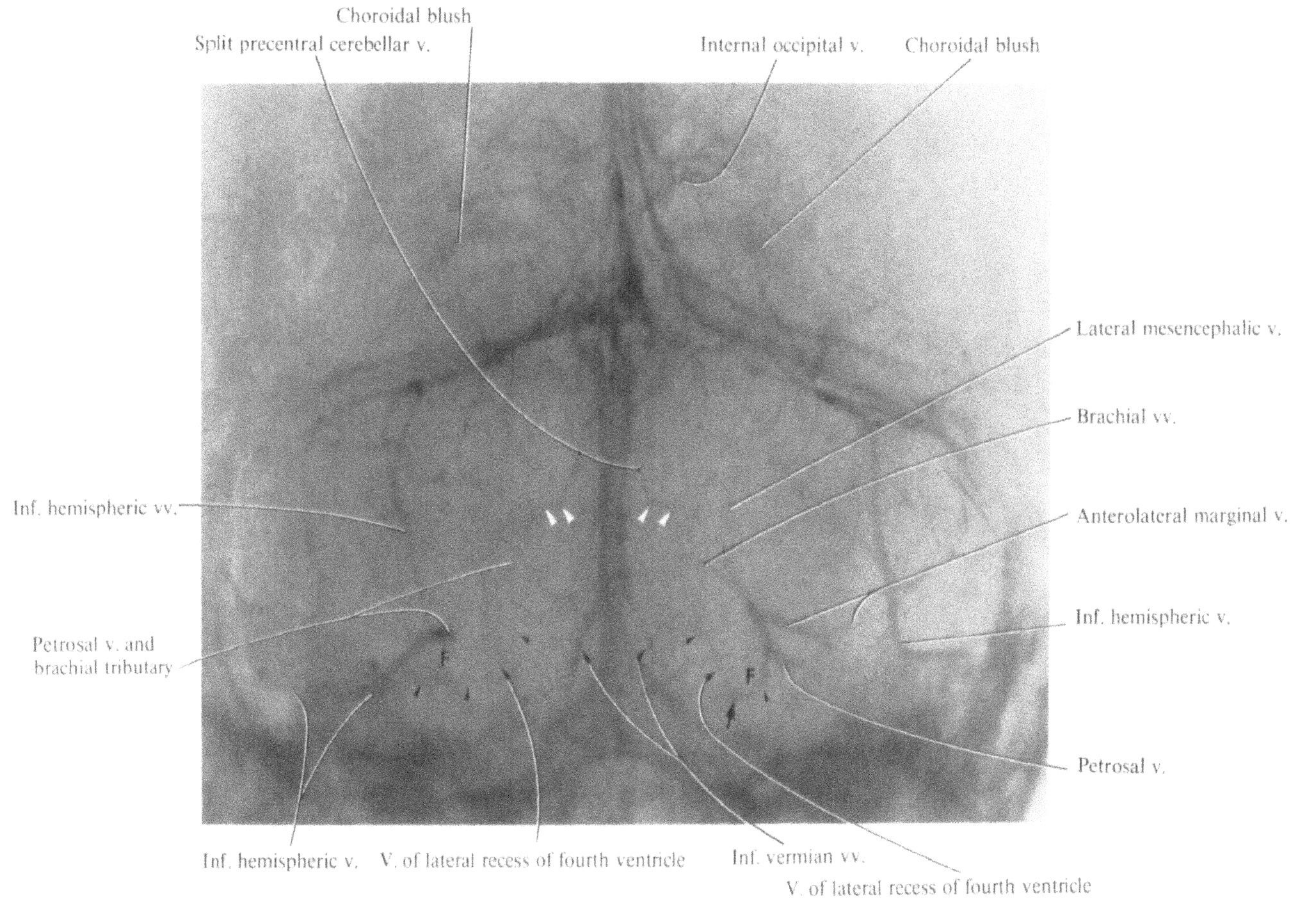

Fig. 270 B. The zigzag course of the brachial tributaries of the split precentral cerebellar vein, running posteriorly, medially and superiorly around the lateral and posterior aspects of the brachia conjunctiva (white arrowheads), outlines indirectly the roof of the upper part of the fourth ventricle. The peduncular and floccular segments of the vein of the lateral recess of the fourth ventricle (row of black arrowheads) mark the location of the anterolateral reccess, the cerebellopontomedullary angle (unlabelled arrow) and the flocculus (*F*) on each side. The distance between the peduncular segment of the petrosal vein and its brachial tributary indicates the thickness of the brachium pontis and the restiform body in the semiaxial projection

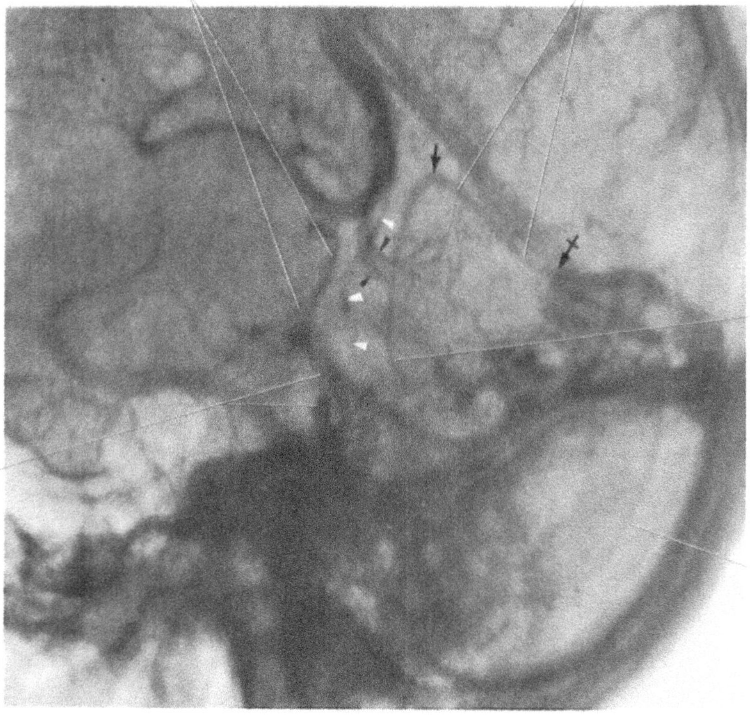

Fig. 271 A

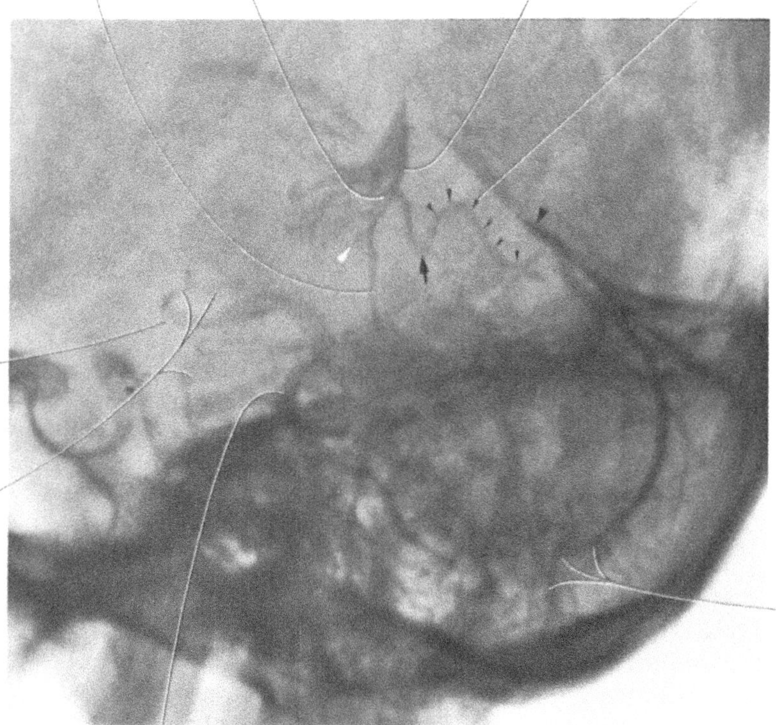

Fig. 271 B

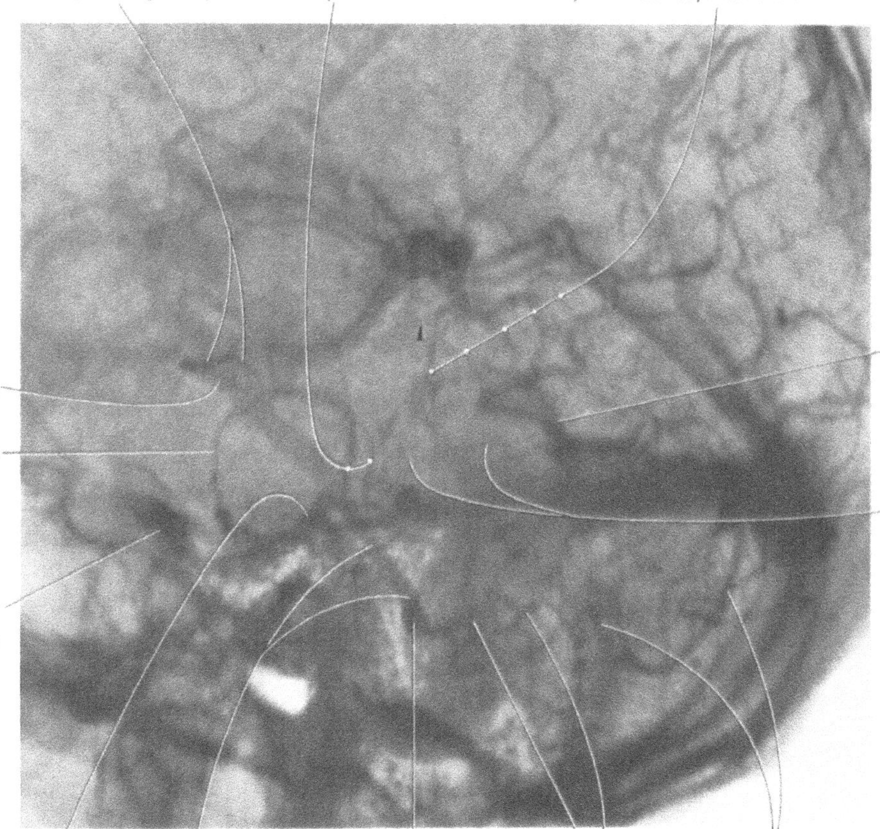

Fig. 272. Prominent anterior draining group of veins. Cerebral angiogram, venous phase, lateral view
The petrosal vein is prominent, receiving the vein of the lateral recess, the superior hemispheric vein and the brachial vein. One of the anastomotic lateral mesencephalic veins is prominent and runs rather low, linking the peduncular and lateral mesencephalic veins. The angular course of the vein of the lateral recess of the fourth ventricle, at the cerebellopontomedullary angle, is typical. The tectal vein (arrowhead) can be identified

◁
Fig. 271. Variations of the superior draining group of veins. Cerebral angiogram, venous phase, lateral views 2 cases

Fig. 271 A. The precentral cerebellar vein originates from the depths of the precentral cerebellar fissure. Instead of joining the great cerebral vein, after travelling in front of the culmen, it passes over the apex (↑) of the cerebellum and descends on the posterior aspect of the culmen and declive to open into the straight sinus (⇞). The internal occipital veins (black arrowheads) and an accessory galenopetrosal vein (white arrowheads) are also opacified

Fig. 271 B. The superior vermian vein originates as a superior hemispheric vein (row of small arrowheads) and runs upwards and forwards on the superior aspect of a cerebellar hemisphere. The vein dips down (↑) into the precentral cerebellar fissure, before running upwards to join the anterior portion of the great cerebral vein. On the other hand, the precentral cerebellar vein, receiving the quadrigeminal (or tectal) vein (white arrowhead), travels posterosuperiorly to open into the posterior portion of the great cerebral vein. The precentral cerebellar and superior vermian veins therefore cross each other in the lateral view. The junction between the inferior vermian vein and the straight sinus is unusually high (large black arrowhead)

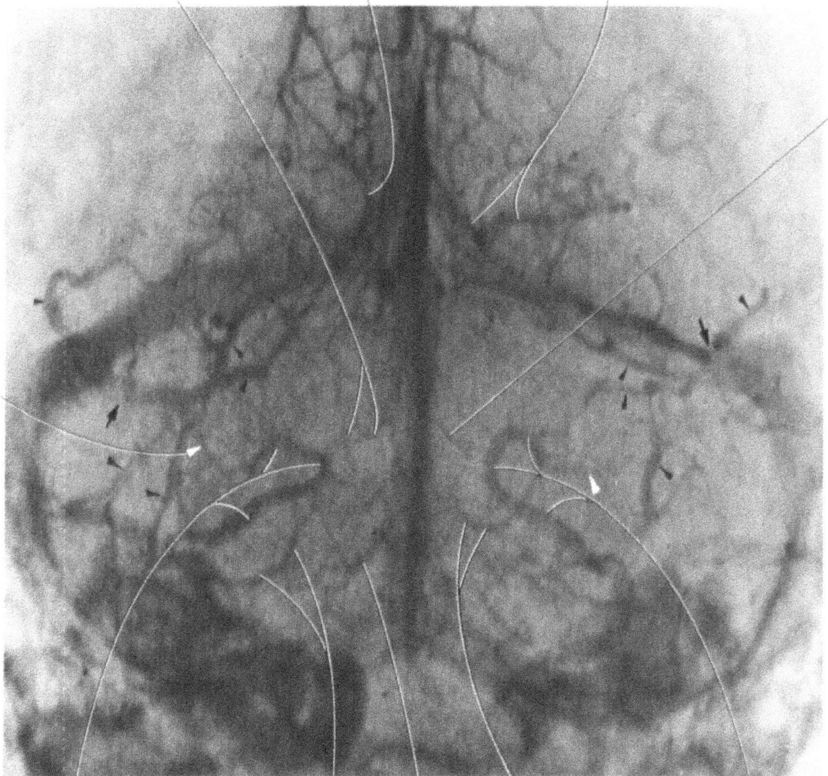

Fig. 273 A

Fig. 273. Prominent lateral mesencephalic veins. Vertebral angiogram, venous phase, semiaxial views, 2 cases

Fig. 273 A. The lateral mesencephalic vein receives the inferior ventricular vein (white arrowhead) on each side. It is connected superomedially to the brachial tributary of the precentral cerebellar vein and inferolaterally to the brachial tributary of the petrosal vein. On the left side, it receives, in addition, the peduncular (or interpeduncular) vein. The vein of the lateral recess of the fourth ventricle is identified on the right (reader's left). The distance between the two lateral mesencephalic veins indicates the transverse width of the tegmentum of the mesencephalon at the level of the lateral mesencephalic sulci. Several supratentorial veins (black arrowheads) draining into the tentorial sinuses (arrows) are seen

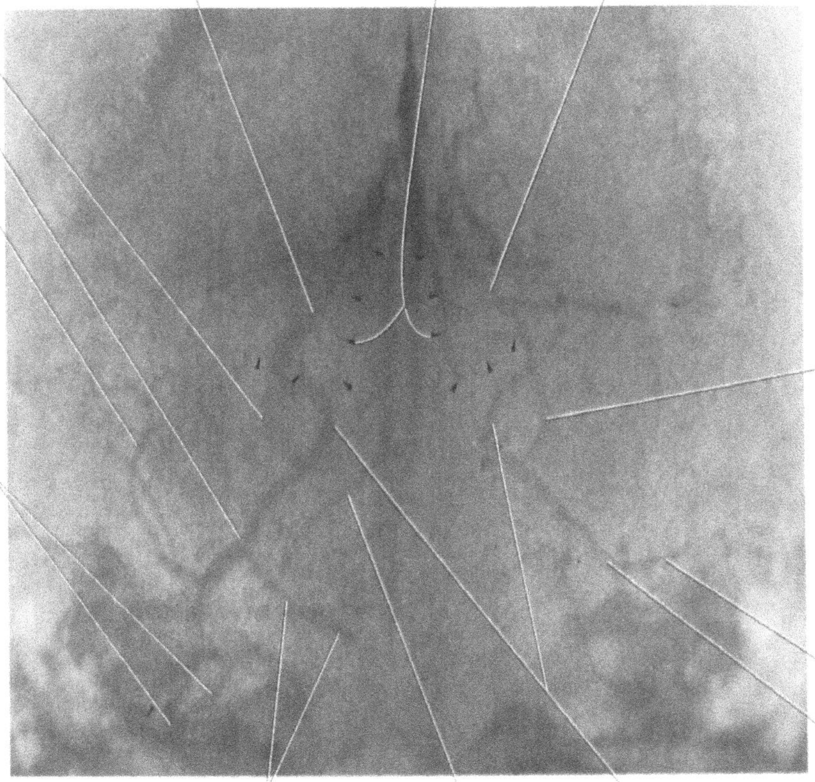

Fig. 273 B. Drainage of tributaries of the right petrosal vein into the great cerebral vein via the anastomotic lateral mesencephalic and posterior mesencephalic veins. On the left (reader's right), the anastomotic lateral mesencephalic vein links the supratentorial posterior mesencephalic vein and the infratentorial petrosal vein. On the right, the petrosal vein receives the superior and the inferior cerebellar hemispheric veins and the transverse pontine vein.

Instead of draining into the superior petrosal sinus, the right petrosal vein runs upwards and backwards. It is joined by the peduncular vein and opens into the great cerebral vein via the brachial, anastomotic lateral mesencephalic and posterior mesencephalic veins. The split precentral cerebellar vein (rows of arrowheads) begins on each side as a superior hemispheric vein that runs medially and dips into the precentral cerebellar fissure, before running superiorly, medially, and posteriorly to join the posterior portion of the internal cerebral vein

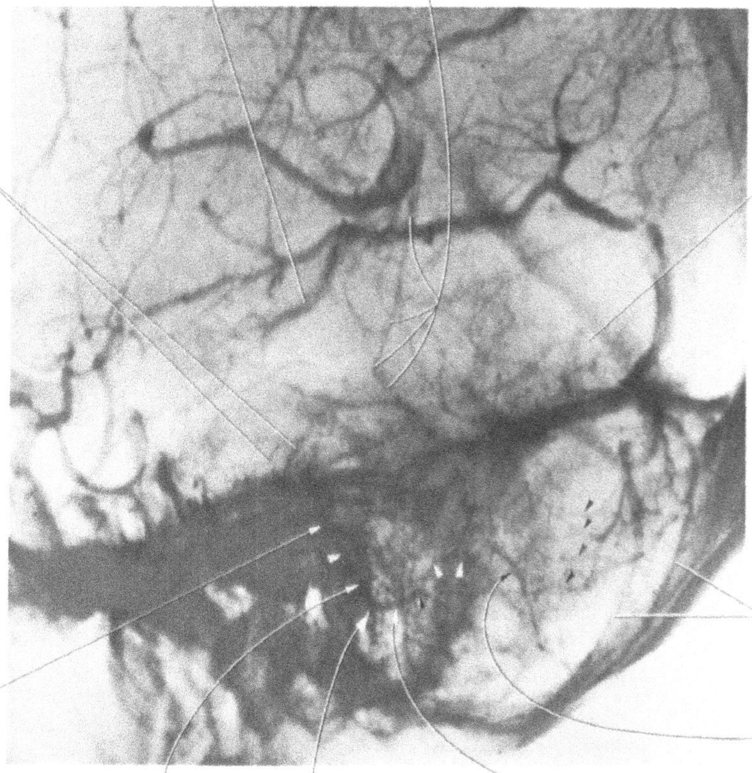

Fig. 274A

Fig. 274. Vein of the lateral recess of the fourth ventricle. Cerebral angiogram, venous phase

Fig 274A. Lateral view. All three segments of the vein of the lateral recess of the fourth ventricle (white arrowheads) can be identified. The peduncular segment of this vein indicates the position and course of the anterolateral recess of the fourth ventricle. Its anterior end marks the location of the cerebellopontomedullary angle, while its posterior end (single black arrowhead) reveals the location of the tonsillar incisura. The superior retrotonsillar vein runs postero-inferiorly and emerges from the posterior cerebellar notch. It then runs superiorly (and laterally) to join the lateral sinus. Many short veins, emerging from the great horizontal fissure (four black arrowheads) join the inferior hemispheric veins

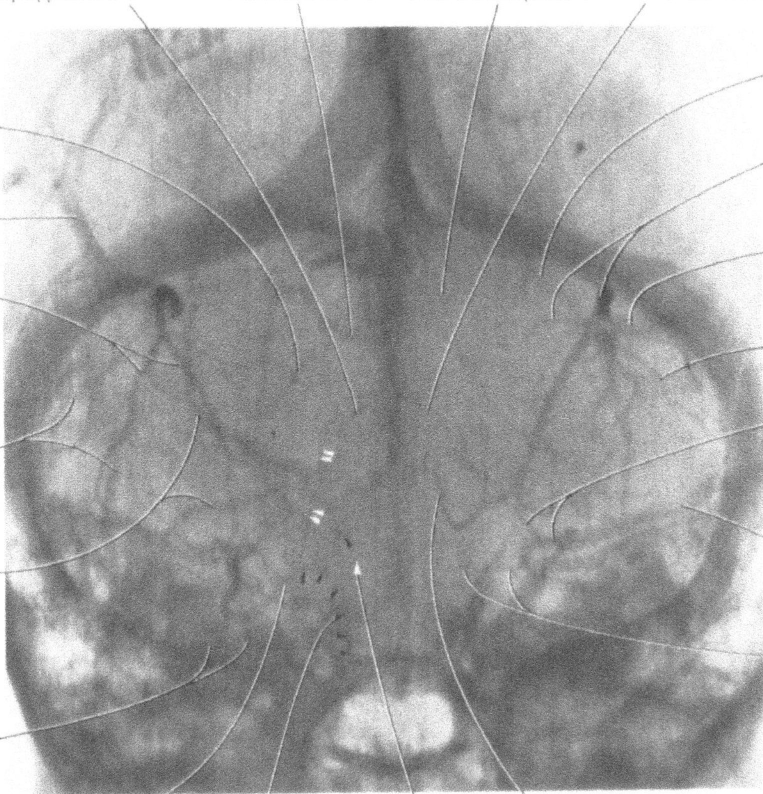

Fig. 274 B. Semiaxial view (same case). The vein of the lateral recess of the fourth ventricle, which receives the lateral supratonsillar (white double arrowhead), medial tonsillar (white single arrowhead) and retro-olivary tributaries (row of black arrowheads), runs below the flocculus and over the adjacent biventral lobule, before turning upwards to join the petrosal vein. The superior retrotonsillar vein joins the lateral sinus on the left, via an inferior hemispheric vein and a short tentorial sinus. The copular point of the right inferior vermian vein can be identified (single black arrowhead). The precentral cerebellar vein and its brachial tributaries outline the roof of the upper part of the fourth ventricle

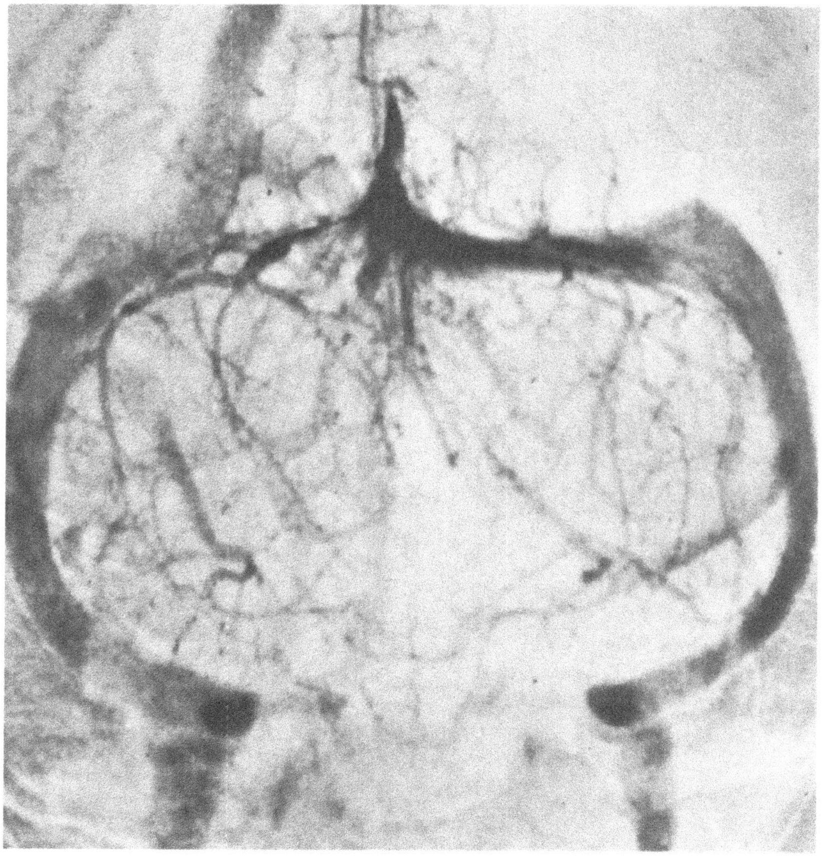

Fig. 275A. Radiograph

Fig. 275. Anterior draining group of veins. Cerebral angiogram, venous phase, semiaxial view
Labelled structures are the anastomotic lateral mesencephalic vein (*ALM*), anterior medullary (or median anterior medullary) vein (*AM*), brachial vein (*B*), copular point (*CP*), flocculus (*F*), tributaries within the great horizontal fissure (*GHF*), inferior foramen caecum (*IFC*), inferior hemispheric veins (*IH*), internal jugular vein (*IJ*), interpeduncular fossa (*IPF*), inferior petrosal sinus (*IPS*), inferior vermian vein (*IV*), jugular bulb (*JB*), lateral pontine vein (*LP*), vein of the lateral recess (*LR*), lateral sinus (*LS*), petrosal vein (*P*), precentral cerebellar vein (*Pc*), postclival vein (*Pcl*), peduncular vein (*Pd*), posterior mesencephalic vein (*PM*), vein of the pontomedullary sulcus (*PMS*), vein of the primary fissure (*1° F*), retro-olivary vein (*Ro*), superior hemispheric vein (*SH*), superior petrosal sinus (*SPS*), sigmoid sinus (*SS*), superior sagittal sinus (*SSS*), supratentorial vein (*ST*), transverse medullary vein (*TM*), transverse pontine vein (*TP*) and tentorial sinus (*TS*).

The vein of the lateral recess of the fourth ventricle (*LR*), receives several inferior hemispheric veins (*IH*) in the floccular segment of the posterolateral fissure, below the flocculus (*F*). Some of the hemispheric tributaries lie deep in the sulci and some are located superficially. In the region of the anterior angle of the cerebellum, the vein of the lateral recess of the fourth ventricle (*LR*) joins the petrosal vein (*P*), together with the brachial (*B*), transverse pontine (*TP*) and lateral pontine veins (*LP*). The latter vein receives the retro-olivary vein (*Ro*). These veins, together with the anterior medullary (*AM*), transverse medullary (*TM*), and perforating veins emerging from the inferior foramen caecum (*IFC*), delineate the anatomic configuration of the lower brain stem. The retrotonsillar vein joins the inferior vermian vein on the left side in the usual fashion. On the right, the retrotonsillar vein unites with an inferior hemispheric vein, which, in turn, opens into a tentorial sinus together with other inferior hemispheric veins. The tentorial sinus then opens into the torcular

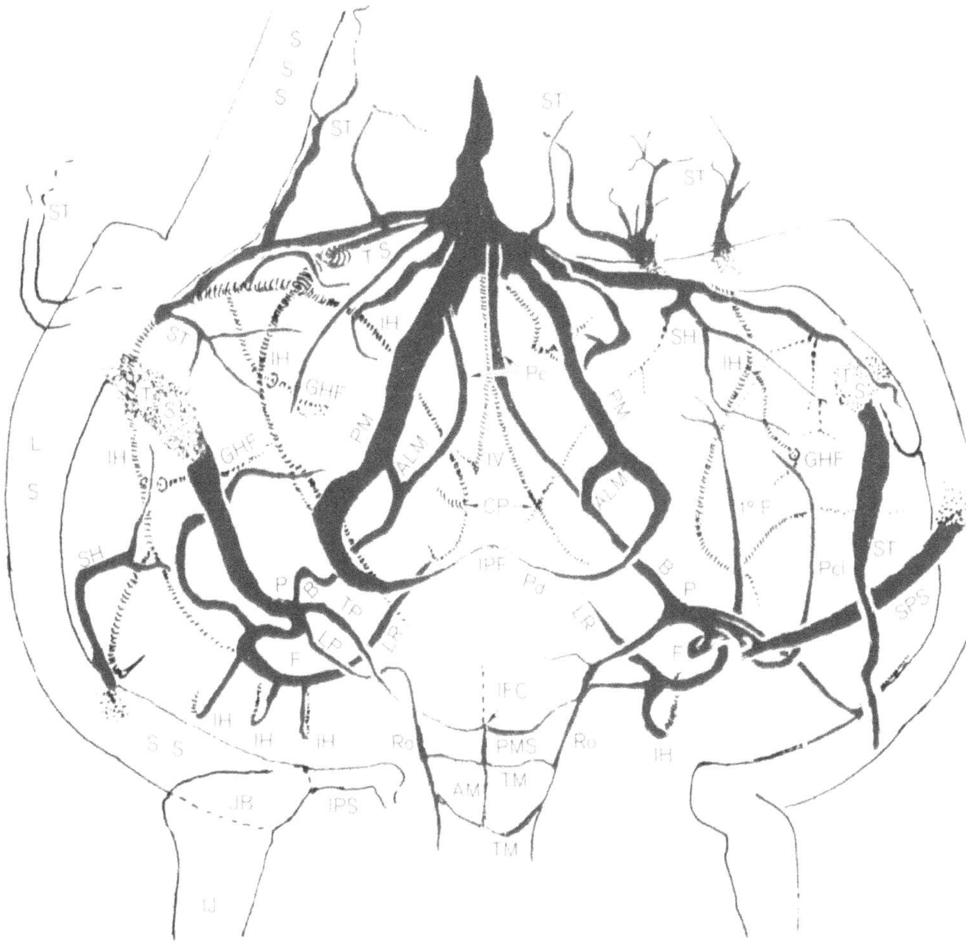

Fig. 275 B. Tracing

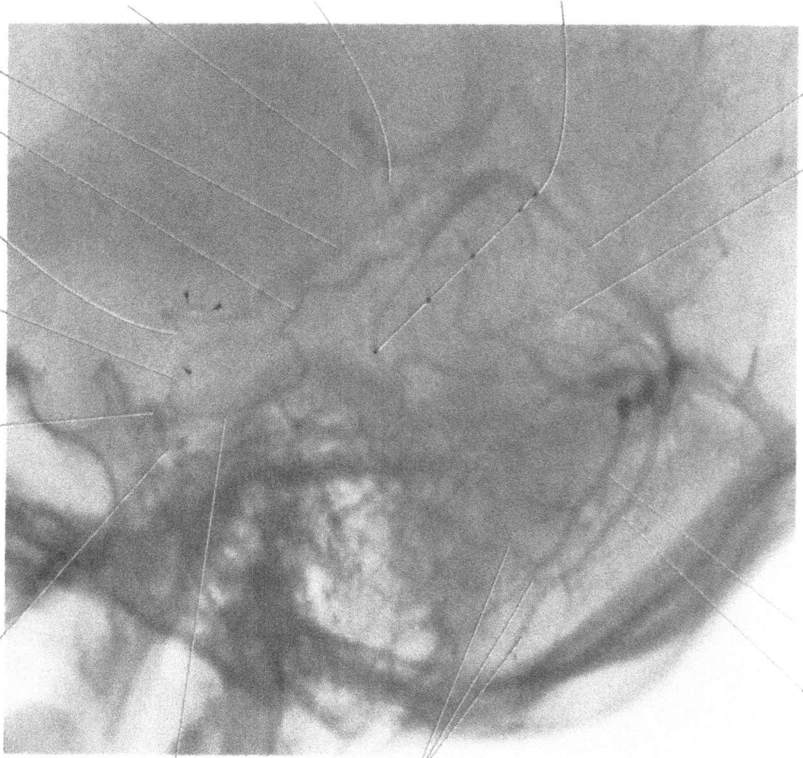

Fig. 276A

Fig. 276. Inferior vermian vein. Cerebral angiogram, venous phase, lateral views, 2 cases

Fig. 276A. The retrotonsillar tributary and copular point of the inferior vermian vein, partly obscured by the inferior hemispheric vein, mark the posterior border of the cerebellar tonsil. The vein of the primary fissure and the paradeclival vein form an obtuse angle, since the former vein originates more laterally in the hemispheric portion of the primary fissure of the cerebellum. The vein that passes over the superior vermis and receives the precentral, preculminate, intraculminate and supraculminate veins runs first upwards and then downwards over the culmen and declive, to open into the lower part of the straight sinus (precentrovermorectal vein). This vein is also connected to the posterior portion of the internal cerebral vein. Note the communication between the lateral mesencephalic and the superior cerebellar vein, above the superior vermis (vermopetrosal vein). The anterior pontomesencephalic vein is also seen (arrowheads).

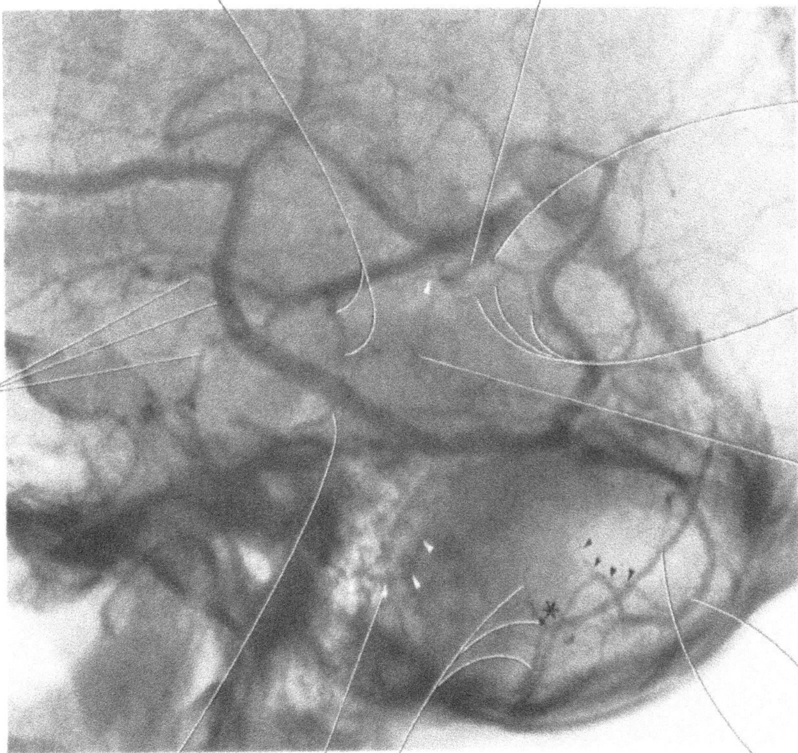

Fig. 276 B. The supratonsillar tributary of the vein of the lateral recess of the fourth ventricle (four white arrowheads) and the superior retrotonsillar tributary of the inferior vermian vein outline the superior pole of the cerebellar tonsil. The pyramid of the inferior vermis is delineated anteriorly by the superior retrotonsillar tributary and posteriorly by the suprapyramidal tributary (four black arrowheads) of the inferior vermian vein. The latter is partly obscured by the tortuous inferior hemispheric vein. The copular point, seen on the course of the superior retrotonsillar vein, marks the antero-inferior border of the copula pyramidis (*). The tectal vein (single white arrowhead) can also be identified

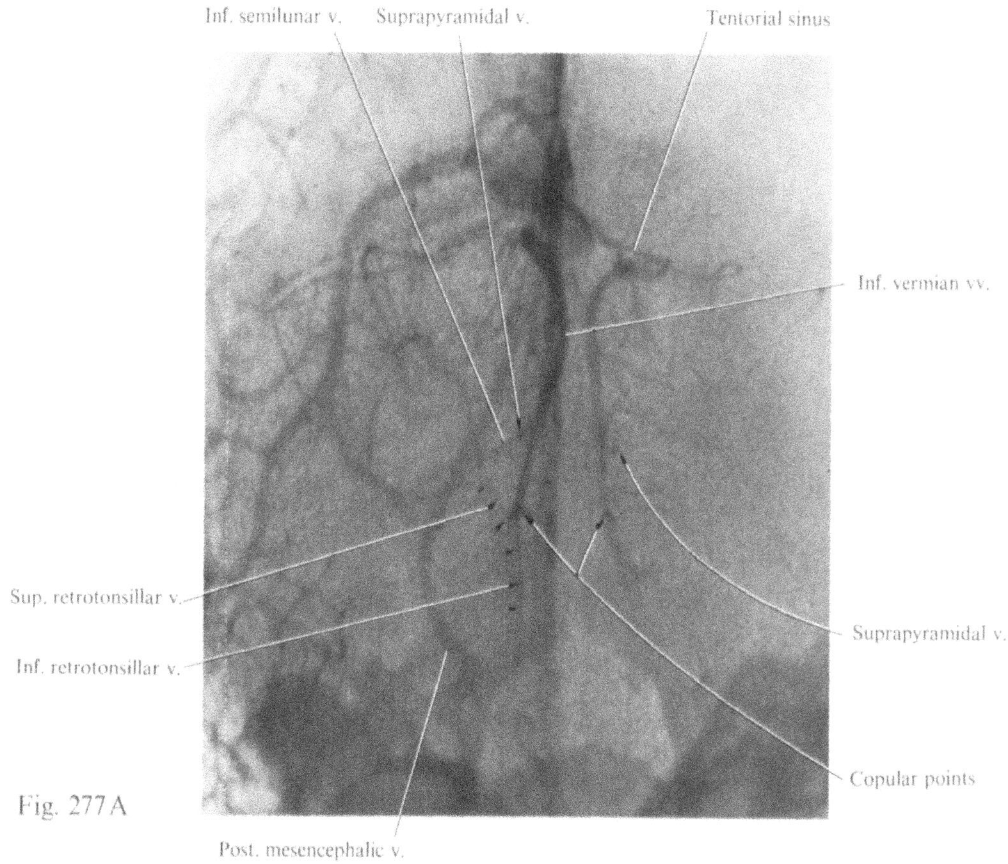

Fig. 277 A

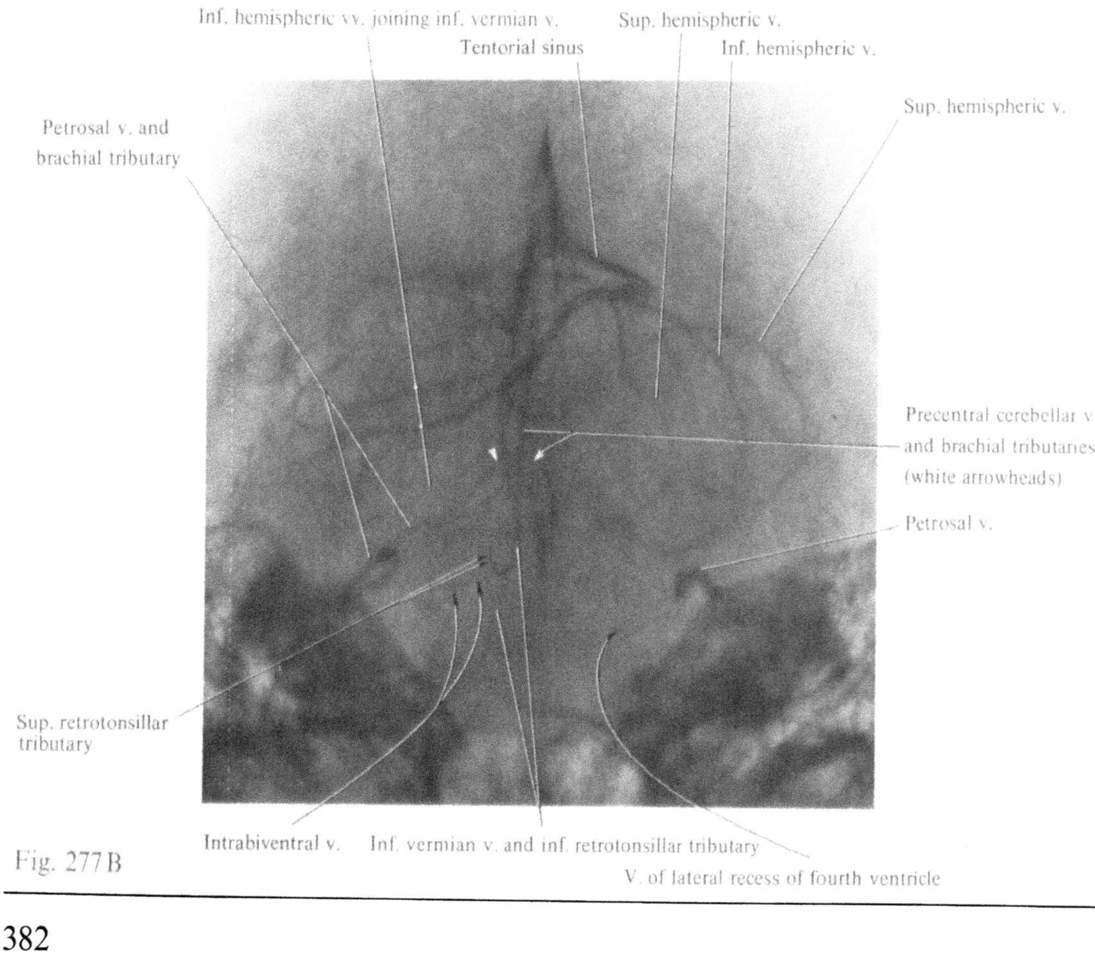

Fig. 277 B

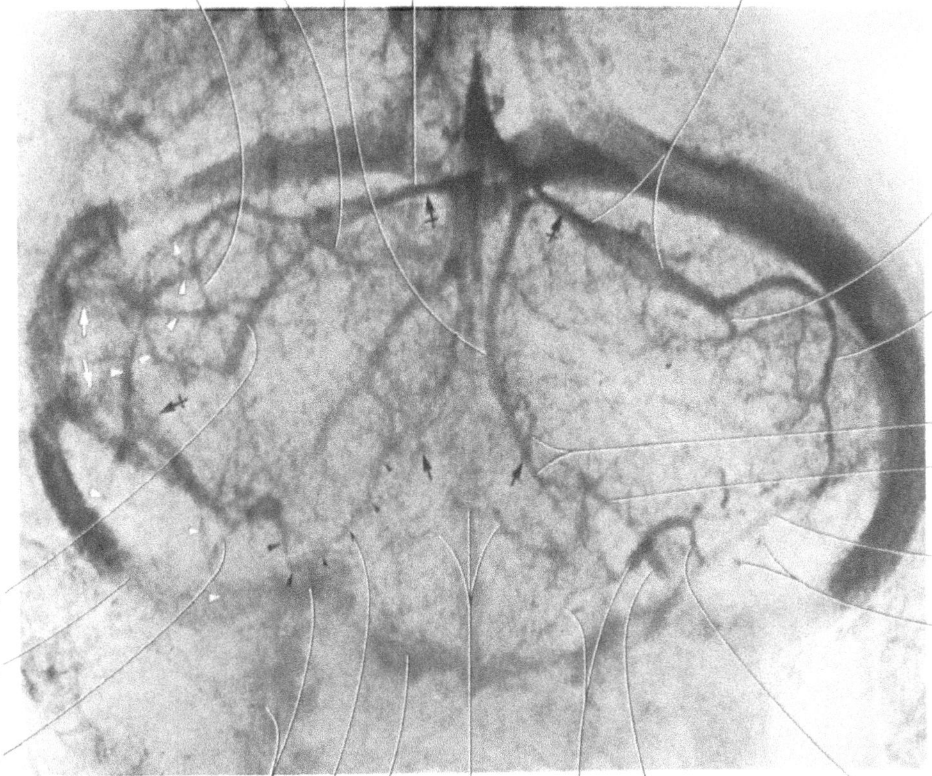

Fig. 278. Tentorial sinuses. Cerebral angiograms, venous phase, semiaxial view
Three tentorial sinuses, two located posteriorly and one anteriorly, can be identified (⇞). Each of the posterior two receives a small superior hemispheric vein, a prominent inferior hemispheric vein and the inferior vermian vein on each side. The left one joins the straight sinus some distance anteriorly to the torcular, whereas the right one opens into the torcular itself. The anterior tentorial sinus, receives supratentorial veins of the middle fossa (white arrowheads), and drains laterally to open into the right lateral sinus, in several places (white arrows). Note that the cavernous sinus is located lower than the jugular bulb in this projection. The copular points (↑) and the vein of the lateral recess of the fourth ventricle (row of black arrowheads) can also be identified

◁
Fig. 277. Inferior vermian vein. Cerebral angiogram, venous phase, semiaxial views, 2 cases

Fig. 277 A. Prominent inferior vermian veins. The inferior vermian vein and its retrotonsillar tributaries (row of arrowheads) are best visualized on the right. The copular point, which marks the location of the tonsillobiventral notch, is seen as a dense dot on each side. The distance between the two copular points corresponds roughly to the transverse width of the cisterna magna at this level. The suprapyramidal veins on both sides mark the posterior border of the pyramid, whereas the copular points indicate its anterior border

Fig. 277 B. Anomalous drainage of the inferior vermian vein and its inferior hemispheric tributary. The inferior retrotonsillar tributaries run upwards and are joined by several hemispheric veins that travel medially and superiorly. The combined stem then crosses the posterior cerebellar notch to run superiorly and laterally on the inferior surface of the left cerebellar hemisphere. It then takes a short course medially, within the tentorium, and flows into the torcular. The brachial tributaries (white arrowheads) of the precentral cerebellar vein mark the location of the roof of the upper part of the fourth ventricle

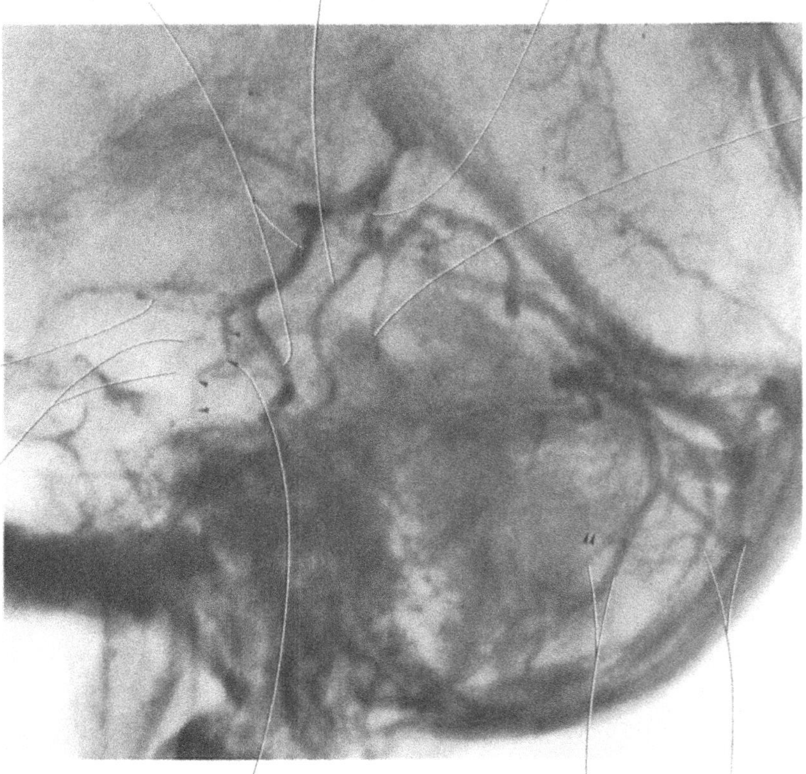

Fig. 279A

Fig. 279. Anomalous drainage of the posterior draining groups. Cerebral angiogram, venous phase, lateral views, 2 cases

Fig. 279A. Inferior vermian vein draining into the great cerebral vein. The inferior vermian vein, receiving the retrotonsillar, suprapyramidal (double arrowheads) and inferior hemispheric tributaries, runs upwards on the posterior aspect of the inferior vermis and then onto the superior aspect of the superior vermis. After it crosses the apex of the cerebellum, the vein is joined by the precentral cerebellar vein and runs upwards as the superior cerebellar vein, to join the great cerebral vein. Note the large anastomotic channel between the superior cerebellar vein and the petrosal vein, above the vermis (vermopetrosal vein). The great cerebral vein and the superior petrosal sinus are connected by the posterior mesencephalic and anastomotic lateral mesencephalic veins (galenopetrosal vein). More anteriorly, the lateral pontomesencephalic vein runs on the lateral aspect of the mesencephalon and pons (row of arrowheads)

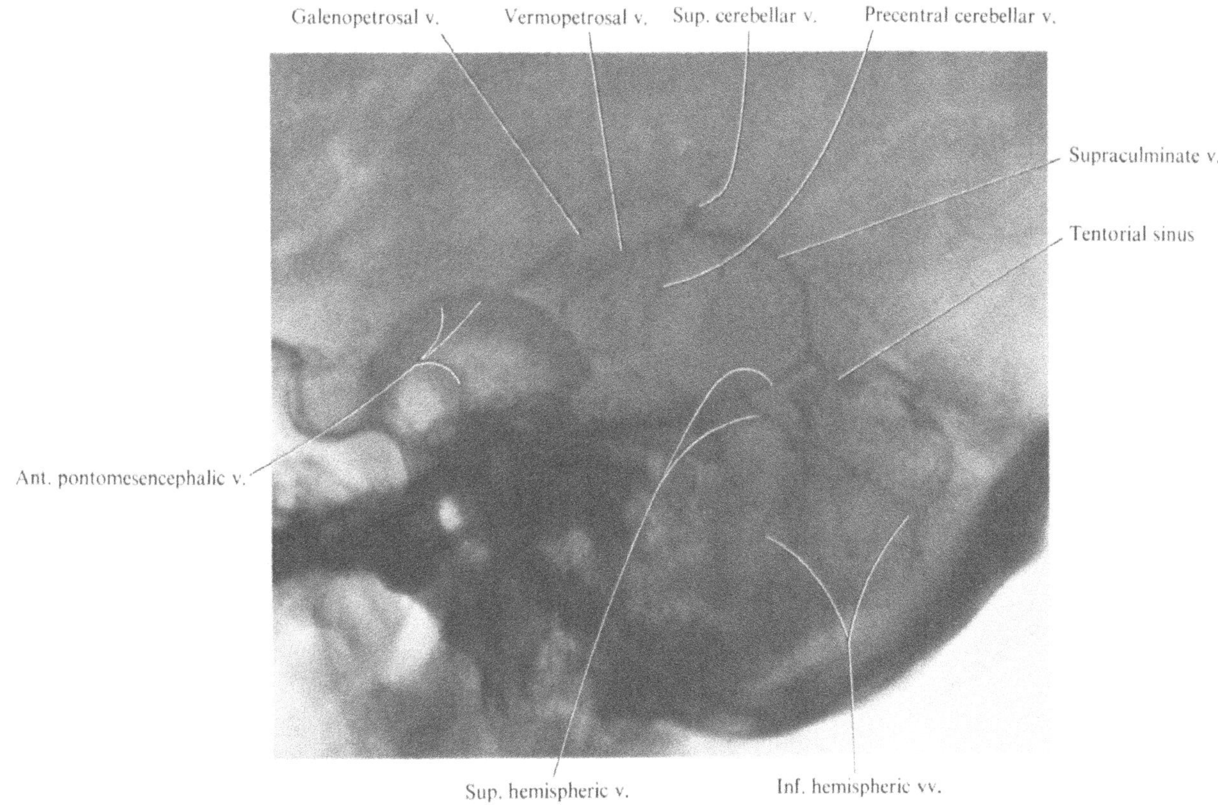

Fig. 279 B. Inferior hemispheric vein joining the upper end of the straight sinus. One of the inferior hemispheric veins runs upwards, crossing the posterolateral margin of the cerebellar hemisphere, to run onto its superior surface. The vein travels further superiorly and medially, flowing into the supraculminate vein. The latter vein reaches the apex of the cerebellum and is joined by the precentral cerebellar and vermopetrosal veins, to open into the upper end of the straight sinus. Note the unusual angular course of the galenopetrosal vein (on the opposite side)

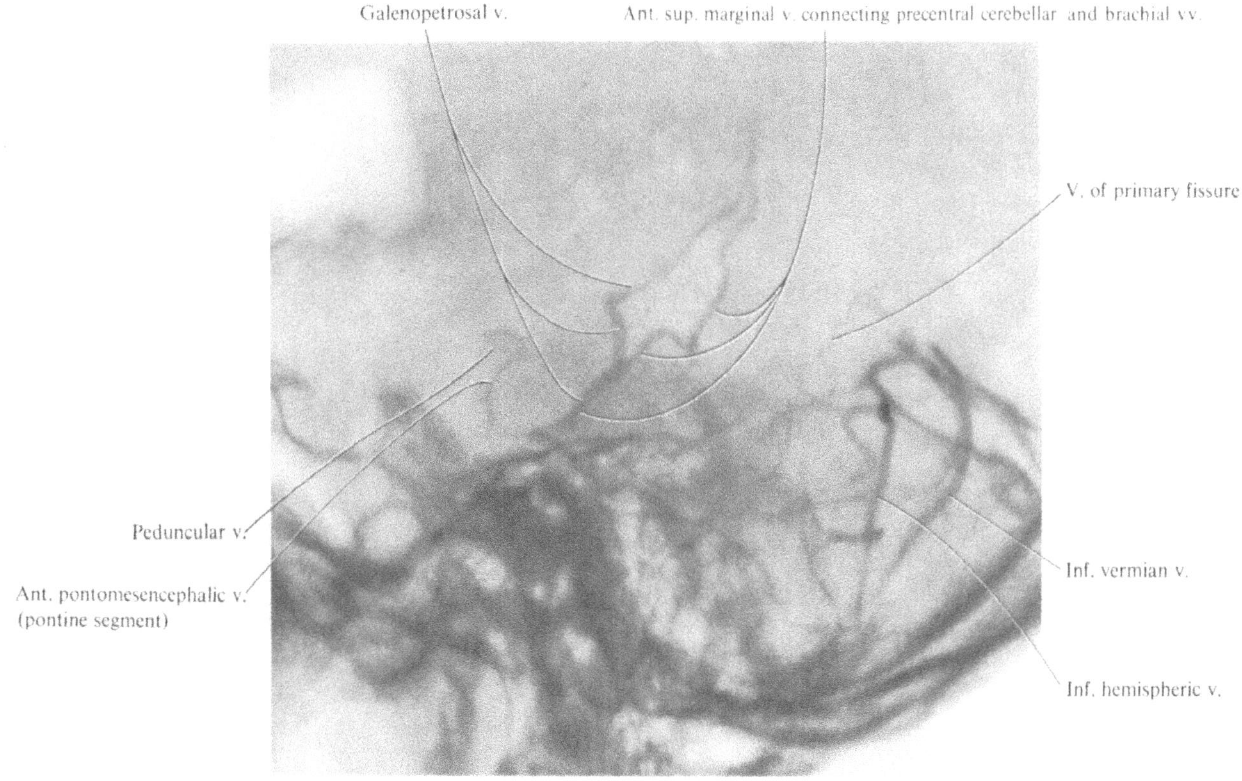

Fig. 280A

Fig. 280. Anastomotic channels connecting the various groups of veins of the posterior fossa. Cerebral angiogram, venous phase, lateral views, 2 cases

Fig. 280A. Anastomosis between the superior and anterior draining groups. The great cerebral vein is connected to the petrosal vein by the posterior mesencephalic vein, the anastomotic lateral mesencephalic vein and the brachial tributary of the petrosal vein (galenopetrosal vein). In addition, there is a communication between the precentral cerebellar vein and the petrosal vein, via the anterosuperior marginal vein

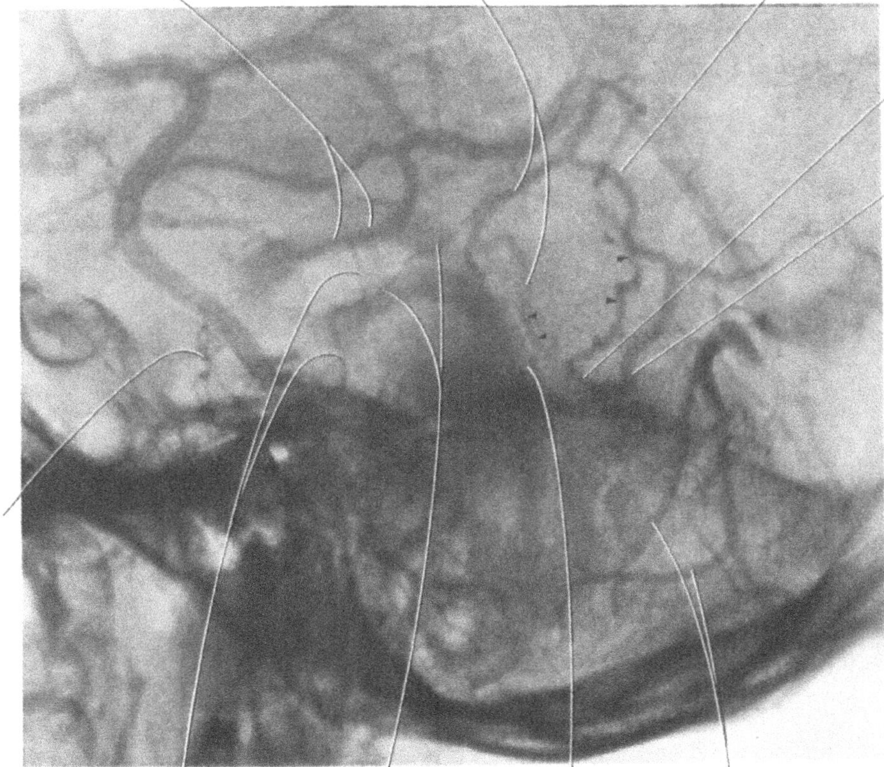

Fig. 280 B. Anastomosis between the superior and posterior draining groups. The superior hemispheric tributaries of the supraculminate and precentral cerebellar veins connect (arrowheads) the superior with posterior groups of veins of the posterior fossa

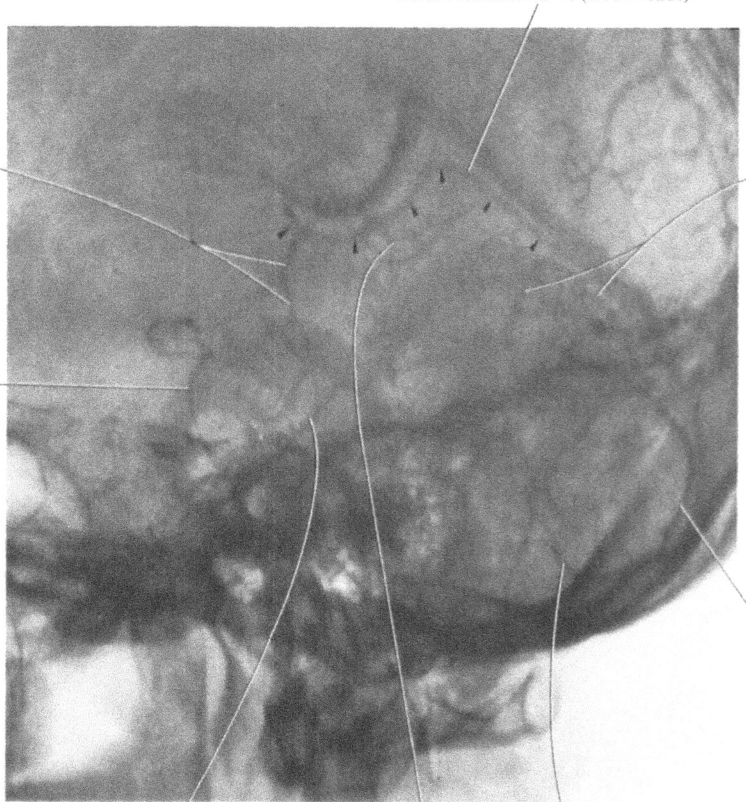

Fig. 281 A

Fig. 281. Galenovermorectal vein. Cerebral angiogram, venous phase, lateral views, 2 cases

Fig. 281 A. A long vein(arrowheads) bridges between the posterior part of the internal cerebral vein and the distal portion of the straight sinus. This galenovermorectal vein runs over the superior vermis. Inferiorly, the superior retrotonsillar vein emerges from the retrotonsillar fissure, leaves the posterior cerebellar notch, and then runs superolaterally as an inferior hemispheric vein, before draining into the lateral sinus

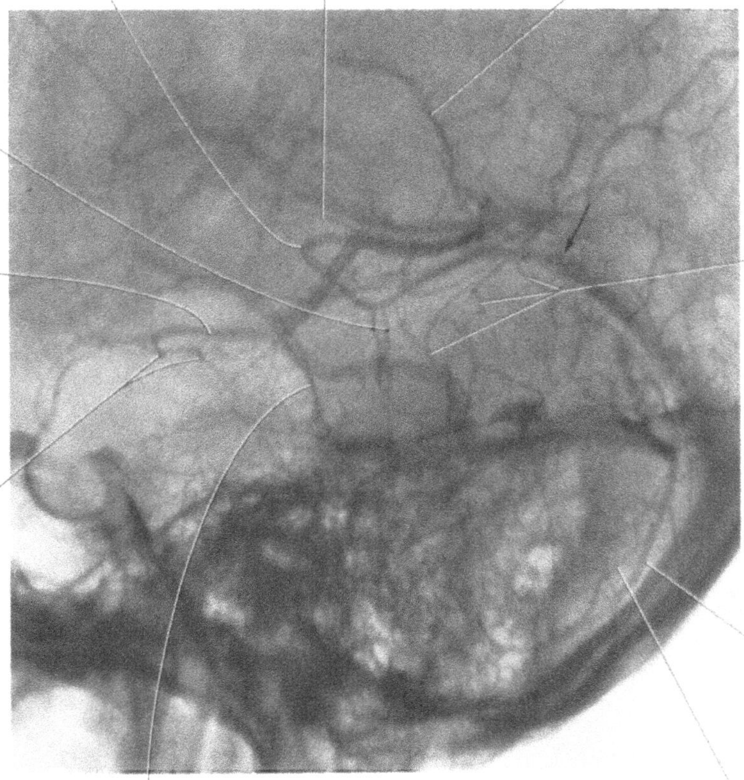

Fig. 281 B. Unlike the galenovermorectal vein seen in Fig. A, this vein loops forwards considerably. The vein receives anteriorly the split precentral cerebellar vein and posteriorly the superior vermian vein. The latter vein receives various culminate tributaries

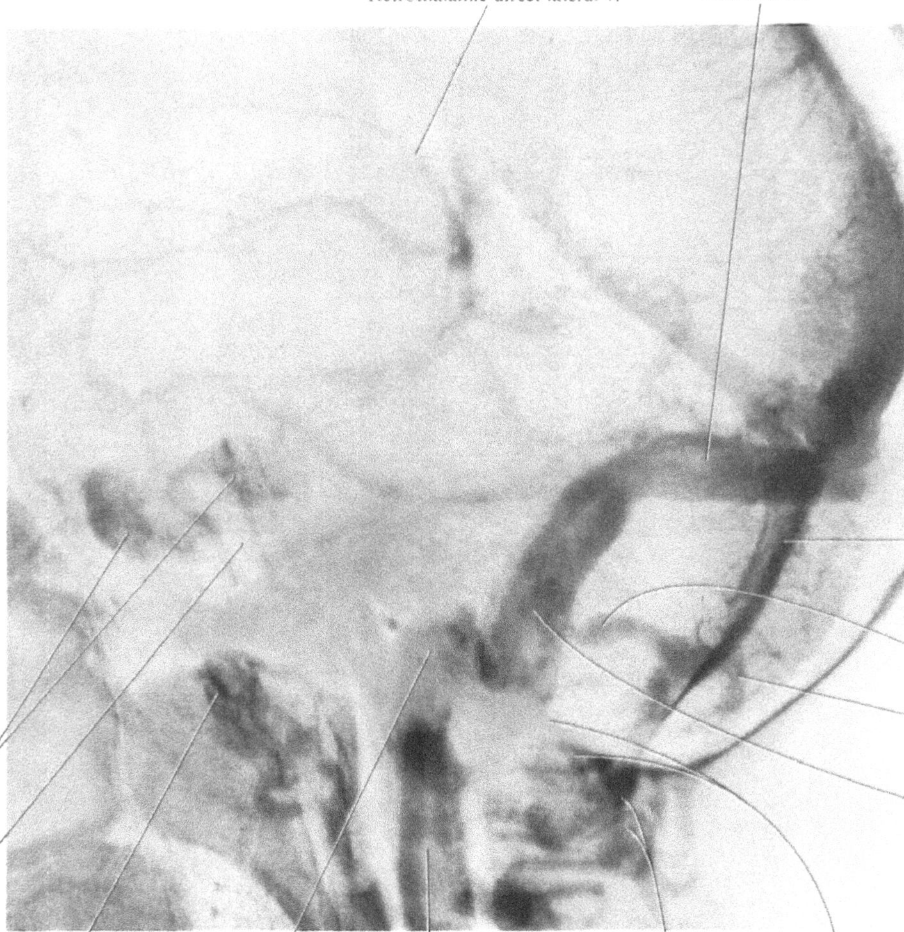

Fig. 282. Occipital sinus, mastoid and condyloid emissary veins. Carotid angiogram, venous phase, lateral view
The occipital sinus is unusually prominent. The mastoid emissary vein connects the sigmoid sinus with the occipital vein, through the mastoid foramen, while the condyloid emissary vein bridges between the jugular bulb and the suboccipital veins. The pterygoid venous plexus is filled via emissary veins from the middle fossa

References

Abbie, A.A.: The clinical significance of the anterior choroidal artery. Brain **56**, 233–246 (1933)

Abbie, A.A.: Blood supply of the lateral geniculate body with a note on the morphology of the choroidal arteries. J. Anat. (Lond.) **67**, 491–521 (1933)

Aitken, H.F.: Diagram of arterial circulation of basal ganglia. New Engl. J. Med. **199**, 1084 (1929)

Alexander, L.: Vascular supply of the stria-pallidum. A. Res. Nerv. Ment. Dis. Proc. **21**, 77–132 (1942)

Amundsen, P., Grimsrud, O.K.: Height of fourth ventricle in normal encephalograms. Acta radiol. (Stockh.) **4**, 257–261 (1966)

Andersen, P.E.: Angiographic localization of small intra-cerebral hematomas. Acta radiol. (Stockh.) **1**, 173–181 (1963)

Andersen, P.E.: The lenticulostriate arteries and their diagnostic value: a preliminary report. Acta radiol. (Stockh.) **50**, 84–91 (1958)

Angevine, J.B., Jr., Mancall, E.L., Yakolev, P.I.: The human cerebellum: an atlas of gross topography in serial sections. Boston: Little, Brown and Co. 1961

Atkinson, W.J.: The anterior inferior cerebellar artery: "its variations, pontine distribution, and significance in the surgery of cerebello-pontine angle tumours". J. Neurol. Neurosurg. Psychiat. **12**, 137–151 (1949)

Azambuja, N., Arana, I.R., Sande, M.T., Garcia: Central ventriculography. Acta neurol. lat.-amer. **1**, 58–64 (1956)

Babin, E.: Contribution à l'étude radio-anatomique de la veine basilaire normale et de ses affluents. Diplôme d'électroradiologie, Strasbourg 1971

Baker, H.L.: Cerebellopontine angle myelography. J. Neurosurg. **36**, 614–624 (1972)

Baker, H.L.: Myelographic examination of the posterior fossa with positive contrast medium. Radiology **81**, 791–801 (1963)

Baptista, A.P.: Study on the arteries of the brain. (II) The anterior cerebral artery: some anatomic features and their clinical implications. Neurology (Minneap.) **13**, 825–835 (1963)

Bassett, D.L.: A stereoscopic atlas of human anatomy. Baltimore: Williams and Wilkins 1954

Baucaud, J., Talairach, J., Geier, S., Scarabin, J.M.: E.E.G et S.E.E.G. dans les tumeurs cérébrales et l'épilepsie. Paris: Edifor 1973

Beau, A., Rabischong, P.: Les veines internes du cerveau. C. R. Ass. Anat. **102**, 175–181 (1959)

Beevor, C.E.: On the distribution of different arteries supplying the human brain. Proc. R. Soc. London (Ser. B.) **80**, 25–28 (1908); **200**, 1–56 (1909)

Bekov, D.B.: Atlas of the venous system of the brain of man (in Russian). Moscow: Izdatelstvo "Meditsina" 1965

Bekov, D.B.: Some structural differences among posterolateral tributaries of the great cerebral vein. Fed. Proc. Suppl. 24T, 166–170 (1965)

Belloni, G.B.: La pneumografia degli spazi arachnoidei encefalici. Boll. Soc. Ital. Biolog. Sper. **16**, 2–10 (1941)

Ben-Amor, M., Marion, C.H., Heldt, N.: Normal and pathological radioanatomy of the superior choroid vein. Neuroradiology **3**, 16–19 (1971)

Ben-Amor, M., Wackenheim, A.: Les veines cérébrales profondes sustentorielles. I. Radioanatomie normale. Ann. Radiol. **16**, 731–757 (1973)

Ben-Amor, M., Wackenheim, A.: Les veines cérébrales profondes sustentorielles. II. Radioanatomie pathologique tumorale. Ann. Radiol. **17**, 71–99 (1974)

Billewicz, O., Ben-Amor, M.: The posterior ventricular branches of the internal cerebral and basilar vein. Neuroradiology **2**, 37–45 (1971)

Bonnal, J., Legré, J.: L'angiographie cérébrale. Paris: Masson 1958

Bories, J.: L'artériographie vertébrale. Monographie médicale et scientifique. Paris 1958

Bories, J., Fredy, D., Rosier, J.: Tomo-encéphalography. Technique and normal images. Neuroradiology **1**, 200–210 (1970)

Bories, J., Fredy, D., Rosier, J., Merland, J.: Etude tomoencéphalographique de la fosse postérieure. Technique et anatomie radiologique. Ann. Radiol. **14**, 649–656 (1971)

Bouchet, A., Lapras, C., Goutelle, A.: Les voies de drainage veineux à l'intérieur de la fosse cérébrale postérieure. C. R. Ass. Anat. **48**, 336–345 (1963–1964)

Bradac, G.B.: The ponto-mesencephalic veins (radio-anatomical study). Neuroradiology **1**, 52–57 (1970)

Bricout, J., Guiot, G.: Atlas stéréotaxique du réseau artériel des noyaux gris centraux. Ann. Radiol. **7**, 701–722 (1964)

Browning, W.: The veins of the brain and its envelopes. Brocklyn-New York: F.B. O'Connor 1884

Bull, J.W.D.: The normal variations in the position of the optic recess of the third ventricle. Acta radiol. (Stockh.) **46**, 72–80 (1956)

Bull, J.W.D.: The volume of the cerebral ventricles. Neurology (Minneap.) **11**, 1–9 (1961)

Bull, J.W.D., Kozlowski, P.: The angiographic pattern of the petrosal veins in the normal and pathological. Neuroradiology **1**, 20–26 (1970)

Carlsson, B., Lodin, H.: Size of interpeduncular, pontine, ponto-cerebellar cisterns and cisterna magna in childhood. Acta radiol. (Stockh.) **8**, 65–73 (1969)

Carpenter, M.B., Noback, C.R., Moss, M.L.: The anterior choroidal artery. Its origins, course, distribution and variations. Arch. Neurol. Psychiat. (Chic.) **71**, 714–722 (1954)

Chrzanowski, R., Wackenheim, A.: Pneumostratigraphie frontale du tronc cérébral. Ann. Radiol. **9**, 872–880 (1966)

Childe, A. E., Penfield, W.: Anatomic and pneumographic study of the temporal horn. Arch. Neurol. Psychiat. (Chic.) **101**, 30 (1944)

COOPER, I. S.: Surgical occlusion of the anterior choroidal artery in Parkinsonism. Surg. Gynec. Obstet. **99**, 207–219 (1954)

CORRALÈS, M., GREITZ, T.: Fourth ventricle. I: A morphologic and radiologic investigation of the normal anatomy. Acta radiol. (Stockh.) **12**, 113–133 (1972)

CORRALÈS, M., GREITZ, T.: Fourth ventricle. II: Tumours of the cerebellum. Acta radiol. (Stockh.) **12**, 241–270 (1972)

CORRALÈS, M., GREITZ, T.: Fourth ventricle. III: Intra and extra cranial tumours. Acta radiol. (Stockh.) **13**, 370–381 (1972)

COUSSEMENT, A.: Repères et mesures en radiodiagnostic. Monographie des Annales de Radiologie. L'Expansion scientifique française. Paris 1974

CRITCHLEY, M.: The anterior cerebral artery and its syndromes. Brain **53**, 121–162 (1930)

DAHLSTRÖM, L., FAGERBERT, G., LANNER, L., STATTIN, S.: Anatomical and angiographic study of arteries supplying anterior part of temporal lobe. A preliminary report. Acta radiol. (Stockh.) **9**, 257–263 (1969)

DANDY, W.E.: An operation for the cure of tic douloureux. Arch. Surg. **18**, 687–734 (1929)

DANDY, W.E.: Roentgenography of the brain after injection of air into the spinal canal. Reprinted in Neurosurgical classics, J. Neurosurg. **20**, 531–536 (1963)

DAVIDOFF, L.M., DYKE, C.G.: The normal encephalogram. Philadelphia: Lea and Fibiger 1951

DECK, M.D.F., POTTS, G.D.: Movements of ventricular fluid levels due to cerebrospinal fluid formation. Amer. J. Roentgenol. **106**, 2, 354–368 (1969)

DECKER, K.: The displacement of the posterior cerebral artery in the cerebral angiogram. Acta radiol. (Stockh.) **40**, 91–95 (1953)

DECKER, K.: Clinical Neuroradiology. New York: Macgraw Hill 1969

DE JERINE, J.: Anatomie des centres nerveux. Paris: Rueff 1895

DI CHIRO, G.: An atlas of detailed normal pneumo-encephalographic anatomy. Springfield/Ill.: Ch. Thomas 1961

DILENGE, D.: Anatomie radiologique de la citerne opto-chiasmatique. Rev. Neurochir. **1**, 257–267 (1955)

DILENGE, D.: L'angiographie de l'artère carotide interne. Paris: Masson 1962

DILENGE, D.: In: Neurochirurgie (DAVID, M., POURPRE, H., LEPOIRE, J., DILENGE, D., Eds.) 1. Vol., p. 49–104. Paris: Flammarion 1965

DILENGE, D., CONSTANS, J.: Séméiologie angiographique de l'artère cérébrale antérieure. Acta radiol. (Stockh.) **1**, 248–256 (1963)

DJINDJIAN, R.: L'angiographie de la moelle épinière. Angiography of the spinal cord. Paris: Masson 1970

DOW, R.S.: The evolution and anatomy of the cerebellum. Biol. Rev. **17**, 179–220 (1942)

DOYEN: In: Precis d'anatomie médicochirurgicale (PATEL, M., CREYSSEL, J., DARGENT, Eds.). Paris: Librairie Maloine 1951

DOYON, D., RAMÉE, A.: Artériographie carotidienne. In: Traité de Radiodiagnostic. Neuroradiologie XIII (FISCHGOLD, H. et coll., Eds.), p. 201–257. Paris: Masson 1972

DURET, H.: Recherches anatomiques sur la circulation de l'encéphale. Arch. physiol. norm. path. **1**, 919–957 (1874)

DUROUX, P.E., PUJOL, H., BOSSY, J.: Contribution à l'étude de l'artère sylvienne et de ses territoires vasculaires. In: XXXIXe Réunion Ass. Anatomistes, p. 135–145 (1952)

DUVERNOY, H.M.: The superficial veins of the human brain. Veins of the brain stem and of the base of the brain. Berlin-Heidelberg-New York: Springer-Verlag 1975

ECONOMOS, D., PROSALENTIS, A.: L'artère cérébelleuse supérieure dans les tumeurs de la fosse postérieure. Acta radiol. (Stockh.) **1**, 267–277 (1963)

EECKEN, VAN DER, H.M.: The anastomose between the leptomeningeal arteries of the brain. Springfield/Ill.: Ch.C. Thomas 1959

EECKEN, VAN DER, H.M., ADAMS, R.D.: The anatomy and functional significance of the meningeal arterial anastomoses of the human brain. J. Neuropath. exp. Neurol. **12**, 132–157 (1953)

ENGESET, A., SKRAASTAD, E.: Methods of measurement in encephalography. Neurology (Minneap.) **14**, 381–385 (1964)

EPSTEIN, B.S.: A pneumoencephalographic study of the normal third and fourth cerebral ventricles and aqueduct of Sylvius. Amer. J. Roentgenol. **63**, 204–209 (1950)

EVANS, W.A.: An encephalographic radio for estimating the size of the cerebral ventricles. Amer. J. Dis. Child. **64**, 820–830 (1942)

FARNARIER, PH.: Les branches corticales et calleuses de l'artère cérébrale antérieure. Thèse Médecine, Marseille 1974

FERNER, H.: Anatomische und phlebographische Studien der inneren Hirnvenen des Menschen. Z. Anat. Entwickl.-Gesch. **120**, 481–491 (1958)

FIELDS, W.S., BRUETMAN, M.E., WEIBEL, J.: Collateral circulation of the brain. Monogr. surg. Sci. **2**, 183–259 (1965)

FISCHER, E.: Lageabweichungen der vorderen Hirnarterie im genlabilld. Z. Neurochir. **3**, 300–313 (1938)

FISCHER, E.: Eine neue Methode zur Lokalization des Angulus Venosus der tiefen Hirnvenen unter Berücksichtigung der Form des Schädels. Acta neurochir. (Wien) **14**, 53–68 (1966)

FISCHER, E.: Roentgenologische Untersuchungen zur Lageabhängigkeit der tiefen Hirnvenen, insbesondere des Angulus Venosus, von der Form des Schädels. Acta neurochir. (Wien) **14**, 25–52 (1966)

FISCHGOLD, H., BONNEMAZOU, A., FREDY, D., METZGER, J.: La citerne optochiasmatique et son contenu. J. Radiol. **50**, 121–134 (1969)

FISCHGOLD, H. et coll.: Traité de Radiodiagnostic. Neuroradiologie XIII. Radio-anatomie et méthodes d'exploration du système nerveux central. Paris: Masson 1972

FOIX, CH., HILLEMAND, P.: Les artères de l'arc encéphalique jusqu'au diencéphale inclusivement. Rev. Neurol. **2**, 705–739 (1925)

FOIX, CH., HILLEMAND, P.: Note sur la disposition générale des artères de l'axe encéphalique. C. R. Soc. Biol. (Paris) **42**, 31–33 (1925)

FOIX, CH., LÉVY, M.: Les ramollissements sylviens; syndromes des lésions en foyer du territoire de l'artère sylvienne et de ses branches. Rev. Neurol. **11**, 1–51 (1927)

GABRIELLE, H., LATARJET, M., LECUIRE, J., DUROUX, P.E.: Contribution à l'étude du tronc de l'artère sylvienne et de la vascularisation artérielle du lobe de l'insula chez l'homme. XXXVIe Réunion Ass. Anat. (Lyon) 291–298 (1949)

GABRIELLE, H., LATARJET, M., LECUIRE, J., EICHLIOTZ, L.: Contribution à l'étude de l'anatomie macroscopique de l'artère cérébrale postérieure et de la vascularisation du lobe occipital chez l'homme. XXXVIe Réunion Ass. Anat. (Lyon) 336–338 (1949)

GABRIELLE, H., LATARJET, M., LECUIRE, J., MILLERET, P.: Contribution à l'étude macroscopique de la vascularisation du lobe temporal chez l'homme. XXXVIe Réunion Ass. Anat. (Lyon) 339–354 (1949)

GALLOWAY, J.R., GREITZ, T.: The medial and lateral choroidal arteries. An anatomic and roentgenographic study. Acta radiol. (Stockh.) **53**, 353–366 (1960)

GASS, H.: Pantopaque anterior basal cisternography of the posterior fossa. Amer. J. Roentgenol. **90**, 1197–1204 (1963)

GASTAUT, H., LAMMERS, H.J.: Anatomie du rhinencéphale. In: Les Grandes activités du rhinencéphale (sous la direction de Th. Alajouanine). Paris: Masson 1961

GAWLER, J., BULL, J.W.D., DU BOULAY, G.H.: The Emi scanner (Computer Assisted Tomography). Its place in investigation of intra cranial tumours. Lancet **2**, 419–423 (1974)

GEORGE, A.E., SALAMON, G., KRICHEFF, I.: Angiography of the thalamoperforate artery, with special emphasis on arteriography of the third ventricle. In: Advances in Cerebral Angiography (SALAMON, G., Ed.). Berlin-Heidelberg-New York: Springer 1975

GILLILAN, L.A.: Blood vessels, Meninges, Cerebro-spinal fluid. In: CROSBY, H.L.: Correlative anatomy of the nervous system. New York: Mac Millan 1962

GIUDICELLI, G., FAURE, J., SALAMON, G.: The veins of the thalamus. Neuroradiology **1**, 92–98 (1970)

GOUAZÉ, A., CASTAING, J.: Tissue marking by fluorescent organic compound in vivo. Med. Biol. **47**, 112–113 (1967)

GRATIOLET: Anatomie Comparée du Système nerveux. Paris 1839–1857

GREITZ, T.: Evaluation of Circulation time in angiography of the vertebral artery. Acta radiol. diagn. **9**, 300–309 (1969)

GREITZ, T.: Technical aspects of the pneumoencephalographic and ventriculographic examination of the fourth ventricle. Neuroradiology **6**, 259–269 (1974)

GREITZ, T., LINDGREN, E.: In Angiography (ABRAMS, H.L., Ed.). Boston: Little, Brown & Co. 1961

GREITZ, T., LÖFSTEDT, S.: The relationship between the third ventricle and the basilar artery. Acta radiol. (Stockh.) **42**, 85–100 (1954)

GREITZ, T., SJÖGREN, S.E.: The posterior inferior cerebellar artery. Acta radiol. (Stockh.) **1**, 284–297 (1963)

GREPE, A.: Examination of intracranial basal cisterns with watersoluble contrast medium. Experimental, anatomic and preliminary clinical investigations. Thesis, Stockholm 1974

GUYOT, J.F., PHILIPPON, J.: Scissure de Sylvius et des repères artériographiques. Acta radiol. (Stockh.) **9**, 317–321 (1969)

HARA, K., FUJINO, J.: The thalamoperforate artery. Acta radiol. (Stockh.) **5**, 192–200 (1966)

HASSLER, O.: Deep cerebral venous system in man. A microangiographic study on its areas of drainage and its anastomoses with the superficial cerebral veins. Neurology (Chic.) **16**, 505–511 (1966)

HASSLER, O.: Venous anatomy of human hindbrain. A stereomicroangiographic study of the venous angio-architecture and the venous areas of drainage. Arch. Neurol. Psych. **16**, 404–409 (1967)

HASSLER, O., SALTZMAN, G.F.: Angiographic and histologic changes in infundibular widening of the posterior communicating artery. Acta radiol. (Stockh.) **1**, 321–327 (1963)

HASTINGS-JAMES, R.: The anatomy of the posterior fossa in relation to positive contrast cisternography. Radiology **92**, 1065–1072 (1969)

HAUGE, T.: Catheter vertebral angiography. Acta radiol. (Stockh.) Suppl. **109** (1954)

HEDON, C.: Etude anatomique sur la circulation veineuse de l'encéphale. Thèse Bordeaux **79**, 1–96 (1888)

HELIAS, A., METZGER, J.: Encéphalographie gazeuse fractionnée. In: Traité de Radiodiagnostic XIII, Neuroradiologie. (FISCHGOLD, H. et coll., Eds.), p. 119–191. Paris: Masson 1972

HERMAN, L.H., OSTROWSKI, A.Z., GURDJIAN, E.S.: Perforating branches of the middle cerebral artery. Anatomical study. Arch. Neurol. Psych. (Chic.) **8**, 32–34 (1963)

HEUBNER, A.: Zur Topographie der Ernährungsgebiete der einzelnen Hirnarterien. Zbl. med. Wiss. **52**, 817–821 (1872)

HILLEMAND, P., SCHIFF-WERTHEIMER, S., CHAVANY: Le syndrome de l'artère choroidienne antérieure. In: Science Médicale Pratique, p. 295–297. Paris 1935

HOCHSTETTER, F.: Über eine Varietät der Vena Cerebralis basialis des Menschen nebst Bemerkungen über die Entwicklung bestimmter Hirnvenen. Z. Anat. Entwickl.-Gesch. **108**, 311–336 (1938)

HOOSHMAND, I., ROSENBAUM, A.E., STEIN, R.L.: Radiographic anatomy of normal cerebral deep medullary veins. Criteria for distinguishing them from their abnormal counterparts. Neuroradiology **7**, 75–84 (1974)

HUANG, Y.P., ITO, J., PINNER, J.: Angiographic anatomy and circulation time of the veins of the posterior fossa. In: Symposium on recent advances in neuroradiology (KITAMURA, K., NEWTON, T.H., Eds.). Tokyo: Igaku Shoin 1975

HUANG, Y.P., ITO, J.S.: Olfactory arteries and veins. The angiographic visualization of the olfactory cistern. Presented at the 11th annual meeting of the American Society of Neuroradiology (April 1973)

HUANG, Y.P., WOLF, B.S.: Veins of the white matter of the cerebral hemispheres (the medullary veins): diagnostic importance in carotid angiography. Amer. J. Roentgenol. **92**, 739–755 (1964)

HUANG, Y.P., WOLF, B.S.: The veins of the posterior-fossa superior or Galenic draining group. Amer. J. Roentgenol. **95**, 808–821 (1965)

HUANG, Y.P., WOLF, B.S.: Precentral cerebellar vein in angiography. Acta radiol. (Stockh.) **5**, 250–262 (1966)

HUANG, Y.P., WOLF, B.S.: The vein of the lateral recess of the fourth ventricle and its tributaries: roentgen appearance and anatomic relationships. Amer. J. Roentgenol. **101**, 1–21 (1967)

HUANG, Y.P., WOLF, B.S.: Veins of the posterior fossa. In: Radiology of the skull and brain (NEWTON, T.H., POTTS, D.B., Eds.), Vol. 2, Book 3, p. 2155–2216. St. Louis: Mosby 1974

HUANG, Y.P., WOLF, B.S.: The basal cerebral vein and its tributaries. In: Radiology of the skull and brain (NEWTON, T.H., POTTS, D.G., Eds.), Vol. 2, Book 4, p. 2111–2154. St. Louis: Mosby 1974

HUANG, Y.P., WOLF, B.S., ANTIN, S.P., OKUDERA, T.: The veins of the posterior fossa – anterior or petrosal draining group. Amer. J. Roentgenol. **104**, 36–56 (1968)

HUANG, Y.P., WOLF, B.S., OKUDERA, T.: Angiographic anatomy of the inferior vermian vein of the cerebellum. Acta radiol. (Stockh.) **9**, 327–344 (1969)

JAIN, K.K.: Some observations on the anatomy of the middle cerebral artery. Canad. J. Surg. **7**, 134–139 (1964)

JOHANSON, C.: Central veins and deep dural sinuses of the brain: anatomical and angiographic study. Acta radiol. (Stockh.) Suppl. **107** (1954)

KAPLAN, H.A.: The trancerebral venous system: an anatomical study. Arch. Neurol. Psych. (Chic.) **1**, 148–152 (1959)

KAPLAN, H.A.: The lateral perforating branches of the anterior and middle cerebral arteries. J. Neurosurgery **23**, 305–310 (1965)

KAPLAN, H.A., FORD, D.H.: The brain vascular system. Amsterdam-New York: Elsevier 1966

KEY, A., RETZIUS, G.: Studien in der Anatomie des Nervensystems und des Bindegewebes. Stockholm: P.A. Norstedt and Soner 1875

KRAYENBÜHL, H.A., RICHTER, H.R.: Die zerebrale Angiographie. Stuttgart: G. Thieme 1952

KRAYENBÜHL, H.A., YASARGIL, M.G.: Die zerebrale Angiographie: Lehrbuch für Klinik und Praxis. Stuttgart: G. Thieme 1965

KRAYENBÜHL, H.A., YASARGIL, M.G.: Les signes artériographiques les plus typiques permettant d'évoquer une néoformation des lobes cérébelleux. Ann. Radiol. **10**, 819–826 (1967)

KRAYENBÜHL, H.A., YASARGIL, M.G.: Cerebral angiography, 2. Ed. London: Butterworth 1968

KRONLEIN: In: Traité d'Anatomie Humaine, IV, Système nerveux (PATURET, G., Ed.). Paris: Masson 1964

LAINE, E.D., DELANDTSHEER, J.M., GALIBERT, P., DELANDTSHEER-ARNOTT, G.: Les données phlébographiques dans les tumeurs des hémisphéres cérébraux et des noyaux gris centraux. J. Radiol. **37**, 368–374 (1956)

LANGELAAN, J.W.: On the development of the external form of the human cerebellum. Brain **42**, 130–170 (1919)

LAZORTHES, G., SALAMON, G.: Etude anatomique et radio-anatomique de la vascularisation artérielle du thalamus. Ann. Radiol. **14**, 905–924 (1971)

LAZORTHES, G.: Vascularisation et circulation cérébrales. Paris: Masson 1961

LAZORTHES, G.: Le système nerveux central. Description. Systématisation. Exploration. Paris: Masson 1967

LAZORTHES, G., GOUAZÉ, A.: Les voies anastomotiques de suppléance de la vascularisation artérielle cérébro-spinale. Bull. Ass. Anat. **139** bis, 1–122 (1968)

LAZORTHES, G., GOUAZÉ, A., SALAMON, G.: Vascularisation et circulation cérébrales. Paris: Masson 1976

LAZORTHES, G., POULHÈS, J.: Les variations de la scissure calcarine et de la corne occipitale des ventricules latéraux. XXXVe Réunion Ass. Anat. (1948)

LAZORTHES, G., POULHÈS, J.: les variations des cornes des ventricules latéraux du cerveau. L'acollement de leurs parois. Etude anatomique et radiologique. Toulouse Médical, 1948

LAZORTHES, G., POULHÈS, J., ESPAGNO, J.: Les artères du cervelet. C. R. Ass. Anat. 279–288 (1950)

LAZORTHES, G., POULHÈS, J., GAUBERT, J.: La distribution centrale et corticale de l'artère cérébrale antérieure. Etude anatomique et incidences neurochirurgicales. Neurochirurgie 1956

LEGRÉ, J., DUFOUR, M., DEBAENE, A.: L'angiographie vertébrale. In: Traité de Radiodiagnostic XIII, Neuroradiologie (FISCHGOLD, H. et coll., Eds.), p. 258–303. Paris: Masson 1972

LEIFER, C.: Artériographie vertébrale. Trajets artériels normaux. Leurs modifications dans les processus expansifs de la fosse postérieure. Thèse Bordeaux 1967

LEMAN, P., COHADON, F., LEIFER, C.: Valeur de l'artériographie vertébrale dans les tumeurs de l'angle ponto-cérébelleux. Ann. Radiol. **10**, 791–802 (1967)

LE MAY, M., NEW, P.F.J.: Radiological diagnosis of occult normal-pressure hydrocephalus. Radiology **96**, 347–358 (1970)

LILIEQUIST, B.: The subarachnoid cisterns. An anatomic and roentgenologic study. Acta radiol. (Stockh.) **1** (1959)

LIMA-ALMEIDA, P.: Cerebral angiography. London: Oxford University Press 1950

LIN, P.M., MOKROHISKY, J.F., STAUFFER, H.M., SCOTT, M.: The importance of the deep cerebral veins in cerebral angiography, with special emphasis on the orientation of the foramen of Monro through visualization of the "venous angle" of the brain. J. Neurosurg. **12**, 256–277 (1955)

LINDGREN, E.: A pneumographic study of the temporal horn. Acta radiol. (Stockh.) Suppl. **69** (1948)

LINDGREN, E.: Percutaneous angiography of the vertebral artery. Acta radiol. (Stockh.) **33**, 389–405 (1950)

LINDGREN, E.: Pneumographie des Schädels. In: Lehrbuch der Roentgendiagnostik (SCHINZ, BAENSCH, FRIEDL, VEHLINGER, Hrsg.). Stuttgart: G. Thieme 1951

LINDGREN, E.: Handbuch der Neurochirurgie Roentgenologie. Berlin-Göttingen-Heidelberg: Springer-Verlag 1954

LINDGREN, E.: Radiologic examination of the brain and spinal cord. Acta radiol. (Stockh.) Suppl. **151**, (1957)

LINDGREN, E., DI CHIRO, G.: The roentgenologic appearance of the aqueduct of Sylvius. Acta radiol. (Stockh.) **39**, 117–121 (1953)

LODIN, H.: Size and development of the cerebral ventricular system in childhood. Acta radiol. (Stockh.) **7**, 385–392 (1968)

LÖFGREN, F.O.: Vertebral angiography in the diagnosis of tumours in the pineal region. Acta radiol. (Stockh.) **50**, 108–124 (1958)

LUCAS CHAMPIONNIÈRE: In: Traité d'Anatomie humaine II. Angéiologie, Système nerveux central (TESTUT, L., LATARJET, A., Eds.), p. 1222. Paris: G. Doin 1948

LUSTED, L.B., KEATS, TH.E.: Atlas of Roentgenographic measurement. Chicago: Year Book Medical Publishers 1967

LYSHOLM, E.: Das ventriculogram. Acta radiol. (Stockh.) Suppl. **24**, **25**, **26** (1935)

MARGOLIS, M.T., HOFFMAN, H.B., NEWTON, T.H.: The Choroidal arteries in the diagnosis of thalamic tumors. J. Neurosurg. **36**, 287–298 (1972)

MARGOLIS, M.T., NEWTON, T.H., HOYT, W.H.: Cortical branches of the posterior cerebral artery. Anatomic-radiologic correlation. Neuroradiology **2**, 127–135 (1971)

MARIE, P., FOIX, CH., BERTRAND: Topographie crânio-encéphalique. Rev. Neurol. (1915)

MEGRET, M.: Repérage des artèries choroidiennes de l'artère cérébelleuse postéroinférieure. Thèse Dijon 1972

METTLER, F.A.: Neuroanatomy. St. Louis: Mosby 1948

METZGER, J.: Le signe du chiasma de face en pneumotomographie hypocycloide. Rev. Neurol. **117**, 666–672 (1967)

MICHOTEY, P.: Les branches corticales de l'artère sylvienne. Etude anatomique. Etude radiologique. Procédé de repérage. Thèse Médecine Marseille 1972

MICHOTEY, P., GRISOLI, F., RAYBAUD, CH., SALAMON, G.: Etude anatomique et radiologique de l'artère cérébrale moyenne. Procédé de repérage. Ann. Radiol. **17**, 721–741 (1974)

MOKROHISKY, J.F., PAUL, R.E., LIN, P.M., STAUFFER, H.M.: The diagnostic importance of normal variants in deep cerebral phlebography. Radiology **67**, 34–47 (1956)

MONIZ, E.: L'encéphalographie artérielle, son importance dans la localisation des tumeurs cérébrales. Rev. Neurol. **34**, 72–89 (1927)

MONIZ, E.: L'angiographie cérébrale: ses applications et résultats en anatomie, physiologie et clinique. Paris: Masson 1934

MORELLO, A., COOPER, I.S.: Arteriographic anatomy of the anterior choroidal artery. Amer. J. Roentgenol. **73**, 748–751 (1955)

MOSCOW, N.P., MICHOTEY, P., SALAMON, G.: Anatomy of the cortical branches of the anterior cerebral artery. In: Radiology of the Skull and Brain (NEWTON, T.H., POTTS, D.G., Eds.), p. 1411–1420. St. Louis: Mosby 1974

MOUCHET, A.: Etude radiographique des artères du cerveau. Thèse Toulouse 1911

MOUNIER-KUHN, A., BOUCHET, A., COSTAZ, G.: Contribution à l'étude anatomique, radiologique et chirurgicale de l'artère choroidienne antérieure. Neurochirurgie **1**, 354–370 (1955)

MOUTIER, F.: L'aphasie de Broca. Thèse Médecine, Paris 1908

NOMURA, T.: Atlas of cerebral angiography. Berlin-Heidelberg-New York: Springer-Verlag 1970

OBERSON, R.: Morphologie radiologique normale du IVe ventricule. Radiol. Clin. Biol. Suppl. **38**, 372–382 (1969)

OTOMO, E.: The anterior choroidal artery. Arch. Neurol. Psych. (Chic.) **13**, 656–658 (1965)

OSTROWSKI, A., WEBER, J.E., GURDJIAN, E.S.: The proximal anterior cerebral artery; an anatomic study. Arch. Neurol. Psych. (Chic.) **3**, 661–664 (1960)

PACHTMAN, H., HILAL, S.K., WOOD, E.H.: The posterior choroidal arteries. Normal measurement and displacement by hydrocephalus or tumors of the pineal region or brainstem. Radiology **112**, 343–352 (1974)

PADGET, D.H.: The cranial venous system in man in reference to development, adult configuration, and relation to the arteries. Amer. J. Anat. **98**, 307–355 (1956)

PADGET, D.H.: The development of the cranial venous system in man from the viewpoint of comparative anatomy. Contrib. Embryol. Carneg. Instn. **36**, 79–140 (1957)

PATURET, G.: Traité d'Anatomie humaine, IV, Système nerveux. Paris: Masson 1964

PENFIELD, W.G.: Cerebral pneumography, its danger and its uses. Arch. Neurol. Psych. (Chic.) **13**, 1580–1590 (1925)

PERCHERON, G.: The anatomy of the arterial supply of the human thalamus and its use for the interpretation of the thalamic vascular pathology. Z. Neurol. **205**, 1–13 (1973)

PERESE, D.M.: Superficial veins of the brain from a surgical point of view. J. Neurosurg. **17**, 402–412 (1960)

PFEIFFER, R.A.: Grundlegende Untersuchungen über die Angioarchitektonik des Menschlichen Gehirns. Berlin: Springer 1930

PLETS, C., BERGH, VAN DEN, R.: Contribution des artères choroidiennes dans la vascularisation du thalamus humain. Bull. Ass. Anat. **58**, 163–173 (1974)

PLETS, C., REUCK, DE, J., EECKEN, VAN DER, H., BERGH, VAN DEN, R.: The vascularization of the human thalamus. Acta neurol. belg. **70**, 687–770 (1970)

POIRIER, P.: In: Traité d'Anatomie Humaine, II, Angéiologie, Système nerveux central. (TESTUT, L., LATARJET, A.G., Eds.), p. 1222. Paris: Doin 1948

POIRIER, P., CHARPY, A., NICOLAS, A.: Traité d'Anatomie Humaine, Vol. 3. Paris: Masson 1921

POTTS, D.G., BERGLAND, R.M.: Roentgenologic studies of small cerebrospinal fluid formation in the dog. Amer. J. Roentgenol. **105**, 4, 756–762 (1969)

POTTS, D.G., TAVERAS, J.M.: Differential diagnosis of space-occupying lesions in the region of the thalamus by cerebral angiography. Acta radiol. (Stockh.) **1**, 373–384 (1963)

REESE, D.F., BULL, J.W.D.: Positive contrast demonstration of normal internal acoustic meatus, Meckel's cave and jugular foramen. Amer. J. Roentgenol. **100**, 650–655 (1967)

RING, B.A.: Variations in the striate and other cerebral veins affecting measurements of the "venous angle". Acta radiol. (Stockh.) **52**, 433–447 (1959)

RING, B.A.: Middle cerebral artery: anatomy and radiographic study. Acta radiol. (Stockh.) **57**, 289–300 (1962)

RING, B.A.: The neglected cause of stroke. St. Louis: Warren H. Green 1969

RING, B.A., WADDINGTON, M.M.: Angiographic identification of the motor strip. J. Neurosurg. **26**, 249–254 (1967)

RING, B.A., WADDINGTON, M.M.: Ascending frontal branch of middle cerebral artery. Acta radiol. (Stockh.) **6**, 209–220 (1967)

RING, B.A., WADDINGTON, M.M.: Roentgenographic anatomy of the pericallosal arteries. Amer. J. Roentgenol. **104**, 109–118 (1968)

ROBERTSON, E.G.: Encephalography. Melbourne: Mac Millan 1941

ROBERTSON, E.G.: Pneumoencephalography. Springfield/Ill.: Ch. C. Thomas 1957

ROBERTSON, E.G.: Pneumoencephalography. Oxford: Blackwell Scientific 1957

ROSA, M., BORZONE, M.: The venous system of the corpus striatum. Angiographic study. Neuroradiology **6**, 219–230 (1973)

ROSA, M., VIALE, G.L.: Subependymal veins in the angiographic diagnosis of brain tumours. Neuroradiology **2**, 90–93 (1971)

RUGGIERO, G.: L'encéphalographie fractionnée. Paris: Masson 1957

RUGGIERO, G.: In: Traité Technique Chirurgicale (crâne, rachis, moelle) (DAVID, M., Ed.). Paris: Masson 1961

RUGGIERO, G.: Encephalography today. Acta radiol. (Stockh.) **5**, 705–715 (1966)

RUGGIERO, G., BORIES, J., CALABRO, A., CRISTI, G., SCIALFA, G., SMALTINO, F., THIBAUT, A.: Radiological exploration of the ventricles and subarachnoid space. Berlin-Heidelberg-New York: Springer-Verlag 1974

RUGGIERO, G., CASTELLANO, F.: Upward displacement of the posterior part of the third ventricle. A method for its evaluation. Acta radiol. (Stockh.) **39**, 377–384 (1953)

SALAMON, G.: Repères fixes de système vertébro-basilaire. Ann. Radiol. **10**, 765–780 (1967)

SALAMON, G.: Atlas de la vascularisation artérielle du cerveau chez l'homme. Paris: Sandoz 1973

SALAMON, G.: Advances in Cerebral angiography. Anatomy, Stereotaxy, Embolization, Computerized Axial Tomography. Berlin-Heidelberg-New York: Springer-Verlag 1976

SALAMON, G., BOUDOURESQUES, J., COMBALBERT, A., KHALIL, R., FAURE, J., GIUDICELLI, G.: Les artères lenticulo-striées. Etude artériographique. Leur intérêt dans le diagnostic des hématomes intra-cérébraux. Rev. Neurol. **114**, 361–373 (1966)

SALAMON, G., GONZALÈS, J., FAURE, J., GUIDICELLI, G.: Etude topographique des branches corticales de l'artère sylvienne. Procédé de repérage angiographique. Acta radiol. (Stockh.) **13**, 226–232 (1972)

SALAMON, G., GONZALÈS, J., RAYBAUD, CH., GRISOLI, F., MICHOTEY, P.: Analyse angiographique des branches corticales de l'artère sylvienne. A propos d'un nouveau procédé de repérage. Neurochirurgie **17**, 177–189 (1971)

SALAMON, G., GRISOLI, J., PAILLAS, J.E., FAURE, J., GIUDICELLI, G.: Etude artériographique des artères méningées. Intérêt des injections sélectives, de la soustraction et des corrélations radio-anatomiques. Neurochirurgie **10**, 1–19 (1967)

SALAMON, G., GUÉRINEL, G., LOUIS, R. et coll.: Etude anatomique du système nerveux central. Vascularisation cérébrale, citernes et ventricules cérébraux. In: Traité de Radiodiagnostic, XIII, Neuroradiologie (FISCHGOLD, H. et coll., Eds.), p. 3–54. Paris: Masson 1972

SALAMON, G., LAZORTHES, G.: Tumours of the basal ganglia. An angiographic study. Neuroradiology **2**, 80–89 (1971).

SALAMON, G., RAYBAUD, CH., MICHOTEY, P., GRISOLI, F., FARNARIER, PH.: Etude angiographique des circonvolutions cérébrales et de leur territoire de vascularisation Rev. Neurol. **131**, 259–284 (1975)

SALAMON, G., ROGER, J., SOULAYROL, R.: L'examen des cornes temporales 24 heures après encéphalographie fractionnée. Ann. Radiol. **6**, 101–110 (1963)

SALTZMAN, G.F.: Angiographic demonstration of the posterior communicating and posterior cerebral arteries. Acta radiol. (Stockh.) **54**, 114–122 (1959)

SCHECHTER, M.M.: Recent advances in neuroradiologic diagnostic methods and techniques. In: Neurological Diagnostic Techniques (FIELDS, W.S., Ed.). Springfield/Ill.: Ch. C. Thomas 1966

SCHECHTER, M.M., ZINGESSER, L.H.: The anterior spinal artery. Acta radiol. (Stockh.) **5**, 489–496 (1966)

SCHIPPS, F.C., MADEIRA, J.T., HUNTINGTON, H.W., WING, R.D.: Atlas of brainanatomy for Emi Scans. Springfield/Ill.: Ch. C. Thomas 1975

SCHLESINGER, B.: The venous drainage of the brain, with special reference to the Galenic system. Brain **62**, 274–291 (1939)

SCHLESINGER, B.: The insulo-opercular arteries of the brain with special reference to angiography of strio-thalamic tumor. Amer. J. Roentgenol. **70**, 555–563 (1953)

SCIALFA, G., BANK, W., MEGRET, M., CORBAZ, J.M.: The posterior fossa arteries: the morphology and variations of the anterior inferior cerebellar artery. The arteriographic localization of the fourth ventricle. In: Advances in Cerebral Angiography (SALAMON, G., Ed.). Berlin-Heidelberg-New York: Springer-Verlag 1976

SHELLSHEAR, J.L.: A contribution to the knowledge of the arterial supply of the cerebral cortex in man. Brain **50**, 236–253 (1927)

SICARD, J.A., FORESTIER, J.: Diagnostic et thérapeutique par le lipiodol. Clinique et radiologie. Paris: Masson 1928

SIGNARGROUT, Y.: La veine basilaire. Thèse Médicine, Rennes 1971

SJÖGREN, S.E.: Percutaneous vertebral angiography. Acta radiol. (Stockh.) **40**, 113–127 (1953)

SJÖRGEN, S.E.: The anterior choroidal artery. Acta radiol. (Stockh.) **46**, 143–157 (1956)

STEIN, R.L., ROSENBAUM, A.E.: Normal deep cerebral venous system and abnormal supratentorial deep venous system. In: Radiology of the Skull and Brain (NEWTON, T.H., POTTS, D.G., Eds.), Vol. 2, Book 3, p. 1904–2110. St. Louis: Mosby 1974

STEPHENS, R.B., STILLWELL, D.L.: Arteries and veins of the human brain. Springfield/Ill.: Ch. C. Thomas 1969

STOPFORD, J.S.B.: The arteries of the pons and medulla oblongata. J. Anat. Physiol. **50**, 131–164; **50**, 225–280 (1915); **51**, 250–277 (1917)

SUTTON, D.: Radiological assessment of the normal aqueduct and fourth ventricle. Brit. J. Radiol. **23**, 208–218 (1950)

SZIKLA, G. et coll.: Atlas des artères cérébrales. Heidelberg-Berlin-New York: Springer Verlag 1975

TAKAHASHI, M., OKUDERA, T.: The choroid plexus and the choroid vein of the lateral ventricle. Radiology **103**, 113–120 (1972)

TAKAHASHI, M., WILSON, G., HANAFEE, W.: The significance of the petrosal vein in the diagnosis of cerebellopontine angle tumors. Radiology **89**, 834–840 (1967)

TALAIRACH, J., DAVID, M., TOURNOUX, P.: L'exploration chirurgicale stéréotaxique du lobe temporal dans l'épilepsie temporale. Paris: Masson 1958

TALAIRACH, J., SZIKLA, G.: Atlas d'anatomie stéréotaxique du télencéphale. Paris: Masson 1967

TAMAKI, N., FUJIWARA, K., MATSUMOTO, S., TAKEDA, H.: Veins draining the pineal body. An anatomical and neuroradiological study of pineal veins. J. Neurosurg. **39**, 448–454 (1973)

TAVERAS, J.M., WOOD, E.H.: Diagnostic neuroradiology. Baltimore: Williams and Wilkins 1964

TAYLOR, E.H., HAUGHTON, W.S.: Some recent researches on the topography of the convolutions and fissures of the brain. Trans. Roy. Acad. Ireland **18** (1900)

TESTUT, L., LATARJET, A.: Traité d'Anatomie humaine, II, Angéiologie, Système nerveux central. Paris: G. Doin 1948

TEXIER, J.: Artère sylvienne. Branches corticales et réseau pie mérien. Thèse Paris 1912

THÉRON, J.: L'artère choroidienne antérieure. Ann. Radiol. 1976

THÉRON, J., DJINDJIAN, R.: Cervicovertebral phlebography using catheterization; a preliminary report. Radiology **108**, 325–331 (1973)

THÉRON, J., DJINDJIAN, R.: Comparison of the venous phase of carotid angiography with direct intracranial venography in the evaluation of lesions at the base of the skull. Neuroradiology **5**, 43–48 (1973)

THIÉBAUT, F., WACKENHEIM, A., VROUSOS, C.: Radio-anatomie normale et pathologique de la fosse postérieure. La pneumostratigraphic sagittale médiane. Ann. Radiol. **3**, 11–12 (1960)

THIÉBAUT, F., WACKENHEIM, A., VROUSOS, C.: Nouvelles données de la pneumostratigraphie sagittale médiane de la fosse postérieure. Radiol. **42**, 1–7 (1961)

THIÉBAUT, F., WACKENHEIM, A., VROUSOS, C.: Pneumostratigraphie sagittale médiane de la fosse postérieure. Acta radiol. (Stockh.) **1**, 638–640 (1963)

TIWISINA, TH.: Die vertebralis angiographie. Heidelberg: Alfred Hüttig 1964

TOMPSETT, D.A.: Anatomical technique. London: E.S. Livingstone 1956

TONNIS, W., SCHIEFER, W.: Zirkulationsstörungen des Gehirns im Serien-Angiogramm. Berlin-Heidelberg-New York: Springer-Verlag 1959

TWINNING, E.W.: Radiology of the third and fourth ventricle. Brit. J. Radiol. **12**, 385–395 (1939)

VLAHOVITCH, B.: Les repères de l'insula dans la pratique de l'angiographie carotidienne. L'expansion scientifique française. Paris 1973

VLAHOVITCH, B., FREREBEAU, PH., KUNHER, A., BILLET, M., GROS, C.: Etude des lignes supra et infra-insulaires dans l'angiographie carotidienne normale et pathologique. Neurochirurgie **16**, 127–138 (1970)

VLAHOVITCH, B., FREREBEAU, PH., QUAKNINE, G., BILLET, M.: Etude anatomoartériographique des branches artérielles du territoire sylvien supra et infrainsulaire. C. R. Ass. Anat., 1749–1758 (1968)

VLAHOVICH, B., GROS, C., ADIB-YAZDI, I.S., FERNADEZ-SERRATS, A., BILLET, M.: Repérage du sillon insulaire supérieur dans l'angiographie carotidienne de profil. Neurochirurgie **10**, 91–99 (1964)

VLAHOVITCH, B., GROS, C., FERNANDEZ-SERRATS, A.: Les repéres insulaires dans l'interprétation angiographique des masses de l'hémisphère cérébral. Neurochirurgie **11**, 461–470 (1965)

VLAHOVITCH, B., GROS, C., FREREBEAU, PH., BILLET, M.: Les repéres insulaires dans l'angiographie carotidienne du nourrisson et de l'enfant. Neurochirurgie **12**, 817–823 (1966)

WACKENHEIM, A., BEN-AMOR, M.: Phlebographic location of the inferior vermis. Neuroradiology **3**, 12–15 (1971)

WACKENHEIM, A., BRAUN, J.-P.: Angiography of the mesencephalon. Normal and pathological findings. Berlin-Heidelberg-New York: Springer-Verlag 1970

WESTBERG, G.: Arteries of the basal ganglia. Acta radiol. (Stockh.) **5**, 581–597 (1966)

WICKBOM, I.: Angiography of the carotid arteries. Acta radiol. (Stockh.) Suppl. **72** (1948)

WHITE, E., GREITZ, T.: The influence of white and gray matter distribution in the drainage area of the subependymal venous filling sequence at cerebral angiography. Acta radiol. (Stockh.) **13**, 272–285 (1972)

WILLIAMS, D.J.: The origin of the posterior cerebral artery. Brain **59**, 175–180 (1936)

WOLF, B.S., HUANG, Y.P.: The insula and deep middle cerebral venous drainage system. Normal antomy and angiography. Amer. J. Roentgenol. **90**, 472–489 (1963)

WOLF, B.S., HUANG, Y.P.: The subependymal veins of the lateral ventricle. Amer. J. Roentgenol. **91**, 406–426 (1964)

WOLF, B.S., HUANG, Y.P., NEWMAN, C.M.: The lateral anastomotic mesencephalic vein and other variations in drainage of the basal cerebral vein. Amer. J. Roentgenol. **89**, 411–422 (1963)

WOLF, B.S., HUANG, Y.P., NEWMAN, C.M.: The superficial sylvian venous drainage system. Amer. J. Roentgenol. **89**, 398–410 (1963)

WOLF, B.S., NEWMAN, C.M., KHILNANI, M.T.: The posterior inferior cerebellar artery on vertebral angiography. Amer. J. Roentgenol. **87**, 322–337 (1962)

WOLF, B.S., NEWMAN, C.M., SCHLESINGER, B.: The diagnostic value of the deep cerebral veins in cerebral angiography. Radiology **64**, 161–177 (1955)

YASARGIL, M.G.: Die Vertebralisangiographie ihre Bedeutung für die Diagnose der Tumoren. Acta neurochir. (Wien) Suppl. **9**, (1962)

ZIEDSES DES PLANTES, B.G.: Examen du IIIe et du IVe ventricule au moyen de petites quantités d'air. Acta radiol. (Stockh.) **34**, 399–405 (1950)

ZIMMER, A.E., ANNES, G.P.: The septal vein: an indicator of space-occupying lesions in the anterior cranial fossa. Radiology **87**, 813–823 (1966)

Subject Index

GPSR Compliance
The European Union's (EU) General Product Safety Regulation (GPSR) is a set of rules that requires consumer products to be safe and our obligations to ensure this.

If you have any concerns about our products, you can contact us on

ProductSafety@springernature.com

In case Publisher is established outside the EU, the EU authorized representative is:

Springer Nature Customer Service Center GmbH
Europaplatz 3
69115 Heidelberg, Germany

www.ingramcontent.com/pod-product-compliance
Ingram Content Group UK Ltd.
Pitfield, Milton Keynes, MK11 3LW, UK
UKHW051004220926
475831UK00003B/113

9783642662751